Clinical Features, Pathogenesis and Treatment of Blistering Diseases

Clinical Features, Pathogenesis and Treatment of Blistering Diseases

Editor: Chris Firestone

FOSTER ACADEMICS
www.fosteracademics.com

www.fosteracademics.com

FOSTER ACADEMICS

Cataloging-in-Publication Data

Clinical features, pathogenesis and treatment of blistering diseases / edited by Chris Firestone.
p. cm.
Includes bibliographical references and index.
ISBN 978-1-64646-590-3
1. Blisters. 2. Skin--Diseases. 3. Skin--Diseases--Pathogenesis.
4. Skin--Diseases--Treatment. I. Firestone, Chris.
RL221 .C55 2023
616.523--dc23

Foster Academics,
118-35 Queens Blvd., Suite 400,
Forest Hills, NY 11375, USA

ISBN 978-1-64646-590-3 (Hardback)

Contents

Preface

Blister is the rounded elevation of the skin that contains clear fluid, caused by a separation between the epidermis and the dermis layers of the skin. Blistering diseases are a heterogenous group of disorders that are characterized by the formation of blisters and bullae in the skin and mucous membranes. Some of the blistering diseases are pemphigus, paraneoplastic pemphigus, bullous pemphigoid, cicatricial pemphigoid, linear IgA bullous disease, porphyria cutanea tarda, and subcorneal pustular dermatitis. Pemphigus is a rare group of blistering autoimmune diseases that are characterized by a loss of normal cell-cell adhesion (acantholysis), and by the presence of disease causing autoantibodies reacting against epithelial adhesion molecules. Examination of skin or mucous membrane biopsy helps in diagnosing blistering diseases. They can be treated by the administration of oral steroids such as prednisone. This book contains some path-breaking studies related to the clinical features, pathogenesis and treatment of blistering diseases. It will serve as a reference to a broad spectrum of readers.

After months of intensive research and writing, this book is the end result of all who devoted their time and efforts in the initiation and progress of this book. It will surely be a source of reference in enhancing the required knowledge of the new developments in the area. During the course of developing this book, certain measures such as accuracy, authenticity and research focused analytical studies were given preference in order to produce a comprehensive book in the area of study.

This book would not have been possible without the efforts of the authors and the publisher. I extend my sincere thanks to them. Secondly, I express my gratitude to my family and well-wishers. And most importantly, I thank my students for constantly expressing their willingness and curiosity in enhancing their knowledge in the field, which encourages me to take up further research projects for the advancement of the area.

Editor

1

Pemphigus Foliaceus—Repeated Treatment With Rituximab 7 Years After Initial Response

Magdalena Kraft and Margitta Worm*

Department of Dermatology, Venerology and Allergology, Allergy-Center-Charité, Charité–Universitätsmedizin Berlin, Berlin, Germany

***Correspondence:**
Margitta Worm
margitta.worm@charite.de

Pemphigus foliaceus is an autoimmune skin disease mediated by autoantibodies directed against desmoglein-1 located in the upper epidermal layer. Rituximab, a monoclonal anit-CD20 antibody depleting b-cells, offers an effective treatment possibility for therapy-resistant pemphigus foliaceus. Here, we present the case of 55-year-old man who did not respond sufficiently to conventional treatment with prednisolone, azathioprine, and cyclophosphamide, but underwent almost complete remission after rituximab treatment. The patient relapsed 7 years later, and a repeated course of rituximab infusions led to a partial remission.

Keywords: pemphigus foliaceus, rituximab, anti-CD20, b-cell depletion, autoimmune blistering diseases

INTRODUCTION

Pemphigus foliaceus is a rare, autoimmune blistering skin disease with an estimated incidence of <1 million individuals in the USA and Europe (1). It is caused by autoantibodies directed against desmoglein-1 (Dsg-1), a glycoprotein important for intercellular adhesion between keratinocytes (2, 3). The disease manifests as erythematous papules, plaques, and erosions with scaly crusts. The involvement of seborrheic skin areas is typical for the disease. The loss of adhesion occurs in the upper epidermal layers and is limited to the skin with no mucosal involvement; this is attributable to the expression pattern of Dsg-1 and distinguishes pemphigus foliaceus from the more common pemphigus vulgaris (4, 5).

Glucocorticoids are the first-line treatment for pemphigus foliaceus. Treatment with other immunosuppressants such as azathioprine, mycophenolate mofetil or methotrexate, is also well-established (6). Recent data suggest that a b-cell-depleting therapy with rituximab is highly effective in treating pemphigus vulgaris, but also pemphigus foliaceus (7–10). Here, we describe the case of a patient suffering from a therapy-resistant pemphigus foliaceus; the patient was in remission for 7 years after initial rituximab treatment and responded well to the repeated treatment.

CASE PRESENTATION

A 55-year-old man with a history of progressing skin lesions over the past 8 months visited our department for the first time in spring 2011. The clinical examination revealed multiple erythematous papules and plaques with crusts on his back, chest, face, and scalp (about 40% of body surface area was involved) with no mucosal involvement (**Figure 1**). The patient presented no other symptoms and had no chronic diseases or allergies. His blood tests revealed a highly elevated Dsg1 antibody level (130 U/ml; normal range < 20 U/ml) and a slightly elevated γ-glutamyltransferase level. Differential blood count, liver enzymes, creatinine, and Dsg3 antibody level were within the normal range. Histological examination of the patient's skin biopsy revealed an inflammatory infiltrate, eosinophilic spongiosis, and superficial epidermal blister formation.

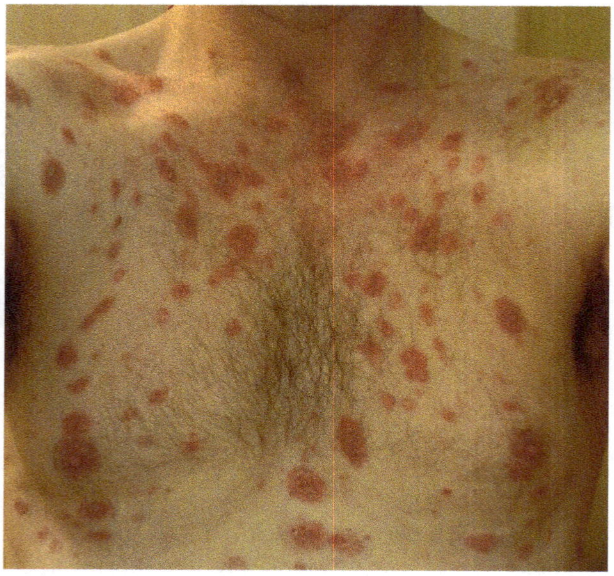

FIGURE 1 | Skin lesions before rituximab treatment.

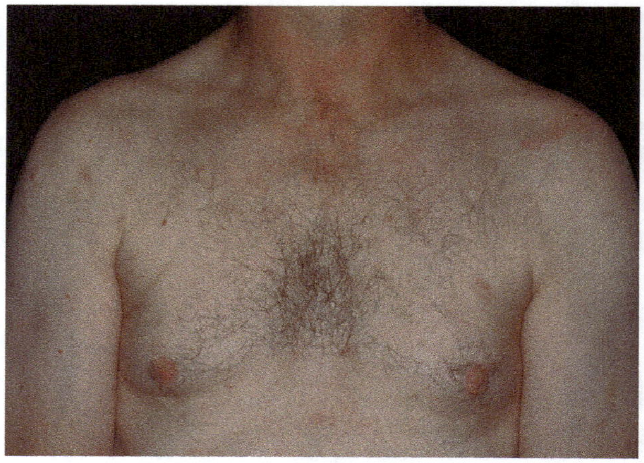

FIGURE 2 | Clinical picture eight months after initial rituximab treatment.

Based on the findings, pemphigus foliaceus was diagnosed and a treatment with prednisolone (10 mg/day) and azathioprine (100 mg/day) was started. Topical therapy with clobetasol propionate and chlorhexidine was also initiated. Furthermore, methylprednisolone infusions (750 mg) were administered once a month for 3 months. This treatment did not result in complete remission; thus, methylprednisolone was replaced with dexamethasone (300 mg) and cyclophosphamide infusions (500 mg) once a month. Azathioprine had to be discontinued due to increasing liver enzymes. The treatment with cyclophosphamide and glucocorticoids was discontinued after 5 months without achieving remission. Hence, we next treated the patient with rituximab. Therefore, two rituximab infusions (1 g each) were administered 2 weeks apart leading to a near-complete b-cell depletion in peripheral blood, a decrease in Dsg1 antibody levels (below the detection range), and an almost complete remission of the skin lesions within the next year (**Figure 2**). Consecutively, therapy with prednisolone (10 mg/day) and topical mometasone furoate was continued and in the following 2 years, the prednisolone dose was reduced to 5 mg/day. The patient remained in remission for 7 years with this therapy (with Dsg1 antibody levels continuously within the normal range). However, in autumn 2017, skin lesions reappeared, which was accompanied by an increase in the Dsg1 antibody levels (75 U/ml). The prednisolone dosage was increased (temporarily up to 60 mg/day), but it was not sufficient to control the disease. Therefore, rituximab infusions (2 × 1 g within 14 days) were readministered, which led to slow continuous healing of the skin lesions.

DISCUSSION

Numerous case reports and studies have reported on the efficacy of rituximab in treating pemphigus vulgaris but also pemphigus foliaceus (1, 7–11). Recently, Joly et al. (10) published a randomized, multi-center, open-labeled clinical study comparing rituximab and prednisolone as the first line of treatment for pemphigus. The study subjects were treated with 1,000 mg rituximab on days 0 and 14, followed by 500 mg rituximab after 12 and 18 months and 0.5–1 mg/kg prednisolone tapered over 3–6 months. The control group was treated with 1–1.5 mg/kg prednisolone tapered over 12–18 months. After 2 years, the achieved remission rates were 89 and 34% for the rituximab and the control group, respectively. In the control group, the rate of serious adverse events was twice as high as that among the rituximab-treated group.

Thus, rituximab is effective in treating pemphigus foliaceus; however, its ideal dosage regimen is still unknown. In most cases, either 375 mg/m^2 rituximab is administered once a week for 4 weeks (lymphoma protocol) or two doses of 1,000 mg rituximab are administered 2 weeks apart (rheumatoid arthritis protocol). In their comprehensive review, Ahmed and Shetty (11) reported that responder rates (in pemphigus vulgaris) for both protocols were similar. Because of the low B-cell burden in autoimmune diseases, some authors proposed a low dosage regimen (12–14).

Relapse of pemphigus after rituximab treatment is common (15). In majority of the patients, remission can be maintained up to a few years. A 7-year remission duration, as observed in the current study, is not frequent. Joly et al. reported that 25% of rituximab treated patients relapsed within 2 years (10). Colliou et al. followed 21 rituximab treated patients for 7 years (16). The relapse occurred in 81% of patients and was associated with either persisting or, as in our case, reincreasing Dsg antibody levels. The factors influencing the remission time are not well-characterized (17). The associations between prolonged time to relapse and either higher number of rituximab cycles or a high-dose regiment were described (7, 15, 17, 18). On the other hand, prophylactic administration of an additional rituximab infusion in patients in remission was shown not to be beneficial (19). Saleh (20) reported a correlation between Dsg1 antibody levels at baseline and time to relapse: patients with high levels of Dsg1 antibodies relapsed usually within one year after rituximab treatment, while patients with low Dsg1 antibody levels stayed in remission for about 2 years. Interestingly there was no association between time to relapse and Dsg3 antibody levels or clinical severity at the time of rituximab treatment.

In a recent small study, Keeley et al. reported that a low-dose maintenance immunomodulatory treatment after rituximab therapy might prevent a relapse (21). Ahmed et al. observed no relapses in ten patients treated with immunoglobulins and rituximab (22). The adjuvant immunoglobulins were administered in average for 34 months following the rituximab treatment and a long-lasting remission was achieved in all patients [average follow up was 7 years after the initial rituximab treatment (22)]. In our patient, it is probable that the prolonged remission was supported by the continuous low-dose prednisolone therapy.

As here observed, treatment with rituximab is successful in the majority of the patients after relapse (15, 18, 23) so that repeated treatment can be recommended for these patients.

Serious adverse event following rituximab treatment are rare. Those are mostly infections (e.g., viral hepatitis reactivation, or herpes virus infections) (24). Few cases of infections with lethal outcomes after rituximab treatment have been reported (24); thus, patients and physicians should be aware of this risk and immediately act in case of suspected adverse event.

CONCLUDING REMARKS

Our case report demonstrates that rituximab can be effective in treating therapy-resistant pemphigus and long-lasting remission may be achieved. A low-dose maintenance immunomodulatory treatment after rituximab therapy may prolong the remission stage. In case of a relapse, repeated treatment with rituximab is usually successful. However, this therapy is limited due to the high cost of rituximab and the risk of rare but severe side effects.

AUTHOR CONTRIBUTIONS

MK wrote the manuscript. MW contributed to conception of the manuscript and revised it critically.

ACKNOWLEDGMENTS

We acknowledge support from the German Research Foundation (DFG) and the Open Access Publication Fund of Charité – Universitätsmedizin Berlin.

REFERENCES

1. Kridin K. Pemphigus group: overview, epidemiology, mortality, and comorbidities. *Immunol Res.* (2018) 66:255–70. doi: 10.1007/s12026-018-8986-7
2. Koulu L, Kusumi A, Steinberg MS, Klaus-Kovtun V, Stanley JR. Human autoantibodies against a desmosomal core protein in pemphigus foliaceus. *J Exp Med.* (1984) 160:1509–18. doi: 10.1084/jem.160.5.1509
3. Ludwig RJ, Vanhoorelbeke K, Leypoldt F, Kaya Z, Bieber K, McLachlan S. M, et al. Mechanisms of autoantibody-induced pathology. *Front Immunol.* (2017) 31:603. doi: 10.3389/fimmu.2017.00603
4. Mahoney MG, Wang Z, Rothenberger K, Koch PJ, Amagai M, Stanley JR. Explanations for the clinical and microscopic localization of lesions in pemphigus foliaceus and vulgaris. *J Clin Invest.* (1999) 103:461–68. doi: 10.1172/JCI5252
5. Pollmann R, Schmidt T, Eming R, Hertl M. Pemphigus: a comprehensive review on pathogenesis, clinical presentation and novel therapeutic approaches. *Clin Rev Allergy Immunol.* (2018) 54:1–25. doi: 10.1007/s12016-017-8662-z
6. Eming R, Sticherling M, Hofmann SC, Hunzelmann N, Kern JS, Kramer H, et al. S2k guidelines for the treatment of pemphigus vulgaris/foliaceus and bullous pemphigoid. *J Dtsch Dermatol Ges.* (2015) 13:833–44. doi: 10.1111/ddg.12606
7. de Sena Nogueira Maehara L, Huizinga J, Jonkman MF. Rituximab therapy in pemphigus foliaceus: report of 12 cases and review of recent literature. *Br J Dermatol.* (2015) 172:1420–3. doi: 10.1111/bjd.13586
8. Tomsitz D, Stefaniak R, Worm M. Rituximab in patients with recalcitrant autoimmune blistering diseases: experience in a cohort of 22 patients. *Br J Dermatol.* (2015) 172:829–31. doi: 10.1111/bjd.13307
9. Palacios-Álvarez I, Riquelme-Mc Loughlin C, Curto-Barredo L, Iranzo P, García-Díez I, España A. Rituximab treatment of pemphigus foliaceus - a retrospective study of 12 patients. *J Am Acad Dermatol.* (2018). doi: 10.1016/j.jaad.2018.05.1252. [Epub ahead of print].
10. Joly P, Maho-Vaillant M, Prost-Squarcioni C, Hebert V, Houivet E, Calbo S, et al. First-line rituximab combined with short-term prednisone versus prednisone alone for the treatment of pemphigus (ritux 3): a prospective, multicentre, parallel-group, open-label randomised trial. *Lancet* (2017) 389:2031–40. doi: 10.1016/S0140-6736(17)30070-3
11. Ahmed AR, Shetty S. A comprehensive analysis of treatment outcomes in patients with pemphigus vulgaris treated with rituximab. *Autoimmun Rev.* (2015) 14:323–31. doi: 10.1016/j.autrev.2014.12.002
12. Horvath B, Huizinga J, Pas HH, Mulder AB, Jonkman MF. Low dose rituximab is effective in pemphigus. *Br J Dermatol.* (2012) 166:405–12. doi: 10.1111/j.1365-2133.2011.10663.x
13. Alaibac M. Ultra-low dosage regimen of rituximab in autoimmune blistering skin conditions. *Front Immunol.* (2018) 9:810. doi: 10.3389/fimmu.2018.00810
14. Schoergenhofer C, Schwameis M, Firbas C, Bartko J, Derhaschnig U, Mader RM, et al. Single, very low rituximab doses in healthy volunteers – a pilot and a randomized trial: implications for dosing and biosimilarity testing. *Sci Rep.* (2018) 8:124. doi: 10.1038/s41598-017-17934-6
15. Wang HH, Liu CW, Li YC, Huang YC. Efficacy of rituximab for pemphigus: a systematic review and meta-analysis of different regimens. *Acta Derm Venereol.* (2015) 95:928–32. doi: 10.2340/00015555-2116
16. Colliou N, Picard D, Caillot F, Calbo S, Le Corre S, Lim, A., et al. Long-term remissions of severe pemphigus after rituximab therapy are associated with prolonged failure of desmoglein B cell response. *Sci Transl Med.* (2013) 5:175ra30. doi: 10.1126/scitranslmed.3005166
17. Heelan K, Al-Mohammedi F, Smith MJ, Knowles S, Lansang P, Walsh S, et al. Durable remission of pemphigus with a fixed-dose rituximab protocol. *JAMA Dermatol.* (2014) 150:703–8. doi: 10.1001/jamadermatol.2013.6739
18. Kim TH, Choi Y, Lee SE, Lim JM, Kim SC. Adjuvant rituximab treatment for pemphigus: a retrospective study of 45 patients at a single center with long-term follow up. *J Dermatol.* (2017) 44:615–20. doi: 10.1111/1346-8138.13757
19. Gregoriou S, Giatrakou S, Theodoropoulos K, Katoulis A, Loumou P, Toumbis-Ioannou E, et al. Pilot study of 19 patients with severe pemphigus: prophylactic treatment with rituximab does not appear to be beneficial. *Dermatology* (2014) 228:158–65. doi: 10.1159/000357031
20. Saleh MA. A prospective study comparing patients with early and late relapsing pemphigus treated with rituximab. *J Am Acad Dermatol.* (2018) 79:97–103. doi: 10.1016/j.jaad.2018.01.029
21. Keeley JM, Bevans SL, Jaleel T, Sami N. Rituximab and low dose oral immune modulating treatment to maintain a sustained response in severe pemphigus patients. *J Dermatolog Treat.* (2018). doi: 10.1080/09546634.2018.1510173. [Epub ahead of print].

22. Ahmed AR, Nguyen T, Kaveri S, Spigelman ZS. First line treatment of pemphigus vulgaris with a novel protocol in patients with contraindications to systemic corticosteroids and immunosuppressive agents: Preliminary retrospective study with a seven year follow-up. *Int Immunopharmacol.* (2016) 34:25–31. doi: 10.1016/j.intimp.2016.02.013
23. Cianchini G, Lupi F, Masini C, Corona R, Puddu P, De Pità O. Therapy with rituximab for autoimmune pemphigus: results from a single-center observational study on 42 cases with long-term follow-up. *J Am Acad Dermatol.* (2012) 67:617–22. doi: 10.1016/j.jaad.2011.11.007
24. Tavakolpour S, Mahmoudi H, Balighi K, Abedini R, Daneshpazhooh M. Sixteen-year history of rituximab therapy for 1085 pemphigus vulgaris patients: a systematic review. *Int Immunopharmacol.* (2018) 54:131–8. doi: 10.1016/j.intimp.2017.11.005

2

Dermatitis Herpetiformis: Novel Perspectives

***Emiliano Antiga*[†]*, Roberto Maglie*[*†]*, Lavinia Quintarelli, Alice Verdelli, Diletta Bonciani, Veronica Bonciolini and Marzia Caproni*[*]**

Section of Dermatology, Department of Health Sciences, University of Florence, Florence, Italy

Correspondence:
Roberto Maglie
robertomaglie.med@libero.it
Marzia Caproni
marzia.caproni@unifi.it

[†]These authors have contributed equally to this work

Dermatitis herpetiformis (DH) is an inflammatory disease of the skin, considered the specific cutaneous manifestation of celiac disease (CD). Both DH and CD occur in gluten-sensitive individuals, share the same Human Leukocyte Antigen (HLA) haplotypes (DQ2 and DQ8), and improve following the administration of a gluten-free diet. Moreover, almost all DH patients show typical CD alterations at the small bowel biopsy, ranging from villous atrophy to augmented presence of intraepithelial lymphocytes, as well as the generation of circulating autoantibodies against tissue transglutaminase (tTG). Clinically, DH presents with polymorphic lesions, including papules, vesicles, and small blisters, symmetrically distributed in typical anatomical sites including the extensor aspects of the limbs, the elbows, the sacral regions, and the buttocks. Intense pruritus is almost the rule. However, many atypical presentations of DH have also been reported. Moreover, recent evidence suggested that DH is changing. Firstly, some studies reported a reduced incidence of DH, probably due to early recognition of CD, so that there is not enough time for DH to develop. Moreover, data from Japanese literature highlighted the absence of intestinal involvement as well as of the typical serological markers of CD (i.e., anti-tTG antibodies) in Japanese patients with DH. Similar cases may also occur in Caucasian patients, complicating DH diagnosis. The latter relies on the combination of clinical, histopathologic, and immunopathologic findings. Detecting granular IgA deposits at the dermal-epidermal junction by direct immunofluorescence (DIF) from perilesional skin represents the most specific diagnostic tool. Further, assessing serum titers of autoantibodies against epidermal transglutaminase (eTG), the supposed autoantigen of DH, may also serve as a clue for the diagnosis. However, a study from our group has recently demonstrated that granular IgA deposits may also occur in celiac patients with non-DH inflammatory skin diseases, raising questions about the effective role of eTG IgA autoantibodies in DH and suggesting the need of revising diagnostic criteria, conceivably emphasizing clinical aspects of the disease along with DIF. DH usually responds to the gluten-free diet. Topical clobetasol ointment or dapsone may be also applied to favor rapid disease control. Our review will focus on novel pathogenic insights, controversies, and management aspects of DH.

Keywords: dermatitis herpetiformis, epidermal transglutaminase, coeliac disease, non-coeliac gluten sensitivity, direct immunofluorescence

INTRODUCTION

About 135 years ago, the American dermatologist Luis Duhring reported for the first time an itching and multiform skin eruption with erythema, papules, bullae, pustules, and above all, grouped vesicles localized at typical areas (1). At that time, he had seen 15 cases of such a disease, and he decided to name it "dermatitis herpetiformis," due to its clinical similarity to herpes virus infection (1). After the identification of dermatitis herpetiformis, several years passed before the second important step in its early story until 1950, when dapsone was accidentally found to be effective for the treatment of the disease (2). Then, 50 years ago, Van der Meer described the typical IgA deposits at the papillary tips, which represent the immunological hallmark of DH as well as the clue for the diagnosis of the disease (3).

However, it was only in the 60s and, above all, in the 70s that DH was clearly related to gluten intolerance, allowing to consider the disease as the specific cutaneous manifestation of celiac disease (CD). In fact, patients with DH were shown to have in most cases intestinal changes similar to those found in CD (4) and to share the same genetic background of CD (5), and gluten-free diet (GFD) was demonstrated to improve skin symptoms (6), although more slowly than the gastrointestinal ones.

Since then, several issues about the pathogenesis and the management of DH have been pointed out (7). Among them, the identification of reliable serologic markers of the disease (8) and the discovery of epidermal transglutaminase (eTG) as the autoantigen of DH were some of the most remarkable steps (9).

DH can be defined as a disease presenting with: (i) symmetrical polymorphic lesions involving typical areas such as the extensor aspects of the limbs and sacral region, (ii) a predominant neutrophilic infiltrate at the dermal papillae at histopathology, (iii) granular IgA deposits along the dermal-epidermal junction, (iv) an invariable association with CD, and (v) a response to a lifelong GFD (7).

However, despite the growing knowledge about the disease, several issues have to be clarified yet, and some of the cornerstones of DH need further discussion. For example, the specificity of IgA deposits in the perilesional skin of patients with DH could be questioned and the diagnostic algorithm should be revised (10), taking also into account the identification of non-coeliac gluten sensitivity (NCGS) as a new entity among the spectrum of gluten-related disorders (11); moreover, the pathogenic role of IgA anti-eTG antibodies needs further demonstration, since they may also occur in patients without DH (12). Finally, even the therapeutic role of GFD is discussed, since some authors suggest that it can be interrupted in the (rare) case of DH remission (13).

The current review will try to address or at least to focus on these and other issues that are still under debate in the context of DH. The picture that hopefully will come out would be that of a lively disease that represents both a pathogenic model of autoimmunity and a paradigmatic example of how the skin can be the mirror of an internal condition such as CD.

THE EPIDEMIOLOGY OF DERMATITIS HERPETIFORMIS: A (RARE) DISEASE OF THE WESTERN COUNTRIES

DH is a rare disease that occurs prevalently in Caucasian individuals. In Europe and USA, the prevalence of DH ranges from 11.2 to 75.3 per 100.000, with the highest reported in Finland; whereas, the incidence ranges from 0.4 to 2.6 per 100.000 people per year (14–16). DH is extremely rare among African and Asian populations. Reasons explaining the low prevalence of DH among such populations include the absence of DH predisposing human leukocyte haplotypes (HLA) DQ2 and DQ8, which are always found in Caucasian DH patients, and the low wheat consumption in these geographic areas (17). However, in the Asians, including Chinese and Japanese populations, the association between DH and CD seems to be weaker than in Western countries, despite DH presents with similar clinical and immunopathological features. The extreme rarity of CD in these populations may have led, indeed, to overlook the diagnosis of DH and possibly underestimate the prevalence of the disease (17, 18).

During the last decades, the overall incidence of DH is significantly decreased, although the incidence of CD is increasing (19–22). One plausible explanation for the opposite trends in the epidemiology of CD and DH could be the increased awareness of CD among physicians and patients and the wide prescription of CD screening tests even in patients without typical gastrointestinal manifestations, leading to identify early patients with latent or potential CD.

DH can occur at any age, but typically occurs during adulthood, and mostly between the third and the fourth decade of life (14). Interestingly, in one Finnish study including 477 patients diagnosed with DH over a 40 year period, the patients' age at DH diagnosis was shown to significantly increase over time. This is presumably related to a parallel decrease of the annual consumption of wheat during the same period, leading to a lower lifetime gluten load (16).

DH has been also reported to occur in pediatric patients, but the exact incidence of DH during childhood is unknown. In one study by our group in 2013 including 159 DH patients, about 36% were diagnosed below the age of 20 (23). Other authors have suggested a possible underestimation of pediatric DH due to clinical overlapping features with atopic dermatitis, which still accounts for the most prevalent dermatologic disease among children (24). Unlike CD, DH seems to occur most commonly in man, although the male/female ratio has reportedly ranging from 2:1 to 1:1 according to different studies (16, 19, 24). Interestingly, a Finnish study found that in females there is a longer diagnostic delay compared to male (25).

Associated Diseases

Like CD, DH has been found to be associated with several autoimmune disorders, including type I diabetes mellitus, autoimmune thyroid diseases, and connective tissue diseases, such as Sjögren syndrome (24). Of interest is also the reported association between DH and bullous pemphigoid (BP), a subepidermal autoimmune blistering disease characterized by autoimmunity against the hemidesmosomal antigens BP180 and BP230 (26, 27). Accordingly, in a retrospective case-control study, diagnosis of DH was found to increase of 22 folds the risk of BP, compared to only a 2-fold higher risk of developing BP amongst coeliac patients. The mean time between the diagnosis of DH and BP development was about 3 years (27).

Since virtually all patients with DH have CD, DH patients also carry an increased risk of non-Hodgkin lymphomas and gastrointestinal malignancies (28). However, unlike CD, mortality of DH patients is not increased (29–31). Accordingly, in a large population-based study including 476 patients with DH, a reduced mortality for all the causes of death compared to the general population and a significantly reduced mortality related to cerebrovascular diseases were shown. Mortality due to non-Hodgkin lymphomas was increased only during the first 5 years following the diagnosis but not thereafter. DH patients were also found to have less hypercholesterolemia, and there were fewer smoker compared to the control population (32). Ali and Lear speculated that smoking might have a protective effect against DH, since it suppresses natural killer (NK) lymphocytes and reduces intestinal IgA secretion (33–36). Finally, an association between DH and higher social class have been reported, and may contribute to the observed reduced mortality reflecting the "many facets of better living" of a high socioeconomic status (33).

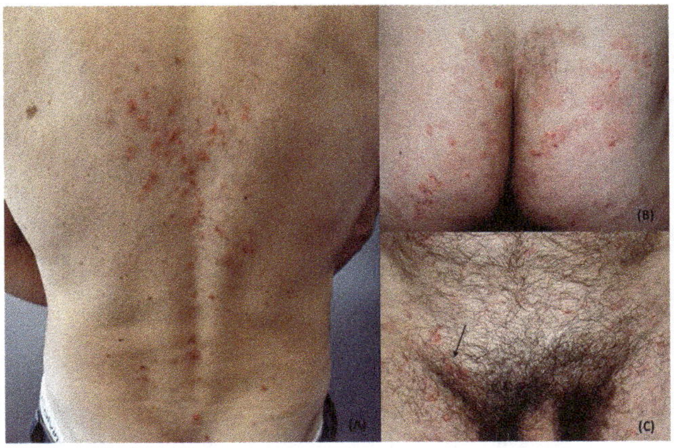

FIGURE 1 | Clinical presentation of dermatitis herpetiformis (DH): erythematous grouped papules and vesicles associated with excoriations and crusts at the back **(A)**, sacral region and buttocks **(B)**. Rarely, DH may also affect the groin and pubis (arrow) **(C)**. The patient gave written informed consent for the publication of these pictures.

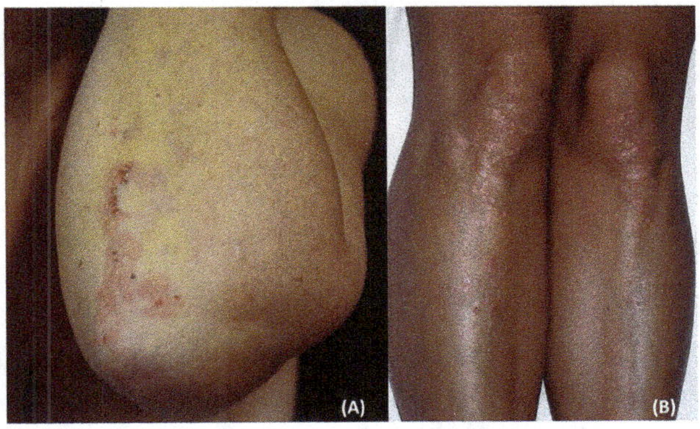

FIGURE 2 | Clinical presentation of dermatitis herpetiformis: grouped papules and vesicles associated with excoriations and crusts at the elbows **(A)** and lower limbs **(B)**. Post-inflammatory pigmentary changes such as hypo-pigmentation could be also appreciated **(B)**. The patient gave written informed consent for the publication of these pictures.

Clinical Manifestations

The polymorphism and the symmetrical distribution of the lesions represent the major clinical hallmarks of DH (37, 38).

The disease usually presents with grouped erythematous papules and urticarial plaques with overwhelming vesicles. The latter may then coalesce into small tense blisters with sero-hemorrhagic content, which are characterized by a centrifugal growth pattern. Erosions, excoriations, and crusts are likely to occur because of blisters rupture and because of the scratching secondary to the associated pruritus (15, 38, 39). Lesions eventually heal leaving post-inflammatory hypo- and hyper-pigmentation (**Figures 1, 2**).

Typically, DH lesions symmetrically localized at the extensor surfaces of upper and lower limbs, mostly at the elbows and knees, buttocks, and the sacral region; the abdomen, upper back, shoulders, nuchal area, and the scalp may also be involved, whereas the face and groin are rarely affected.

Likewise, mucosal involvement has sporadically been reported. Oral manifestations of DH mainly consist of erosions affecting both the oral mucosa and the tongue; associated symptoms include pain and burning sensation (15, 40). However, it is not clear whether oral involvement has to be considered as a specific manifestation of DH or, rather, a sign of the underlying CD; accordingly, oral aphthosis, erosions, and/or ulcerations are also frequently found in CD (40–44).

Pruritus is the leading symptom of DH and its absence is a strong argument against the diagnosis (45). In one study by our group including a cohort of 159 patients, almost all complained of severe pruritus, which had a significantly negative impact on the patient's quality of life. Moreover, in many cases, pruritus along with a stinging and burning sensation of the skin was shown to be the presenting sign of DH, preceding of 12–24 h the appearance of the cutaneous lesions (46). Notably, pruritus has reportedly occurred even months before the onset of skin lesions (47, 48).

Atypical Cases of Dermatitis Herpetiformis: Are They Always Dermatitis Herpetiformis?

Several atypical cases of DH have been reported in the literature. Asymptomatic palmoplantar petechiae, occurring either alone or in association with characteristic DH clinical findings, have been reported in some cases of pediatric DH. Petechiae were found to occur prevalently at the dominant hand or foot, suggesting repeated microtraumatism as a possible trigger (44, 49–55).

Moreover, Naylor et al. reported a case of DH presenting with a diffuse petechial rush and microscopic changes consistent with both DH and vasculitis (56). Kern et al. reported a patient with DH presenting as pseudovasculitis, characterized by a diffuse petechial rush and a large ulcer at his extensor forearm, and histopathologic and direct immunofluorescence (DIF) findings consistent with DH without additional signs of small-vessel inflammation (57). A possible hypothesis of the association between DH and vascular damage might be the presence of perivascular IgA immune complexes leading to small vessel inflammation.

Finally, cases of DH presenting as palmoplantar keratosis (58), purpuric lesions with chronic urticaria (59), and prurigo pigmentosa-like lesions (60) have been also reported.

PATHOGENESIS

DH represents a paradigmatic model of autoimmune disease, owing that it can be switched on or off by a known external trigger: the gluten. The pathogenesis of DH, which relies on a complex inflammatory network along the gut-skin axis, remains at present only partly understood. Over the past 30 years, major efforts have led to the identification of eTG as the main autoantigen of DH and to well-characterize the inflammatory microenviroment underlying skin lesions development. However, controversies still persist about the mechanisms by which (i) anti-eTG autoantibodies develop, (ii) they form the typical granular aggregates at the dermal papillary tips, and (iii) eventually induce the appearance of the skin lesions. Herein, we summarized the current knowledge of DH pathogenesis, highlighting the major controversial issues that may represent the starting point for future researches (**Figure 3**).

HLA DQ2/DQ8 and Gluten Are Required for the Occurrence of Dermatitis Herpetiformis

About 5–10% of DH patients have a first-degree relative affected by either DH or CD (61–63), suggesting that genetic factors play a major pathogenic role in the disease. Previous studies have found an association between DH and both HLA class I and II molecules, including HLA A1, B8, DR3, and DPB1 (64). However, the closest association occurs with HLA-DQ2 (combination of the DQA1*0501 and DQB1*02 alleles) and DQ8 (combination of the DQA1*03 and DQB1*0302 alleles), which can be found in roughly 85 and 15% of the patients, respectively (65). Other studies have tried to investigate the role of more than 40 other non-HLA gene polymorphisms in the pathogenesis of both CD and DH, but none has yielded convincing results (66–69).

Both HLA-DQ2 and DQ8, whose genes map on the chromosome 6, are crucially involved in processing the gluten antigen gliadin (70), corresponding to the same predisposing haplotypes found in coeliac patients (71, 72). In CD, tissue TG (tTG) catalyze deamidation of gliadin, creating epitopes that increase gluten-peptide binding affinity to HLA-DQ2 and DQ8 expressed on the surface of antigen presenting cells, leading to an adaptive immune reaction against both tTG and gliadin. In parallel, activation of innate immunity leads to characteristic small bowel alterations, including reversible villous atrophy in the upper part of the jejunum, crypt hyperplasia on small bowel mucosal samples and prominent intraepithelial lymphocytosis (73–75). Virtually all DH patients show evidence of a potential or manifest, usually mild, CD, suggesting that DH represents a specific cutaneous manifestation of CD (76). The pathogenic relevance of HLA-DQ and gluten intake in DH has been further demonstrated experimentally by Marietta and coworkers. Firstly, they observed that, unlike other autoimmune blistering dermatoses, passive transfer of DH serum into athymic mice with human skin engrafts did not induce DH lesions. However, DH lesions developed in about 17% of HLA-DQ8 positive autoimmune prone NOD mice when they were exposed to gluten through periodic intraperitoneal injections. This suggests that DH develops only in the presence of predisposing HLA-DQ antigens together with gluten exposure (77, 78).

An exception to what aforementioned is DH occurring in Japanese populations. To date, only two studies have delineated the clinical and immunological features of Japanese DH, including a total of 116 patients, suggesting the extreme rarity of DH in Japan. Although these studies were biased by the fact that the results of some analyzed parameters, including the presence of villous atrophy, circulating antibodies, and response to a GFD, were available only for a few patients, some peculiar characteristics of Japanese DH have emerged, including (i) the absence of HLA DQ2/DQ8 haplotypes, (ii) the absence of an underlying CD, (iii) a higher clinical involvement of non-predilection sites such as the extremities and trunk, (iv) fibrillar rather than granular IgA deposits in the papillary dermis of a substantial proportion of patients, and (v) a lower incidence of CD-associated autoimmune diseases and non-Hodgkin lymphomas (**Table 1**) (18, 79). Even in some Chinese DH patients, the disease was shown to occur outside the setting of CD, which is also very rare in China (80). Altogether, these observations raise speculation on the existence of a subgroup of DH that may be not elicited by gluten, although showing some clinic-pathologic features like in gluten-related DH.

Triggers Other Than Gluten Possibly Involved in the Pathogenesis of Dermatitis Herpetiformis

There is evidence that external triggers other than gluten may induce or worsen DH. For example, potassium iodide, a common compound of expectorants, has reportedly been a trigger of DH both after oral ingestion and when applied topically (81). Similarly, Snider et al. described two cases of DH elicited by a cleaning solution (82).

Kovaleski et al. reported on two cases of DH following a gastric stapling procedure and a gastrectomy with partial pancreatectomy and colectomy, respectively (83). Similarly, a non-coeliac patient developing DH after a mini-gastric bypass surgery was reported (84). In these cases, the authors hypothesized that the surgery-induced enteral inflammation promoted a cross-reaction between cutaneous and intestinal anti-TG antibodies, that seems to be in accordance with the recent demonstration of the intestinal origin of anti-eTG IgA autoantibodies (85).

Hormonal factors, and specifically the hypothalamic-pituitary-gonadal axis, may play a role in DH. Accordingly,

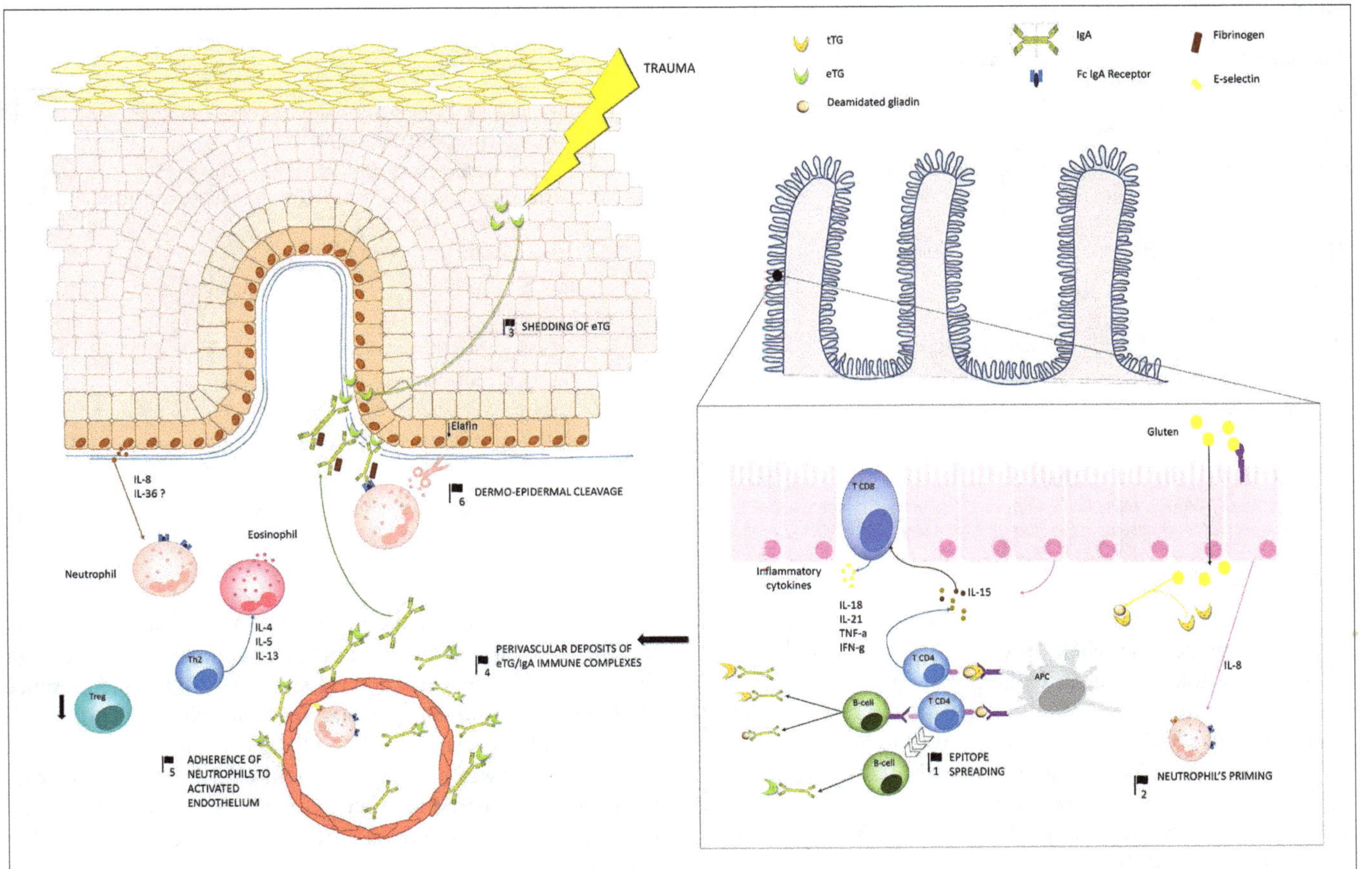

FIGURE 3 | Pathogenesis of dermatitis herpetiformis (DH): Production of IgA autoantibodies against eTG occurs in the gut, probably as a result of an epitope spreading phenomenon (1), due to the high sequence homology between tissue TG, which is a major autoantigen in coeliac disease, and eTG. Activation of innate immunity in the gut leads to increased release of IL-8, which is thought to be responsible for the initial priming of neutrophils (2). One theory suggests that, in region of trauma, keratinocyte damage leads to shedding of eTG to the dermal-epidermal junction (3), where it binds to anti-eTG IgA. An alternative hypothesis suggests that eTG/IgA complexes exists as circulating immune complexes, which can deposit both at the dermal-epidermal junction and around dermal vessels (4). A complex interplay between inflammatory cytokines and the activation of fibrinogen stimulate neutrophil adherence to the activated endothelium (5) and migration to the dermal papillae. Herein neutrophils, which probably bind to IgA aggregates through the Fc IgA receptor, release proteases, which finally induce the cleavage of the dermal-epidermal junction (6). In parallel, hyper-activation of Th2 cells activate eosinophils, which also co-operate with neutrophils to the cleavage of the dermal-epidermal junction. Down-regulation of Treg cells do also occur, favoring the maintenance of a pro-inflammatory microenvironment in DH skin. Abbreviations in the figure: eTG, epidermal transglutaminase; tTG, tissue transglutaminase; IL, interleukin; Th, T helper cell; Treg, regulatory T cell; APC, antigen presenting cell.

hormone replacement therapy for panhypopituitarism has been reported to cure DH (86). One study reported DH following progesterone contraception (87). Other two studies reported DH occurrence after a therapy with leuprolide acetate, an analog of the gonadotropin-releasing hormone (GnRH). In both cases, lesions resolved upon drug discontinuation. However, in one case, skin lesions recurred once the patient was started on biculatamide, another GnRH analog (88, 89).

Intriguingly, drugs may be also a potential trigger of DH. Marakli et al. described a patient who developed DH while on therapy with the Tumor Necrosis Factor-alfa inhibitor infliximab for an ankylosing spondylitis (90); whereas, Mochel et al. recently illustrated a patient who developed DH after several weeks of ipilimumab treatment for a metastatic melanoma. Interestingly, the patient had a positive result of anti tTG IgA antibodies prior to the diagnosis of the metastatic cancer but neither a confirmed diagnosis of coeliac disease nor active skin rush before taking ipilimumab (91). The latter is a monoclonal antibody targeting CTLA-4 and is thought to exert its anti-tumor activity by promoting T-cell activation and down-regulation of Treg function (92). It is arguable that the reported patient had a latent or silent gluten-sensitive enteropathy with an immunological reaction against tTG and eTG, and that inhibition of Tregs precipitated the manifestation of DH, in agreement with the critical role of Treg in the disease pathogenesis (93).

Finally, DH has reportedly been occurred close to a diagnosis of an adenocarcinoma of the lung and an autoimmune pancreatitis in two Japanese patients, who had neither serum IgA antibodies against eTG nor signs of an underlying CD (94).

Interestingly, a gastrointestinal infection appears to be an essential factor for the induction of CD. Several pathogenes have been suggested to trigger CD, including rotavirus, Epstein Bar Virus, Cytomegalovirus, HCV, HBV, *Bacteroides* species, *C. jejuni*, *Pneumococcus*, *M. tuberculosis*, and *H. pylori* (95).

TABLE 1 | Different characteristics between Caucasian and Japanese patients with dermatitis herpetiformis.

Characteristics	Caucasian DH	Japanese DH
HLA	HLA-DQ2 (DQB1*02:01)–85% HLA-DQ8 (DQB1*03:02)–15%	HLA-DQ2 (DQB1*02:01)–0% HLA-DQ8 (DQB1*03:02)–37%*
Sites of involvement	Elbow, buttock, knee, face, ear, neck, scalp, groin	Elbow, buttock, knee, face, ear, neck, scalp, groin Non-predilection sites, including the extremities and trunk. Whole body
Villous atrophy	Most of the patients	Not known**
Circulating anti-tTG IgA	50–95%	38%
Circulating anti-eTG IgA	50–95%	43%
DIF	Granular IgA deposits	Granular and fibrillar IgA deposits
Response to the GFD	Most of the patients	Lack of consistent data
Association with autoimmune diseases	Frequent	Rare

HLA, Human Leucocyte Antigen; DIF, Direct Immunofluorescent; GFD, gluten-free diet.
**The frequency of HLA-DQ8 refers to the study by Ohata et al. (18), where the allele was found in six (37%) out of 16 Japanese patients with DH (19).*
***Found in three out of six patients in the study by Ohata et al. (79), including a total of 91 patients in 2012.*

A recent study demonstrated a link between Reovirus, an avirulent pathogen that elicit protective immunity, and the loss of peripheral tolerance against dietary antigens, resulting in a Th1-type immunity to dietary antigens. Moreover, the study found an increased titer of antibodies against Reovirus in patients with active CD and elevated serum anti-tTG autoantibodies, suggesting a direct link between the pathogen and the induction of CD (96). Whether there might be an infectious trigger also for DH is far less clear (97).

To conclude, complex endocrine and immunologic factors seem to play a role in modulating the inflammatory response in DH, suggesting that its pathogenesis is much more complex than a simple interaction between HLA-DQ antigens and gluten.

Epidermal Transglutaminase Is the Main Autoantigen of Dermatitis Herpetiformis

Epidermal transglutaminase (eTG) belongs to a nine-member Ca^{2+}-dependent enzyme family that promotes the formation of covalent cross-links between proteins (98). eTG is physiologically expressed in the spinous layer of the epidermis, and contribute to epidermal terminal differentiation, formation of the cornified cell envelop, and protection of keratinocytes against UVB-induced apoptosis (99–102).

While tTG was shown to be a major autoantigen of CD, Sardy et al. identified eTG as the main autoantigen of DH (9). Specifically, they observed that CD and DH patients had autoantibodies targeting both tTG and eTG; however, IgA autoantibodies binding selectively and with high avidity to eTG were found only in DH patients. Moreover, eTG, but not tTG, was found to co-localize with IgA in the granular deposits at the papillary tips of DH skin (9). The mechanism by which both CD and DH patients develop an autoimmune response against eTG remains still obscure. One suggested hypothesis is related to epitope spreading (99). The phenomenon of epitope spreading involves the development over time of a humoral or cell-mediated immune response from an initial dominant epitope to a secondary one, belonging to the same (intramolecular) or a distinct (intermolecular) antigen (103). Evidence supporting the theory of epitope spreading in DH include: (i) the high sequence homology between tTG and eTG (9); (ii) the presence of an autoimmunity also against neuronal TG (or TG6), which is also highly similar to tTG and eTG, in both CD and DH (99); (iii) the lower prevalence of anti-eTG IgA autoantibodies in pediatric compared to adult CD patients, which (iv) parallels the decreased, albeit not abolished, incidence of DH during childhood (23, 104).

One recent study demonstrated that patients with active DH secreted considerably high amounts of anti-eTG IgA in the organ culture medium of small bowel mucosal biopsies, and had eTG-binding IgA-positive cells in the lamina propria, thereby suggesting that autoimmunity against eTG possibly develops in the gut (85). Interestingly, small bowel secretion of eTG-targeting IgA did not occur in CD patients, despite they showed elevated levels of such autoantibodies in the serum (85).

An unmet issue concerns the mechanism underlying the formation of eTG/IgA aggregates in the skin. One theory suggests that, in regions of trauma, where DH lesions classically occurs, epidermal damage leads to eTG shedding from the spinous layer to the upper dermis, where it binds to circulating anti-eTG IgA. A study by Zone et al. supports this hypothesis, showing that passive transfer of goat anti-eTG IgG or DH serum into mice with human skin grafts reproduced DH-like deposits only in the engrafted skin, the only source of human eTG (105). An alternative hypothesis is that eTG/IgA aggregates exists as circulating immune complexes. Accordingly, DH patients may show asymptomatic IgA immune complex deposition in the kidney (106); Preisz et al. described deposits of eTG/IgA1 complexes in both upper and deep dermal vessels in roughly 64% of DH patients (107); rare clinical manifestations of DH include digital purpura and ecchymosis, that show evidence of small vessels vasculitis on microscopic examination (49, 108); circulating eTG/IgA immune complexes can be found in patients with DH and their concentrations decrease under the GFD (109).

TABLE 2 | Evidence which seem to support or point against the pathogenic relevance of eTG/IgA deposits which are typically found in the perilesional skin of patients with DH.

Evidence supporting the pathogenic role of eTG/IgA aggregates in DH
1) Circulating eTG IgA correlate with disease activity and disappear after a GFD
2) eTG/IgA complexes are enzimatically active, and activate fibrinogen at the tips of the papillary dermis
3) Circulating and skin resident neutrophils express Fc IgA receptor (CD89), suggesting a direct interaction between neutrophils and IgA.
Evidence against the pathogenic role of eTG/IgA aggregates in DH
1) eTG/IgA complexes can be found in the healthy skin of patients with DH
2) eTG/IgA complexes can be detected in the skin of coealic patients without DH
3) eTG/IgA complexes disappears even years after the introduction of the GFD and the resolution of the skin rash
4) Passive transfer of goat anti-eTG IgG or human DH sera in mice with human skin grafts reproduces DH-like granular deposits in the engrafted skin, but not DH lesions

DH, dermatitis herpetiformis; eTG, epidermal transglutaminase; IgA, immunoglobulin A; GFD, gluten free diet.

Pathogenic Relevance of IgA Autoantibodies Against Epidermal Transglutaminase

A major controversial issue concerns the role of eTG/IgA aggregates in DH, since some studies clearly support their pathogenic relevance, whilst others did not (**Table 2**). For example, serum anti-eTG IgA autoantibodies has proven to correlate positively with disease activity (110): along with anti-tTG IgA and anti-endomysium autoantibodies (EmA), they significantly decrease in patients achieving clinical remission owing to the GFD, while increasing in patients who suffer a relapse (111). However, passive transfer of goat anti-eTG autoantibodies or DH human serum into SCID mice with human skin grafts fails to induce DH lesions, despite the formation of the typical granular eTG/IgA deposits into the engrafted skin (105, 112).

In the skin, eTG/IgA aggregates have been shown to activate fibrinogen, which can be found at the tips of the papillary dermis in a pattern similar to that of eTG/IgA aggregates (113). Fibrinolysis directly contributes to the blister formation in DH, and it is also believed to function as a chemoattractant for neutrophis, T-cells and macrophages, which are major components of the inflammatory infiltrate of DH (114). Both circulating and skin resident neutrophils in DH have been shown to highly express Fc IgA receptors, suggesting activation dependent on the interaction with the eTG/IgA complexes (115, 116). However, Donaldson et al. observed that granular IgA deposits could be also detected in the non-affected skin of DH patients (114). More intriguingly, Cannistraci et al. documented eTG/IgA co-localization in the papillary dermis, at the dermal-epidermal junction and in the vessel walls of coeliac patients without skin manifestations both before and during a GFD (10, 117, 118). It is also worth of mention that disappearance of eTG/IgA deposits from the skin occurs only in a subset of patients despite a long and strict GFD and no active skin rash, and takes much longer than serum autoantibodies or immune complexes (76, 119).

Recently, Taylor and Zone found that Potassium Iodide, a known precipitating factor of DH, increases the capacity of eTG/IgA complexes to bind the substrate cadaverin in normal skin cryosections from DH patients on dapsone or on a GFD. Thus, one could speculate that, during disease remission, eTG/IgA complexes preserve a baseline enzymatic activity, allowing tight binding with anchoring fibrils of the BMZ but not the activation of fibrinogen (76, 120).

Cytokine Network in Dermatitis Herpetiformis and Mechanisms of Blister Formation

The mechanisms leading to tissue damage in DH are only partly understood. The microscopic finding of neutrophil accumulation at the papillary dermis and the responsiveness of skin lesions to dapsone support the key role of neutrophils in DH inflammation. Circulating neutrophils in DH show an increased expression of CD11b, decreased cell surface L-selectin, and increased Fc IgA receptor function, suggesting that they have already been primed before migrating into the skin (115). Indeed, neutrophils priming is likely to occur in the gut under the influx of gut-derived IL-8 (121). Accordingly, IL-8 mRNA was shown to be significantly increased in the small bowel of DH patients on a normal diet compared to that on a GFD. Circulating IL-8 decreases following the GFD, while persists elevated in DH patients who take a normal diet. A positive correlation between serum IL-8 and anti-tTG IgA antibodies has been also demonstrated, suggesting that the cytokine levels parallel the ongoing mucosal inflammation in the gut and depend directly on gluten ingestion (121). Likewise, the underlying mucosal inflammation leads to enhanced expression of the adhesion molecule E-selectin in endothelial cells from both lesional and non-lesional skin (122). Local production of cytokines and chemokines, including IL-8 and GM-CSF, in the presence of eTG/IgA deposits eventually allow migration of adhered neutrophils to the papillary dermis (121, 123). A recent study demonstrated a down-regulation of elafin, a serine protease inhibitor that inhibits a neutrophil mediated inflammatory response, in keratinocytes from DH skin. A similar finding could be also found in the epithelial cells from the small bowel of patients with active CD (124).

Activated neutrophils release neutrophil elastase and granzyme B, which induce subepidermal split by cleaving adhesion molecules of the BMZ, such as collagen VII (125). Accordingly, immunomapping studies have shown that dermal-epidermal detachment in DH mainly occurs within the lamina lucida, between collagen VII and laminin 332, and probably involves destruction of laminin 332 (126, 127). In addition, basal keratinocytes over-expresses collagenase, stromelysin-1, and urokinase-type plasminogen activator, which contribute to degrading basement membrane zone proteins (128).

The activation of the coagulation cascade is thought to be an additional pathomechanism of DH. Accordingly, Bognar et al. found a high prevalence of criofibrinogenaemia in untreated DH patients (129). Another study demonstrated an impaired fibrinogen/fibrin turnover in the disease. More in detail, untreated DH patients showed significantly prolonged clot lysis time and thicker fibrin fibers, which could be normalized by the *in vitro* adjunct of dapsone (130). Conversely, unlike BP, no studies demonstrated significant skin expression of tissue factor as well as elevation of serum D-dimer in patients with DH compared to healthy individuals (131, 132).

Previous studies have also suggested that other inflammatory cells participate to the pathogenesis of DH (133). In particular, T-lymphocytes, mononuclear phagocytes and B-cells were shown to accumulate around dermal vessels during the early phases of DH lesion formation (134). Other studies found increased Th2-related cytokines in the skin but not in the serum of DH patients (133, 135). By comparison, Makino et al. recently reported a significant elevation of IL-4, IL-5, IL-13, and eotaxin in fibrillary-type DH, whereas Th1-related cytokines, including IL-12 and IFN-γ, did not show significant differences compared to healthy controls (136).

In another study, our group demonstrated that, in DH skin, Tregs and IL-10 were significantly reduced compared to the skin of healthy subjects, whereas both coeliac and DH patients had a similar number of Tregs in duodenal biopsies, suggesting that the down-regulation of Tregs in the skin may be critical for the development of DH lesions (93).

The Pathogenesis of Pruritus in Dermatitis Herpetiformis

While over the recent years different studies have gradually shed light on the major pathogenic mechanisms of DH, the pathogenesis of pruritus is far less clear. Probably, different pathways are involved, including neurogenic inflammation, mechanical itch dysesthesias, and release of inflammatory cytokines. Accordingly, Cynkier et al. demonstrated an over-expression of neuropeptides, including corticotropin releasing factor and the receptor for endotelin B in DH lesional skin, which may be released by activated keratinocytes (137). In DH, pruritus may be evoked or worsened by mechanical stimuli (allokinesis), such as clothing. Moreover, the intensity of the perceived pruritus is also enhanced (hyperkinesis).

Among inflammatory cytokines involved in pruritogenesis, IL-31 has gained a major interest. IL-31 belongs to the cytokine family of IL-6. IL-31 interacts with a heterodimeric receptor, which comprises the IL-31 receptor A (IL-31RA) and the oncostatin M receptor (138), and is expressed on various immune cells including T cells, keratinocytes, dendritic cells, eosinophils, basophils, macrophages, and dorsal root ganglia (139–145). In mice, over-expression of IL-31 was shown to evoke pruritus and induce inflammatory cells accumulation with increased number of mast cells. Injection of IL-31 in the dog also triggers a scratching behavior. Several studies have demonstrated an over-expression of IL-31 in the skin of different pruritic dermatoses, including atopic dermatitis (146), psoriasis (147), cutaneous T-cell lymphomas (148), nephrogenic pruritus (149), and mastocytosis (145).

IL-31 seems to be particularly implicated in pruritic dermatoses related to a prevalent Th2 type inflammation (150). A recent study demonstrated that eosinophils are the major source of IL-31 in BP, a prototype of highly pruritic Th2-mediated autoimmune blistering dermatoses (151). We have previously shown that Th2 type cytokines are also elevated in the skin of DH patients, thereby allowing speculation about a possible role of IL-31 in the associated pruritus. Interestingly, while a previous paper did not show significant elevation of serum IL-31 concentration in DH patients (152), a recent study by our group demonstrated that IL-31 was not only elevated in DH serum, but also significantly over-expressed in the skin, where it co-localized with IL-31RA (153).

Intriguingly, a monoclonal antibody targeting IL-31 is currently under clinical investigation in atopic dermatitis (154). If the role of IL-31 in DH pruritus were to be confirmed, IL-31 monoclonal antibodies will open interesting therapeutic perspectives, potentially allowing a faster control of DH pruritus, which is typically refractory to either topical or systemic treatments and improve only after months following a GFD.

GLUTEN AND THE SKIN: NOT ALWAYS DERMATITIS HERPETIFORMIS

Although DH is the specific cutaneous manifestation of CD, several other skin diseases secondary to gluten ingestion are increasingly reported, especially in the last years, when the focus on gluten intolerance has grown steadily. In fact, despite the exclusion of gluten from the diet is even becoming a fashion, data from the literature demonstrate a higher incidence of skin diseases in patients with gluten-related disorders (14).

In 2012, Sapone et al. reviewed the spectrum of gluten-related disorders, including CD, DH, wheat allergy, gluten ataxia, and non-celiac gluten sensitivity (NCGS) (155). In their review, the authors highlighted that gluten ingestion could cause the involvement of different organs (such as bowel, nervous system, and skin), via the activation of different pathogenic mechanisms.

Accordingly, in recent years, several studies focused on skin manifestations different from DH that occurred in patients with both CD and NCGS.

The Skin in Celiac Patients

According to the classification proposed by Humbert et al. (156), our group recently reviewed in detail the cutaneous and mucosal manifestations associated with CD (43). As a result, different groups of CD-related skin diseases were identified; however, the main distinction was between those that improve after a GFD and those that are just occasionally associated with CD.

In general, common dermatological diseases such as psoriasis, atopic dermatitis, urticaria, aphtous stomatitis, and rosacea are more frequently diagnosed in celiac patients than in the general population (157). Notably, their diagnosis is often difficult because of atypical clinical presentation, and their course is sometimes characterized by the resistance to standard therapies and the response (or at least the improvement) after the introduction of a GFD.

In this regard, the relationship between psoriasis and CD has been studied in depth, and patients with psoriasis seem to have a 3-fold increased risk of CD (158). Moreover, in a recent meta-analysis, patients with psoriasis were demonstrated to have an increased risk of positivity for serologic markers of CD and GFD was suggested to be of potential benefit for celiac antibody-positive patients with psoriasis (159).

Despite the association between the aforementioned skin diseases, testing patients having psoriasis, atopic dermatitis, or other dermatologic diseases for CD is not advisable, since the relative risk is low. There are only few conditions in which the screening is recommended, such as type 1 diabetes mellitus, autoimmune thyroiditis, autoimmune liver disease, juvenile chronic arthritis, Down syndrome, Turner syndrome, Williams syndrome, IgA deficiency, as well as patients having first-degree relatives with CD (160); among them, no skin disorders have been included yet.

Non-celiac Gluten Sensitivity: The Skin as a Major Target

NCGS is a new entity within the group of gluten-related disorders that is being increasingly reported in the medical literature. Despite the lack of specific biomarkers, that makes the diagnosis of NCGS one of exclusion, the reported high frequency of the disease and its potential impact on the quality of life make NCGS a health challenge.

NCGS mainly affects the bowel; however, extra-intestinal manifestations are common, being the skin one of the major target of the disease.

To date, only two studies have investigated the cutaneous manifestations of NCGS, including one by our group. In general, skin lesions were found to be predominantly located on the extensor surfaces of the upper and lower limbs, and consisted of erythema, papules, crusts, and sometimes, vesicles, resembling subacute eczema, or even DH. Some patients had hyperkeratotic scales overlying mild erythematous plaques similar to psoriasis, while others showed urticarial plaques or wheals (161, 162). Besides the prevalent clinical phenotype, all the patients suffered from intense pruritus, that in about 10% of the cases represented the only symptom.

Interestingly, in both studies, patients were shown to respond well to a GFD, with some patients achieving disease remission within only 1 month following the GFD (161). It is worth mentioning that about 80% of the patient included in our study showed at DIF the presence of DH-like granular C3 deposits at the dermal-epidermal junction, but none showed the presence of IgA.

This immunopathologic profile, together with itching and the resolution of the skin lesions after the introduction of a GFD were considered as the main features of this new entity, referred to as "cutaneous gluten sensitivity."

Despite the low number of enrolled patients, suggesting that further studies are required to confirm these data, the introduction of the concept of specific skin manifestations related to NCGS may be helpful for the management of the patients, as is for DH and CD.

In fact, the main issue of NCGS is represented by the diagnosis, that relies on a procedure that is impractical to be implemented in the clinical setting (i.e., double blind placebo controlled challenge with duodenal biopsy) (163). Accordingly, the identification of specific skin features such as cutaneous gluten sensitivity might allow the diagnosis of NCGS without the need of invasive investigations.

DIAGNOSIS OF DERMATITIS HERPETIFORMIS

DH is a difficult disease to be diagnosed. Accordingly, the delay from the occurrence of the first symptoms or clinical signs to the diagnosis is usually of several months or even years, although it is reported to be decreasing in the last decades, probably due to a major awareness both of DH itself and of coeliac disease (25).

This diagnostic delay is caused by the rarity of DH and the polymorphic cutaneous manifestations, which can be misdiagnosed as other chronic pruritic dermatoses including autoimmune blistering diseases such as BP or Linear IgA bullous dermatosis but also atopic dermatitis, eczema, prurigo, urticaria, or scabies (7). Moreover, in the last years skin manifestations of NCGS have emerged as a novel diagnostic challenge in patients with gluten intolerance, since they can clinically resemble DH and can share similar intestinal involvement (161, 162).

The Role of Skin Biopsy: Are IgA Deposits Still Pathognomonic of Dermatitis Herpetiformis?

After taking patient's history and clinical examination, the first step to make a diagnosis of DH is to perform a skin biopsy. The biopsy specimen can be investigated for histopathological examination, which may show typical features such as subepidermal vesicles and blisters associated with accumulation of neutrophils at the papillary tips (7). However, in a third of the cases (164), histopathology is non-specific; atypical findings have been also reported, including acantholysis, leading to a possible histopathologic overlap with pemphigus (165).

Therefore, although histopathological examination may be helpful, DIF from the perilesional skin is still considered the gold standard for the diagnosis. The main finding is the presence of granular IgA deposits at the dermal papillae and/or at the dermal-epidermal junction (**Figure 4**) (7); in some cases, and in up to 50% of Japanese patients (79), a fibrillar deposition of IgA could be found.

Besides IgA, other immunoreactants can be found at the dermal-epidermal junction or at the dermal papillae in the perilesional skin. Among them, IgG granular deposits are infrequently detected, while IgM and C3 granular deposits are present in more cases.

In some cases, patients may show only granular deposition of C3 in the absence of IgA, IgG, or IgM. Recently, a case series of 20 patients showing these findings at DIF has been reported (166). Half of them had clinical features mimicking DH and very few of them showed low titres of anti-eTG, anti-tTG, anti-gliadin, and anti-BP180 antibodies. The authors proposed the

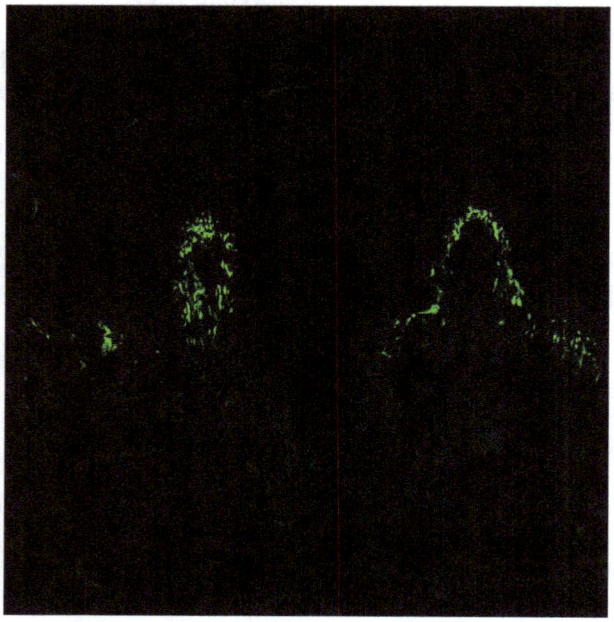

FIGURE 4 | Direct immunofluorescence of perilesional skin specimens from patients with dermatitis herpetiformis (DH). Granular IgA deposits at the dermal papillary tips are considered a pathognomonic finding of DH (magnification 400×).

term granular C3 dermatosis to describe this condition (166), that might be considered as an umbrella concept including different diseases (DH, cutaneous gluten sensitivity, non-DH dermatoses occurring in patients with CD) rather than a distinct clinical entity.

Although its prominent role in the diagnostic algorithm for DH, due to its high sensitivity and specificity, DIF can have some limitations. As an example, several papers reported patients diagnosed with DH according to compatible clinical features, histopathology, concomitant presence of CD, the response to the GFD or dapsone, and the recurrence of cutaneous lesions after a gluten challenge, but showing negative DIF results (167, 168).

In some instances, DIF may result negative because of the site of the biopsy; in fact, when the skin specimen is taken in lesional skin or too far from the skin lesions, it may lack the presence of IgA deposits (7). However, in some confirmed DH cases, even repeated biopsies performed at different times gave negative DIF results, suggesting that false-negative patients are possible (169, 170).

Another pitfall can be related to the interpretation of DIF. On this point, a recent paper from our group reported a case-series of six celiac patients presenting with skin diseases different from DH, such as contact eczema, dermatophytosis, granuloma annulare, pytiriasis rosea, lichenoid dermatitis, and psoriasis. Notably, all these patients showed a granular deposit of IgA at the dermal-epidermal junction and/or at the papillary tips (10). As previously mentioned, Cannistraci et al. observed granular IgA deposits in the healthy skin of nine celiac patients without any cutaneous manifestation (117). Both these studies raise the hypothesis that granular IgA deposits may occur also as a cutaneous marker of CD. Interestingly, while in study by Cannistraci et al. coeliac patients showed IgA/eTG co-localization in the granular deposits, no IgA/eTG co-localization was documented in any case from our study.

To conclude, the diagnosis of DH should be the result of an overall assessment, including clinical, histological, and immunopathological findings and could not rely only on DIF findings. Whether assessing the co-localization between IgA and eTG deposits in the perilesional skin might be helpful to confirm the diagnosis of DH in doubtful cases warrants further investigation.

Beyond Direct Immunofluorescence: Serology and Other Investigations

Among other examinations that can help in the diagnosis of DH, serology plays a primary role, mainly as a screening tool. In fact, as happens for CD, patients with DH test positive in the majority of cases for anti-tTG, anti-EMA and anti-deamidated synthetic gliadin-derived peptides, that overall showed a sensitivity ranging from 50 to 95%, and a specificity higher than 90% (171). Moreover, in the last years, after the demonstration of eTG as the main autoantigen for DH, anti-eTG antibodies have been shown to be a promising tool for the diagnosis of DH (12, 104, 111). Unfortunately, although their sensitivity and specificity for DH are close to those of anti-tTG antibodies, anti-eTG antibodies can be found in about 30 to 50% of the patients with CD (12, 172), and therefore, are not helpful to differentiate between DH and other dermatoses occurring in celiac patients.

Other antibodies have been tested in patients with DH showing promising results, such as anti-neo epitope tissue TG (173) and anti-GAF3X antibodies (174); however they were no further tested and their high sensitivity and specificity values should be confirmed.

A comprehensive assessment of patients with DH can include other investigations that may be helpful in doubtful cases. Duodenal biopsy is usually not required but, since it is the gold standard for the diagnosis of CD, it should be performed if the clinical picture or other findings are highly evocative for the diagnosis of DH but DIF results negative (7). In that case, the presence of villous atrophy at histopathology is important to confirm (or to exclude) the diagnosis of CD and to support the introduction of a GFD, at least in the Caucasians. Accordingly, it is worth noting that duodenal biopsy might be not helpful in Japanese DH patients, because of the weaker association of DH with CD in that population and because diseases other than CD represent a more frequent cause of villous atrophy in Asia, including tropical sprue, parasitic infections, immunoproliferative small intestinal diseases and combined variable immunodeficiency disease (175).

Since virtually all the patients with CD and DH, at least in western countries, have HLA-DQ2 or DQ8 aplotypes, HLA testing may be helpful for its high negative predictive value in order to exclude a diagnosis of DH and to avoid repetition of unnecessary investigations (171).

Finally, in the last years, other potential diagnostic tools have been proposed for DH. As an example, dermoscopy was found to be helpful in the differential diagnosis of autoimmune bullous diseases involving the scalp. In particular, patients with DH usually show the absence of yellow scales, that are more typical of pemphigus patients, but display extravasation and clustered dotted vessels (176), that seem to be a specific finding of the disease and are found even in the petechial lesions of palms and soles (177).

Other more complex investigations, such as the analysis of microbiota and of metabolic signature of the patients, may provide some information on the patients with DH. However, although they were investigated in detail in patients with CD, paving the way for their potential use in the clinical setting (178, 179), very scarce data are available for DH (180), and further studies are needed to address the questions that are still open in this field.

TREATMENT

The Central Role of Gluten: What's Beyond Gluten-Free Diet?

Since DH is the specific cutaneous manifestation of CD, at least in the Caucasians, all the patients require a GFD. Although some authors suggested that a subgroup of the patients with DH can go into remission and, therefore, gluten-free diet may be stopped (13), other studies demonstrated that DH is associated with an increased risk of associated diseases, such as non-Hodgkin lymphomas (28). Moreover, although this risk is higher in the first 5 years after the diagnosis, it overlaps that of the general population thereafter (32). As a result, since GFD in DH is a way to prevent complications rather just a symptomatic treatment for skin lesions, it should be maintained for all the life (181).

Gluten-free diet requires strict monitoring of all ingested foods, it is time-consuming, and socially restricting (182), and patient compliance depends on different individual and environmental factors, with a self-reported diet adherence in adult patients with CD ranging from 36 to 96%(183). By contrast, patients with DH seem to have a better compliance to gluten-free diet, with an overall adherence of 98% (percentage that decreases to 72% for strict adherence) (32). However, since gluten contamination is possible even in supposed gluten-free food, nutritional monitoring, and participation in support groups are recommended for both patients with CD and DH (184). Moreover, some patients that adhere to gluten-free diet are refractory even several years after the introduction of the diet (185).

According to the limitations of gluten-free diet reported above, novel approaches to treat patients with CD and DH are currently under investigation. Such new therapies rely on blocking at different steps the pathogenic process occurring in gluten-sensitive disorders.

For example, the reduction of gluten immunogenicity via the production of genetically modified grains may lead to a decrease of the number of patients that are able to develop autoimmunity to gliadin-tissue TG complexes (186). RNA interference is another way that could be applied in order to reduce gluten toxicity (187). Moreover, gluten exposure could be reduced using some binders that allow its sequestration in the bowel lumen, or by hydrolysis of gluten peptides that are resistant to proteolysis in a physiological setting using orally administered glutenases (188). Finally, the exposure to immunogenic peptides can be prevented by altering gut permeability; in this regard, the blockade of zonulin, a tight junction protein that regulates the epithelial transit of molecules, with inhibitors such as larazotide has proven to ameliorate symptoms of patients with CD (189).

Other steps that can be targeted in patients with CD are related to the activation of the immune response. tTG activity inhibition, HLA-DQ2 blocking with gluten peptide analogs or immune tolerance induction using specific gluten epitopes are under study or are being tested in patients with CD (190, 191).

Pharmacologic Treatment of DH: When Gluten-Free Diet Is Not Enough

All the approaches reported above are being developed for patients with CD but, since they are oriented to prevent gluten sensitization or to restore gluten tolerance, they might work even for DH. The latter, however, has some specific therapeutic issues that differ from those of CD. In fact, while intestinal symptoms usually resolve in few weeks, cutaneous manifestations may last months or even years after the introduction of a GFD. Therefore, in most cases, pharmacologic treatment is required in order to control itching as well as the skin rash (7).

Despite the lack of randomized controlled trials, dapsone has been considered the first line treatment in patients with DH for over 70 years. Dosages of about 50 to 100 mg per day are usually sufficient to clear the skin rash. At these dosages, side effects are usually rare. However, hemolytic anemia and methemoglobinemia, that are dose-dependent side effects, can be seen in some patients. As a result, all the patients taking the drug should be followed up with frequent testing of hemoglobin levels and reticulocytes. In patients with glucose-6-posphate dehydrogenase deficiency dapsone treatment is contraindicated (7).

In two case reports, topical dapsone 5% gel was also shown to be effective as an adjuvant treatment for DH, which is not adequately controlled by GFD or oral dapsone (192, 193). Compared to the oral counterpart, topical dapsone shows a lower incidence of side effects and can be administered safely in patients with glucose-6-posphate dehydrogenase deficiency (192).

Possible alternatives to dapsone are the so-called sulfonamides, including sulfasalazine, sulfapyridine, and sulfamethoxypyridazine, that may potentially cause hemolytic anemia and gastrointestinal upset, but require a less strict monitoring than dapsone (7). Furthermore, a recent report suggested that combination therapy with dapsone and sulfasalazine may be effective in patients who do not tolerate increasing doses of dapsone monotherapy (194).

Several other pharmacologic treatments have been proposed for DH. Case reports do exist showing that cyclosporin A, azathioprine, colchicine, heparin, tetracyclines, nicotinamide, and mycophenolate may control the acute rash in patients with DH (171). Among them, some authors suggested that colchicine may be used as a second choice after dapsone, due to its antineutrophilic and antithrombotic activity (195), since DH was reported to be associated with a decreased fibrinolytic potential (130).

Besides these "old" drugs, biologics may become the next step in DH pharmacologic treatment. Among them, rituximab has been proven to be effective in a patient resistant to GFD, dapsone, sulfasalazine, and conventional immunosuppressive agents such as azathioprine, and was suggested as a viable treatment option for recalcitrant DH (196).

Celiac Disease and Dermatitis Herpetiformis: Is Prevention Possible?

In the last years, some authors focused on the risk factors associated with the development of CD, aiming at the prevention of the disease in genetically at-risk infants or children. Randomized controlled trials investigated the possible role of the age at which gluten is introduced, showing that neither ingestion of small gluten amounts between weeks 16–24, nor delayed introduction of gluten (at 6 or at 12 months) modified the incidence of CD in the studied groups (197, 198).

Besides gluten, microbiota has been suggested to act as a trigger in several autoimmune diseases, including CD. In the latter, both genetic and environmental factors, such as rotavirus infection, may modified the gut microbiota of at-risk patients that, in turn, can affect bowel immunity and permeability (199). In particular, altered gut microbiota increases the production of pro-inflammatory cytokines, impairs the mucosal barrier, and produces microbial TG (199), that is a target of antibodies found in celiac patients (200). Therefore, targeting the gut microbiota via probiotics may be a reasonable approach in order to prevent CD in at-risk individuals, and trials are currently underway (199).

Notably, all these data are available for CD. However, due to the close correlation with CD, it could be assumed that such strategies may work even for the prevention of DH, and studies on these topics would be advisable.

FINAL CONSIDERATIONS AND FUTURE PERSPECTIVES

DH is an autoimmune bullous disease associated with a chronic, usually asymptomatic, autoimmune enteropathy, that arises in genetically susceptible individuals, in the presence of gluten proteins consumed in common grain products.

One of the main concerns of DH is still represented by misdiagnosis, due to its rarity, the growing report of atypical clinical presentations and the possible occurrence of IgA deposits in non-DH skin diseases. In the near future, the diagnostic challenge is expected even to increase, due to the falling incidence of DH (16). This is reflected by the quite long diagnostic delay, found even in high prevalence areas (25).

In the last years, NCGS has emerged as a new entity within the spectrum of gluten-related disorders. Similarities in both clinical and immunopathological findings may enhance the diagnostic challenge and have important therapeutic implications. In fact, although GFD is the first line treatment for both DH and NCGS, patients with DH should be followed up closely for dietary adherence, nutritional deficiencies, and potential complications.

Recent advances in the pathogenesis of DH have paved the way for the development of new treatments to be used in the time window between the beginning of the GFD and the complete resolution of skin lesions. As an example, the recent finding of elevated serum levels of IL-17 and IL-36 in DH patients supported their possible role in the activation of neutrophils and NK cells, making them as possible targets for new therapeutic strategies (201). In addition, the involvement of IL-31 pathway in DH suggests a connection among the immune system, the nervous system and itch, and its targeting holds promise for the treatment of the patients (153).

AUTHOR CONTRIBUTIONS

EA, RM, and MC designed the study and drafted the manuscript. LQ, AV, DB, and VB drafted the manuscript. EA, RM, and MC revised the whole manuscript. All the authors approved the final content of the manuscript.

ACKNOWLEDGMENTS

We thank the Italian Celiac Foundation for the support given to our research group in the field of dermatitis herpetiformis.

REFERENCES

1. Duhring LA. Landmark article, Aug 30, 1884: Dermatitis herpetiformis. *JAMA*. (1983) 250:212–16. doi: 10.1001/jama.250.2.212
2. Esteves J, Brandao FN. Effect of sulfonamides and sulfones on Duhring's disease. *Clin Lat.* (1952) 2:34–9.
3. van der Meer JB. Granular deposits of immunoglobulins in the skin of patients with dermatitis herpetiformis. An immunofluorescent study. *Br J Dermatol.* (1969) 81:493–503. doi: 10.1111/j.1365-2133.1969.tb16024.x
4. Marks J, Shuster S, Watson AJ. Small-bowel changes in dermatitis herpetiformis. *Lancet.* (1966) 2:1280–2. doi: 10.1016/S0140-6736(66)91692-8
5. Katz SI, Falchuk ZM, Dahl MV, Rogentine GN, Strober W. HL-A8: a genetic link between dermatitis herpetiformis and gluten-sensitive enteropathy. *J Clin Invest.* (1972) 51:2977–80. doi: 10.1172/JCI 107123
6. Fry L, Seah PP, Riches DJ, Hoffbrand AV. Clearance of skin lesions in dermatitis herpetiformis after gluten withdrawal. *Lancet.* (1973) 1:288–91. doi: 10.1016/S0140-6736(73)91539-0
7. Caproni M, Antiga E, Melani L, Fabbri P, Italian group for cutaneous I. Guidelines for the diagnosis and treatment of dermatitis herpetiformis. *J Eur Acad Dermatol Venereol.* (2009) 23:633–8. doi: 10.1111/j.1468-3083.2009.03188.x
8. Caproni M, Cardinali C, Renzi D, Calabro A, Fabbri P. Tissue transglutaminase antibody assessment in dermatitis herpetiformis. *Br J Dermatol.* (2001) 144:196–7. doi: 10.1111/j.1365-2133.2001.03981.x
9. Sardy M, Karpati S, Merkl B, Paulsson M, Smyth N. Epidermal transglutaminase (TGase 3) is the autoantigen of dermatitis herpetiformis. *J Exp Med.* (2002) 195:747–57. doi: 10.1084/jem.20011299
10. Bonciolini V, Antiga E, Bianchi B, Del Bianco E, Ninci A, Maio V, et al. Granular IgA deposits in the skin of patients with coeliac disease: is it

always dermatitis herpetiformis? *Acta Derm Venereol.* (2019) 99:78–83. doi: 10.2340/00015555-3001
11. Leonard MM, Sapone A, Catassi C, Fasano A. Celiac disease and non-celiac gluten sensitivity: a review. *JAMA.* (2017) 318:647–56. doi: 10.1001/jama.2017.9730
12. Hull CM, Liddle M, Hansen N, Meyer LJ, Schmidt L, Taylor T, et al. Elevation of IgA anti-epidermal transglutaminase antibodies in dermatitis herpetiformis. *Br J Dermatol.* (2008) 159:120–4. doi: 10.1111/j.1365-2133.2008.08629.x
13. Paek SY, Steinberg SM, Katz SI. Remission in dermatitis herpetiformis: a cohort study. *Arch Dermatol.* (2011) 147:301–5. doi: 10.1001/archdermatol.2010.336
14. Graziano M, Rossi M. An update on the cutaneous manifestations of coeliac disease and non-coeliac gluten sensitivity. *Int Rev Immunol.* (2018) 37:291–300. doi: 10.1080/08830185.2018.1533008
15. Bolotin D, Petronic-Rosic V. Dermatitis herpetiformis. Part I. Epidemiology, pathogenesis, and clinical presentation. *J Am Acad Dermatol.* (2011) 64:1017–24. doi: 10.1016/j.jaad.2010.09.777
16. Salmi TT, Hervonen K, Kautiainen H, Collin P, Reunala T. Prevalence and incidence of dermatitis herpetiformis: a 40-year prospective study from Finland. *Br J Dermatol.* (2011) 165:354–9. doi: 10.1111/j.1365-2133.2011.10385.x
17. Zhang F, Yang B, Lin Y, Chen S, Zhou G, Wang G, et al. Dermatitis herpetiformis in China: a report of 22 cases. *J Eur Acad Dermatol Venereol.* (2012) 26:903–7. doi: 10.1111/j.1468-3083.2011.04204.x
18. Ohata C, Ishii N, Niizeki H, Shimomura Y, Furumura M, Inoko H, et al. Unique characteristics in Japanese dermatitis herpetiformis. *Br J Dermatol.* (2016) 174:180–3. doi: 10.1111/bjd.13965
19. West J, Fleming KM, Tata LJ, Card TR, Crooks CJ. Incidence and prevalence of celiac disease and dermatitis herpetiformis in the UK over two decades: population-based study. *Am J Gastroenterol.* (2014) 109:757–68. doi: 10.1038/ajg.2014.55
20. Smith JB, Tulloch JE, Meyer LJ, Zone JJ. The incidence and prevalence of dermatitis herpetiformis in Utah. *Arch Dermatol.* (1992) 128:1608–10. doi: 10.1001/archderm.1992.04530010046006
21. Virta LJ, Kaukinen K, Collin P. Incidence and prevalence of diagnosed coeliac disease in Finland: results of effective case finding in adults. *Scand J Gastroenterol.* (2009) 44:933–8. doi: 10.1080/00365520903030795
22. Askling J, Linet M, Gridley G, Halstensen TS, Ekstrom K, Ekbom A. Cancer incidence in a population-based cohort of individuals hospitalized with celiac disease or dermatitis herpetiformis. *Gastroenterology.* (2002) 123:1428–35. doi: 10.1053/gast.2002.36585
23. Antiga E, Verdelli A, Calabro A, Fabbri P, Caproni M. Clinical and immunopathological features of 159 patients with dermatitis herpetiformis: an Italian experience. *G Ital Dermatol Venereol.* (2013) 148:163–9.
24. Collin P, Salmi TT, Hervonen K, Kaukinen K, Reunala T. Dermatitis herpetiformis: a cutaneous manifestation of coeliac disease. *Ann Med.* (2017) 49:23–31. doi: 10.1080/07853890.2016.1222450
25. Mansikka E, Salmi T, Kaukinen K, Collin P, Huhtala H, Reunala T, et al. Diagnostic delay in dermatitis herpetiformis in a high-prevalence area. *Acta Derm Venereol.* (2018) 98:195–9. doi: 10.2340/00015555-2818
26. Maglie R, Hertl M. Pharmacological advances in pemphigoid. *Curr Opin Pharmacol.* (2019) 46:34–43. doi: 10.1016/j.coph.2018.12.007
27. Varpuluoma O, Jokelainen J, Forsti AK, Timonen M, Huilaja L, Tasanen K. Dermatitis herpetiformis and celiac disease increase the risk of bullous pemphigoid. *J Invest Dermatol.* (2019) 139:600–4. doi: 10.1016/j.jid.2018.10.010
28. Grainge MJ, West J, Solaymani-Dodaran M, Card TR, Logan RF. The long-term risk of malignancy following a diagnosis of coeliac disease or dermatitis herpetiformis: a cohort study. *Aliment Pharmacol Ther.* (2012) 35:730–9. doi: 10.1111/j.1365-2036.2012.04998.x
29. Swerdlow AJ, Whittaker S, Carpenter LM, English JS. Mortality and cancer incidence in patients with dermatitis herpetiformis: a cohort study. *Br J Dermatol.* (1993) 129:140–4. doi: 10.1111/j.1365-2133.1993.tb03516.x
30. Viljamaa M, Kaukinen K, Pukkala E, Hervonen K, Reunala T, Collin P. Malignancies and mortality in patients with coeliac disease and dermatitis herpetiformis: 30-year population-based study. *Dig Liver Dis.* (2006) 38:374–80. doi: 10.1016/j.dld.2006.03.002
31. Lewis NR, Logan RF, Hubbard RB, West J. No increase in risk of fracture, malignancy or mortality in dermatitis herpetiformis: a cohort study. *Aliment Pharmacol Ther.* (2008) 27:1140–7. doi: 10.1111/j.1365-2036.2008.03660.x
32. Hervonen K, Alakoski A, Salmi TT, Helakorpi S, Kautiainen H, Kaukinen K, et al. Reduced mortality in dermatitis herpetiformis: a population-based study of 476 patients. *Br J Dermatol.* (2012) 167:1331–7. doi: 10.1111/j.1365-2133.2012.11105.x
33. Ali FR, Lear JT. Is dermatitis herpetiformis a proxy of prosperity? *Br J Dermatol.* (2013) 169:231. doi: 10.1111/bjd.12319
34. Lear JT, Neary RH, Jones P, Fitzgerald DA, English JS. Risk factors for ischaemic heart disease in patients with dermatitis herpetiformis. *J R Soc Med.* (1997) 90:247–9. doi: 10.1177/014107689709000504
35. Ferson M, Edwards A, Lind A, Milton GW, Hersey P. Low natural killer-cell activity and immunoglobulin levels associated with smoking in human subjects. *Int J Cancer.* (1979) 23:603–9. doi: 10.1002/ijc.2910230504
36. Barton JR, Riad MA, Gaze MN, Maran AG, Ferguson A. Mucosal immunodeficiency in smokers, and in patients with epithelial head and neck tumours. *Gut.* (1990) 31:378–82. doi: 10.1136/gut.31.4.378
37. Collin P, Reunala T. Recognition and management of the cutaneous manifestations of celiac disease: a guide for dermatologists. *Am J Clin Dermatol.* (2003) 4:13–20. doi: 10.2165/00128071-200304010-00002
38. Zone JJ. Skin manifestations of celiac disease. *Gastroenterology.* (2005) 128(4 Suppl 1):S87–91. doi: 10.1053/j.gastro.2005.02.026
39. Reunala T, Salmi TT, Hervonen K, Kaukinen K, Collin P. Dermatitis herpetiformis: a common extraintestinal manifestation of coeliac disease. *Nutrients.* (2018) 10:E602. doi: 10.3390/nu10050602
40. Nicolas ME, Krause PK, Gibson LE, Murray JA. Dermatitis herpetiformis. *Int J Dermatol.* (2003) 42:588–600. doi: 10.1046/j.1365-4362.2003.01804.x
41. da Silva PC, de Almeida Pdel V, Machado MA, de Lima AA, Gregio AM, Trevilatto PC, et al. Oral manifestations of celiac disease. A case report and review of the literature. *Med Oral Patol Oral Cir Bucal.* (2008) 13:E559–62.
42. Campisi G, Di Liberto C, Iacono G, Compilato D, Di Prima L, Calvino F, et al. Oral pathology in untreated coeliac [corrected] disease. *Aliment Pharmacol Ther.* (2007) 26:1529–36. doi: 10.1111/j.1365-2036.2007.03535.x
43. Caproni M, Bonciolini V, D'Errico A, Antiga E, Fabbri P. Celiac disease and dermatologic manifestations: many skin clue to unfold gluten-sensitive enteropathy. *Gastroenterol Res Pract.* (2012) 2012:952753. doi: 10.1155/2012/952753
44. Lahteenoja H, Toivanen A, Viander M, Maki M, Irjala K, Raiha I, et al. Oral mucosal changes in coeliac patients on a gluten-free diet. *Eur J Oral Sci.* (1998) 106:899–906. doi: 10.1046/j.0909-8836.1998.eos106501.x
45. Reunala TL. Dermatitis herpetiformis. *Clin Dermatol.* (2001) 19:728–36. doi: 10.1016/S0738-081X(00)00184-X
46. Antiga E, Fabbri P, Caproni M. Is dermatitis herpetiformis changing? *G Ital Dermatol Venereol.* (2013) 148:159–62.
47. Mistry A, Mistry N. Persistent pruritic papulovesicles. Dermatitis herpetiformis. *Am Fam Physician.* (2014) 90:407–8.
48. Olson MA, Wieland CN, Newman CC. Diffuse vesicular rash with intractable pruritus. *JAMA.* (2015) 313:1158–9. doi: 10.1001/jama.2014.17575
49. Tu H, Parmentier L, Stieger M, Spanou Z, Horn M, Beltraminelli H, et al. Acral purpura as leading clinical manifestation of dermatitis herpetiformis: report of two adult cases with a review of the literature. *Dermatology.* (2013) 227:1–4. doi: 10.1159/000347108
50. Zone JJ, Egan CA, Taylor TB, Meyer LJ. IgA autoimmune disorders: development of a passive transfer mouse model. *J Investig Dermatol Symp Proc.* (2004) 9:47–51. doi: 10.1111/j.1087-0024.2004.00840.x
51. Marks R, Jones EW. Purpura in dermatitis herpetiformis. *Br J Dermatol.* (1971) 84:386–8.
52. McCleskey PE, Erickson QL, David-Bajar KM, Elston DM. Palmar petechiae in dermatitis herpetiformis: a case report and clinical review. *Cutis.* (2002) 70:217−23.
53. McGovern TW, Bennion SD. Palmar purpura: an atypical presentation of childhood dermatitis herpetiformis. *Pediatr Dermatol.* (1994) 11:319–22. doi: 10.1111/j.1525-1470.1994.tb00096.x
54. Pierce DK, Purcell SM, Spielvogel RL. Purpuric papules and vesicles of the palms in dermatitis herpetiformis. *J Am Acad Dermatol.* (1987) 16:1274–6. doi: 10.1016/S0190-9622(87)80040-3

55. Hofmann SC, Nashan D, Bruckner-Tuderman L. Petechiae on the fingertips as presenting symptom of dermatitis herpetiformis Duhring. *J Eur Acad Dermatol Venereol.* (2009) 23:732–3. doi: 10.1111/j.1468-3083.2009.03200.x
56. Naylor E, Atwater A, Selim MA, Hall R, Puri PK. Leukocytoclastic vasculitis as the presenting feature of dermatitis herpetiformis. *Arch Dermatol.* (2011) 147:1313–6. doi: 10.1001/archdermatol.2011.293
57. Kern M, Kim KH, Johnson G, Hawkins SD, Wong HK. Dermatitis herpetiformis presenting as pseudovasculitis. *JAAD Case Rep.* (2017) 3:444–7. doi: 10.1016/j.jdcr.2017.06.033
58. Ohshima Y, Tamada Y, Matsumoto Y, Hashimoto T. Dermatitis herpetiformis Duhring with palmoplantar keratosis. *Br J Dermatol.* (2003) 149:1300–2. doi: 10.1111/j.1365-2133.2003.05660.x
59. Powell GR, Bruckner AL, Weston WL. Dermatitis herpetiformis presenting as chronic urticaria. *Pediatr Dermatol.* (2004) 21:564–7. doi: 10.1111/j.0736-8046.2004.21509.x
60. Saito M, Boer A, Ishiko A, Nishikawa T. Atypical dermatitis herpetiformis: a Japanese case that presented with initial lesions mimicking prurigo pigmentosa. *Clin Exp Dermatol.* (2006) 31:290–1. doi: 10.1111/j.1365-2230.2005.02009.x
61. Meyer LJ, Zone JJ. Familial incidence of dermatitis herpetiformis. *J Am Acad Dermatol.* (1987) 17:643–7. doi: 10.1016/S0190-9622(87)70250-3
62. Reunala T. Incidence of familial dermatitis herpetiformis. *Br J Dermatol.* (1996) 134:394–8. doi: 10.1111/j.1365-2133.1996.tb16220.x
63. Hervonen K, Hakanen M, Kaukinen K, Collin P, Reunala T. First-degree relatives are frequently affected in coeliac disease and dermatitis herpetiformis. *Scand J Gastroenterol.* (2002) 37:51–5. doi: 10.1080/003655202753387356
64. Hall MA, Lanchbury JS, Ciclitira PJ. HLA class II region genes and susceptibility to dermatitis herpetiformis: DPB1 and TAP2 associations are secondary to those of the DQ subregion. *Eur J Immunogenet.* (1996) 23:285–96. doi: 10.1111/j.1744-313X.1996.tb00124.x
65. Spurkland A, Ingvarsson G, Falk ES, Knutsen I, Sollid LM, Thorsby E. Dermatitis herpetiformis and celiac disease are both primarily associated with the HLA-DQ (alpha 1*0501, beta 1*02) or the HLA-DQ (alpha 1*03, beta 1*0302) heterodimers. *Tissue Antigens.* (1997) 49:29–34. doi: 10.1111/j.1399-0039.1997.tb02706.x
66. Alshiekh S, Zhao LP, Lernmark A, Geraghty DE, Naluai AT, Agardh D. Different DRB1*03:01-DQB1*02:01 haplotypes confer different risk for celiac disease. *HLA.* (2017) 90:95–101. doi: 10.1111/tan.13065
67. Messer G, Kick G, Ranki A, Koskimies S, Reunala T, Meurer M. Polymorphism of the tumor necrosis factor genes in patients with dermatitis herpetiformis. *Dermatology.* (1994) 189(Suppl 1):135–7. doi: 10.1159/000246957
68. Sharma A, Liu X, Hadley D, Hagopian W, Liu E, Chen WM, et al. Identification of non-HLA genes associated with celiac disease and country-specific differences in a large, international pediatric cohort. *PLoS ONE.* (2016) 11:e0152476. doi: 10.1371/journal.pone.0152476
69. Trynka G, Hunt KA, Bockett NA, Romanos J, Mistry V, Szperl A, et al. Dense genotyping identifies and localizes multiple common and rare variant association signals in celiac disease. *Nat Genet.* (2011) 43:1193–201. doi: 10.1038/ng.998
70. Black KE, Murray JA, David CS. HLA-DQ determines the response to exogenous wheat proteins: a model of gluten sensitivity in transgenic knockout mice. *J Immunol.* (2002) 169:5595–600. doi: 10.4049/jimmunol.169.10.5595
71. Sciurti M, Fornaroli F, Gaiani F, Bonaguri C, Leandro G, Di Mario F, et al. Genetic susceptibilty and celiac disease: what role do HLA haplotypes play? *Acta Biomed.* (2018) 89:17–21. doi: 10.23750/abm.v89i9-S.7953
72. Megiorni F, Pizzuti A. HLA-DQA1 and HLA-DQB1 in Celiac disease predisposition: practical implications of the HLA molecular typing. *J Biomed Sci.* (2012) 19:88. doi: 10.1186/1423-0127-19-88
73. Lebwohl B, Sanders DS, Green PHR. Coeliac disease. *Lancet.* (2018) 391:70–81. doi: 10.1016/S0140-6736(17)31796-8
74. Karpati S. Dermatitis herpetiformis: close to unravelling a disease. *J Dermatol Sci.* (2004) 34:83–90. doi: 10.1016/j.jdermsci.2003.11.004
75. Molberg O, McAdam SN, Korner R, Quarsten H, Kristiansen C, Madsen L, et al. Tissue transglutaminase selectively modifies gliadin peptides that are recognized by gut-derived T cells in celiac disease. *Nat Med.* (1998) 4:713–7. doi: 10.1038/nm0698-713
76. Reunala T, Salmi TT, Hervonen K. Dermatitis herpetiformis: pathognomonic transglutaminase IgA deposits in the skin and excellent prognosis on a gluten-free diet. *Acta Derm Venereol.* (2015) 95:917–22. doi: 10.2340/00015555-2162
77. Marietta E, Black K, Camilleri M, Krause P, Rogers RS III, David C, et al. A new model for dermatitis herpetiformis that uses HLA-DQ8 transgenic NOD mice. *J Clin Invest.* (2004) 114:1090–7. doi: 10.1172/JCI200421055
78. Pollmann R, Eming R. Research techniques made simple: mouse models of autoimmune blistering diseases. *J Invest Dermatol.* (2017) 137:e1–6. doi: 10.1016/j.jid.2016.11.003
79. Ohata C, Ishii N, Hamada T, Shimomura Y, Niizeki H, Dainichi T, et al. Distinct characteristics in Japanese dermatitis herpetiformis: a review of all 91 Japanese patients over the last 35 years. *Clin Dev Immunol.* (2012) 2012:562168. doi: 10.1155/2012/562168
80. Sun Y, Lin Y, Yang B, Wang C, Fu X, Bao F, et al. The HLA alleles B*0801 and DRB1*0301 are associated with dermatitis herpetiformis in a chinese population. *J Invest Dermatol.* (2016) 136:530–2. doi: 10.1016/j.jid.2015.10.057
81. Haffenden GP, Blenkinsopp WK, Ring NP, Wojnarowska F, Fry L. The potassium iodide patch test in the dermatitis herpetiformis in relation to treatment with a gluten-free diet and dapsone. *Br J Dermatol.* (1980) 103:313–7. doi: 10.1111/j.1365-2133.1980.tb07250.x
82. Snider RL, Maize JC. Can chemicals precipitate dermatitis herpetiformis? *J Am Acad Dermatol.* (1993) 28:111–2. doi: 10.1016/S0190-9622(08)80847-X
83. Kovaleski CR, Jaliman D, Kumar V, Valeski JE. Dermatitis herpetiformis following gastric surgery. *Arch Dermatol.* (1997) 133:113–4. doi: 10.1001/archderm.1997.03890370125031
84. Stephan F, Haber R, Maalouf D, Tomb R. A case of dermatitis herpetiformis after a mini-gastric bypass surgery. *J Am Acad Dermatol.* (2014) 71:e18–20. doi: 10.1016/j.jaad.2014.01.854
85. Hietikko M, Hervonen K, Ilus T, Salmi T, Huhtala H, Laurila K, et al. *Ex vivo* culture of duodenal biopsies from patients with dermatitis herpetiformis indicates that transglutaminase 3 antibody production occurs in the gut. *Acta Derm Venereol.* (2018) 98:366–72. doi: 10.2340/00015555-2849
86. Spitzweg C, Hofbauer LC, Heufelder AE. Dermatitis herpetiformis cured by hormone replacement for panhypopituitarism. *Endocr J.* (1997) 44:437–40. doi: 10.1507/endocrj.44.437
87. Hassan S, Dalle S, Descloux E, Balme B, Thomas L. Dermatitis herpetiformis associated with progesterone contraception. *Ann Dermatol Venereol.* (2007) 134(Pt 1):385–6. doi: 10.1016/S0151-9638(07)89198-8
88. Grimwood RE, Guevara A. Leuprolide acetate-induced dermatitis herpetiformis. *Cutis.* (2005) 75:49–52.
89. Yu SS, Connolly MK, Berger TG, McCalmont TH. Dermatitis herpetiformis associated with administration of a gonadotropin-releasing hormone analog. *J Am Acad Dermatol.* (2006) 54(2 Suppl):S58–9. doi: 10.1016/j.jaad.2005.08.024
90. Marakli SS, Uzun S, Ozbek S, Tuncer I. Dermatitis herpetiformis in a patient receiving infliximab for ankylosing spondylitis. *Eur J Dermatol.* (2008) 18:88–9. doi: 10.1684/ejd.2007.0323
91. Mochel MC, Ming ME, Imadojemu S, Gangadhar TC, Schuchter LM, Elenitsas R, et al. Cutaneous autoimmune effects in the setting of therapeutic immune checkpoint inhibition for metastatic melanoma. *J Cutan Pathol.* (2016) 43:787–91. doi: 10.1111/cup.12735
92. Vajaitu C, Draghici CC, Solomon I, Lisievici CV, Popa AV, Lupu M, et al. The central role of inflammation associated with checkpoint inhibitor treatments. *J Immunol Res.* (2018) 2018:4625472. doi: 10.1155/2018/4625472
93. Antiga E, Quaglino P, Pierini I, Volpi W, Lami G, Bianchi B, et al. Regulatory T cells as well as IL-10 are reduced in the skin of patients with dermatitis herpetiformis. *J Dermatol Sci.* (2015) 77:54–62. doi: 10.1016/j.jdermsci.2014.11.003
94. Shigeta M, Saiki M, Tsuruta D, Ohata C, Ishii N, Ono F, et al. Two Japanese cases of dermatitis herpetiformis associated each with lung cancer and autoimmune pancreatitis but showing no intestinal symptom or circulating immunoglobulin A antibodies to any known antigens. *J Dermatol.* (2012) 39:1002–5. doi: 10.1111/j.1346-8138.2012.01663.x

95. Lerner A, Arleevskaya M, Schmiedl A, Matthias T. Microbes and viruses are bugging the gut in celiac disease. Are they friends or foes? *Front Microbiol.* (2017) 8:1392. doi: 10.3389/fmicb.2017.01392
96. Bouziat R, Hinterleitner R, Brown JJ, Stencel-Baerenwald JE, Ikizler M, Mayassi T, et al. Reovirus infection triggers inflammatory responses to dietary antigens and development of celiac disease. *Science.* (2017) 356:44–50. doi: 10.1126/science.aah5298
97. Handley J, O'Neill H, Connolly J, Burrows D. Adenovirus 12 and dermatitis herpetiformis. *Acta Derm Venereol.* (1993) 73:430–2.
98. Lorand L, Graham RM. Transglutaminases: crosslinking enzymes with pleiotropic functions. *Nat Rev Mol Cell Biol.* (2003) 4:140–56. doi: 10.1038/nrm1014
99. Karpati S, Sardy M, Nemeth K, Mayer B, Smyth N, Paulsson M, et al. Transglutaminases in autoimmune and inherited skin diseases: the phenomena of epitope spreading and functional compensation. *Exp Dermatol.* (2018) 27:807–14. doi: 10.1111/exd.13449
100. Eckert RL, Sturniolo MT, Broome AM, Ruse M, Rorke EA. Transglutaminase function in epidermis. *J Invest Dermatol.* (2005) 124:481–92. doi: 10.1111/j.0022-202X.2005.23627.x
101. Frezza V, Terrinoni A, Pitolli C, Mauriello A, Melino G, Candi E. Transglutaminase 3 protects against photodamage. *J Invest Dermatol.* (2017) 137:1590–4. doi: 10.1016/j.jid.2017.02.982
102. Caproni M, Torchia D, Antiga E, Degl'Innocenti D, Barletta E, Baroni G, et al. The role of apoptosis in the pathogenesis of dermatitis herpetiformis. *Int J Immunopathol Pharmacol.* (2005) 18:691–9. doi: 10.1177/039463200501800411
103. Didona D, Di Zenzo G. Humoral epitope spreading in autoimmune bullous diseases. *Front Immunol.* (2018) 9:779. doi: 10.3389/fimmu.2018.00779
104. Jaskowski TD, Hamblin T, Wilson AR, Hill HR, Book LS, Meyer LJ, et al. IgA anti-epidermal transglutaminase antibodies in dermatitis herpetiformis and pediatric celiac disease. *J Invest Dermatol.* (2009) 129:2728–30. doi: 10.1038/jid.2009.142
105. Zone JJ, Schmidt LA, Taylor TB, Hull CM, Sotiriou MC, Jaskowski TD, et al. Dermatitis herpetiformis sera or goat anti-transglutaminase-3 transferred to human skin-grafted mice mimics dermatitis herpetiformis immunopathology. *J Immunol.* (2011) 186:4474–80. doi: 10.4049/jimmunol.1003273
106. Reunala T, Helin H, Pasternack A, Linder E, Kalimo K. Renal involvement and circulating immune complexes in dermatitis herpetiformis. *J Am Acad Dermatol.* (1983) 9:219–23. doi: 10.1016/S0190-9622(83)70132-5
107. Preisz K, Sardy M, Horvath A, Karpati S. Immunoglobulin, complement and epidermal transglutaminase deposition in the cutaneous vessels in dermatitis herpetiformis. *J Eur Acad Dermatol Venereol.* (2005) 19:74–9. doi: 10.1111/j.1468-3083.2004.01132.x
108. Heinlin J, Knoppke B, Kohl E, Landthaler M, Karrer S. Dermatitis herpetiformis presenting as digital petechiae. *Pediatr Dermatol.* (2012) 29:209–12. doi: 10.1111/j.1525-1470.2011.01401.x
109. Gorog A, Nemeth K, Kolev K, Zone JJ, Mayer B, Sillo P, et al. Circulating transglutaminase 3-immunoglobulin A immune complexes in dermatitis herpetiformis. *J Invest Dermatol.* (2016) 136:1729–31. doi: 10.1016/j.jid.2016.03.039
110. Rose C, Armbruster FP, Ruppert J, Igl BW, Zillikens D, Shimanovich I. Autoantibodies against epidermal transglutaminase are a sensitive diagnostic marker in patients with dermatitis herpetiformis on a normal or gluten-free diet. *J Am Acad Dermatol.* (2009) 61:39–43. doi: 10.1016/j.jaad.2008.12.037
111. Borroni G, Biagi F, Ciocca O, Vassallo C, Carugno A, Cananzi R, et al. IgA anti-epidermal transglutaminase autoantibodies: a sensible and sensitive marker for diagnosis of dermatitis herpetiformis in adult patients. *J Eur Acad Dermatol Venereol.* (2013) 27:836–41. doi: 10.1111/j.1468-3083.2012.04586.x
112. Antiga E, Caproni M, Fabbri P. Comment on "Dermatitis herpetiformis sera or goat anti-transglutaminase-3 transferred to human skin-grafted mice mimics dermatitis herpetiformis immunopathology". *J Immunol.* (2011) 187:595. doi: 10.4049/jimmunol.1190031
113. Taylor TB, Schmidt LA, Meyer LJ, Zone JJ. Transglutaminase 3 present in the IgA aggregates in dermatitis herpetiformis skin is enzymatically active and binds soluble fibrinogen. *J Invest Dermatol.* (2015) 135:623–5. doi: 10.1038/jid.2014.368
114. Donaldson MR, Zone JJ, Schmidt LA, Taylor TB, Neuhausen SL, Hull CM, et al. Epidermal transglutaminase deposits in perilesional and uninvolved skin in patients with dermatitis herpetiformis. *J Invest Dermatol.* (2007) 127:1268–71. doi: 10.1038/sj.jid.5700682
115. Smith AD, Streilein RD, Hall RP, 3rd. Neutrophil CD11b, L-selectin and Fc IgA receptors in patients with dermatitis herpetiformis. *Br J Dermatol.* (2002) 147:1109–17. doi: 10.1046/j.1365-2133.2002.05004.x
116. Gornowicz-Porowska J, Seraszek-Jaros A, Bowszyc-Dmochowska M, Kaczmarek E, Dmochowski M. Immunoexpression of IgA receptors (CD89, CD71) in dermatitis herpetiformis. *Folia Histochem Cytobiol.* (2017) 55:212–20. doi: 10.5603/FHC.a2017.0024
117. Cannistraci C, Lesnoni La Parola I, Cardinali G, Bolasco G, Aspite N, Stigliano V, et al. Co-localization of IgA and TG3 on healthy skin of coeliac patients. *J Eur Acad Dermatol Venereol.* (2007) 21:509–14. doi: 10.1111/j.1468-3083.2006.02017.x
118. Bonciolini V, Antiga E, Fabbri P, Caproni M. Skin manifestations of celiac disease: not always dermatitis herpetiformis. *Int J Dermatol.* (2014) 53:e352–3. doi: 10.1111/ijd.12350
119. Hietikko M, Hervonen K, Salmi T, Ilus T, Zone JJ, Kaukinen K, et al. Disappearance of epidermal transglutaminase and IgA deposits from the papillary dermis of patients with dermatitis herpetiformis after a long-term gluten-free diet. *Br J Dermatol.* (2018) 178:e198–201. doi: 10.1111/bjd.15995
120. Taylor TB, Zone JJ. Sensitivity of Transglutaminase 3 in the IgA aggregates in dermatitis herpetiformis skin to potassium iodide. *J Invest Dermatol.* (2018) 138:2066–8. doi: 10.1016/j.jid.2018.03.1497
121. Hall RP III, Benbenisty KM, Mickle C, Takeuchi F, Streilein RD. Serum IL-8 in patients with dermatitis herpetiformis is produced in response to dietary gluten. *J Invest Dermatol.* (2007) 127:2158–65. doi: 10.1038/sj.jid.5700929
122. Hall RP III, Takeuchi F, Benbenisty KM, Streilein RD. Cutaneous endothelial cell activation in normal skin of patients with dermatitis herpetiformis associated with increased serum levels of IL-8, sE-Selectin, and TNF-alpha. *J Invest Dermatol.* (2006) 126:1331–7. doi: 10.1038/sj.jid.5700277
123. Graeber M, Baker BS, Garioch JJ, Valdimarsson H, Leonard JN, Fry L. The role of cytokines in the generation of skin lesions in dermatitis herpetiformis. *Br J Dermatol.* (1993) 129:530–2. doi: 10.1111/j.1365-2133.1993.tb00479.x
124. Ollague JE, Nousari CH. Expression of elafin in dermatitis herpetiformis. *Am J Dermatopathol.* (2018) 40:1–6. doi: 10.1097/DAD.0000000000000915
125. Russo V, Klein T, Lim DJ, Solis N, Machado Y, Hiroyasu S, et al. Granzyme B is elevated in autoimmune blistering diseases and cleaves key anchoring proteins of the dermal-epidermal junction. *Sci Rep.* (2018) 8:9690. doi: 10.1038/s41598-018-28070-0
126. Smith JB, Taylor TB, Zone JJ. The site of blister formation in dermatitis herpetiformis is within the lamina lucida. *J Am Acad Dermatol.* (1992) 27(Pt 1):209–13. doi: 10.1016/0190-9622(92)70172-C
127. Suzuki M, Hosoda S, Yamada T, Komine M, Murata S, Yokokura H, et al. A case of dermatitis herpetiformis with blister formation between laminin-332 and type 7 collagen. *J Dermatol.* (2014) 41:1030–1. doi: 10.1111/1346-8138.12630
128. Airola K, Vaalamo M, Reunala T, Saarialho-Kere UK. Enhanced expression of interstitial collagenase, stromelysin-1, and urokinase plasminogen activator in lesions of dermatitis herpetiformis. *J Invest Dermatol.* (1995) 105:184–9. doi: 10.1111/1523-1747.ep12317093
129. Bognar P, Gorog A, Karpati S. High prevalence of cryofibrinogenaemia in dermatitis herpetiformis. *J Eur Acad Dermatol Venereol.* (2016) 30:517–8. doi: 10.1111/jdv.12913
130. Gorog A, Nemeth K, Szabo L, Mayer B, Sillo P, Kolev K, et al. Decreased fibrinolytic potential and morphological changes of fibrin structure in dermatitis herpetiformis. *J Dermatol Sci.* (2016) 84:17–23. doi: 10.1016/j.jdermsci.2016.07.005
131. Marzano AV, Tedeschi A, Berti E, Fanoni D, Crosti C, Cugno M. Activation of coagulation in bullous pemphigoid and other eosinophil-related inflammatory skin diseases. *Clin Exp Immunol.* (2011) 165:44–50. doi: 10.1111/j.1365-2249.2011.04391.x
132. Zebrowska A, Wagrowska-Danilewicz M, Danilewicz M, Wieczfinska J, Pniewska E, Zebrowski M, et al. Tissue factor in dermatitis herpetiformis and bullous pemphigoid: link between immune and coagulation system in subepidermal autoimmune bullous diseases. *Mediators Inflamm.* (2015) 2015:870428. doi: 10.1155/2015/870428

133. Caproni M, Feliciani C, Fuligni A, Salvatore E, Atani L, Bianchi B, et al. Th2-like cytokine activity in dermatitis herpetiformis. *Br J Dermatol.* (1998) 138:242–7. doi: 10.1046/j.1365-2133.1998.02068.x
134. Reitamo S, Reunala T, Konttinen YT, Saksela O, Salo OP. Inflammatory cells, IgA, C3, fibrin and fibronectin in skin lesions in dermatitis herpetiformis. *Br J Dermatol.* (1981) 105:167–77. doi: 10.1111/j.1365-2133.1981.tb01202.x
135. Caproni M, Cardinali C, D'Agata A, Selvaggi W, Fabbri P. Serum eosinophil cationic protein, myeloperoxidase, tryptase, eotaxin and Th2-L-like cytokines in Dermatitis herpetiformis. *Int Arch Allergy Immunol.* (2002) 128:67–72. doi: 10.1159/000058005
136. Makino T, Yoshihisa Y, Mizawa M, Tsutsui K, Nishijima C, Inaoki M, et al. Increased serum levels of Th2-type cytokines and eotaxin in fibrillar-type dermatitis herpetiformis. *Acta Derm Venereol.* (2017) 97:642–3. doi: 10.2340/00015555-2604
137. Cynkier A, Zebrowska A, Wagrowska-Danilewicz M, Danilewicz M, Erkiert-Polguj A, Stasikowska-Kanicka O, et al. Expression of selected neuropeptides in pathogenesis of bullous pemphigoid and dermatitis herpetiformis. *Pol J Pathol.* (2012) 63:31–9.
138. Sokolowska-Wojdylo M, Glen J, Zablotna M, Rebala K, Trzeciak M, Sikorska M, et al. The frequencies of haplotypes defined by three polymorphisms of the IL-31 gene:−1066,−2057, and IVS2+12 in Polish patients with atopic dermatitis. *Int J Dermatol.* (2015) 54:62–7. doi: 10.1111/ijd.12666
139. Ishii T, Wang J, Zhang W, Mascarenhas J, Hoffman R, Dai Y, et al. Pivotal role of mast cells in pruritogenesis in patients with myeloproliferative disorders. *Blood.* (2009) 113:5942–50. doi: 10.1182/blood-2008-09-179416
140. Malek M, Glen J, Rebala K, Kowalczyk A, Sobjanek M, Nowicki R, et al. Il-31 does not correlate to pruritus related to early stage cutaneous T-cell lymphomas but is involved in pathogenesis of the disease. *Acta Derm Venereol.* (2015) 95:283–8. doi: 10.2340/00015555-1958
141. Rabenhorst A, Hartmann K. Interleukin-31: a novel diagnostic marker of allergic diseases. *Curr Allergy Asthma Rep.* (2014) 14:423. doi: 10.1007/s11882-014-0423-y
142. Schulz F, Marenholz I, Folster-Holst R, Chen C, Sternjak A, Baumgrass R, et al. A common haplotype of the IL-31 gene influencing gene expression is associated with nonatopic eczema. *J Allergy Clin Immunol.* (2007) 120:1097–102. doi: 10.1016/j.jaci.2007.07.065
143. Hartmann K, Wagner N, Rabenhorst A, Pflanz L, Leja S, Forster A, et al. Serum IL-31 levels are increased in a subset of patients with mastocytosis and correlate with disease severity in adult patients. *J Allergy Clin Immunol.* (2013) 132:232–5. doi: 10.1016/j.jaci.2012.11.008
144. Dillon SR, Sprecher C, Hammond A, Bilsborough J, Rosenfeld-Franklin M, Presnell SR, et al. Interleukin 31, a cytokine produced by activated T cells, induces dermatitis in mice. *Nat Immunol.* (2004) 5:752–60. doi: 10.1038/ni1084
145. Lange M, Glen J, Zablotna M, Nedoszytko B, Sokolowska-Wojdylo M, Rebala K, et al. Interleukin-31 polymorphisms and serum IL-31 level in patients with mastocytosis: correlation with clinical presen-tation and pruritus. *Acta Derm Venereol.* (2017) 97:47–53. doi: 10.2340/00015555-2474
146. Nobbe S, Dziunycz P, Muhleisen B, Bilsborough J, Dillon SR, French LE, et al. IL-31 expression by inflammatory cells is preferentially elevated in atopic dermatitis. *Acta Derm Venereol.* (2012) 92:24–8. doi: 10.2340/00015 555-1191
147. Nattkemper LA, Tey HL, Valdes-Rodriguez R, Lee H, Mollanazar NK, Albornoz C, et al. The genetics of chronic itch: gene expression in the skin of patients with atopic dermatitis and psoriasis with severe itch. *J Invest Dermatol.* (2018) 138:1311–7. doi: 10.1016/j.jid.2017.12.029
148. Nattkemper LA, Martinez-Escala ME, Gelman AB, Singer EM, Rook AH, Guitart J, et al. Cutaneous T-cell lymphoma and pruritus: the expression of IL-31 and its receptors in the skin. *Acta Derm Venereol.* (2016) 96:894–8. doi: 10.2340/00015555-2417
149. Ko MJ, Peng YS, Chen HY, Hsu SP, Pai MF, Yang JY, et al. Interleukin-31 is associated with uremic pruritus in patients receiving hemodialysis. *J Am Acad Dermatol.* (2014) 71:1151–9.e1. doi: 10.1016/j.jaad.2014.08.004
150. Cornelissen C, Luscher-Firzlaff J, Baron JM, Luscher B. Signaling by IL-31 and functional consequences. *Eur J Cell Biol.* (2012) 91:552–66. doi: 10.1016/j.ejcb.2011.07.006
151. Amber KT, Valdebran M, Kridin K, Grando SA. The role of eosinophils in bullous pemphigoid: a developing model of eosinophil pathogenicity in mucocutaneous disease. *Front Med (Lausanne).* (2018) 5:201. doi: 10.3389/fmed.2018.00201
152. Kulczycka-Siennicka L, Cynkier A, Waszczykowska E, Wozniacka A, Zebrowska A. The role of intereukin-31 in pathogenesis of itch and its intensity in a course of bullous pemphigoid and dermatitis herpetiformis. *Biomed Res Int.* (2017) 2017:5965492. doi: 10.1155/2017/5965492
153. Bonciani D, Quintarelli L, Del Bianco E, Bianchi B, Caproni M. Serum levels and tissue expression of interleukin-31 in dermatitis herpetiformis and bullous pemphigoid. *J Dermatol Sci.* (2017) 87:210–2. doi: 10.1016/j.jdermsci.2017.04.008
154. Ruzicka T, Mihara R. Anti-interleukin-31 receptor A antibody for atopic dermatitis. *N Engl J Med.* (2017) 376:2093. doi: 10.1056/NEJMoa1606490
155. Sapone A, Bai JC, Ciacci C, Dolinsek J, Green PH, Hadjivassiliou M, et al. Spectrum of gluten-related disorders: consensus on new nomenclature and classification. *BMC Med.* (2012) 10:13. doi: 10.1186/1741-7015-10-13
156. Humbert P, Pelletier F, Dreno B, Puzenat E, Aubin F. Gluten intolerance and skin diseases. *Eur J Dermatol.* (2006) 16:4–11.
157. Rodrigo L, Beteta-Gorriti V, Alvarez N, Gomez de Castro C, de Dios A, Palacios L, et al. Cutaneous and mucosal manifestations associated with celiac disease. *Nutrients.* (2018) 10:E800. doi: 10.3390/nu10070800
158. Ungprasert P, Wijarnpreecha K, Kittanamongkolchai W. Psoriasis and risk of celiac disease: a systematic review and meta-analysis. *Indian J Dermatol.* (2017) 62:41–6. doi: 10.4103/0019-5154.198031
159. Bhatia BK, Millsop JW, Debbaneh M, Koo J, Linos E, Liao W. Diet and psoriasis, part II: celiac disease and role of a gluten-free diet. *J Am Acad Dermatol.* (2014) 71:350–8. doi: 10.1016/j.jaad.2014.03.017
160. Kaplan L, Castelo-Soccio L. When your patient's parent asks: "My child's alopecia areata is not getting better. Should he or she get tested for celiac disease?" *Pediatr Dermatol.* (2018) 35:535–8. doi: 10.1111/pde.13542
161. Bonciolini V, Bianchi B, Del Bianco E, Verdelli A, Caproni M. Cutaneous manifestations of non-celiac gluten sensitivity: clinical histological and immunopathological features. *Nutrients.* (2015) 7:7798–805. doi: 10.3390/nu7095368
162. Faina V, Paolino G, Bavastrelli M, Calvieri S, Grieco T. Classification of cutaneous manifestations in patients with non-celiac gluten sensitivity (NCGS) and wheat allergy (WA). *J Am Acad Dermatol.* (2017). doi: 10.1016/j.jaad.2017.12.013. [Epub ahead of print].
163. Catassi C, Elli L, Bonaz B, Bouma G, Carroccio A, Castillejo G, et al. Diagnosis of non-celiac gluten sensitivity (NCGS): the salerno experts' criteria. *Nutrients.* (2015) 7:4966–77. doi: 10.3390/nu7064966
164. Warren SJ, Cockerell CJ. Characterization of a subgroup of patients with dermatitis herpetiformis with nonclassical histologic features. *Am J Dermatopathol.* (2002) 24:305–8. doi: 10.1097/00000372-200208000-00003
165. Ziemer M, Pemler S, Simon JC, Treudler R. Acantholytic variant of Duhring's disease. *J Dtsch Dermatol Ges.* (2016) 14:186–8. doi: 10.1111/ddg.12746
166. Hashimoto T, Tsuruta D, Yasukochi A, Imanishi H, Sekine H, Fujita T, et al. Granular C3 dermatosis. *Acta Derm Venereol.* (2016) 96:748–53. doi: 10.2340/00015555-2379
167. Alonso-Llamazares J, Gibson LE, Rogers RS, 3rd. Clinical, pathologic, and immunopathologic features of dermatitis herpetiformis: review of the Mayo Clinic experience. *Int J Dermatol.* (2007) 46:910–9. doi: 10.1111/j.1365-4632.2007.03214.x
168. Bresler SC, Granter SR. Utility of direct immunofluorescence testing for IgA in patients with high and low clinical suspicion for dermatitis herpetiformis. *Am J Clin Pathol.* (2015) 144:880–4. doi: 10.1309/AJCPXIVSR6OZK1HU
169. Beutner EH, Baughman RD, Austin BM, Plunkett RW, Binder WL. A case of dermatitis herpetiformis with IgA endomysial antibodies but negative direct immunofluorescent findings. *J Am Acad Dermatol.* (2000) 43(Pt 2):329–32. doi: 10.1016/S0190-9622(00)70284-2
170. Huber C, Trueb RM, French LE, Hafner J. Negative direct immunofluorescence and nonspecific histology do not exclude the diagnosis of dermatitis herpetiformis Duhring. *Int J Dermatol.* (2013) 52:248–9. doi: 10.1111/j.1365-4632.2011.04909.x
171. Antiga E, Caproni M. The diagnosis and treatment of dermatitis herpetiformis. *Clin Cosmet Investig Dermatol.* (2015) 8:257–65. doi: 10.2147/CCID.S69127

172. Salmi TT, Kurppa K, Hervonen K, Laurila K, Collin P, Huhtala H, et al. Serum transglutaminase 3 antibodies correlate with age at celiac disease diagnosis. *Dig Liver Dis.* (2016) 48:632–7. doi: 10.1016/j.dld.2016.03.003
173. Lytton SD, Antiga E, Pfeiffer S, Matthias T, Szaflarska-Poplawska A, Ulaganathan VK, et al. Neo-epitope tissue transglutaminase autoantibodies as a biomarker of the gluten sensitive skin disease–dermatitis herpetiformis. *Clin Chim Acta.* (2013) 415:346–9. doi: 10.1016/j.cca.2012.10.051
174. Kasperkiewicz M, Dahnrich C, Probst C, Komorowski L, Stocker W, Schlumberger W, et al. Novel assay for detecting celiac disease-associated autoantibodies in dermatitis herpetiformis using deamidated gliadin-analogous fusion peptides. *J Am Acad Dermatol.* (2012) 66:583–8. doi: 10.1016/j.jaad.2011.02.025
175. Makharia GK, Mulder CJ, Goh KL, Ahuja V, Bai JC, Catassi C, et al. Issues associated with the emergence of coeliac disease in the Asia-Pacific region: a working party report of the World Gastroenterology Organization and the Asian Pacific Association of Gastroenterology. *J Gastroenterol Hepatol.* (2014) 29:666–77. doi: 10.1111/jgh.12514
176. Sar-Pomian M, Rudnicka L, Olszewska M. Trichoscopy - a useful tool in the preliminary differential diagnosis of autoimmune bullous diseases. *Int J Dermatol.* (2017) 56:996–1002. doi: 10.1111/ijd.13725
177. Criado PR, Criado RF, Aoki V, Belda W, Jr., Halpern I, Landman G, et al. Dermatitis herpetiformis: relevance of the physical examination to diagnosis suspicion. *Can Fam Physician.* (2012) 58:843–7.
178. Calabro A, Gralka E, Luchinat C, Saccenti E, Tenori L. A metabolomic perspective on coeliac disease. *Autoimmune Dis.* (2014) 2014:756138. doi: 10.1155/2014/756138
179. Chander AM, Yadav H, Jain S, Bhadada SK, Dhawan DK. Cross-talk between gluten, intestinal microbiota and intestinal mucosa in celiac disease: recent advances and basis of autoimmunity. *Front Microbiol.* (2018) 9:2597. doi: 10.3389/fmicb.2018.02597
180. Wacklin P, Kaukinen K, Tuovinen E, Collin P, Lindfors K, Partanen J, et al. The duodenal microbiota composition of adult celiac disease patients is associated with the clinical manifestation of the disease. *Inflamm Bowel Dis.* (2013) 19:934–41. doi: 10.1097/MIB.0b013e31828029a9
181. Antiga E, Caproni M, Pierini I, Bonciani D, Fabbri P. Gluten-free diet in patients with dermatitis herpetiformis: not only a matter of skin. *Arch Dermatol.* (2011) 147:988–9. doi: 10.1001/archdermatol.2011.221
182. Turchin I, Barankin B. Dermatitis herpetiformis and gluten-free diet. *Dermatol Online J.* (2005) 11:6.
183. Elli L, Ferretti F, Orlando S, Vecchi M, Monguzzi E, Roncoroni L, et al. Management of celiac disease in daily clinical practice. *Eur J Intern Med.* (2018) 61:15–24. doi: 10.1016/j.ejim.2018.11.012.
184. Clarindo MV, Possebon AT, Soligo EM, Uyeda H, Ruaro RT, Empinotti JC. Dermatitis herpetiformis: pathophysiology, clinical presentation, diagnosis and treatment. *An Bras Dermatol.* (2014) 89:865–75. doi: 10.1590/abd1806-4841.20142966
185. Hervonen K, Salmi TT, Ilus T, Paasikivi K, Vornanen M, Laurila K, et al. Dermatitis herpetiformis refractory to gluten-free dietary treatment. *Acta Derm Venereol.* (2016) 96:82–6. doi: 10.2340/00015555-2184
186. Makharia GK. Current and emerging therapy for celiac disease. *Front Med (Lausanne).* (2014) 1:6. doi: 10.3389/fmed.2014.00006
187. Gil-Humanes J, Piston F, Tollefsen S, Sollid LM, Barro F. Effective shutdown in the expression of celiac disease-related wheat gliadin T-cell epitopes by RNA interference. *Proc Natl Acad Sci USA.* (2010) 107:17023–8. doi: 10.1073/pnas.1007773107
188. Freeman HJ. Celiac disease: a disorder emerging from antiquity, its evolving classification and risk, and potential new treatment paradigms. *Gut Liver.* (2015) 9:28–37. doi: 10.5009/gnl14288
189. Leffler DA, Kelly CP, Green PH, Fedorak RN, DiMarino A, Perrow W, et al. Larazotide acetate for persistent symptoms of celiac disease despite a gluten-free diet: a randomized controlled trial. *Gastroenterology.* (2015) 148:1311–9.e6. doi: 10.1053/j.gastro.2015.02.008
190. Daveson AJM, Ee HC, Andrews JM, King T, Goldstein KE, Dzuris JL, et al. Epitope-specific immunotherapy targeting CD4-positive T cells in celiac disease: safety, pharmacokinetics, and effects on intestinal histology and plasma cytokines with escalating dose regimens of nexvax2 in a randomized, double-blind, placebo-controlled phase 1 study. *EBioMedicine.* (2017) 26:78–90. doi: 10.1016/j.ebiom.2017.11.018
191. Tye-Din JA, Galipeau HJ, Agardh D. Celiac *Disease: A Review of Current Concepts in Pathogenesis, Prevention, and Novel Therapies. Front Pediatr.* (2018) 6:350. doi: 10.3389/fped.2018.00350
192. Burbidge T, Haber RM. Topical dapsone 5% gel as an effective therapy in dermatitis herpetiformis. *J Cutan Med Surg.* (2016) 20:600–1. doi: 10.1177/1203475416651053
193. Handler MZ, Chacon AH, Shiman MI, Schachner LA. Letter to the editor: Application of dapsone 5% gel in a patient with dermatitis herpetiformis. *J Dermatol Case Rep.* (2012) 6:132–3. doi: 10.3315/jdcr.2012.1124
194. Bevans SL, Sami N. Dapsone and sulfasalazine combination therapy in dermatitis herpetiformis. *Int J Dermatol.* (2017) 56:e90–2. doi: 10.1111/ijd.13542
195. Abdelmaksoud A. Dermatitis herpetiformis (Duhring's disease): a therapeutic challenge. *Int J Dermatol.* (2017) 56:e192–3. doi: 10.1111/ijd.13641
196. Albers LN, Zone JJ, Stoff BK, Feldman RJ. Rituximab treatment for recalcitrant dermatitis herpetiformis. *JAMA Dermatol.* (2017) 153:315–8. doi: 10.1001/jamadermatol.2016.4676
197. Vriezinga SL, Auricchio R, Bravi E, Castillejo G, Chmielewska A, Crespo Escobar P, et al. Randomized feeding intervention in infants at high risk for celiac disease. *N Engl J Med.* (2014) 371:1304–15. doi: 10.1056/NEJMoa1404172
198. Lionetti E, Castellaneta S, Francavilla R, Pulvirenti A, Tonutti E, Amarri S, et al. Introduction of gluten, HLA status, and the risk of celiac disease in children. *N Engl J Med.* (2014) 371:1295–303. doi: 10.1056/NEJMoa1400697
199. Kho ZY, Lal SK. The human gut microbiome - a potential controller of wellness and disease. *Front Microbiol.* (2018) 9:1835. doi: 10.3389/fmicb.2018.01835
200. Lerner A, Matthias T. Changes in intestinal tight junction permeability associated with industrial food additives explain the rising incidence of autoimmune disease. *Autoimmun Rev.* (2015) 14:479–89. doi: 10.1016/j.autrev.2015.01.009
201. Zebrowska A, Wozniacka A, Juczynska K, Ociepa K, Waszczykowska E, Szymczak I, et al. Correlation between IL36alpha and IL17 and activity of the disease in selected autoimmune blistering diseases. *Mediators Inflamm.* (2017) 2017:8980534. doi: 10.1155/2017/8980534

3

Diagnosis of Autoimmune Blistering Diseases

Mareike Witte*, Detlef Zillikens and Enno Schmidt

Department of Dermatology, University of Lübeck, Lübeck, Germany

***Correspondence:**
Mareike Witte
mareike.witte@uksh.de

Autoimmune skin blistering diseases (AIBD) are characterized by autoantibodies that are directed against structural proteins in the skin and adjacent mucous membranes. Some clinical signs are typical for a specific AIBD, however, correct diagnosis requires the detection of tissue-bound or circulating autoantibodies. The gold standard for diagnosis of AIBD is the detection of autoantibodies or complement component 3 by direct immunofluorescence (DIF) microscopy of a perilesional biopsy. Circulating antibodies can be detected via indirect immunofluorescence (IIF) microscopy of different tissue substrates including human skin, monkey esophagus, and more recently, recombinant forms of the different target antigens. Latter are also employed in various commercial ELISA systems and by immunoblotting in in-house assays available in specialized laboratories. ELISA systems are also particularly valuable for monitoring of the disease activity during the disease course which can be helpful for treatment decisions. Exact diagnosis is essential for both treatment and prognosis, since some AIBD are associated with malign tumors such as paraneoplastic pemphigus and anti-laminin 332 mucous membrane pemphigoid. This review presents clinical and immunopathological features of AIBD for the state-of the art diagnosis of these disorders.

Keywords: autoantibody, biochip, immunofluorescence, ELISA, pemphigus, pemphigoid, epidermolysis bullosa acquisita, dermatitis herpetiformis

INTRODUCTION

Autoimmune skin blistering diseases (AIBD) are a diverse group of dermatoses that are characterized by autoantibodies binding to antigens in the skin and mucous membranes. They can be subdivided into pemphigoid diseases (PD), with subepidermal split formation and autoantibody binding to structural components of the dermal-epidermal junction (DEJ), and pemphigus, with autoantibodies directed against desmosomal proteins that connect neighboring keratinocytes (1, 2). A special type of AIBD is dermatitis herpetiformis, with autoantibodies directed against the tissue and epidermal transglutaminase. In this review, we will provide a comprehensive overview about the clinical features and current diagnosis of AIBD extending and updating previous work (3, 4).

EPIDEMIOLOGY

Bullous pemphigoid (BP) is the most frequent AIBD in Central Europe. Its incidence reaches around 20/million/year. BP is followed by mucous membrane pemphigoid (MMP) and pemphigoid gestationis, with incidences of 2/million/year, respectively (5–8). Higher incidences of BP have been reported in Great Britain (9). In contrast to other autoimmune diseases, the incidence of BP is increasing with age. Regarding this matter, its annual incidence in people older than 80 years reaches 150–180/million/year (5, 6). Like other autoimmune diseases, the incidence of BP is constantly increasing and has nearly doubled in the last decade (7–11). This is partly due to the rising life expectancy of the general population, increasing awareness, and enhanced diagnostic tests. Further, the close association between BP and neurological diseases [reviewed in (12)], whose incidences are also rising, may contribute to the increased occurrence of BP. This rise in BP incidence is reflected by hospitalization numbers of BP patients that increased by 26% for a primary diagnosis and by 62% for a secondary diagnosis to 3,260/million inpatients between 2002 and 2012 in the USA (13).

In pemphigus, the incidence depends on the geographical region. In Central Europe and the United States, its incidence is estimated between 1 and 7 new patients/million/year (9, 14). Generally, PV is more common than pemphigus foliaceus (PF), with ratios ranging from 4:1 to 9:1 (15). In Tunisia and Brazil, endemic forms of PF with much higher incidences are present (16, 17).

The prevalence of AIBD in Germany have recently been calculated based on the ICD-coding-based dataset of the country's largest health insurance. The study revealed about 40,000 AIBD patients including 21,000 patients with BP, 7,700 with PV, and around 2,000 with MMP (18).

HISTORICAL BACKGROUND

The term pemphigus was first used by Hippocrates in 460–370 B.C. (19). However, the differentiation between pemphigus and BP was first made by Walter Lever in 1953 based on lesional histopathology (20). In 1964 and 1967, detection of autoantibodies in serum and skin were reported for pemphigus and BP (21, 22), providing milestones for the diagnosis of AIBD. Diagnosis of the different AIBD entities became subsequently possible by the molecular identification of target antigens (23). In parallel it became clear that the autoantibodies used for the diagnosis of AIBDs may be directly pathogenic (24–29), reviewed in (1, 30–34).

DIRECT IMMUNOFLUORESCENCE MICROSCOPY

The diagnosis of AIBDs is based on the combination of the clinical presentation and detection of tissue-bound and/or circulating autoantibodies. Tissue-bound autoantibodies can be detected via direct immunofluorescence (DIF) microscopy, which is the diagnostic gold standard for AIBD. For DIF microscopy, cryosections of perilesional biopsies are required and need to be snap frozen and stored at −20°C or conserved in isotonic NaCl or modified Michels medium until processed (35, 36).

DIF microscopy only provides limited information about the target antigen(s), however the diagnosis can be narrowed down according to the immunoglobulin subclass and binding pattern. In pemphigus, DIF microscopy reveals intercellular binding of IgG and/or C3 within the epidermis and/or epithelium. In pemphigoid diseases, a linear deposition of IgG and/or C3 at the DEJ can be observed (**Figures 1, 2**). Linear staining at the DEJ can further be differentiated into n-serrated and u-serrated patterns. In an n-serration pattern, arches are closed at the top (**Figure 3** left) and in a u-serrated staining pattern, arches are closed at the bottom appearing like "growing grass" (**Figure 3** right). While u-serration is unique for antibody binding to type VII collagen and can been seen in epidermolysis bullosa acquisita (EBA), n-serration is found in all other pemphigoid diseases (37–39). Serration pattern analysis can be performed in any routine immunofluorescence (IF) laboratory and is best performed in 6 μm sections and 400- or 600-fold magnification without oil (38, 39). IF pictures for training of serration pattern analysis are freely available (www.nversusu.umcg.nl).

In dermatitis herpetiformis, DIF microscopy reveals granular deposition of IgA at the dermal papillae and along the DEJ. An automated staining for DIF microscopy sections has recently been developed and revealed more intensive IF staining and reduced background compared to the manual procedure due to continuous movement and overhead incubation (40). A flowchart navigating through differential diagnoses using DIF microscopy is shown in **Figure 1**. For further differentiation of the target antigen(s) serological analyses is required.

INDIRECT IMMUNOFLUORESCENCE MICROSCOPY USING TISSUE SUBSTRATES

Several tissues can be employed by indirect IF (IIF) microscopy to screen for serum autoantibodies in AIBD including monkey, rabbit, guinea pig, and human esophagus (for pemphigus and pemphigoid diseases), monkey and rat bladder (for paraneoplastic pemphigus), and amnion epithelium (for BP and PV). In one study, monkey esophagus was the most sensitive substrate for pemphigus; another study showed that monkey esophagus is more sensitive for PV and human esophagus is more sensitive for PF (41–44). The most frequently used substrates are monkey esophagus and human split skin. On monkey esophagus, autoantibodies in pemphigus reveal intercellular labeling of the epithelium and linear staining of the DEJ in pemphigoid diseases (**Figure 2**). Sensitivities of 90% and 73.2% have been reported for pemphigus and BP, respectively (41, 43). In dermatitis herpetiformis, IgA binds to the endomysium. The tissue substrate with the highest sensitivity for autoantibodies in pemphigoid diseases is 1M NaCl split human skin. Here, antibodies bind either to the epidermal ("roof") or dermal ("floor") side of the artificial blister (**Figure 2**, left and right panel, respectively). "Floor"-binding antibodies can be detected in EBA, anti-p200/laminin γ1 pemphigoid, and anti-laminin 332 MMP. "Roof"-binding antibodies target BP180 and BP230 and are observed in BP, linear IgA-disease, pemphigoid gestationis, and anti-BP180-type mucous membrane pemphigoid. Sensitivities for BP range between 73 and 84% (41, 45).

The most sensitive substrates for the detection of anti-plakin reactivity are monkey and rat bladder epithelium. In pemphigoid

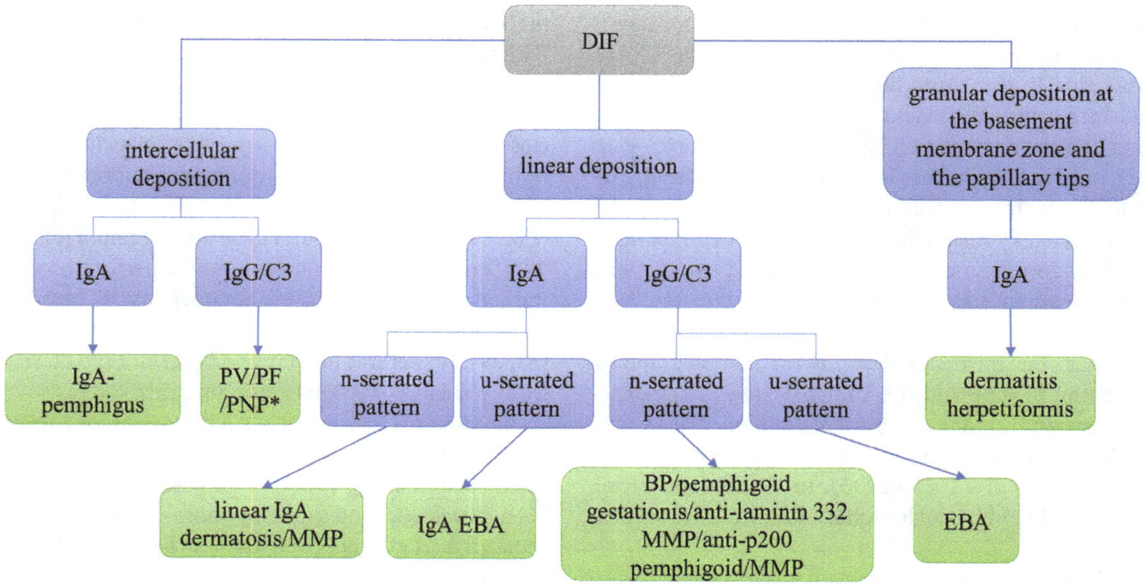

FIGURE 1 | Differential diagnosis of autoimmune skin blistering diseases based on direct immunofluorescence (DIF) microscopy of a perilesional biopsy. BP, bullous pemphigoid; EBA, epidermolysis bullosa acquisita; MMP, mucous membrane pemphigoid; PF, pemphigus foliaceus; PNP, paraneoplastic pemphigus; PV, pemphigus vulgaris; *may be combined with linear deposition.

gestationis, the complement fixation test detects complement-fixing IgG on human salt-split skin. For definite diagnosis of most AIBD refined analysis of serum autoantibodies can be performed, employing recombinant or cell-derived antigens. A flowchart depicting the serological diagnosis of autoimmune blistering diseases is shown in **Figure 4**.

TARGET ANTIGEN-SPECIFIC ANALYSIS OF SERUM AUTOANTIBODIES

For the identification of the target antigen, three main systems have been described: (i) Enzyme-linked immunosorbent assay (ELISA), (ii) IIF microscopy, and (iii) immunoblot/immunoprecipitation.

(i) ELISA systems allow the identification and quantification of autoantibodies against specific autoantigens. They are applied for both diagnosis and monitoring of the activity of the disease during the disease process (46). For pemphigoid diseases, commercial ELISA systems include BP180 NC16A, BP230, and type VII collagen, which employ recombinant protein, respectively (MBL, Euroimmun) (47–52). The sensitivity of the BP180 NC16A ELISA ranges between 84 and 89% in BP (47, 49, 53) and between 96 and 97% in pemphigoid gestations (54, 55). The sensitivity in BP can be increased by the additional use of the BP230 ELISA by about 5% (52, 56, 57). For pemphigus, ELISA systems employ the ectodomains of Dsg1 and Dsg3 recombinantly expressed in HEK293 cells (Euroimmun) or baculovirus (MBL, Nagoya, Japan) (46, 58, 59). For paraneoplastic pemphigus, an ELISA system for autoantibodies against envoplakin has been developed (Euroimmun) (60). For dermatitis herpetiformis, ELISA systems for the detection of coeliac-specific gliadin IgG and IgA autoantibodies as well as anti-transglutaminase 2 and 3-antibodies are available (61). ELISA systems that are less standardized and only available in specialized laboratories include desmocollin (62, 63), laminin $\gamma1$ (64, 65), the ectodomain of BP180 (66), full-length BP180 (67), laminin 332 (68, 69) and BP180 NC16A-IgE-ELISA (70–72) as well as other forms of BP180 (73, 74).

In addition, two multivariant ELISA systems compiled of the individual assays include recombinant Dsg 1 and 3, BP180 NC16A, BP230, type VII collagen, and only in one system, envoplakin, are widely available (75, 76).

(ii) IIF-based assays employing recombinant forms of the target antigens are available as multivariant assays and thus, offer a single-step method for the diagnosis of AIBDs. These assays are based on the BIOCHIP® mosaic technology using normally-sized laboratory slides with 5–10 incubation fields. The serum sample is loaded onto an incubation field, consisting of several miniature biochips coated with different substrates (e.g., monkey esophagus, salt-split skin, recombinant BP180 NC16A or HEK293 cells recombinantly expressing Dsg1, Dsg3, or BP230). We have shown that the sensitivity and specificity of BIOCHIP® mosaic analysis is comparable to that of ELISA systems regarding AIBDs (77). Meanwhile, this technology has been applied in different routine laboratories worldwide (78–80). More recently, a mosaic comprising 4 biochips coated with recombinant BP180 NC16A, HEK cells expressing BP230, salt-split skin and monkey esophagus, respectively, showed a sensitivity

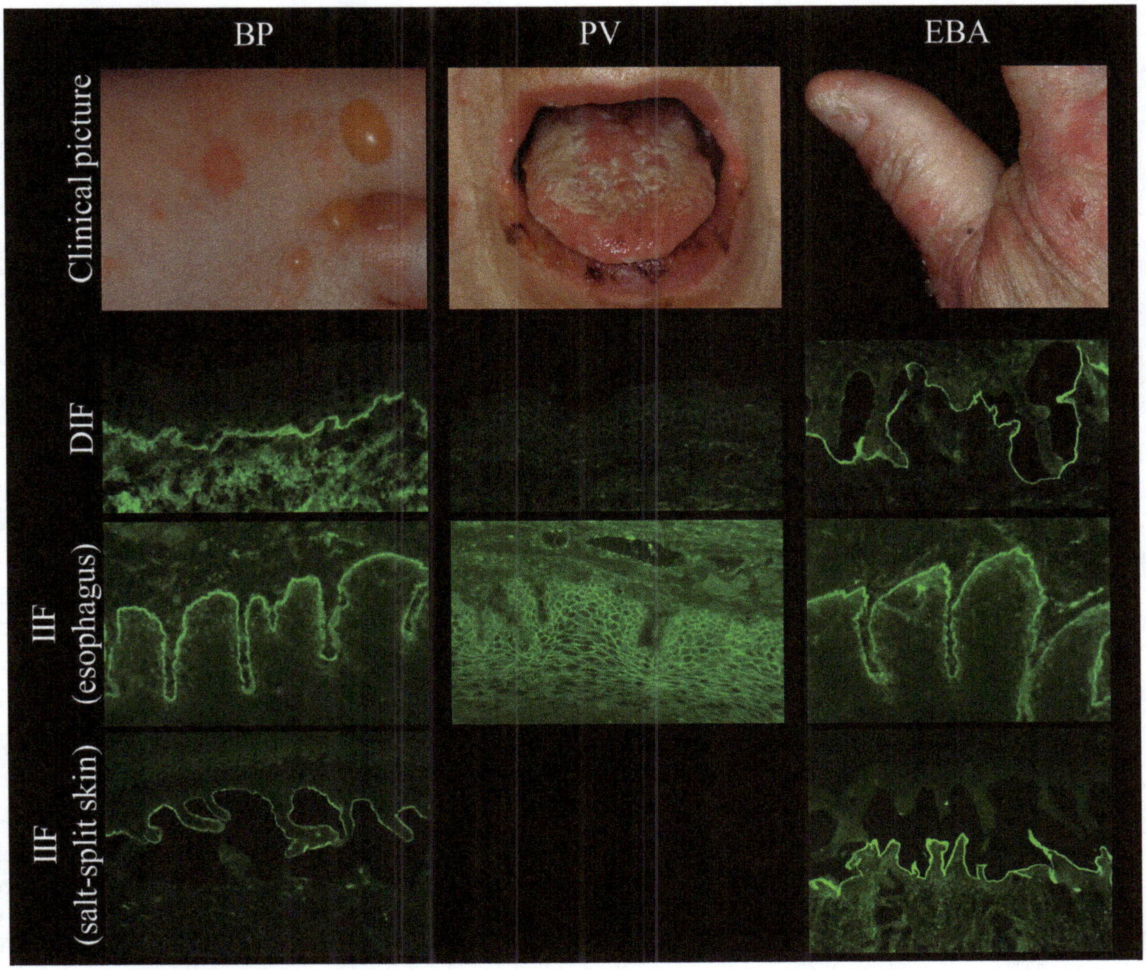

FIGURE 2 | Clinical and immunopathological characteristics in bullous pemphigoid (BP, **left**), pemphigus vulgaris (PV, **middle**), and epidermolysis bullosa acquisita (EBA, **right**).

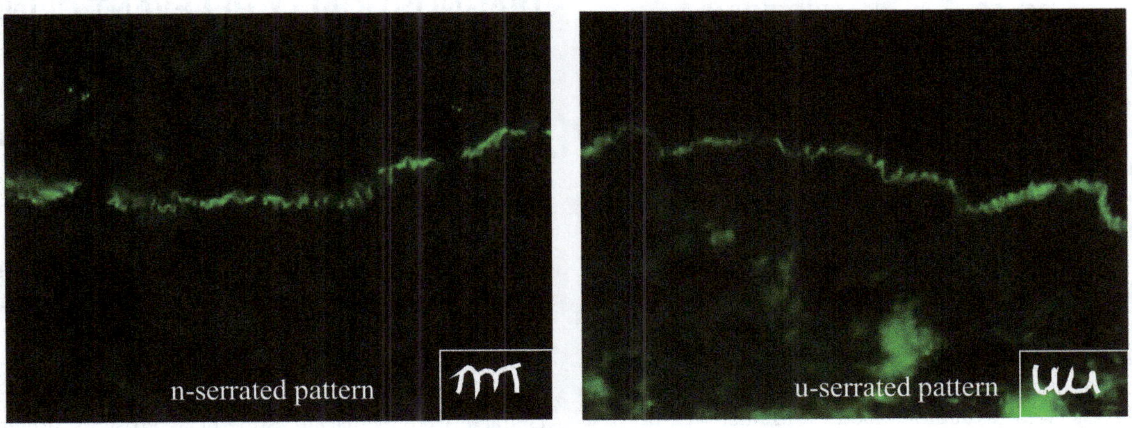

FIGURE 3 | n-serrated **(left)** and u-serrated pattern **(right)** of basement membrane zone staining in pemphigoid diseases detected by direct immunofluorescence microscopy. While an u-serrated pattern is exclusively seen in epidermolysis bullosa acquisita, an n-serrated pattern can be detected in all other pemphigoid diseases.

of 100% when testing with pemphigoid gestationis sera (79). A BIOCHIP® mosaic including the immunodominant NC1 domain of type VII collagen yielded sensitivities of 92 and 100% (50, 81), indicating that BIOCHIP® technology is a valuable tool in the routine diagnosis of pemphigoid gestationis and EBA. As for desmocollins, anti-desmocollin

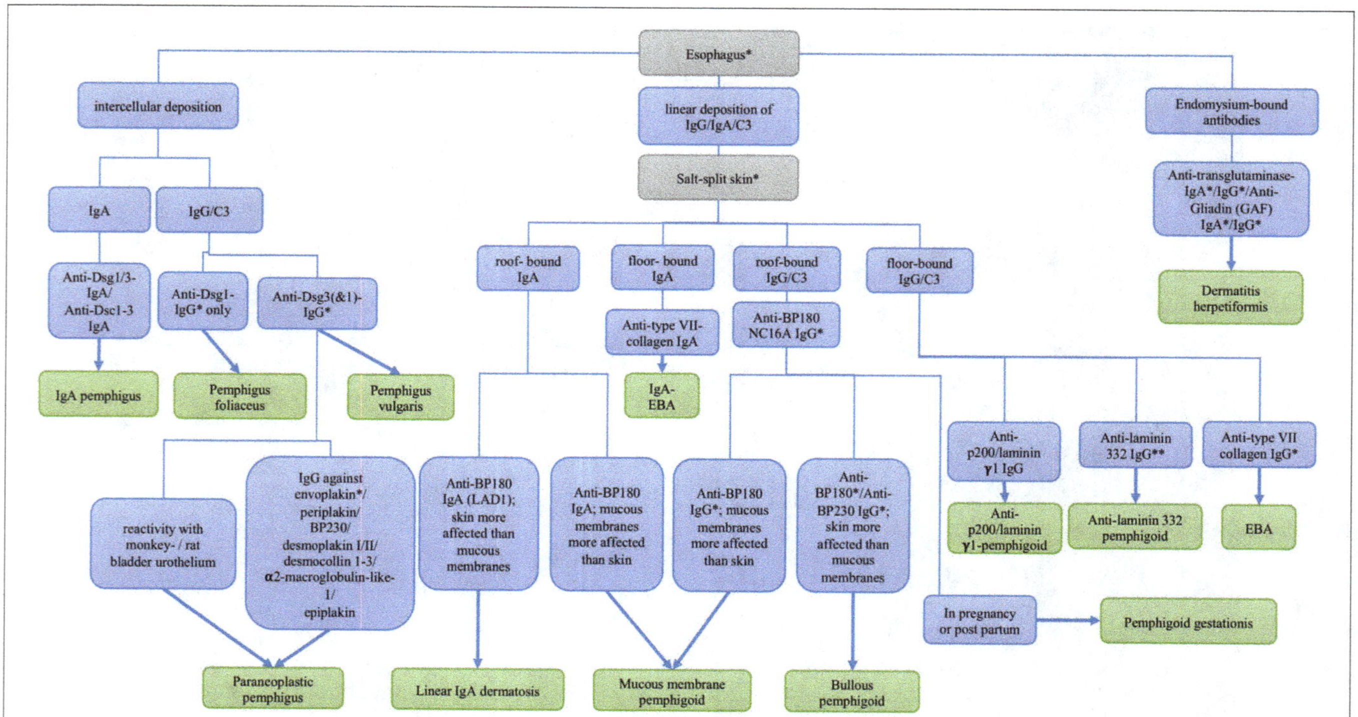

FIGURE 4 | Differential diagnosis of autoimmune skin blistering diseases based on the serological detection of autoantibodies. Dsc, desmocollin; Dsg, desmoglein; EBA, epidermolysis bullosa acquisita; * commercial assays are available; ** available by the end of 2018.

IgG and/or IgA reactivity was only found in about 3% of around 400 pemphigus sera, using a BIOCHIP® mosaic containing recombinant forms of desmocollin 1, −2, and −3 (82). Therefore, according to the guidelines of the German Dermatological Society, the analysis for anti-desmocollin reactivity is only recommended in patients with IgA pemphigus, pemphigus vegetans, atypical pemphigus, and the rare patients with pemphigus vulgaris/foliaceus without anti-Dsg reactivity (36). Most recently, a BIOCHIP® mosaic was developed containing recombinant chains of laminin 332 for the diagnosis of anti-laminin 332-pemphigoid (83) (**Figure 5**). This BIOCHIP® mosaic yields sensitivities between 75 and 85% with a specificity of nearly 100% (83).

(iii) Immunoblotting and immunoprecipitation are performed using recombinant proteins or extracts of dermis, epidermis, bovine gingiva, amnion membrane or cultured keratinocytes (80–86). These systems are part of the diagnostic algorithm for AIBD in some laboratories. They can be used for the detection of anti-p200 autoantibodies (**Figure 6**), anti-laminin γ1 autoantibodies, antibodies against C-terminal stretches of BP180, and the soluble ectodomain of BP180 (LAD-1; **Figure 7**), as well as autoantibodies against cell-derived forms of envoplakin, periplakin, desmoplakin, BP180, BP230, α4β6-integrin, laminin 332, and type VII collagen (**Figure 6**) (87). Latter test systems are, however, only available in specialized laboratories including the autoimmune laboratory of the Department of Dermatology, Lübeck, Germany (88). The laboratory has been accredited by Deutsche Akkreditierungsstelle (DAkkS D-ML-13069-06-00) and is also involved in the development of novel assay systems (www.uksh.de/dermatologie-luebeck/Infos+für+Ärzte+und+Einsender/Autoimmunlabor.html). The main diagnostic algorithm of our laboratory is shown in **Figure 4** and further detailed in Schmidt et al. (3).

DIAGNOSTICALLY RELEVANT CLINICAL AND IMMUNOPATHOLOGICAL CHARACTERISTICS OF MAJOR AIBD

Pemphigus Vulgaris and Pemphigus Foliaceus

Pemphigus can be divided in two major clinical subtypes, PV and PF. Autoantibodies in pemphigus are directed against epidermal desmosomes, mainly desmoglein (Dsg) 1 and 3. A common clinical finding is a positive Nikolsky sign. Here, mechanical friction of perilesional skin results in exfoliation of the outermost skin layer. The Nikolsky sign moderately sensitive, but highly specific in the diagnosis of pemphigus (89). PF is clinically characterized by flaccid, superficial erosions preferentially in seborrheic areas. The erosions are usually covered by scaling, which is due to the detachment of the superficial layers of the epidermis (90). In PF, mucous membranes are completely spared (3). Autoantibodies in PF are directed against Dsg1 and can be detected by ELISA or IIF microscopy (46, 88, 91) (**Figure 4**). In nearly all PF patients, anti-Dsg1 serum levels closely correlate with disease activity (46).

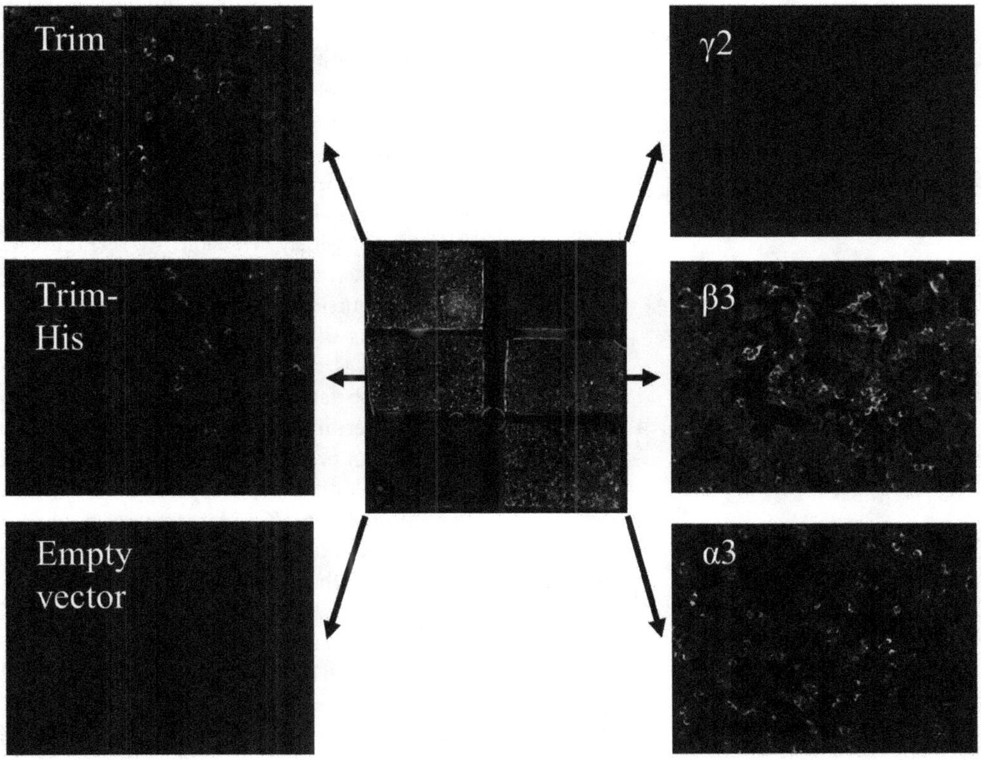

FIGURE 5 | Anti-laminin 332 BIOCHIP® mosaic. The mosaic contains HEK293 cells expressing the recombinant laminin 332 heterotrimer (Trim; upper left and middle left), the recombinant γ2- t β3-, and α3-chains of laminin 332 as well as negative control, cells transfected with the empty vector. Here, antibody binding is seen with the heterotrimer and the β3- and α3-chains in a patient with anti-laminin 332 mucous membrane pemphigoid.

In contrast to PF, patients with PV always suffer from mucous membrane lesions (**Figure 2** middle). These are accompanied to a variable extent with blisters and/or erosions of the skin. Autoantibodies in PV are directed against Dsg 3 (92). When in addition to mucosal involvement, lesions are also present on the skin, patients with PV also have autoantibodies against Dsgl (1). According to the extent of affected skin, three types of PV can be distinguished: (i) the mucosal-dominant type with limited cutaneous involvement (Dsg 3-autoantibodies are predominant), (ii) the mucocutaneous type with both mucosal and cutaneous involvement (Dsg3- and Dsgl-autoantibodies are equally predominant) and the cutaneous type with predominant anti-Dsgl and pathogenically weak anti-Dsg3 autoantibodies (1). Alike Dsgl-specific autoantibodies, anti-Dsg3-autoantibodies can be detected by ELISA (46). Both Dsgl- and 3-autoantibody levels correlate with the disease activity and can therefore be used as disease activity marker (30, 46).

Paraneoplastic Pemphigus

Paraneoplastic pemphigus (PNP) is an AIBD that is characterized by its association with malignant (or rarely benign) neoplasms. The most frequently associated neoplasms are B-cell lymphoma, Castleman disease, chronic lymphocytic leukemia, thymoma, and Waldenstrom macroglobulinemia (84, 93, 94). The clinical phenotype is diverse. First, PNP mainly affects the oral mucosa with other mucous membranes less frequently involved (95–97). Cutaneous lesions may arise on any part of the skin and may include: (i) pemphigus-like lesions with flaccid blisters, erosions, erythema and crusts; (ii) BP-like lesions such as urticarial lesions and tense blisters (96); (iii) erythema multiforme-like lesions and (iv) lichen planus-like lesions presenting as flat scaly papules and intense mucous membrane involvement (95). Furthermore, pulmonary destruction leading to bronchiolitis obliterans was noticed in many PNP-patients (98).

Apart from Dsg3, the autoantibodies may be directed against plakins such as BP230, periplakin, envoplakin, desmoplakin 1 and 2, and plectin (84). More recently, antibodies against desmocollins, α2 macroglobulin-like 1, and epiplakin have been described (62, 99, 100) (**Figure 4**). Antibodies against envoplakin and periplakin are most frequent (60, 101, 102). They can be detected via Western blotting or immunoprecipitation of extracts from keratinocytes (84), and, more conveniently, by a commercial ELISA employing the recombinant N-terminus of envoplakin (60).

Bullous Pemphigoid

In BP, autoantibodies are directed against a 180 kDa-sized (BP180/BPAG2/XVII collagen) and/or a 230 kDa-sized (BP230/BPAG1) antigen, which are essential for dermal-epidermal adhesion (103) (**Figure 2** left). The disease is mainly diagnosed in people aged between 75 and 80 years (18). It rarely occurs in people under the age of 50 years with few children

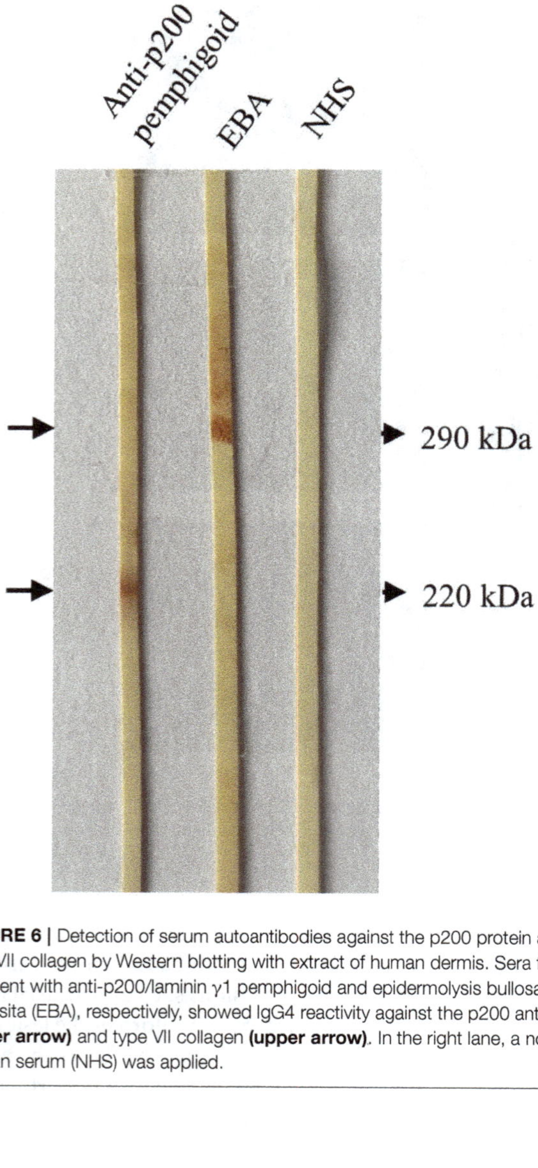

FIGURE 6 | Detection of serum autoantibodies against the p200 protein and type VII collagen by Western blotting with extract of human dermis. Sera from a patient with anti-p200/laminin γ1 pemphigoid and epidermolysis bullosa acquisita (EBA), respectively, showed IgG4 reactivity against the p200 antigen **(lower arrow)** and type VII collagen **(upper arrow)**. In the right lane, a normal human serum (NHS) was applied.

described with BP (104). In nearly all patients with BP, intense pruritus is present (105). Classically, BP presents with tense blisters and erosions. In contrast to pemphigus, the Nikolsky sign is negative. Alternatively or additionally, urticarial and erythematous non-bullous lesions are present (106). In fact, about 20% of patients present with non-bullous variants with excoriations, erythematous, or urticarial lesions (107). Non-bullous lesions also usually develop during a prodromal stage that may last for several months. Mucosal lesions, which occur in 15–20% of the BP patients, are associated with high disease severity and with absence of anti-BP230 antibodies (108).

BP180 is a collagen-type transmembrane glycoprotein of about 1,500 amino acids. It is a heterotrimer, consisting of a globular intracellular domain, a short transmembranous segment, and an extracellular C-terminal domain composed of 15 collagen repeats that are separated by 16 noncollagenous (NC) subdomains (109). The C-terminal domain forms a loop structure as it goes through the lamina lucida, spans the lamina densa, and then bends back into the lamina lucida (110). The 16th of the extracellular non-collagenous subdomains, NC16A, is the immunodominant region in BP (111). It is used in two ELISA systems (47, 48) (**Figure 4**), which on the one hand provide a sensitive and specific diagnostic tool for the routine diagnosis of BP and on the other hand are used to monitor the serum levels of anti-BP180 NC16A antibodies during the course of the disease (112). Alternatively, an IIF test using recombinant NC16A is widely available (77) (**Figure 4**). In most of the BP patients, autoantibodies are also directed against BP180-epitopes outside the NC16A-domain (113). In the 10–15% of BP patients with no reactivity against NC16A, testing for those antibodies is recommended; however, no commercial assay is available so far. In addition to several recombinant fragments of the C-terminal part of BP180, the cell-derived 120 kDa shed ectodomain present in the conditioned concentrated medium of cultures keratinocytes can be applied by immunoblotting for the detection of non-NC16A-reactive sera.

The major immunoglobulin class in BP is IgG. However, it has been shown that some patients also develop anti-BP180 IgA and IgE autoantibodies (114). In fact, most of the BP sera contain both IgG and IgA autoantibodies to BP180 (114, 115). Anti-BP180 IgE antibodies can be detected in 30–95% of the BP patients, and their detection corresponds to a high disease severity (70, 116).

BP230 is an intracellular component of the hemidesmosomal anchoring complex. It is a member of the plakin family. Anti-BP230 IgG can be detected in the serum of 40–60% of the BP patients. Like for BP180, commercial ELISA systems are available for the detection of anti-BP230 antibodies, which can be used for the diagnosis of BP (49, 52) (**Figure 4**). 80% of the anti-BP230 autoantibodies found in the sera of BP patients most frequently target the globular C-terminal domain of BP230 that interacts with keratin filaments (117, 118). However, it remains unclear whether anti-BP230 antibodies are directly pathogenic (119). Also, unlike anti-BP180, serum levels of anti-BP230-antibodies do not correlate with the disease activity in BP patients (120). However, the detection of anti-BP230 autoantibodies remains a useful tool for the diagnosis of BP. Regarding this matter, the combined use of the BP180 and BP230 ELISA system provides a sensitivity of around 90% for the detection of circulating autoantibodies (52, 56, 57).

Pemphigoid Gestationis

Pemphigoid gestationis (previously called herpes gestationis) is a dermatosis of pregnancy. It usually occurs during the third trimenon and less commonly, in the second trimenon or post partal period (121, 122). In contrast to BP, blisters are infrequent and usually small with predominating urticarial erythema frequently initiating around the umbilicus. Pemphigoid gestationis tends to recur in subsequent pregnancies, appearing earlier and with a more severe course. Serum autoantibodies to BP180 NC16A can be detected in >95% of the patients by ELISA, having a sensitivity of 97% (**Figure 4**) (47, 55). Recently, Sadik et al. detected NC16A reactivity in all of a large cohort of 65 pemphigoid gestationis sera using an IIF test based on the Biochip® mosaic technology (123). The main IgG subclasses are IgG1 and IgG3, explaining their high potential

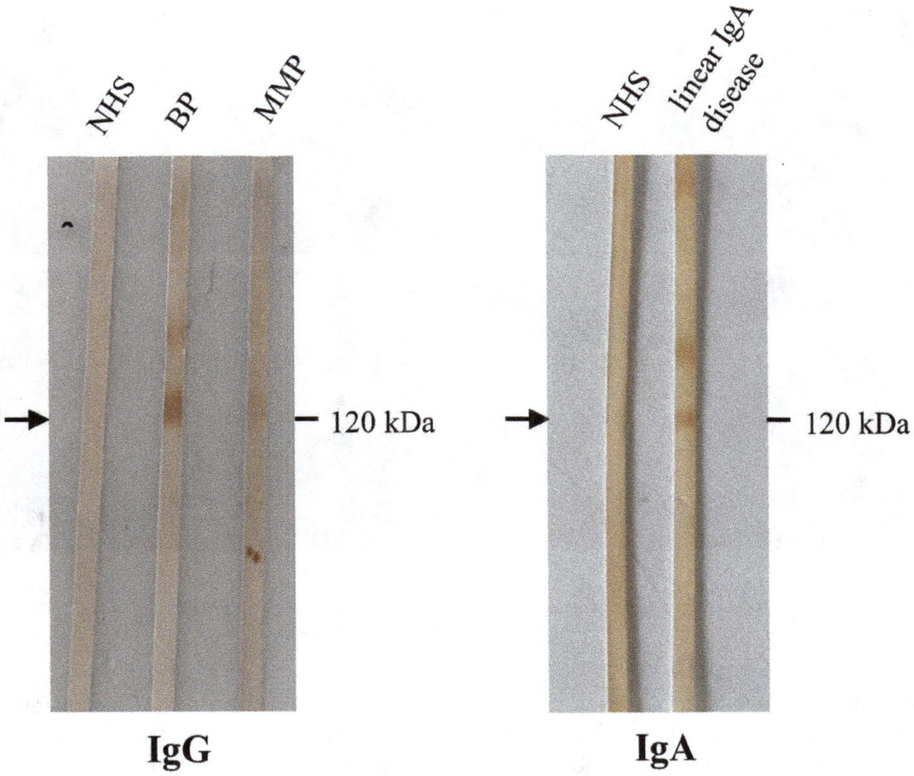

FIGURE 7 | Detection of IgG and IgA autoantibodies against LAD-1 by Western blotting with the concentrated conditioned medium of cultured human keratinocytes. Sera from patients with bullous pemphigoid (BP), mucous membrane pemphigoid (MMP), both without BP180 NC16A IgG by ELISA, showed IgG reactivity with the soluble ectodomain of BP180 (LAD-1; **left**, arrow). In serum of a patient with linear IgA disease, IgA antibodies against LAD-1 were present **(right)**. NHS, normal human serum.

for the fixation of complement (124), a feature that is exploited by the IIF complement binding test that visualizes complement-binding anti-basement membrane antibodies (**Figure 4**). Anti-BP230 reactivity is found in only 10% of sera (123).

Mucous Membrane Pemphigoid

MMP is defined as pemphigoid disease with predominant involvement of mucous membranes (125). It usually affects the mucous membranes of the mouth, eyes and genitals. Complications of the disease are conjunctival involvement and blindness, which may cause serious morbidity (**Figure 8**) (126, 127). Diagnosis is made by DIF microscopy of a perilesional biopsy, showing linear deposition of IgG and/or IgA and/or C3 along the DEJ (**Figure 1**) (126). In IIF microscopy, autoantibodies can only be detected in 50% of the MMP patients. Therefore, immunoprecipitation, Western blotting, and ELISA systems that employ cell-derived and recombinant proteins are essential diagnostic tests for MMP (**Figure 4**) (126). The main target antigen in MMP is BP180. However, in contrast to BP, the NC16A domain is only targeted in around 50%. More commonly, the autoantibodies target C-terminal epitopes of BP180 such as LAD-1, the soluble ectodomain of BP180 (128, 129). Those autoantibodies can be detected by Western blotting, using the respective recombinant fragments of the C-terminus of BP180. Both anti-BP180 IgG and IgA are predominant in anti-BP180-type MMP. Therefore, it is necessary to test for both isotypes (**Figure 4**) (128). Further antigens in MMP are laminin 332 as well as α6 and β4 integrin. Anti-laminin 332 antibodies can be detected in around 25% of the MMP-patients (128, 130). Laminin 332, which was formerly known as epiligrin or laminin 5, is a heterotrimeric protein composed of an α3, β3, and γ2 subunit. Anti-laminin 332 autoantibodies typically target the α3 chain (131). Since the presence of anti-laminin 332 autoantibodies is associated with development of malignancies in 25% (38, 132, 133), screening for anti-laminin 332 reactivity is strongly recommended in every MMP patient and in case of positivity, a tumor search is mandatory. Unfortunately, no detection system for serum antibodies against laminin 332 is widely available. A sensitive and highly specific assay for serum anti-laminin 332 IgG based on the Biochip® mosaic technology has recently been developed (83) and will be commercialized later in 2018. Antibodies against α6 and β4 integrin were detected in a few cases of oral and conjunctival MMP, respectively (134).

Linear IgA Disease

Linear IgA disease (LAD) is characterized by subepidermal blistering and linear deposition of predominantly IgA at the DEJ. The disease is characterized by its heterogenous phenotype that

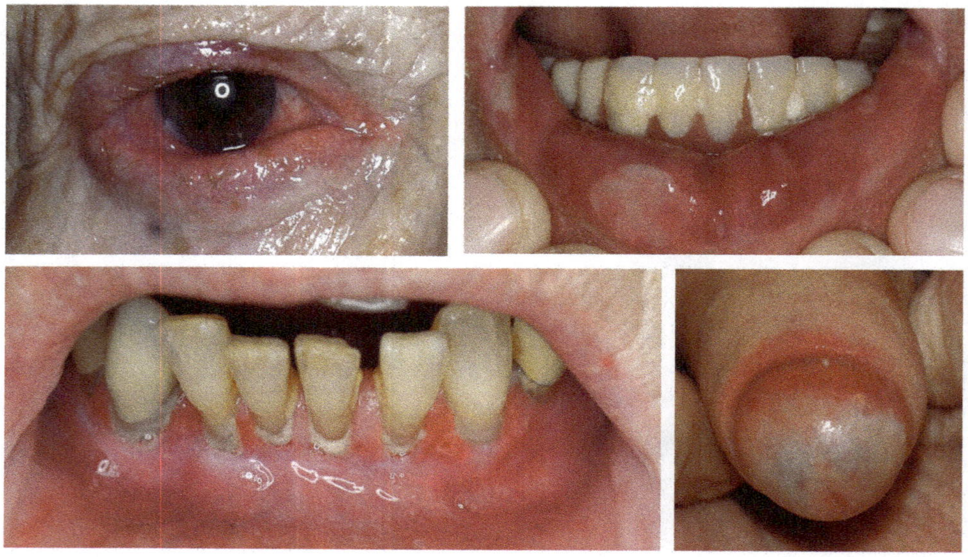

FIGURE 8 | Clinical findings in mucous membrane pemphigoid affecting the conjunctiva, lips, gingiva, and glans penis.

may be similar to other autoimmune skin blistering diseases. Mostly, the patients present with vesiculobullous lesions on the skin and adjacent mucous membranes (135, 136). Using DIF microscopy of a perilesional biopsy, a linear deposition of IgA autoantibodies along the DEJ can be detected (**Figure 1**). The autoantibodies bind to antigens of different molecular weights, including 97-, 120-, 180-, 200-, 230-, 280-, 285-, and 290-kDa proteins (137–139). According to the IIF findings, LAD can be divided into the lamina lucida type, where sera react with the epidermal side of salt-split skin and mostly with LAD-1 (140), and the sublamina densa type, that reveals serum antibodies against the dermal side of salt-split skin recognizing type VII collagen (138, 141, 142) (**Figure 4**). Interestingly, a recent study showed that type VII collagen is also the most common target antigen in vancomycine-induced LAD (143). Due to sematic overlap, patients with IgA reactivity against type VII collagen can also be classified as IgA EBA, a view that is supported by a recent consensus of an international expert panel (144).

Anti-P200/Anti-laminin γ 1 Pemphigoid

Anti-p200 pemphigoid is an autoimmune skin blistering disease with antibodies directed against a 200 kDa protein of the DEJ (145). Since laminin γ1 is the target antigen in 90% of the cases, it is also known as anti-laminin γ1 pemphigoid (65). Like LAD, the clinical presentation is heterogeneous and in most of the cases resembles BP and the inflammatory variant of EBA. The lesions heal without scarring or milia formation. Mucous membranes are involved in about 20% of the patients (146). Palmoplantar involvement seems to be more frequent compared to BP and a high association with psoriasis is seen in Japanese patients with anti-laminin 332 pemphigoid (146, 147). Antibodies against p200 bind to the floor of the artificial blister of salt-split skin using IIF microscopy (**Figure 4**). They can be detected by Western blotting with extracts of human dermis (**Figure 6**) (145). However, the preparation of those extracts is challenging and problematic. Therefore, an ELISA system was developed, using the recombinant C-terminus of laminin γ1, with a sensitivity of around 70% and a specificity of nearly 99% (64).

Epidermolysis Bullosa Acquisita

EBA affects skin and, to less extent, mucous membranes and is characterized by autoantibodies against type VII collagen (**Figure 2** right) (31, 148). There are two main clinical forms of EBA (144, 149, 150). The mechanobullous form represents the classical form of EBA. It is clinically characterized by skin fragility, tense blisters, vesicles, and erosions on non-inflamed skin in trauma-prone sites. Lesions may heal with scarring and milia formation (149, 151). In about two thirds of EBA, the inflammatory variant develops resembling BP, MMP, or LAD (149, 152). The diagnostic gold standards are direct immunogold electron microscopy, a methods nowadays only performed for this purpose in handful of centers, and more conveniently, DIF microscopy (144). By latter method, diagnosis of EBA can be made when a u-serrated binding pattern is present as detailed above (**Figures 1, 3**). Type VII collagen-specific autoantibodies are deposited at the floor of the artificial blister of salt-split human skin using IIF microscopy (**Figure 2** right) and are mostly directed against the noncollagenous (NC)1 domain (153, 154). Autoantibodies can be detected via Western blotting, using an extract of the human dermis (**Figure 6**). Three assays for the diagnostic detection of serum IgG against type VII collagen are available; two ELISA system using the NC1 domain or both the NC1 and NC2 domains as well as an IIF test based on the Biochip mosaic technology employing human cells that express the recombinant NC1 domain (**Figure 4**) (50, 51, 75). Anti-type VII collagen ELISA values were shown to correlate with disease activity (155), thus, like in PV, PF, and BP, the respective

ELISA systems are useful tools not only for the diagnosis of the disease but also to guide treatment decisions during the course of the diseases. Patients with predominant or exclusive IgA reactivity against type VII collagen are usually classified as IgA EBA following the consensus of an international expert panel (144, 149, 152, 156, 157).

Dermatitis Herpetiformis

Dermatitis herpetiformis is an autoimmune disease that always occurs in combination with glutensensitive enteropathy (celiac disease). It is clinically characterized by grouped vesicles and papules and predominantly affects the elbows, buttocks, and knees (146, 147, 149, 158–160). The autoantigen is the epidermal transglutaminase, however antibodies against gliadin, endomysium, tissue transglutaminase (TG2), and epidermal transglutaminase (TG3) can be detected (161). The main antibody-subclass is IgA but can be IgG in some patients. In patients under treatment with dapsone or on gluten-restricted diet, autoantibodies against the epidermal transglutaminase are found more frequently than autoantibodies to tissue transglutaminase (162). The diagnosis is based on the DIF and IIF microscopy findings as well as commercial ELISA systems. Here, IgA (or IgG)-autoantibodies against the epidermal and tissue transglutaminase as well as the deaminated gliadin-analogous fusion (GAF) peptides can be detected (61, 162).

AUTHOR CONTRIBUTIONS

MW and ES performed the literature research, acquired and designed the figures and wrote the manuscript. DZ performed literature research and critically revised the manuscript.

ACKNOWLEDGMENTS

We thank Inge Atefi, Dr. Stephanie Freyher, and Marina Kongsbak-Reim, Lübeck, for technical assistance. This work was supported by grants from the Deutsche Forschungsgemeinschaft through CRU 303 *Pemphigoid Diseases* (to DZ and ES) and Excellence Cluster 306/2 *Inflammation at Interfaces.*

REFERENCES

1. Kasperkiewicz M, Ellebrecht CT, Takahashi H, Yamagami J, Zillikens D, Payne AS, et al. Pemphigus. *Nat Rev Dis Primer* (2017) 3:17026. doi: 10.1038/nrdp.2017.26
2. Schmidt E, Zillikens D. Pemphigoid diseases. *Lancet Lond Engl.* (2013) 381:320–32. doi: 10.1016/S0140-6736(12)61140-4
3. Schmidt E, Zillikens D. The diagnosis and treatment of autoimmune blistering skin diseases. *Dtsch Arzteblatt Int.* (2011) 108:399–405. doi: 10.3238/arztebl.2011.0405
4. Schmidt E, Zillikens D. Modern diagnosis of autoimmune blistering skin diseases. *Autoimmun Rev.* (2010) 10:84–9. doi: 10.1016/j.autrev.2010.08.007
5. Bertram F, Bröcker E-B, Zillikens D, Schmidt E. Prospective analysis of the incidence of autoimmune bullous disorders in Lower Franconia, Germany. *J Dtsch Dermatol Ges J Ger Soc Dermatol.* (2009) 7:434–40. doi: 10.1111/j.1610-0387.2008.06976.x
6. Marazza G, Pham HC, Schärer L, Pedrazzetti PP, Hunziker T, Trüeb RM, et al. Incidence of bullous pemphigoid and pemphigus in Switzerland: a 2-year prospective study. *Br J Dermatol.* (2009) 161:861–8. doi: 10.1111/j.1365-2133.2009.09300.x
7. Joly P, Baricault S, Sparsa A, Bernard P, Bédane C, Duvert-Lehembre S, et al. Incidence and mortality of bullous pemphigoid in France. *J Invest Dermatol.* (2012) 132:1998–2004. doi: 10.1038/jid.2012.35
8. Försti A-K, Jokelainen J, Timonen M, Tasanen K. Increasing incidence of bullous pemphigoid in Northern Finland: a retrospective database study in Oulu University Hospital. *Br J Dermatol.* (2014) 171:1223–6. doi: 10.1111/bjd.13189
9. Langan SM, Smeeth L, Hubbard R, Fleming KM, Smith CJP, West J. Bullous pemphigoid and pemphigus vulgaris–incidence and mortality in the UK: population based cohort study. *BMJ* (2008) 337:a180. doi: 10.1136/bmj.a180
10. Thorslund K, Seifert O, Nilzén K, Grönhagen C. Incidence of bullous pemphigoid in Sweden 2005-2012: a nationwide population-based cohort study of 3761 patients. *Arch Dermatol Res.* (2017) 309:721–7. doi: 10.1007/s00403-017-1778-4
11. Bertram F, BrÄcker E-B, Zillikens D, Schmidt E. Prospektive Untersuchung der Inzidenz blasenbildender Autoimmundermatosen in Unterfranken. *J Dtsch Dermatol Ges.* (2009) 7:434–40. doi: 10.1111/j.1610-0387.2008.06976_supp.x
12. Försti A-K, Huilaja L, Schmidt E, Tasanen K. Neurological and psychiatric associations in bullous pemphigoid-more than skin deep? *Exp Dermatol.* (2017) 26:1228–34. doi: 10.1111/exd.13401
13. Ren Z, Hsu DY, Brieva J, Silverberg NB, Langan SM, Silverberg JI. Hospitalization, inpatient burden and comorbidities associated with bullous pemphigoid in the U.S.A. *Br J Dermatol.* (2017) 176:87–99. doi: 10.1111/bjd.14821
14. Meyer N, Misery L. Geoepidemiologic considerations of auto-immune pemphigus. *Autoimmun Rev.* (2010) 9:A379–82. doi: 10.1016/j.autrev.2009.10.009
15. Kridin K. Pemphigus group: overview, epidemiology, mortality, and comorbidities. *Immunol Res.* (2018) 66:255–70. doi: 10.1007/s12026-018-8986-7
16. Bastuji-Garin S, Souissi R, Blum L, Turki H, Nouira R, Jomaa B, et al. Comparative epidemiology of pemphigus in Tunisia and France: unusual incidence of pemphigus foliaceus in young Tunisian women. *J Invest Dermatol.* (1995) 104:302–405.
17. Culton DA, Qian Y, Li N, Rubenstein D, Aoki V, Filhio GH, et al. Advances in pemphigus and its endemic pemphigus foliaceus (Fogo Selvagem) phenotype: a paradigm of human autoimmunity. *J Autoimmun.* (2008) 31:311–24. doi: 10.1016/j.jaut.2008.08.003
18. Hübner F, Recke A, Zillikens D, Linder R, Schmidt E. Prevalence and age distribution of pemphigus and pemphigoid diseases in Germany. *J Invest Dermatol.* (2016) 136:2495–8. doi: 10.1016/j.jid.2016.07.013
19. Lever WF. Pemphigus: a historical study. *Arch Dermatol Syphilol.* (1942) 46:800. doi: 10.1001/archderm.1942.01500180020004
20. Lever WF. Pemphigus. *Medicine* (1953) 32:1–123.
21. Beutner EH, Jordon RE. Demonstration of skin antibodies in sera of pemphigus vulgaris patients by indirect immunofluorescent staining. *Proc Soc Exp Biol Med.* (1964) 117:505–10.
22. Jordon RE, Beutner EH, Witebsky E, Blumental G, Hale WL, Lever WF. Basement zone antibodies in bullous pemphigoid. *JAMA* (1967) 200:751–6.
23. Mihai S, Sitaru C. Immunopathology and molecular diagnosis of autoimmune bullous diseases. *J Cell Mol Med.* (2007) 11:462–81. doi: 10.1111/j.1582-4934.2007.00033.x
24. Anhalt GJ, Labib RS, Voorhees JJ, Beals TF, Diaz LA. Induction of pemphigus in neonatal mice by passive transfer of IgG from patients with the disease. *N Engl J Med.* (1982) 306:1189–96. doi: 10.1056/NEJM198205203062001
25. Liu Z, Diaz LA, Troy JL, Taylor AF, Emery DJ, Fairley JA, et al. A passive transfer model of the organ-specific autoimmune disease, bullous pemphigoid, using antibodies generated against the hemidesmosomal antigen, BP180. *J Clin Invest.* (1993) 92:2480–8. doi: 10.1172/JCI116856

26. Lazarova Z, Hsu R, Yee C, Yancey KB. Antiepiligrin cicatricial pemphigoid represents an autoimmune response to subunits present in laminin 5 (alpha3beta3gamma2). *Br J Dermatol.* (1998) 139:791–7.
27. Nishie W, Sawamura D, Goto M, Ito K, Shibaki A, McMillan JR, et al. Humanization of autoantigen. *Nat Med.* (2007) 13:378–83. doi: 10.1038/nm1496
28. Schulze FS, Beckmann T, Nimmerjahn F, Ishiko A, Collin M, Köhl J, et al. Fcγ receptors III and IV mediate tissue destruction in a novel adult mouse model of bullous pemphigoid. *Am J Pathol.* (2014) 184:2185–96. doi: 10.1016/j.ajpath.2014.05.007
29. Heppe EN, Tofern S, Schulze FS, Ishiko A, Shimizu A, Sina C, et al. Experimental laminin 332 mucous membrane pemphigoid critically involves C5aR1 and reflects clinical and immunopathological characteristics of the human disease. *J Invest Dermatol.* (2017) 137:1709–18. doi: 10.1016/j.jid.2017.03.037
30. Stanley JR, Amagai M. Pemphigus, bullous impetigo, and the staphylococcal scalded-skin syndrome. *N Engl J Med.* (2006) 355:1800–10. doi: 10.1056/NEJMra061111
31. Witte M, Koga H, Hashimoto T, Ludwig RJ, Bieber K. Discovering potential drug-targets for personalized treatment of autoimmune disorders-what we learn from epidermolysis bullosa acquisita. *Expert Opin Ther Targets* (2016) 20:985–98. doi: 10.1517/14728222.2016.1148686
32. Liu Z, Sui W, Zhao M, Li Z, Li N, Thresher R, et al. Subepidermal blistering induced by human autoantibodies to BP180 requires innate immune players in a humanized bullous pemphigoid mouse model. *J Autoimmun.* (2008) 31:331–8. doi: 10.1016/j.jaut.2008.08.009
33. Spindler V, Waschke J. Pemphigus-A disease of desmosome dysfunction caused by multiple mechanisms. *Front Immunol.* (2018) 9:136. doi: 10.3389/fimmu.2018.00136
34. Spindler V, Eming R, Schmidt E, Amagai M, Grando S, Jonkman MF, et al. Mechanisms causing loss of keratinocyte cohesion in pemphigus. *J Invest Dermatol.* (2018) 138:32–7. doi: 10.1016/j.jid.2017.06.022
35. Boraiy L, Fontao L. Michel's transport medium as an alternative to liquid nitrogen for PCR analysis of skin biopsy specimens. *Dermatopathology* (2014) 1:70–4. doi: 10.1159/000368347
36. Schmidt E, Goebeler M, Hertl M, Sárdy M, Sitaru C, Eming R, et al. S2k guideline for the diagnosis of pemphigus vulgaris/foliaceus and bullous pemphigoid. *J Dtsch Dermatol Ges.* (2015) 13:713–27. doi: 10.1111/ddg.12612
37. Vodegel RM, Jonkman MF, Pas HH, de Jong MCJM. U-serrated immunodeposition pattern differentiates type VII collagen targeting bullous diseases from other subepidermal bullous autoimmune diseases. *Br J Dermatol.* (2004) 151:112–8. doi: 10.1111/j.1365-2133.2004.06006.x
38. Terra JB, Pas HH, Hertl M, Dikkers FG, Kamminga N, Jonkman MF. Immunofluorescence serration pattern analysis as a diagnostic criterion in antilaminin-332 mucous membrane pemphigoid: immunopathological findings and clinical experience in 10 Dutch patients. *Br J Dermatol.* (2011) 165:815–22. doi: 10.1111/j.1365-2133.2011.10474.x
39. Meijer JM, Atefi I, Diercks GFH, Vorobyev A, Zuiderveen J, Meijer HJ, et al. Serration pattern analysis for differentiating epidermolysis bullosa acquisita from other pemphigoid diseases. *J Am Acad Dermatol.* (2018) 78:754–9.e6. doi: 10.1016/j.jaad.2017.11.029
40. Lemcke S, Sokolowski S, Rieckhoff N, Buschtez M, Kaffka C, Winter-Keil A, et al. Automated direct immunofluorescence analyses of skin biopsies. *J Cutan Pathol.* (2016) 43:227–35. doi: 10.1111/cup.12637
41. Sárdy M, Kostaki D, Varga R, Peris K, Ruzicka T. Comparative study of direct and indirect immunofluorescence and of bullous pemphigoid 180 and 230 enzyme-linked immunosorbent assays for diagnosis of bullous pemphigoid. *J Am Acad Dermatol.* (2013) 69:748–53. doi: 10.1016/j.jaad.2013.07.009
42. Ng PPL, Thng STG, Mohamed K, Tan SH. Comparison of desmoglein ELISA and indirect immunofluorescence using two substrates (monkey oesophagus and normal human skin) in the diagnosis of pemphigus. *Australas J Dermatol.* (2005) 46:239–41. doi: 10.1111/j.1440-0960.2005.00191.x
43. Harman KE, Gratian MJ, Bhogal BS, Challacombe SJ, Black MM. The use of two substrates to improve the sensitivity of indirect immunofluorescence in the diagnosis of pemphigus. *Br J Dermatol.* (2000) 142:1135–9. doi: 10.1046/j.1365-2133.2000.03538.x
44. Oyama N, Bhogal BS, Carrington P, Gratian MJ, Black MM. Human placental amnion is a novel substrate for detecting autoantibodies in autoimmune bullous diseases by immunoblotting. *Br J Dermatol.* (2003) 148:939–44. doi: 10.1046/j.1365-2133.2003.05316.x
45. Machado P, Michalaki H, Roche P, Gaucherand M, Thivolet J, Nicolas JF. Serological diagnosis of bullous pemphigoid (BP): comparison of the sensitivity of indirect immunofluorescence on salt-split skin to immunoblotting. *Br J Dermatol* (1992) 126:236–241.
46. Schmidt E, Dähnrich C, Rosemann A, Probst C, Komorowski L, Saschenbrecker S, et al. Novel ELISA systems for antibodies to desmoglein 1 and 3: correlation of disease activity with serum autoantibody levels in individual pemphigus patients. *Exp Dermatol.* (2010) 19:458–63. doi: 10.1111/j.1600-0625.2010.01069.x
47. Sitaru C, Dähnrich C, Probst C, Komorowski L, Blöcker I, Schmidt E, et al. Enzyme-linked immunosorbent assay using multimers of the 16th non-collagenous domain of the BP180 antigen for sensitive and specific detection of pemphigoid autoantibodies. *Exp Dermatol.* (2007) 16:770–7. doi: 10.1111/j.1600-0625.2007.00592.x
48. Kobayashi M, Amagai M, Kuroda-Kinoshita K, Hashimoto T, Shirakata Y, Hashimoto K, et al. BP180 ELISA using bacterial recombinant NC16a protein as a diagnostic and monitoring tool for bullous pemphigoid. *J Dermatol Sci.* (2002) 30:224–32. doi: 10.1016/S0923-1811(02)00109-3
49. Yoshida M, Hamada T, Amagai M, Hashimoto K, Uehara R, Yamaguchi K, et al. Enzyme-linked immunosorbent assay using bacterial recombinant proteins of human BP230 as a diagnostic tool for bullous pemphigoid. *J Dermatol Sci.* (2006) 41:21–30. doi: 10.1016/j.jdermsci.2005.11.002
50. Komorowski L, Müller R, Vorobyev A, Probst C, Recke A, Jonkman MF, et al. Sensitive and specific assays for routine serological diagnosis of epidermolysis bullosa acquisita. *J Am Acad Dermatol.* (2013) 68:e89–95. doi: 10.1016/j.jaad.2011.12.032
51. Saleh MA, Ishii K, Kim Y-J, Murakami A, Ishii N, Hashimoto T, et al. Development of NC1 and NC2 domains of type VII collagen ELISA for the diagnosis and analysis of the time course of epidermolysis bullosa acquisita patients. *J Dermatol Sci.* (2011) 62:169–75. doi: 10.1016/j.jdermsci.2011.03.003
52. Blöcker IM, Dähnrich C, Probst C, Komorowski L, Saschenbrecker S, Schlumberger W, et al. Epitope mapping of BP230 leading to a novel enzyme-linked immunosorbent assay for autoantibodies in bullous pemphigoid. *Br J Dermatol* (2012) 166:964–970. doi: 10.1111/j.1365-2133.2012.10820.x
53. Tampoia M, Giavarina D, Di Giorgio C, Bizzaro N. Diagnostic accuracy of enzyme-linked immunosorbent assays (ELISA) to detect anti-skin autoantibodies in autoimmune blistering skin diseases: a systematic review and meta-analysis. *Autoimmun Rev.* (2012) 12:121–6. doi: 10.1016/j.autrev.2012.07.006
54. Powell AM, Sakuma-Oyama Y, Oyama N, Albert S, Bhogal B, Kaneko F, et al. Usefulness of BP180 NC16a enzyme-linked immunosorbent assay in the serodiagnosis of pemphigoid gestationis and in differentiating between pemphigoid gestationis and pruritic urticarial papules and plaques of pregnancy. *Arch Dermatol.* (2005) 141:705–10. doi: 10.1001/archderm.141.6.705
55. Al Saif F, Jouen F, Hebert V, Chiavelli H, Darwish B, Duvert-Lehembre S, et al, French Study Group on Autoimmune Bullous Skin Diseases. Sensitivity and specificity of BP180 NC16A enzyme-linked immunosorbent assay for the diagnosis of pemphigoid gestationis. *J Am Acad Dermatol.* (2017) 76:560–2. doi: 10.1016/j.jaad.2016.09.030
56. Charneux J, Lorin J, Vitry F, Antonicelli F, Reguiai Z, Barbe C, et al. Usefulness of BP230 and BP180-NC16a enzyme-linked immunosorbent assays in the initial diagnosis of bullous pemphigoid: a retrospective study of 138 patients. *Arch Dermatol.* (2011) 147:286–91. doi: 10.1001/archdermatol.2011.23
57. Roussel A, Benichou J, Randriamanantany ZA, Gilbert D, Drenovska K, Houivet E, et al. Enzyme-linked immunosorbent assay for the combination of bullous pemphigoid antigens 1 and 2 in the diagnosis of bullous pemphigoid. *Arch Dermatol.* (2011) 147:293–8. doi: 10.1001/archdermatol.2011.21
58. Ishii K, Amagai M, Hall RP, Hashimoto T, Takayanagi A, Gamou S, et al. Characterization of autoantibodies in pemphigus using antigen-specific enzyme-linked immunosorbent assays with baculovirus-expressed recombinant desmogleins. *J Immunol.* (1997) 159:2010–7.

59. Harman KE, Seed PT, Gratian MJ, Bhogal BS, Challacombe SJ, Black MM. The severity of cutaneous and oral pemphigus is related to desmoglein 1 and 3 antibody levels. *Br J Dermatol.* (2001) 144:775–80. doi: 10.1046/j.1365-2133.2001.04132.x
60. Probst C, Schlumberger W, Stöcker W, Recke A, Schmidt E, Hashimoto T, et al. Development of ELISA for the specific determination of autoantibodies against envoplakin and periplakin in paraneoplastic pemphigus. *Clin Chim Acta* (2009) 410:13–8. doi: 10.1016/j.cca.2009.08.022
61. Kasperkiewicz M, Dähnrich C, Probst C, Komorowski L, Stöcker W, Schlumberger W, et al Novel assay for detecting celiac disease-associated autoantibodies in dermatitis herpetiformis using deamidated gliadin-analogous fusion peptides. *J Am Acad Dermatol.* (2012) 66:583–8. doi: 10.1016/j.jaad.2011.02.025
62. Müller R, Heber B, Hashimoto T, Messer G, Müllegger R, Niedermeier A, et al. Autoantibodies against desmocollins in European patients with pemphigus. *Clin Exp Dermatol.* (2009) 34:898–903. doi: 10.1111/j.1365-2230.2009.03241.x
63. Ishii N, Teye K, Fukuda S, Uehara R, Hachiya T, Koga H, et al. Anti-desmocollin autoantibodies in nonclassical pemphigus. *Br J Dermatol.* (2015) 173:59–68. doi: 10.1111/bjd.13711
64. Groth S, Recke A, Vafia K, Ludwig RJ, Hashimoto T, Zillikens D, et al. Development of a simple enzyme-linked immunosorbent assay for the detection of autoantibodies in anti-p200 pemphigoid. *Br J Dermatol.* (2011) 164:76–82. doi: 10.1111/j.1365-2133.2010.10056.x
65. Dainichi T, Kurono S, Ohyama B, Ishii N, Sanzen N, Hayashi M, et al. Anti-laminin gamma-1 pemphigoid. *Proc Natl Acad Sci USA.* (2009) 106:2800–5. doi: 10.1073/pnas.0809230106
66. Csorba K, Schmidt S, Florea F, Ishii N, Hashimoto T, Hertl M, et al. Development of an ELISA for sensitive and specific detection of IgA autoantibodies against BP180 in pemphigoid diseases. *Orphanet J Rare Dis.* (2011) 6:31. doi: 10.1186/1750-1172-6-31
67. Izumi K, Nishie W, Mai Y, Wada M, Natsuga K, Ujiie H, et al. Autoantibody Profile Differentiates between Inflammatory and noninflammatory bullous pemphigoid. *J Invest Dermatol.* (2016) 136:2201–10. doi: 10.1016/j.jid.2016.06.622
68. Bekou V, Thoma-Uszynski S, Wendler O, Uter W, Schwietzke S, Hunziker T, et al. Detection of laminin 5-specific auto-antibodies in mucous membrane and bullous pemphigoid sera by ELISA. *J Invest Dermatol.* (2005) 124:732–40. doi: 10.1111/j.0022-202X.2005.23646.x
69. Bernard P, Antonicelli F, Bedane C, Joly P, Le Roux-Villet C, Duvert-Lehembre S, et al. Prevalence and clinical significance of anti-laminin 332 autoantibodies detected by a novel enzyme-linked immunosorbent assay in mucous membrane pemphigoid. *JAMA Dermatol.* (2013) 149:533–40. doi: 10.1001/jamadermatol.2013.1434
70. Hashimoto T, Ohzono A, Teye K, Numata S, Hiroyasu S, Tsuruta D, et al. Detection of IgE autoantibodies to BP180 and BP230 and their relationship to clinical features in bullous pemphigoid. *Br J Dermatol.* (2017) 177:141–51. doi: 10.1111/bjd.15114
71. van Beek N, Lüttmann N, Huebner F, Recke A, Karl I, Schulze FS, et al. Correlation of serum levels of IgE autoantibodies against BP180 with bullous pemphigoid disease activity. *JAMA Dermatol.* (2017) 153:30–8. doi: 10.1001/jamadermatol.2016.3357
72. Messingham KAN, Noe MH, Chapman MA, Giudice GJ, Fairley JA. A novel ELISA reveals high frequencies of BP180-specific IgE production in bullous pemphigoid. *J Immunol Methods* (2009) 346:18–25. doi: 10.1016/j.jim.2009.04.013
73. Di Zenzo G, Thoma-Uszynski S, Fontao L, Calabresi V, Hofmann SC, Hellmark T, et al. Multicenter prospective study of the humoral autoimmune response in bullous pemphigoid. *Clin Immunol.* (2008) 128:415–26. doi: 10.1016/j.clim.2008.04.012
74. Hofmann S, Thoma-Uszynski S, Hunziker T, Bernard P, Koebnick C, Stauber A, et al. Severity and phenotype of bullous pemphigoid relate to autoantibody profile against the NH2- and COOH-terminal regions of the BP180 ectodomain. *J Invest Dermatol.* (2002) 119:1065–73. doi: 10.1046/j.1523-1747.2002.19529.x
75. van Beek N, Dähnrich C, Johannsen N, Lemcke S, Goletz S, Hübner F, et al. Prospective studies on the routine use of a novel multivariant enzyme-linked immunosorbent assay for the diagnosis of autoimmune bullous diseases. *J Am Acad Dermatol.* (2017) 76:889–94.e5. doi: 10.1016/j.jaad.2016.11.002
76. Horváth ON, Varga R, Kaneda M, Schmidt E, Ruzicka T, Sárdy M. Diagnostic performance of the "MESACUP anti-Skin profile TEST." *Eur J Dermatol.* (2016) 26:56–63. doi: 10.1684/ejd.2015.2692
77. van Beek N, Rentzsch K, Probst C, Komorowski L, Kasperkiewicz M, Fechner K, et al. Serological diagnosis of autoimmune bullous skin diseases: prospective comparison of the BIOCHIP mosaic-based indirect immunofluorescence technique with the conventional multi-step single test strategy. *Orphanet J Rare Dis.* (2012) 7:49. doi: 10.1186/1750-1172-7-49
78. Tampoia M, Zucano A, Villalta D, Antico A, Bizzaro N. Anti-skin specific autoantibodies detected by a new immunofluorescence multiplex biochip method in patients with autoimmune bullous diseases. *Dermatology* (2012) 225:37–44. doi: 10.1159/000339776
79. Russo I, Saponeri A, Peserico A, Alaibac M. The use of biochip immunofluorescence microscopy for the diagnosis of Pemphigus vulgaris. *Acta Histochem.* (2014) 116:713–6. doi: 10.1016/j.acthis.2013.12.012
80. Xuan RR, Yang A, Murrell DF. New biochip immunofluorescence test for the serological diagnosis of pemphigus vulgaris and foliaceus: a review of the literature. *Int J Womens Dermatol.* (2018) 4:102–8. doi: 10.1016/j.ijwd.2017.10.001
81. Marzano AV, Cozzani E, Biasin M, Russo I, Alaibac M. The use of Biochip immunofluorescence microscopy for the serological diagnosis of epidermolysis bullosa acquisita. *Arch Dermatol Res.* (2016) 308:273–6. doi: 10.1007/s00403-016-1632-0
82. Mindorf S, Dettmann IM, Krüger S, Fuhrmann T, Rentzsch K, Karl I, et al. Routine detection of serum antidesmocollin autoantibodies is only useful in patients with atypical pemphigus. *Exp Dermatol.* (2017) 26:1267–70. doi: 10.1111/exd.13409
83. Goletz S, Probst C, Komorowski L, Schlumberger W, Fechner K, van Beek N, et al. Sensitive and specific assay for the serological diagnosis of anti-laminin 332 mucous membrane pemphigoid. *Br J Dermatol.* (2018) doi: 10.1111/bjd.17202. [Epub ahead of print].
84. Zimmermann J, Bahmer F, Rose C, Zillikens D, Schmidt E. Clinical and immunopathological spectrum of paraneoplastic pemphigus. *J Dtsch Dermatol Ges.* (2010) 8:598–606. doi: 10.1111/j.1610-0387.2010.07380.x
85. Grootenboer-Mignot S, Descamps V, Picard-Dahan C, Nicaise-Roland P, Prost-Squarcioni C, Leroux-Villet C, et al. Place of human amniotic membrane immunoblotting in the diagnosis of autoimmune bullous dermatoses. *Br J Dermatol.* (2010) 162:743–50. doi: 10.1111/j.1365-2133.2009.09566.x
86. Rashid KA, Stern JNH, Ahmed AR. Identification of an epitope within human integrin alpha 6 subunit for the binding of autoantibody and its role in basement membrane separation in oral pemphigoid. *J Immunol.* (2006) 176:1968–77. doi: 10.4049/jimmunol.176.3.1968
87. Vodegel RM, Kiss M, Cjm De Jong M, Pas HH, Altmayer A, Molnar K, et al. The use of skin substrates deficient in basement membrane molecules for the diagnosis of subepidermal autoimmune bullous disease. *Eur J Dermatol EJD.* (1998) 8:83–5.
88. van Beek N, Knuth-Rehr D, Altmeyer P, Assaf C, Babilas P, Bayerl C, et al. Diagnostics of autoimmune bullous diseases in German dermatology departments. *J Dtsch Dermatol Ges.* (2012) 10:492–9. doi: 10.1111/j.1610-0387.2011.07840.x
89. Uzun S, Durdu M. The specificity and sensitivity of nikolskiy sign in the diagnosis of pemphigus. *J Am Acad Dermatol.* (2006) 54:411–5. doi: 10.1016/j.jaad.2005.10.019
90. James KA, Culton DA, Diaz LA. Diagnosis and clinical features of pemphigus foliaceus. *Dermatol Clin.* (2011) 29:405–12. doi: 10.1016/j.det.2011.03.012
91. Stanley JR, Koulu L, Klaus-Kovtun V, Steinberg MS. A monoclonal antibody to the desmosomal glycoprotein desmoglein I binds the same polypeptide as human autoantibodies in pemphigus foliaceus. *J Immunol.* (1986) 136:1227–30.
92. Kárpáti S, Amagai M, Prussick R, Stanley JR. Pemphigus vulgaris antigen is a desmosomal desmoglein. *Dermatolology* (1994) 189 (Suppl. 1):24–6. doi: 10.1159/000246923
93. Anhalt GJ. Paraneoplastic pemphigus. *Adv Dermatol.* (1997) 12:77–96; discussion 97.

94. Anhalt GJ. Paraneoplastic pemphigus. *J Invest Dermatol Symp Proc.* (2004) 9:29–33. doi: 10.1111/j.1087-0024.2004.00832.x
95. Czernik A, Wieczorek M. Paraneoplastic pemphigus: a short review. *Clin Cosmet Investig Dermatol.* (2016) 9:291–5. doi: 10.2147/CCID.S100802
96. Akel R, Fakhri G, Salem R, Boulos F, Habib K, Tfayli A. Paraneoplastic pemphigus as a first manifestation of an intra-abdominal follicular dendritic cell sarcoma: rare case and review of the literature. *Case Rep Oncol.* (2018) 353–9. doi: 10.1159/000489602
97. Adaszewska A, Ishii N, Dwilewicz-Trojaczek J, Wozniak K, Hashimoto T, Kowalewski C. Paraneoplastic pemphigus with anti-desmocollin 3 autoantibodies and chronic lymphocytic leukemia. *Adv Dermatol Allergol.* (2018) 35:113–5. doi: 10.5114/ada.2018.73171
98. Nikolskaia OV, Nousari CH, Anhalt GJ. Paraneoplastic pemphigus in association with Castleman's disease. *Br J Dermatol.* (2003) 149:1143–51. doi: 10.1111/j.1365-2133.2003.05659.x
99. Tsuchisaka A, Numata S, Teye K, Natsuaki Y, Kawakami T, Takeda Y, et al. Epiplakin is a paraneoplastic pemphigus autoantigen and related to bronchiolitis obliterans in Japanese patients. *J Invest Dermatol.* (2016) 136:399–408. doi: 10.1038/JID.2015.408
100. Schepens I, Jaunin F, Begre N, Läderach U, Marcus K, Hashimoto T, et al. The protease inhibitor alpha-2-macroglobulin-like-1 is the p170 antigen recognized by paraneoplastic pemphigus autoantibodies in human. *PLoS ONE* (2010) 5:e12250. doi: 10.1371/journal.pone.0012250
101. Zhang B, Zheng R, Wang J, Bu D, Zhu X. Epitopes in the linker subdomain region of envoplakin recognized by autoantibodies in paraneoplastic pemphigus patients. *J Invest Dermatol.* (2006) 126:832–40. doi: 10.1038/sj.jid.5700198
102. Nagata Y, Karashima T, Watt FM, Salmhofer W, Kanzaki T, Hashimoto T. Paraneoplastic pemphigus sera react strongly with multiple epitopes on the various regions of envoplakin and periplakin, except for the c-terminal homologous domain of periplakin. *J Invest Dermatol.* (2001) 116:556–63. doi: 10.1046/j.1523-1747.2001.01263.x
103. Stanley JR, Hawley-Nelson P, Yuspa SH, Shevach EM, Katz SI. Characterization of bullous pemphigoid antigen: a unique basement membrane protein of stratified squamous epithelia. *Cell* (1981) 24:897–903.
104. Schwieger-Briel A, Moellmann C, Mattulat B, Schauer F, Kiritsi D, Schmidt E, et al. Bullous pemphigoid in infants: characteristics, diagnosis and treatment. *Orphanet J Rare Dis.* (2014) 9:185. doi: 10.1186/s13023-014-0185-6
105. Kippes W, Schmidt E, Roth A, Rzany B, Bröcker EB, Zillikens D. Immunopathologic changes in 115 patients with bullous pemphigoid. *Hautarzt Z Dermatol Venerol Verwandte Geb.* (1999) 50:866–72.
106. Schmidt E, della Torre R, Borradori L. Clinical features and practical diagnosis of bullous pemphigoid. *Dermatol Clin.* (2011) 29:427–38. doi: 10.1016/j.det.2011.03.010
107. della Torre R, Combescure C, Cortés B, Marazza G, Beltraminelli H, Naldi L, et al. Clinical presentation and diagnostic delay in bullous pemphigoid: a prospective nationwide cohort. *Br J Dermatol.* (2012) 167:1111–7. doi: 10.1111/j.1365-2133.2012.11108.x
108. Clapé A, Muller C, Gatouillat G, Le Jan S, Barbe C, Pham B-N, et al. Mucosal involvement in bullous pemphigoid is mostly associated with disease severity and to absence of anti-BP230 autoantibody. *Front Immunol.* (2018) 9:479. doi: 10.3389/fimmu.2018.00479
109. Giudice GJ, Emery DJ, Diaz LA. Cloning and primary structural analysis of the bullous pemphigoid autoantigen BP180. *J Invest Dermatol.* (1992) 99:243–50.
110. Masunaga T, Shimizu H, Yee C, Borradori L, Lazarova Z, Nishikawa T, et al. The extracellular domain of BPAG2 localizes to anchoring filaments and its carboxyl terminus extends to the lamina densa of normal human epidermal basement membrane. *J Invest Dermatol.* (1997) 109:200–6.
111. Zillikens D, Rose PA, Balding SD, Liu Z, Olague-Marchan M, Diaz LA, et al. Tight clustering of extracellular BP180 epitopes recognized by bullous pemphigoid autoantibodies. *J Invest Dermatol.* (1997) 109:573–9.
112. Schmidt E, Obe K, Bröcker EB, Zillikens D. Serum levels of autoantibodies to BP180 correlate with disease activity in patients with bullous pemphigoid. *Arch Dermatol.* (2000) 136:174–8. doi: 10.1001/archderm.136.2.174
113. Di Zenzo G, Grosso F, Terracina M, Mariotti F, De Pità O, Owaribe K, et al. Characterization of the anti-BP180 autoantibody reactivity profile and epitope mapping in bullous pemphigoid patients. *J Invest Dermatol.* (2004) 122:103–10. doi: 10.1046/j.0022-202X.2003.22126.x
114. Horváth B, Niedermeier A, Podstawa E, Müller R, Hunzelmann N, Kárpáti S, et al. IgA autoantibodies in the pemphigoids and linear IgA bullous dermatosis. *Exp Dermatol.* (2010) 19:648–53. doi: 10.1111/j.1600-0625.2010.01080.x
115. Kromminga A, Scheckenbach C, Georgi M, Hagel C, Arndt R, Christophers E, et al. Patients with bullous pemphigoid and linear IgA disease show a dual IgA and IgG autoimmune response to BP180. *J Autoimmun.* (2000) 15:293–300. doi: 10.1006/jaut.2000.0437
116. van Beek N, Schulze FS, Zillikens D, Schmidt E. IgE-mediated mechanisms in bullous pemphigoid and other autoimmune bullous diseases. *Expert Rev Clin Immunol.* (2016) 12:267–77. doi: 10.1586/1744666X.2016.1123092
117. Skaria M, Jaunin F, Hunziker T, Riou S, Schumann H, Bruckner-Tuderman L, et al. IgG autoantibodies from bullous pemphigoid patients recognize multiple antigenic reactive sites located predominantly within the B and C subdomains of the COOH-terminus of BP230. *J Invest Dermatol.* (2000) 114:998–1004. doi: 10.1046/j.1523-1747.2000.00893.x
118. Hamada T, Nagata Y, Tomita M, Salmhofer W, Hashimoto T. Bullous pemphigoid sera react specifically with various domains of BP230, most frequently with C-terminal domain, by immunoblot analyses using bacterial recombinant proteins covering the entire molecule. *Exp Dermatol.* (2001) 10:256–63. doi: 10.1034/j.1600-0625.2001.100405.x
119. Hayakawa T, Teye K, Hachiya T, Uehara R, Hashiguchi M, Kawakami T, et al. Clinical and immunological profiles of anti-BP230-type bullous pemphigoid: restriction of epitopes to the C-terminal domain of BP230, shown by novel ELISAs of BP230-domain specific recombinant proteins. *Eur J Dermatol.* 26:155–63. doi: 10.1684/ejd.2015.2719
120. Daneshpazhooh M, Ghiasi M, Lajevardi V, Nasiri N, Balighi K, Teimourpour A, et al. BPDAI and ABSIS correlate with serum anti-BP180 NC16A IgG but not with anti-BP230 IgG in patients with bullous pemphigoid. *Arch Dermatol Res.* (2018) 310:255–9. doi: 10.1007/s00403-018-1817-9
121. Intong LRA, Murrell DF. Pemphigoid gestationis: pathogenesis and clinical features. *Dermatol Clin.* (2011) 29:447–52. doi: 10.1016/j.det.2011.03.002
122. Huilaja L, Mäkikallio K, Tasanen K. Gestational pemphigoid. *Orphanet J Rare Dis.* (2014) 9:136. doi: 10.1186/s13023-014-0136-2
123. Sadik CD, Pas HH, Bohlmann MK, Mousavi S, Benoit S, Sárdy M, et al. Value of BIOCHIP technology in the serological diagnosis of pemphigoid gestationis. *Acta Derm Venereol.* (2017) 97:128–30. doi: 10.2340/00015555-2460
124. Chimanovitch I, Schmidt E, Messer G, Döpp R, Partscht K, Bröcker EB, et al. IgG1 and IgG3 are the major immunoglobulin subclasses targeting epitopes within the NC16A domain of BP180 in pemphigoid gestationis. *J Invest Dermatol.* (1999) 113:140–2. doi: 10.1046/j.1523-1747.1999.00622.x
125. Chan LS, Ahmed AR, Anhalt GJ, Bernauer W, Cooper KD, Elder MJ, et al. The first international consensus on mucous membrane pemphigoid: definition, diagnostic criteria, pathogenic factors, medical treatment, and prognostic indicators. *Arch Dermatol.* (2002) 138:370–9. doi: 10.1001/archderm.138.3.370
126. Holtsche MM, Zillikens D, Schmidt E. Mucous membrane pemphigoid. *Hautarzt Z Dermatol Venerol Verwandte Geb.* (2018) 69:67–83. doi: 10.1007/s00105-017-4089-y
127. Witte M, Zillikens D, Shimanovich I. Intravenous immunoglobulins for rituximab-resistant mucous membrane pemphigoid. *J Eur Acad Dermatol Venereol.* (2018) 32:e321–4. doi: 10.1111/jdv.14873
128. Schmidt E, Skrobek C, Kromminga A, Hashimoto T, Messer G, Bröcker EB, et al. Cicatricial pemphigoid: IgA and IgG autoantibodies target epitopes on both intra- and extracellular domains of bullous pemphigoid antigen 180. *Br J Dermatol.* (2001) 145:778–83. doi: 10.1046/j.1365-2133.2001.04471.x
129. Oyama N, Setterfield JF, Powell AM, Sakuma-Oyama Y, Albert S, Bhogal BS, et al. Bullous pemphigoid antigen II (BP180) and its soluble extracellular domains are major autoantigens in mucous membrane pemphigoid: the pathogenic relevance to HLA class II alleles and disease severity. *Br J Dermatol.* (2006) 154:90–8. doi: 10.1111/j.1365-2133.2005.06998.x
130. Domloge-Hultsch N, Gammon WR, Briggaman RA, Gil SG, Carter WG, Yancey KB. Epiligrin, the major human keratinocyte integrin ligand, is a target in both an acquired autoimmune and an inherited

subepidermal blistering skin disease. *J Clin Invest.* (1992) 90:1628–33. doi: 10.1172/JCI116033

131. Kirtschig G, Marinkovich MP, Burgeson RE, Yancey KB. Anti-basement membrane autoantibodies in patients with anti-epiligrin cicatricial pemphigoid bind the alpha subunit of laminin 5. *J Invest Dermatol.* (1995) 105:543–8.
132. Egan CA, Lazarova Z, Darling TN, Yee C, Coté T, Yancey KB. Anti-epiligrin cicatricial pemphigoid and relative risk for cancer. *Lancet Lond Engl.* (2001) 357:1850–1. doi: 10.1016/S0140-6736(00)04971-0
133. Leverkus M, Schmidt E, Lazarova Z, Bröcker EB, Yancey KB, Zillikens D. Antiepiligrin cicatricial pemphigoid: an underdiagnosed entity within the spectrum of scarring autoimmune subepidermal bullous diseases? *Arch Dermatol.* (1999) 135:1091–8.
134. Rashid KA, Gürcan HM, Ahmed AR. Antigen specificity in subsets of mucous membrane pemphigoid. *J Invest Dermatol.* (2006) 126:2631–6. doi: 10.1038/sj.jid.5700465
135. Kasperkiewicz M, Meier M, Zillikens D, Schmidt E. Linear IgA disease: successful application of immunoadsorption and review of the literature. *Dermatology* (2010) 220:259–63. doi: 10.1159/000279318
136. Mintz EM, Morel KD. Clinical features, diagnosis, and pathogenesis of chronic bullous disease of childhood. *Dermatol Clin.* (2011) 29:459–62. doi: 10.1016/j.det.2011.03.022
137. Wojnarowska F, Whitehead P, Leigh IM, Bhogal BS, Black MM. Identification of the target antigen in chronic bullous disease of childhood and linear IgA disease of adults. *Br J Dermatol.* (1991) 124:157–62.
138. Marinkovich MP, Taylor TB, Keene DR, Burgeson RE, Zone JJ. LAD-1, the linear IgA bullous dermatosis autoantigen, is a novel 120-kDa anchoring filament protein synthesized by epidermal cells. *J Invest Dermatol.* (1996) 106:734–8.
139. Zone JJ, Taylor TB, Meyer LJ, Petersen MJ. The 97 kDa linear IgA bullous disease antigen is identical to a portion of the extracellular domain of the 180 kDa bullous pemphigoid antigen, BPAg2. *J Invest Dermatol.* (1998) 110:207–10. doi: 10.1046/j.1523-1747.1998.00129.x
140. Willsteed E, Bhogal BS, Black MM, McKee P, Wojnarowska F. Use of 1M NaCl split skin in the indirect immunofluorescence of the linear IgA bullous dermatoses. *J Cutan Pathol.* (1990) 17:144–8.
141. Zillikens D, Herzele K, Georgi M, Schmidt E, Chimanovitch I, Schumann H, et al. Autoantibodies in a subgroup of patients with linear IgA disease react with the NC16A domain of BP1801. *J Invest Dermatol.* (1999) 113:947–53. doi: 10.1046/j.1523-1747.1999.00808.x
142. Tsuchisaka A, Ohara K, Ishii N, Nguyen NT, Marinkovich MP, Hashimoto T. Type VII collagen is the major autoantigen for sublamina densa-type linear IgA bullous dermatosis. *J Invest Dermatol.* (2015) 135:626–9. doi: 10.1038/jid.2014.381
143. Yamagami J, Nakamura Y, Nagao K, Funakoshi T, Takahashi H, Tanikawa A, et al. Vancomycin mediates IgA autoreactivity in drug-induced linear iga bullous dermatosis. *J Invest Dermatol.* (2018) 138:1473–80. doi: 10.1016/j.jid.2017.12.035
144. Prost-Squarcioni C, Caux F, Schmidt E, Jonkman MF, Vassileva S, Kim SC, et al. International bullous diseases group: consensus on diagnostic criteria for epidermolysis bullosa acquisita. *Br J Dermatol.* (2017) 179:30–41. doi: 10.1111/bjd.16138
145. Zillikens D, Kawahara Y, Ishiko A, Shimizu H, Mayer J, Rank CV, et al. A novel subepidermal blistering disease with autoantibodies to a 200-kDa antigen of the basement membrane zone. *J Invest Dermatol.* (1996) 106:1333–8.
146. Goletz S, Hashimoto T, Zillikens D, Schmidt E. Anti-p200 pemphigoid. *J Am Acad Dermatol.* (2014) 71:185–91. doi: 10.1016/j.jaad.2014.02.036
147. Dainichi T, Koga H, Tsuji T, Ishii N, Ohyama B, Ueda A, et al. From anti-p200 pemphigoid to anti-laminin gamma1 pemphigoid. *J Dermatol.* (2010) 37:231–8. doi: 10.1111/j.1346-8138.2009.00793.x
148. Woodley DT, Briggaman RA, O'Keefe EJ, Inman AO, Queen LL, Gammon WR. Identification of the skin basement-membrane autoantigen in epidermolysis bullosa acquisita. *N Engl J Med.* (1984) 310:1007–13. doi: 10.1056/NEJM198404193101602
149. Vorobyev A, Ludwig RJ, Schmidt E. Clinical features and diagnosis of epidermolysis bullosa acquisita. *Expert Rev Clin Immunol.* (2017) 13:157–69. doi: 10.1080/1744666X.2016.1221343
150. Ludwig RJ. Clinical presentation, pathogenesis, diagnosis, and treatment of epidermolysis bullosa acquisita. *ISRN Dermatol.* (2013) 2013:812029. doi: 10.1155/2013/812029
151. Roenigk HH, Ryan JG, Bergfeld WF. Epidermolysis bullosa acquisita. Report of three cases and review of all published cases. *Arch Dermatol.* (1971) 103:1–10.
152. Buijsrogge JJA, Diercks GFH, Pas HH, Jonkman MF. The many faces of epidermolysis bullosa acquisita after serration pattern analysis by direct immunofluorescence microscopy. *Br J Dermatol.* (2011) 165:92–8. doi: 10.1111/j.1365-2133.2011.10346.x
153. Lapiere JC, Woodley DT, Parente MG, Iwasaki T, Wynn KC, Christiano AM, et al. Epitope mapping of type VII collagen. Identification of discrete peptide sequences recognized by sera from patients with acquired epidermolysis bullosa. *J Clin Invest.* (1993) 92:1831–9. doi: 10.1172/JCI116774
154. Ishii N, Yoshida M, Hisamatsu Y, Ishida-Yamamoto A, Nakane H, Iizuka H, et al. Epidermolysis bullosa acquisita sera react with distinct epitopes on the NC1 and NC2 domains of type VII collagen: study using immunoblotting of domain-specific recombinant proteins and postembedding immunoelectron microscopy. *Br J Dermatol.* (2004) 150:843–51. doi: 10.1111/j.1365-2133.2004.05933.x
155. Kim JH, Kim YH, Kim S, Noh EB, Kim S-E, Vorobyev A, et al. Serum levels of anti-type VII collagen antibodies detected by enzyme-linked immunosorbent assay in patients with epidermolysis bullosa acquisita are correlated with the severity of skin lesions. *J Eur Acad Dermatol Venereol.* (2013) 27:e224–30. doi: 10.1111/j.1468-3083.2012.04617.x
156. Cox NH, Bearn MA, Herold J, Ainsworth G, Liu C. Blindness due to the IgA variant of epidermolysis bullosa acquisita, and treatment with osteo-odonto-keratoprosthesis. *Br J Dermatol.* (2007) 156:775–7. doi: 10.1111/j.1365-2133.2006.07739.x
157. Vodegel RM, de Jong MCJM, Pas HH, Jonkman MF. IgA-mediated epidermolysis bullosa acquisita: two cases and review of the literature. *J Am Acad Dermatol.* (2002) 47:919–25. doi: 10.1067/mjd.2002.125079
158. Bonciolini V, Bonciani D, Verdelli A, D'Errico A, Antiga E, Fabbri P, et al. Newly described clinical and immunopathological feature of dermatitis herpetiformis. *Clin Dev Immunol.* (2012) 2012:967974. doi: 10.1155/2012/967974
159. Bolotin D, Petronic-Rosic V. Dermatitis herpetiformis. Part I. epidemiology, pathogenesis, and clinical presentation. *J Am Acad Dermatol.* (2011) 64:1017–24. doi: 10.1016/j.jaad.2010.09.777
160. Bolotin D, Petronic-Rosic V. Dermatitis herpetiformis. Part II. diagnosis, management, and prognosis. *J Am Acad Dermatol.* (2011) 64:1027–33. doi: 10.1016/j.jaad.2010.09.776
161. Sárdy M, Kárpáti S, Merkl B, Paulsson M, Smyth N. Epidermal transglutaminase (TGase 3) is the autoantigen of dermatitis herpetiformis. *J Exp Med.* (2002) 195:747–757. doi: 10.1084/jem.20011299
162. Rose C, Armbruster FP, Ruppert J, Igl B-W, Zillikens D, Shimanovich I. Autoantibodies against epidermal transglutaminase are a sensitive diagnostic marker in patients with dermatitis herpetiformis on a normal or gluten-free diet. *J Am Acad Dermatol.* (2009) 61:39–43. doi: 10.1016/j.jaad.2008.12.037

4

Role of Src and Cortactin in Pemphigus Skin Blistering

Daniela Kugelmann[1], Vera Rötzer[1], Elias Walter[1], Desalegn Tadesse Egu[1], Michael Tobias Fuchs[1], Franziska Vielmuth[1], Hilda Vargas-Robles[2], Michael Schnoor[2], Michael Hertl[3], Rüdiger Eming[3], Klemens Rottner[4,5], Ansgar Schmidt[6], Volker Spindler[1,7] and Jens Waschke[1]*

[1] Chair of Vegetative Anatomy, Institute of Anatomy, Medical Faculty, Ludwig-Maximilians-Universität München, Munich, Germany, [2] Department of Molecular Biomedicine, Cinvestav-IPN, Mexico City, Mexico, [3] Department of Dermatology and Allergology, Philipps-Universität Marburg, Marburg, Germany, [4] Division of Molecular Cell Biology, Zoological Institute, Technische Universität Braunschweig, Braunschweig, Germany, [5] Department of Cell Biology, Helmholtz Centre for Infection Research, Braunschweig, Germany, [6] Instiute of Pathology, Philipps-Universität Marburg, Marburg, Germany, [7] Department of Biomedicine, University of Basel, Basel, Switzerland

***Correspondence:**
Jens Waschke
jens.waschke@med.uni-muenchen.de

Autoantibodies against desmoglein (Dsg) 1 and Dsg3 primarily cause blister formation in the autoimmune disease pemphigus vulgaris (PV). Src was proposed to contribute to loss of keratinocyte cohesion. However, the role and underlying mechanisms are unclear and were studied here. In keratinocytes, cell cohesion in response to autoantibodies was reduced in Src-dependent manner by two patient-derived PV-IgG fractions as well as by AK23 but not by a third PV-IgG fraction, although Src was activated by all autoantibodies. Loss of cell cohesion was progredient in a timeframe of 24 h and AK23, similar to PV-IgG, interfered with reconstitution of cell cohesion after Ca^{2+}-switch, indicating that the autoantibodies also interfered with desmosome assembly. Dsg3 co-localized along cell contacts and interacted with the Src substrate cortactin. In keratinocytes isolated from cortactin-deficient mice, cell adhesion was impaired and Src-mediated inhibition of AK23-induced loss of cell cohesion for 24 h was significantly reduced compared to wild-type (wt) cells. Similarly, AK23 impaired reconstitution of cell adhesion was Src-dependent only in the presence of cortactin. Likewise, Src inhibition significantly reduced AK23-induced skin blistering in wt but not cortactin-deficient mice. These data suggest that the Src-mediated long-term effects of AK23 on loss of cell cohesion and skin blistering are dependent on cortactin-mediated desmosome assembly. However, in human epidermis PV-IgG-induced skin blistering and ultrastructural alterations of desmosomes were not affected by Src inhibition, indicating that Src may not be critical for skin blistering in intact human skin, at least when high levels of autoantibodies targeting Dsg1 are present.

Keywords: src, cortactin, adhesion, skin blistering diseases, pemphigus vulgaris (PV)

INTRODUCTION

Pemphigus vulgaris (PV) is a severe autoimmune skin blistering disease. Patients suffer from mucocutaneous erosions and blisters caused by autoantibody-induced acantholysis (1, 2). It is accepted that loss of keratinocyte cohesion is primarily caused by autoantibodies directed against the desmosomal cadherins desmoglein 3 (Dsg3) and Dsg1 (3). Autoantibodies were proposed to directly interfere with trans-interaction of Dsg3 and to require cellular signaling mechanisms to induce loss of cell adhesion (2). Pemphigus autoantibodies modulate the activity of signaling pathways such as Ca^{2+} -influx, protein kinase C (PKC), p38 mitogen-activated protein kinase (p38MAPK) and sarcoma-associated kinase (Src), and interfere with the turnover of desmosomal components (2). It was shown that Src can be activated by PV-IgG containing antibodies against Dsg3 as well as by AK23, which constitutes a Dsg3-specific monoclonal autoantibody from a pemphigus mouse model (4, 5). However, the role of Src in the loss of keratinocyte cohesion and the underlying mechanisms are not fully understood. Src is a signal-transducing non-receptor protein kinase which is involved in several signaling pathways (6). It is enriched in various cancer diseases and plays an important role in metastasis, cell migration and motility as well as cell survival and proliferation (6–9). Furthermore, Src is located at adherens junctions in various cell types (10), and the inhibition of Src-kinase activity is proposed to stabilize cadherin dependent cell-cell contacts (11). In previous studies we showed that PV-IgG-mediated loss of keratinocyte cohesion can be abrogated by Src inhibition (4), and that the activity of Src in combination with E-cadherin is necessary for the cytoskeletal anchorage of Dsg3 (12). Moreover, Dsg3 forms a complex with Src and regulates its activity (12, 13). All these findings led to the hypothesis that Dsg3 organizes cell contacts coordinating cell adhesion with signaling responses required for cellular behavior (14). Thus, we speculated that Src could be a key regulator of desmosomal adhesion in PV pathogenesis. In this context, it was demonstrated that autoantibodies from pemphigus patients caused Src-dependent phosphorylation of Pkp3 paralleled by Dsg3 translocation to the cytoplasm and destabilization of cell adhesion (15). Since we observed that Src is required for desmosome assembly, which is regulated by actin-binding proteins such as adducin (12, 16), we focused on the actin binding protein cortactin, which was identified as a major substrate for Src (17). Among many other functions, phosphorylation of cortactin is crucial for cadherin-mediated intercellular adhesion strength (18). In the work presented here, we show for the first time that cortactin regulates reconstitution of cell adhesion in pemphigus and provide new insights into the role and function of Src in PV.

MATERIALS AND METHODS

Cell Culture

The immortalized human keratinocyte cell line HaCaT was cultured in Dulbecco's Modified Eagle Medium (DMEM) (Life Technologies, Carlsbad, CA) supplemented with 10% FCS (Biochrom, Berlin, Germany), 50 U/ml penicillin and 50 g/ml streptomycin (both AppliChem, Darmstadt, Germany) in a humidified atmosphere of 5% CO_2 at 37°C.

Preparation of Mouse Keratinocytes

Murine keratinocytes from the epidermis of newborn cortactin-deficient ($CTTN^{-/-}$) and cortactin wildtype ($CTTN^{+/+}$) mice were isolated and immortalized according to the literature for preparation of mouse keratinocytes (19–21). In brief, the skin was taken and incubated for 16 h in 2.4 U/ml dispase II in PBS supplemented with Gentamicin/AmphotericinB (CELLnTEC, Bern, Switzerland) at 4°C. After separating the dermis and epidermis, the epidermis was incubated for 20 min with accutase (CELLnTEC) at room temperature, in order to dissociate the cells. Mouse keratinocytes were resuspended and then grown in complete FAD medium (0.05 mM CaCl) on collagen I-coated culture dishes (rat tail; BD Bioscience, New Jersey, USA). The cells were cultivated in a humidified atmosphere containing 5% CO_2 at 35°C. After reaching confluence, cells were switched to 1.2 mM Ca^{2+} and used for experiments after 48 h.

TABLE 1 | Antibody profiles of pemphigus vulgaris patients' IgG fractions as determined by ELISA for Dsg1 or Dsg3, respectively, and clinical phenotype.

ELISA	Dsg1 (U/ml)	Dsg3 (U/ml)	
PV1-IgG	375	11.55	Mucocutaneous PV
PV2-IgG	212.27	181.44	Mucocutaneous PV
PV3-IgG	101.18	106.72	Mucocutaneous PV
PV4-IgG	5542	711	Mucocutaneous PV

Test Reagents, Antibodies, and Purification of PV-IgG Fractions

The Src-inhibitor PP2 (Calbiochem, Darmstadt, Germany) was used at 10 μM for the respective time periods. For short time-incubations PP2 was preincubated for 2 h. The following commercial primary antibodies were used: anti- cortactin (clone 4F-11; Milipore), anti-phospho-cortactin tyr421 (Milipore), anti-alpha-tubulin (Abcam), anti-desmoplakin (DP) (Abcam), anti-desmoglein 3 (Dsg3) (Clone H154, Santa Cruz), anti-Src (Clone 32G6, Cell Signaling), anti-phospho-Src Tyr 416 (Cell Signaling), anti-plakophilin 3 (Pkp3) (Progen), anti-phospho-plakophilin Tyr 195 (kindly provided by Ansgar Schmidt, Marburg, Germany). Filamentous actin (F-actin) was visualized using an Alexa Fluor™ 488 phalloidin dye (Life Technologies). The corresponding secondary antibodies for immunofluorescence analysis were purchased from Dianova (Hamburg). AK23, a monoclonal pathogenic antibody, derived from a pemphigus mouse model, was purchased from Biozol (Eching, Germany) and used at 75 μg/ml. PV-IgG (all including autoantibodies against both Dsg1 and Dsg3) and IgG fractions pooled from three healthy donors (c-IgG) were purified as described previously (22). The autoantibody profiles were determined using enzyme-linked immunosorbent assay (ELISA), (Euroimmun, Luebeck, Germany). ELISA scores of antibodies against Dsg1 and Dsg3 were determinded before purification (cut-off value: 20 U/ml). The scores are shown in **Table 1**. All patients had mucocutaneous involvement. Patients and donors gave written consent for research use. A positive vote of the Ethics Committee from the Medical Faculty of the University of Marburg was given.

Western Blotting

Cells were washed with PBS, lysed with SDS-lysis buffer (25 mmol/l HEPES, 25 mmol/l NaF and 1% SDS, pH 7.4) and sonicated on ice. Protein amounts were determined using the Pierce^{TM} BCA Protein Assay Kit (Thermo Fisher, USA). Cell lysates were mixed with laemmli buffer containing 50 mM dithiothreitol. Electrophoresis and western blotting were performed according to standard procedures. Membranes were incubated at 4°C overnight with respective primary autoantibody in tris-buffered-saline containing 0.05% tween (TBS-T), and supplemented with 5% bovine serum albumin (BSA).

Triton X-100 Protein Fractionation

Cells were washed with ice-cold PBS and incubated in Triton buffer (0.5% Triton X-100, 50 mM MES, 25 mM EGTA, 5 mM $MgCl_2$) supplemented with 1 mM PMSF (Roth, Germany), Aprotinin, Pepstatin A (both Applichem, Germany), and Leupeptin (VWR, Germany) for 20 min on ice under continuous shaking. Thereafter, cell lysates were centrifuged at 13.000 rpm for 5 min, which leads to separation of the soluble cytosolic and insoluble cytoskeleton bound fraction. Subsequently, the pellets (insoluble fractions) were resuspended in SDS lysis buffer for Western blotting or with RIPA buffer (0.05 M Tris-HCl, 0.15 M NaCl, 0.1% SDS, 1% Nonidet P-40, 0.1 mM EDTA) for immunoprecipitation and followed by sonification. Protein concentrations were calculated as described above and equivalent amounts used for Western blotting or immunoprecipitation analyses.

Immunoprecipitation

Following Triton X-100 mediated solubilization, cell lysates (protein amount of 1,000 μg) were precleared with 25 μl Protein A/G Agarose Beads (Santa Cruz Biotechnology, Santa Cruz, CA, USA) for 1 h at 4°C, thereafter centrifuged at 10,300 rpm for 5 min at 4°C. The supernatant (IP-lysat) was incubated with 1 μg of anti-Dsg3 antibody (Santa Cruz) or IgG control, for 3 h at 4°C with gentle rotation. The lysate was then added to 40 μl of beads and incubated overnight at 4°C under rotation. IP lysates were washed with RIPA buffer and subjected to Western blot analyses.

In situ Proximity Ligation (PLA) Assay

Spatial proximities of Dsg3 and cortactin were investigated using the Duolink *in situ* kit (Olink, Bioscience) as described previously (23).

Histology and Immunostaining

Samples were embedded in Tissue Tec (Leica Biosystems, Nussloch, Germany) and thereafter serial-sectioned at 7 μm thickness using a cryostat microtome (Cyrosstar NX70, Thermo Fisher). Hematoxylin and esoin (H.E.) staining was performed according to standard protocols (24), and mounted in DEPX (Sigma-Aldrich, St. Louis, MO, U.S.A). Images were captured using a Leica DMi8 microscope with a HC PL APO 40x/0.85 dry objective. For immunostaining, cells were seeded on coverslips and grown to confluence. After respective treatment, cell monolayers were washed with PBS and fixed with 2% paraformaldehyde in PBS for 10 min (HaCaT) or fixed with 4% paraformaldehyde in PBS for 20 min ($CTTN^{-/-}$ and $CTTN^{+/+}$ keratinocytes). Next, samples were rinsed several times with PBS, permeabilized with 0,1% Triton X-100 for 5 min and after final washing with PBS, blocked with 3% bovine serum albumin and 1% normal goat serum for 60 min. The primary antibodies were incubated overnight at 4°C. After washing with PBS, respective secondary antibodies were applied for 60 min at room temperature. Subsequently, coverslips were washed and mounted with 1.5% n-propyl gallate in glycerol. Images were taken with a Leica SP5 confocal microscope using a 63x/1.40 PL APO oil objective (Leica, Mannheim, Germany).

Ca^{2+} Switch Assay

Cells were grown to confluence and, after respective treatment, incubated with 2.5 mM EGTA for 30 min (Ca^{2+}-depletion), which leads to a Ca^{2+}-dependent disruption of cell-cell junctions. Reformation of junctions was induced by medium change with corresponding growth medium containing 1.8 mM Ca^{2+} for 8 h (Ca^{2+} repletion).

Dispase-Based Dissociation Assay

After incubation with test reagents, confluent cell monolayers were washed with Hank's buffered saline solution (HBSS; Sigma Aldrich) and subjected to 2.4 U/ml dispase II (Sigma- Aldrich) in HBSS for 20 min at 37°C and 5% CO_2. After detachment of the monolayer the reaction was stopped by replacing the dispase II solution with HBSS. Defined shear stress was applied with an electrical pipette. Resulting fragments were counted using a binocular microscope (Leica, Mannheim, Germany). All independent experiments were performed in duplicates.

Neonatal Mouse Model

The model was used as described before (25). Newborn cortactin-deficient ($CTTN^{-/-}$) and cortactin wt ($CTTN^{+/+}$) mice were injected intra-dermally into the back skin with a total volume of 50 μl containing 2 mg/ml AK23 without or in combination with 10 μM PP2. The area injected was marked. Twenty hours after incubation the injection site was exposed to defined mechanical stress. Skin was explanted, embedded into cryo freezing medium (Leica, Mannheim, Germany), frozen on dry ice, followed by preparation for cryo-cutting. The experimental protocol was approved by the institutional animal care and use committee of Cinvestav (IACUC), Mexico-City.

Ex vivo Human Skin Model

Biopsies of healthy human skin were acquired from cadavers from the human body donor program from the institute of Anatomy and Cell Biology, Ludwig-Maximilians-Universität München, Germany. Written informed consent was given from body donors for the use of research samples. Biopsies were taken only if death occurred <24 h before arrival at the institute. From each body donor, a skin piece of approximately 5 × 5 cm size was removed from the shoulder, gently stripped off fat including excessive connective tissue. The skin was cut into 1 cm^2 pieces and injected intra-dermally with 50 μl of the respective IgG-fraction (PV-IgG and c-IgG) with or without PP2 (10 μM), using a 30G syringe. Samples were incubated floating on DMEM at 37°C and 5% CO_2 for 24 h. After incubation sheer stress was applied using a rubber head with equal frequency and magnitude. Treated samples were cut into two parts and processed for hematoxylin and eosin (HE) stainings and electron microscopy analyses. Blister score of the human samples was measured as described below.

Scoring of Blister Size

Each section was evaluated and sorted into the following score system as published previously (23): absence of intraepidermal separation, score 0; cleft size covering 1–25% of total section length, score 1; cleft size between 26 and 50% of section length, score 2; cleft size between 51 and 75% section length, score 3; cleft size between 76 and 100%, score 4.

Electron Microscopy

The injected and incubated human skin explants were cut into small pieces of approximately 2 mm in diameter and fixed with 2–5% glutaraldehyde (Sigma Aldrich). After washing in PBS, tissue samples were post-fixed with 2% osmium tetroxide (Merk Millipore), and dehydrated through a graded ethanol series followed by clearance in propylene oxide, embedding into EPON 812 (Serva Eletrophoresis GmbH, Heidelberg, Germany) and curing at 80°C for 24 h. Resulting blocks were trimmed and sectioned at 60 nm thick slices with a Reichert-Jung Ultracut E ultra-microtome using a diamond knife (DiATOME Electron Microscopy Sciences, Hatfield, PA, USA). Silver-appearing sections were placed onto a 150 mesh copper/rhodium grid (Plano GmbH, Wetzlar, Germany). Sections were then contrasted with alcoholic uranyl-acetate and lead citrate. For imaging a Libra 120 transmission electron microscope (Carl Zeiss NTS GmbH, Oberkochen, Germany) equipped with a SSCCD camera system (TRS, Olympus, Tokyo, Japan) was used.

Statistical Analysis

Data were analyzed in Exel (Microsoft, Redmond, WA) and compared using one-way ANOVA followed by Bonferroni *post-hoc* test (for Gaussian-distributed samples) using Graphpad Prism (Graphpad Software, LaJolla, CA). Error bars represent SEM. Significance was assumed with $p \leq 0.05$. Data are shown as mean ± SEM. Each n represent one independent experiment.

RESULTS

Role of Src for Autoantibody-Induced Loss of Keratinocyte Cohesion

To investigate the role of Src for loss of cell adhesion in pemphigus, human keratinocytes (HaCaT) were incubated with PV-IgG in combination with the Src family kinase inhibitor PP2 and intercellular cohesion was measured by dispase-based dissociation assay (26). Incubation with PV-IgG from pemphigus vulgaris patient 1 (PV1-IgG) significantly increased the number of fragments in comparison to incubation with control IgG (c-IgG) for all time periods (15 min, 60 min and 24 h). Src inhibition using PP2 abrogated loss of intercellular adhesion after incubation with PV1-IgG for 15 and 60 min. In contrast, after 24 h incubation of PP2 together with PV1, no protective effect was observed (**Figure 1A**). After incubation of PV1-IgG for 15, 30 and 120 min, Western blot analysis showed a phosphorylation of Src at Tyr 416, which is one of the major phosphorylation sites and leads to autophosphorylation (9). In contrast, no activation of Src was detectable after 24 h of incubation, indicating that inhibiton of Src was only protective at time points when Src was activated (**Figure 1B**). To get more insights into the importance of Src in PV, two more IgG fractions from different pemphigus patients (PV2-IgG and PV3-IgG) as well as a monoclonal autoantibody against Dsg3 from a pemphigus mouse model (AK23) (27), were included for respective time points. In dissociation assays, PV2- and PV3-IgG as well as AK23 caused keratinocyte monolayer fragmentation after 15 min (**Figure 1C**), 1 h (**Figure 1D**), 2 h (**Figure 1E**), and 24 h (**Figure 1F**) compared to incubation with c-IgG. PV3-IgG and AK23-induced loss of cell cohesion was significantly reduced by PP2 at all time-points whereas inhibition of Src was not effective to modulate loss of adhesion caused by PV2-IgG (**Figures 1C–F**). Western blot analysis showed that all autoantibody fractions were effective to activate Src (**Figure 1G**).

Cadherin-based adhesion is Ca^{2+}-dependent. *In vitro*, the assembly of intercellular junctions in keratinocytes can be induced by a switch from low to high Ca^{2+} medium (28, 29). Vice versa, reduction of the extracellular Ca^{2+} concentration leads to translocation of cadherins from cell-cell borders to the cytosol, followed by disassembly of adherens junctions and desmosomes (28, 30). Since inhibition of Src was protective for adhesion of kerationcytes after treatment with AK23 and PV3-IgG, we investigated the role of Src for desmosomal reassembly. Ca^{2+}-depleted HaCaTs were re-exposed to Ca^{2+} for 8 h in combination with c-IgG, AK23, and PV3-IgG with or without PP2 and then subjected to a dispase-based dissociation assay. Ca^{2+} repletion in combination with autoantibodies did not restore cell adhesion indicating that autoantibodies interfered with desmosome re-assembly, which likely contributes to loss of cell cohesion when autoantibodies are applied for longer periods such as shown in **Figure 1**. However, PP2 reduced this negative effect of both AK23 and PV3-IgG on reconstitution of cell cohesion (**Figure 2A**).

The Src Target Cortactin Colocalizes and Interacts With Dsg3

The actin binding protein cortactin was identified as a major substrate of Src (17), and is proposed to be activated by Src-mediated tyrosine phosphorylation (31). Therefore, we were interested if cortactin plays a role in Src-mediated effects on desmosomal adhesion. First, we investigated the correlation of cortactin and Dsg3 in desmosomal assembly by immunofluorescence analysis under Ca^{2+} switch conditions. Under control conditions, both proteins are located at cell borders and cortactin was phosphorylated on the Src-dependent phosphorylation site Tyr 421. Depletion of Ca^{2+} resulted in Dsg3 dissociation form the cell borders, accompanied by disruption of cortactin and phospho-cortactin immunostaining. Re-administration of Ca^{2+} led to restored Dsg3, cortactin, and phospho-cortactin staining at cell-cell borders (**Figure 2B**). Moreover, immunostaining showed that cortactin and Dsg3 partially co-localized at the cell membrane (**Figure 2C**) which was validated by a proximity ligation assay (PLA), also revealing a close association with the cortical actin cytoskeleton (**Figure 2D**, upper images) at the cell periphery

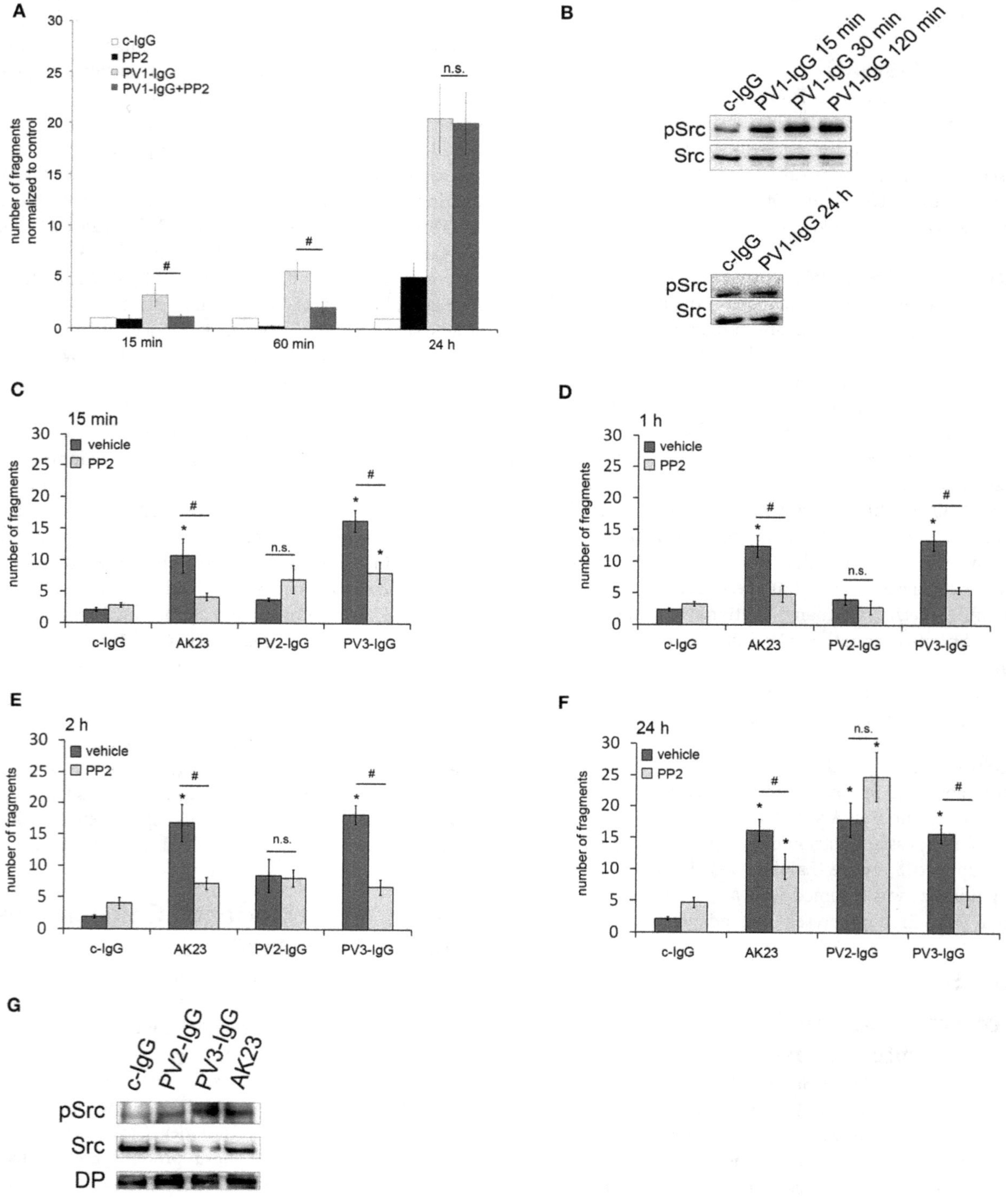

FIGURE 1 | Protective effect of Src inhibition against autoantibody-induced loss of cell cohesion is variable. **(A)** HaCaT cells were incubated with PV1-IgG or with control IgG (c-IgG) and subjected to dispase-based dissociation assays. Inhibition of Src by PP2 prevented fragmentation of cell monolayers after incubation with PV1 for 15 min and 60 min but not for 24 h ($n = 5$; $\#p < 0.05$; $^{*}p < 0.05$ vs. c-IgG). **(B)** Western blot analysis revealed that Src was phosphorylated after 15, 30, and 120 min but not after 24 h of incubation with PV1 ($n = 3$). **(C–F)** PV2- and PV3-IgG as well as AK23 were applied for several time points: 15 min **(C)**, 1 h **(D)**, 2 h **(E)**, and 24 h **(F)**, with keratinocytes being subsequently subjected to dissociation assays. Co-incubation with PP2 led to significantly reduced fragment numbers in PV3-IgG- and AK23- but not PV2-IgG-treated cells ($n > 7$; $\#p < 0.05$; $^{*}p < 0.05$ vs. c-IgG). **(G)** Corresponding Western blot analysis for 2 h revealed that all autoantibody fractions were effective to activate Src ($n = 3$).

(**Figure 2D**, XZ presentation). Next, immunoprecipitation analysis verified that cortactin co-precipitated with Dsg3 in the triton-soluble protein pool but not in the triton-insoluble fraction (**Figure 2E**). This implied that cortactin may play a role in Src-mediated regulation of desmosome assembly. In contrast, phosphorylation of Pkp3 after incubation with AK23 was not detectable (**Supplemental Figure 1**).

Cortactin Is Important for Src-Mediated Reconstitution of Cell Cohesion *in vitro* and in a Pemphigus Mouse Model *in vivo*

To study the role of cortactin in more detail, we isolated primary keratinocytes form newborn cortactin wild type (wt) and cortactin-deficient mice (32). Cortactin-deficient ($CTTN^{-/-}$) mouse keratinocyte mono-layers showed significantly more fragments in a dispase-based dissociation assay, indicating that cortactin is required for cell cohesion (**Figure 3A**). The knockout of cortactin was verified by Western blot analysis (**Figure 3B**), which also showed no changes of desmosomal proteins such as desmoplakin (DP) and Dsg3 in $CTTN^{-/-}$ cells. Next, we subjected cells to a dissociation assay after application of PP2 in combination with AK23 for 2 h (**Figure 3C**) or 24 h (**Figure 3D**). In wt mouse keratinocytes, cell adhesion was rescued by Src inhibition when AK23 was applied for 2 h or for 24 h. In contrast, in $CTTN^{-/-}$ cells, PP2 blocked AK23-induced loss of adhesion only when AK23 was incubated for 2 h but not for 24 h. This suggested that short-term effects auf AK23 were Src- but not cortactin-dependent, whereas long-term effects at least in part required both Src and cortactin. To examine the importance of cortactin for restoring of cell adhesion, Ca^{2+}-switch assay was performed under the same conditions (**Figure 3E**). Again, dissociation assay experiments showed that Src inhibition by PP2 was not effective to restore cell cohesion in $CTTN^{-/-}$ cells in presence of AK23, indicating that reconstitution of cell adhesion is both Src- and cortactin-dependent.

To verify these findings *in vivo*, we used the neonatal passive immuno-transfer mouse model as described previously using AK23 (23). Therefore, we injected AK23 alone and in combination with the Src-inhibitor PP2 into the skin of newborn $CTTN^{+/+}$ and $CTTN^{-/-}$ mice. After incubation for 24 h, defined shear stress was applied. H.E. staining of serial sections showed AK23-induced gross blistering at injection sites of both wt and cortactin-deficient pubs (**Figures 4A–C**). However, in wt animals co-incubation with the Src inhibitor abrogated blister formation almost completely whereas in cortactin-deficient mice, blisters were still observed. These results indicate that AK23-induced skin blistering *in vivo* is Src- and cortactin-dependent, at least, in mice.

Inhibition of Src Was Not Protective Against PV-IgG-Induced Blistering in Human Skin *ex vivo*

Finally, to study the role of Src for skin blistering in intact human skin, we used a human *ex vivo* skin model as reported previously using PV-IgG (22, 33). After injection and incubation of human skin with PV4-IgG alone or in combination with the Src inhibitor PP2 for 24 h, HE-stained serial sections revealed blister formation after treatment with PV-IgG alone as well as in combination with PP2 (**Figures 5A,B**). Analysis of the ultrastructure showed no differences after PV-IgG incubation in conjunction with vehicle or PP2 treatment (**Figure 5A**, lower panel, **Figures 5C–E**). Under both experimental conditions, the number of desmosomes (**Figure 5C**) and desmosome length (**Figure 5D**) were reduced in comparison to control conditions and inter-desmosomal widening was observed (**Figure 5E**). This data show that PP2 was in the long term not protective against PV-IgG-induced skin blistering in human skin.

DISCUSSION

The study provides further insights into the role and mechanisms of Src-mediated epidermal blistering in pemphigus. Inhibition of Src was protective against AK23-induced skin blistering in an *in vivo* mouse model but not against PV-IgG-induced skin blistering in human epidermis. Moreover, the role of Src for loss of cell cohesion appeared to be patient-dependent and to negatively correlate at least in part with autoantibody scores against Dsg1. Src-mediated loss of keratinocyte cohesion engaged mechanisms which were both cortactin-dependent and -independent, the former of which were involved in reconstitution of keratinocyte adhesion.

Role of Src in Pemphigus Autoantibody-Induced Skin Blistering

In accordance with the literature, PV-IgG fractions as well as AK23 led to activation of Src (4, 5, 34, 35). In this context, it was shown that PV-IgG induce Src activation early after application of autoantibodies and thus before other signaling molecules such as p38MAPK or EGFR were activated (5). The first question is by which autoantibodies Src signaling is triggered. It was shown that activation of Src was detectable only when PV-IgG fractions contained antibodies against Dsg3 but not when pemphigus foliaceus (PF) autoantibodies against Dsg1 were applied (4). Since AK23, which is specifically directed against Dsg3, was effective to activate Src it can be concluded that Dsg3 is sufficient to modulate Src signaling (4). Nevertheless, experiments using siRNA-mediated depletion of Dsg1 and Dsg3 suggest that antibodies against other targets may also be capable of activating Src (5).

Consistent with these previous findings, our data confirmed activation of Src after PV-IgG and AK23 treatment for 15 min and up to 2 h. Furthermore, loss of cell adhesion caused by AK23 was completely abolished by PP2 in cell culture *in vitro* as well as in the neonatal mouse model *in vivo*, demonstrating that Src plays an important role in loss of cell cohesion caused by autoantibodies directed against Dsg3. This supports previous findings where either broad-spectrum tyrosin kinase inhibitors or PP2 were efficient to inhibit PV-IgG-induced skin blistering in mice (35, 36).

However, inhibition of Src was not effective to consistently protect against PV-IgG-induced loss of adhesion when autoantibody fractions from different donors were applied.

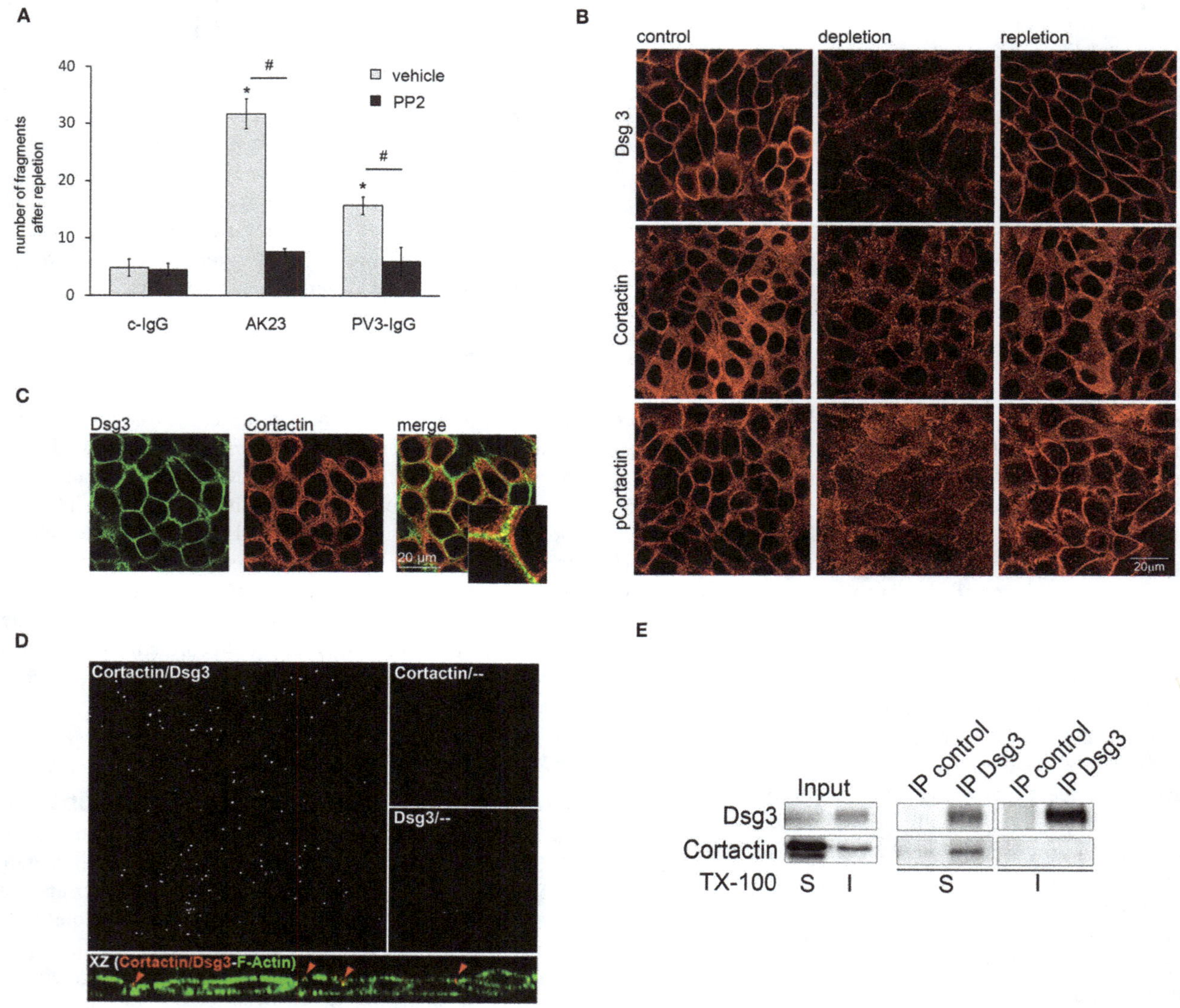

FIGURE 2 | Cortactin colocalizes and interacts with Dsg3. **(A)** Under conditions of desmosome re-assembly (Ca^{2+}-repletion) co-incubation with PP2 significantly reduced PV3-IgG- and AK23-induced monolayer fragmentation ($n > 7$; $\#p < 0.05$; $^*p < 0.05$ vs. c-IgG). **(B)** Immunostaining revealed that under control conditions Dsg3 and cortactin as well as phosphorylated cortactin were in part localized at cell borders, which was reduced by Ca^{2+}-depletion. Following Ca^{2+}-repletion for 8 h, all proteins relocated along the cell-membrane (scale bar 20 μm; $n = 4$). **(C)** Under basal conditions, Dsg3 and cortactin partly co-localized at cell borders (scale bar 20 μm; insets represent 3.2x magnifications of indicated areas; $n = 3$) **(D)** Proximity ligation assay revealed co-localization of Dsg3 and cortactin close to the cell periphery. Cells were illuminated with F-actin to localize cell-structures. Incubation with cortactin or Dsg3 only served as negative control ($n = 3$). **(E)** Immunoprecipitation (IP) of Dsg3 documented a complex of cortactin within the Triton-soluble but not the -insoluble fraction ($n = 3$).

For one fraction, Src inhibition abrogated loss of cell adhesion only when autoantibodies were incubated short-time. Using a second fraction, no protection against loss of cell cohesion was detectable at all (27). Since all autoantibody fractions were equally effective to induce loss of cell cohesion *in vitro*, this suggests that different mechanisms maybe involved in different patients. This is supported by the observation that PP2 was not effective to inhibit PV-IgG-induced skin blistering in human skin *ex vivo*. The data presented here do not allow the conclusion that Src is not involved in human skin at all. Nevertheless, the data show that PP2 under the conditions where it is effective to block AK23-mediated blistering in mice and to prevent loss of keratinocyte cohesion in response to some patients' IgG fractions *in vitro*, is not consistently protective in intact human skin.

A limitation of the study is that the conditions used in the different experimental models do not necessarily reflect the situation in patients. Regarding the inhibition of Dsg3 with the monoclonal autoantibody AK23 derived from a pempighus mouse model (27), it should be considered that the concentration used was supraphysiologic compared to patients' autoantibody levels. This could lead to an excessive direct inhibition of Dsg3 binding and activation of signaling by Src and p38MAPK (37), both of which may not be typical in PV patients. However, in contrast to the neonatal mouse model used here, AK23 in a

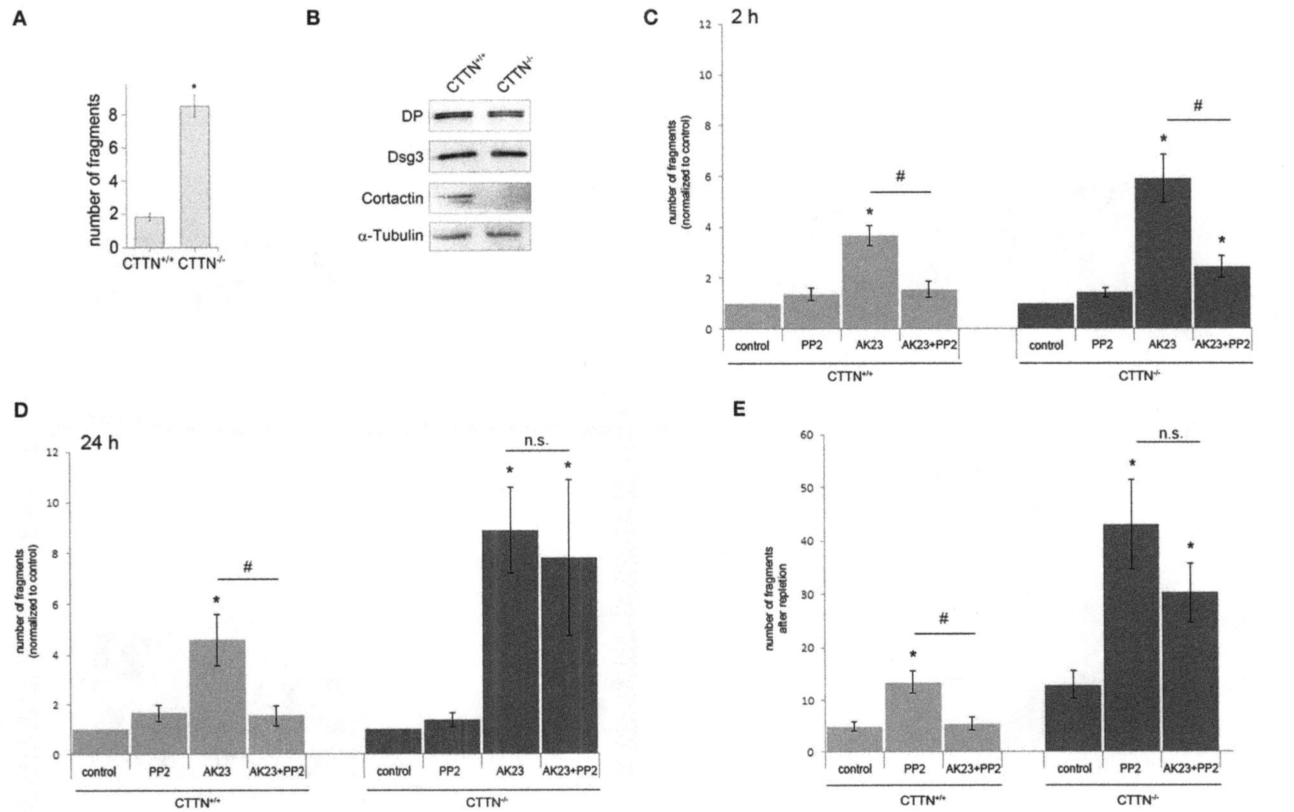

FIGURE 3 | Role of cortactin in Src-mediated modulation of AK23-induced loss of cell cohesion. **(A)** Cortactin is important for cell cohesion, indicated by enhanced fragmentation of cortactin-deficient (CTTN$^{-/-}$) cell monolayers in dispase-based dissociation assay ($n = 5$; $^*p < 0.05$ vs. control). **(B)** Confirmation of cortactin knockout by Western blot, α-Tubulin served as loading control ($n = 3$). **(C,D)** CTTN$^{-/-}$ and wt mouse keratinocytes exposed to a dissociation assay following either short time (2 h) or long time (24 h) incubation with AK23 ($n > 7$, $^{\#}p < 0.05$; $^*p < 0.05$ vs. control). **(E)** Reconstitution of cell adhesion measured by dissociation assay after Ca^{2+} switch in CTTN$^{-/-}$ and wt keratinocytes in absence or presence of Src inhibitor PP2 ($n > 7$, $^{\#}p < 0.05$; $^*p < 0.05$ vs. control).

human skin model was not effective to induce blister formation and reduce desmosome numbers indicating that mechanisms triggered by autoantibodies against Dsg1 may be required for blister formation as well (33). Similarly, the autoantibody profiles of the PV-IgG fractions and the abundance of aDsg1 autoantibodies used in this study may at least in part explain the different roles of Src for loss of keratinocyte adhesion. PV3-IgG, the effects of which were consistently ameliorated by Src-inhibition, contained comparable amounts of autoantibodies against Dsg1 and Dsg3, whereas in all other PV-IgG fractions the relative amount of Dsg1 autoantibodies was higher. Especially, PV4-IgG used for the *ex vivo* human skin model contained excessive levels of autoantibodies against Dsg1. However, for PV2-IgG this explanation falls short because Src inhibition was not protective at all despite comparable levels of antibodies against Dsg1 and Dsg3. Since we have no information about antibodies against other antigens including desmocollin isoforms or others, we cannot rule out that such antibodies may trigger mechanisms others than Src in loss of keratinocyte adhesion.

Nevertheless, the results are in line with the hypothesis that the different clinical phenotypes of pemphigus may at least in part be determined by the mechanisms which are involved in loss of cell cohesion and engaged by antibodies targeting Dsg3 or Dsg1 (4). Moreover, the data indicate that a therapeutic paradigm to modulate Src activity alone unlikely would be effective to treat the majority of patients with epidermal blistering as this usually is associated with antibodies against Dsg1 (1). This may be related to the different mechanisms induced by autoantibodies against Dsg1 in pemphigus pathogenesis.

Mechanisms by Which Src Regulates Cell Cohesion In Pemphigus

For some of the PV-IgG fractions such as PV1-IgG and PV2-IgG, loss of cell cohesion was clearly progressive from 15 min up to 24 h as studied in dispase assays. For other autoantibody fractions such as PV3-IgG and AK23, this effect was less pronounced which is in line with previous observations (37). This may indicate that at early time-points the underlying mechanisms may be different from later stages of adhesion loss. This is supported by the observation that short time co-incubation of AK23 with PP2 in cortactin-deficient cells can abrogate loss of cell cohesion whereas long-term incubation is not affected by Src inhibition. We conclude that short time effects of autoantibodies are in part Src- but not cortactin-dependent whereas cortactin at later stages of cell cohesion loss becomes more relevant.

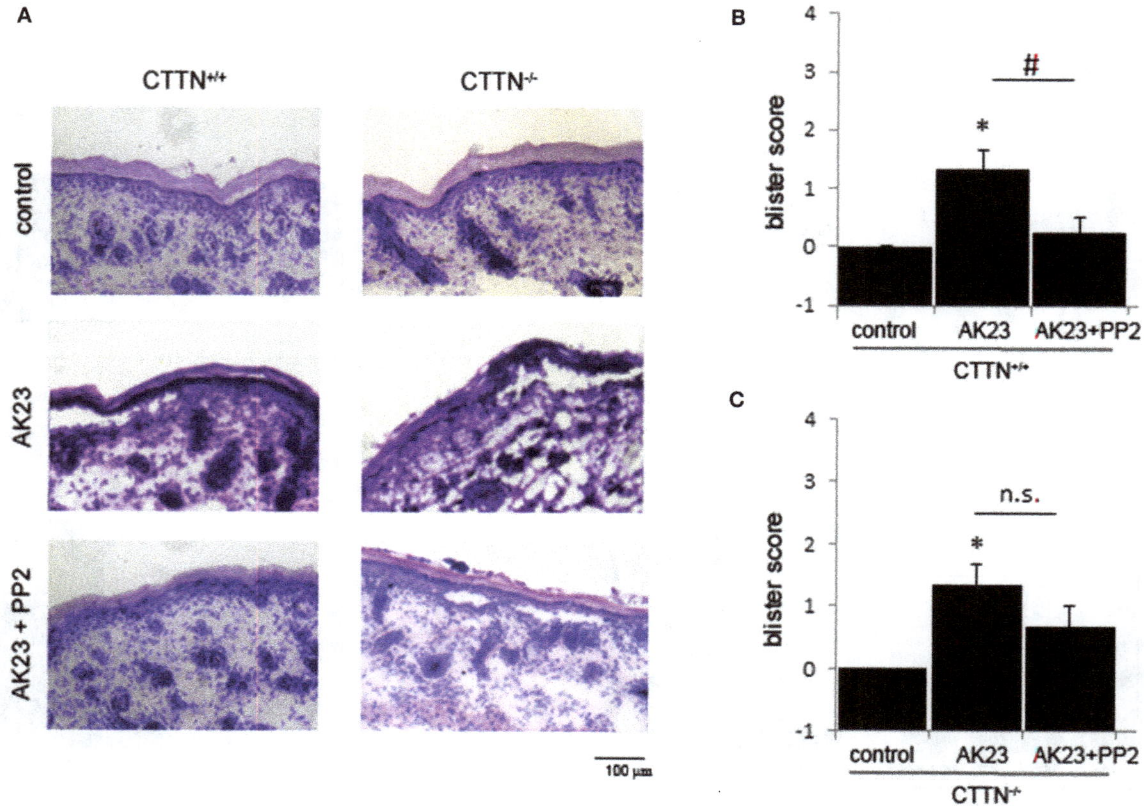

FIGURE 4 | AK23-induced blister formation *in vivo* is Src- and cortactin-dependent. **(A)** H.E.-stained serial sections showed that acantholysis induced by AK23 is almost completely blocked by inhibition of Src in wt but not $CTTN^{-/-}$ mice. Scale bar = 100 µm. **(B,C)** Blister scores for experiments described above ($n = 3$, $^{\#}p < 0.05$; $^{*}p < 0.05$ vs. control).

We observed that autoantibodies indeed interfered with reconstitution of cell adhesion in a manner dependent on Src. Moreover, because phosphorylation of the Src substrate cortactin at cell junctions correlated with junction integrity and cortactin binds to extra-desmosomal Dsg3, we reasoned that cortactin may be involved in desmosome assembly. The interaction of cortactin with desmosomal cadherins recently has been shown for Dsg1 also (38). More detailed studies are required to elucidate how cortactin is important in this context. Here, we observed that short-time effects of autoantibodies cause loss of cell cohesion by mechanisms which do not impair formation of new desmosomes whereas at later stages, impaired reformation of junctions may contribute to adhesion loss. This can be concluded from Ca^{2+}-switch assays in cortactin-deficient monolayers where Src inhibition was no longer protective against autoantibody-induced adhesion reconstitution. These data are in line with the observation that Dsg3 and Src form a complex together with E-cadherin, which appears to be involved in formation of new desmosomes (12). Since both in intact human skin *ex vivo* as well as in neonatal mouse skin *in vivo* autoantibodies were applied for 24 h, it is possible that cell cohesion in neonatal skin is more sensitive to mechanisms impairing formation of new cell contacts.

Since the pathogenesis of pemphigus appears to be complex and to include direct inhibition of Dsg3 binding as well as signaling events (2), the question arises about the role of Src and cortactin for loss of cell cohesion when compared to other mechanisms. Here we show that the short-time effects by which autoantibodies interfere with keratinocyte adhesion are at least in part dependent on Src but are independent of cortactin. Therefore, it is possible that phosphorylation of plakophilin (Pkp) 3 and its dissociation from desmosomes may be involved as has been suggested for experiments with PV-IgG (15). However, for AK23 we did not observe Pkp3 phosphorylation (**Supplemental Figure 1**) indicating that phosphorylation of Pkp3 can be independent of Dsg3. Aside from Src, other signaling molecules likely contribute to loss of cell cohesion in pemphigus. Electron microscopy in *ex vivo* human skin revealed that ultrastructural alterations such as loss of desmosomes, shortening of desmosomes and inter-desmososomal widening, all of which are observed in patients' lesions as well (39), were independent of Src. In contrast, these effects were shown previously to be mediated by p38MAPK (33). This is in line with the observation that pemphigus autoantibody fractions including autoantibodies targeting Dsg3 activate both Src and p38MAPK (4).

Finally, it is well-established that autoantibody titers correlate with the clinical phenotype of pemphigus (1, 3). For pemphigus autoantibodies from patients with muco-cutaneous PV or with PF, influx of Ca^{2+} and activation of ERK were also detected

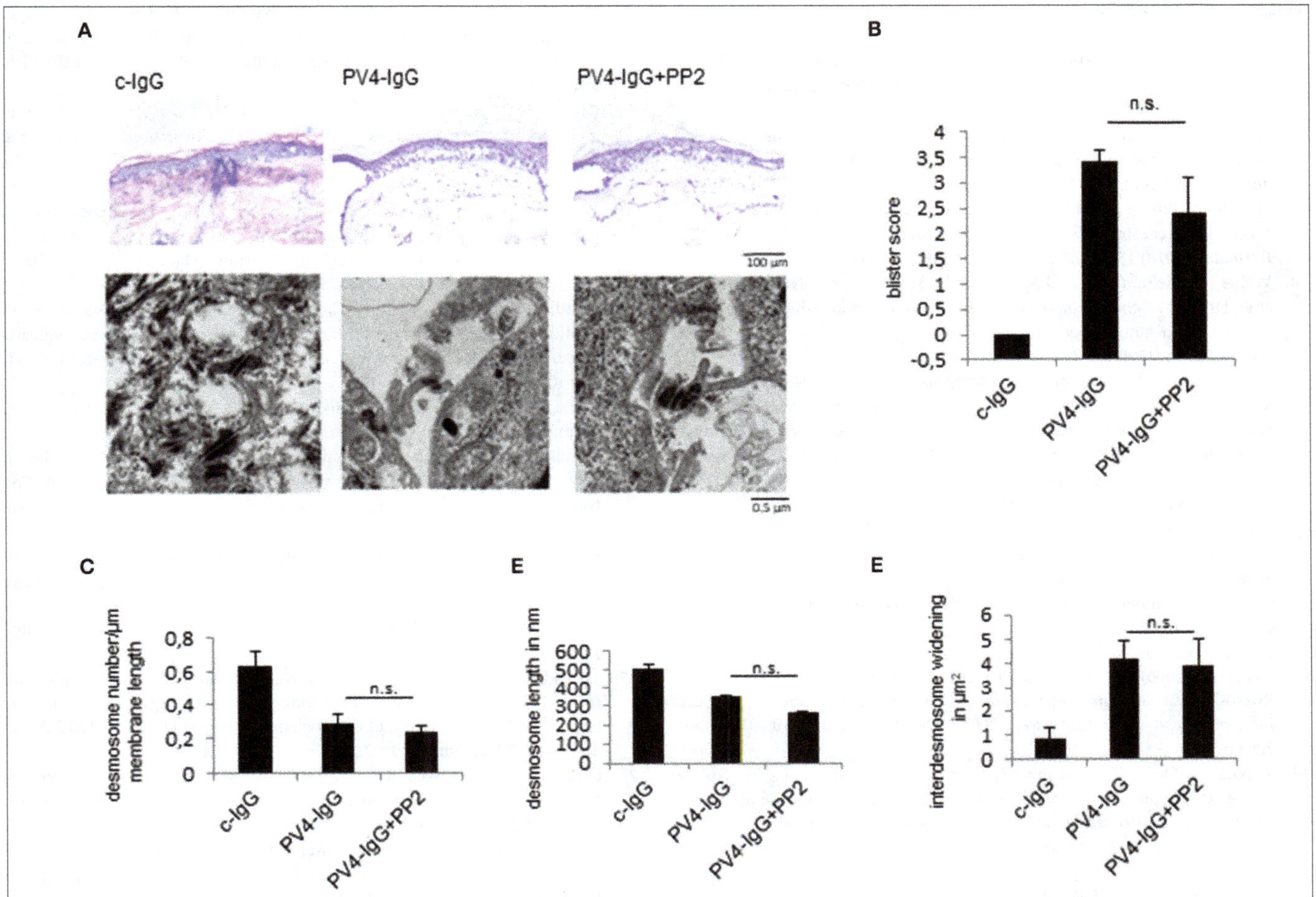

FIGURE 5 | Src inhibition does not prevent PV-IgG-induced skin blistering and desmosome alterations in human skin *ex vivo*. **(A)** upper images, **(B)** H.E.-stained serial sections revealed no change in blister formation after incubation with PV4-IgG in presence of Src-inhibitor PP2 (scale bar = 100 µm). (**A**, lower images) Ultrastructural alterations of desmosomes were evaluated by transmission electron microscopy in absence or presence of PP2 (scale bar = 0.5 µm). **(C–E)** Quantification of number of the desmosomes **(C)**, desmosome length **(D)** and inter-desmosomal widening **(E)** for the conditions described above ($n = 5$).

(4). Since Dsg1 was shown to suppress EGFR/ERK signaling by interacting with the ErbB2 binding protein Erbin (40), it is possible that autoantibodies targeting Dsg1 interfere with ERK signaling via this pathway. Taken together, we show that Src contributes to loss of cell adhesion primarily downstream of antibodies against Dsg3 in pemphigus by mechanisms which are both cortactin-dependent and -independent. The notion that actin-binding proteins such as cortactin and adducin become increasingly recognized to control desmosome function and cell behavior (12, 38), opens a new field for research on desmosome regulation.

AUTHOR CONTRIBUTIONS

DK, VR, EW, DE, MF, and HV-R performed experiments. DK, VR, EW, DE, and MF analyzed data. DK, EW, FV, MS, MH, RE, KR, AS, VS, and JW discussed data and interpreted results. DK and JW designed the study and wrote the manuscript.

ACKNOWLEDGMENTS

We thank Martina Hitzenbichler and Thomas Korbica for their excellent technical assistance, as well as Jessica Plewa, Michael Becker, and Axel Unverzagt for assistance in preparation of human body donors' skins. This work was supported by DFG grants WA 2474/4-3 and FOR2497 (PEGASUS) JW.

REFERENCES

1. Kasperkiewicz M, Ellebrecht CT, Takahashi H, Yamagami J, Zillikens D, Payne AS, et al. Pemphigus. *Nat Rev Dis Primers.* (2017) 3:17026. doi: 10.1038/nrdp.2017.26
2. Spindler V, Waschke J. Pemphigus—a disease of desmosome dysfunction caused by multiple mechanisms. *Front Immunol.* (2018) 9:136. doi: 10.3389/fimmu.2018.00136
3. Spindler V, Eming R, Schmidt E, Amagai M, Grando S, Jonkman MF, et al. Mechanisms causing loss of keratinocyte cohesion in pemphigus. *J Invest Dermatol.* (2018) 138:32–7. doi: 10.1016/j.jid.2017.06.022
4. Walter E, Vielmuth F, Rotkopf L, Sárdy M, Horváth ON, Goebeler M, et al. Different signaling patterns contribute to loss of keratinocyte cohesion dependent on autoantibody profile in pemphigus. *Sci Rep.* (2017) 7:3579. doi: 10.1038/s41598-017-03697-7
5. Chernyavsky AI, Arredondo J, Kitajima Y, Sato-Nagai M, Grando SA. Desmoglein versus non-desmoglein signaling in pemphigus acantholysis: characterization of novel signaling pathways downstream of pemphigus vulgaris antigens. *J Biol Chem.* (2007) 282:13804–12. doi: 10.1074/jbc.M611365200
6. Thomas SM, Brugge JS. Cellular functions regulated by Src family kinases. *Annu Rev Cell Dev Biol.* (1997) 13:513–609. doi: 10.1146/annurev.cellbio.13.1.513
7. Roskoski R. Src protein-tyrosine kinase structure, mechanism, and small molecule inhibitors. *Pharmacol Res.* (2015) 94:9–25. doi: 10.1016/j.phrs.2015.01.003
8. Irby RB, Yeatman TJ. Role of Src expression and activation in human cancer. *Oncogene.* (2000) 19:5636–42. doi: 10.1038/sj.onc.1203912
9. Roskoski R. Src protein-tyrosine kinase structure and regulation. *Biochem Biophys Res Commun.* (2004) 324:1155–64. doi: 10.1016/j.bbrc.2004.09.171
10. Tsukita S, Oishi K, Akiyama T, Yamanashi Y, Yamamoto T, Tsukita S. Specific proto-oncogenic tyrosine kinases of src family are enriched in cell-to-cell adherens junctions where the level of tyrosine phosphorylation is elevated. *J Cell Biol.* (1991) 113:867–79. doi: 10.1083/jcb.113.4.867
11. Owens DW, McLean GW, Wyke AW, Paraskeva C, Parkinson EK, Frame MC, et al. The catalytic activity of the Src family kinases is required to disrupt cadherin-dependent cell-cell contacts. *Mol Biol Cell.* (2000) 11:51–64. doi: 10.1091/mbc.11.1.51
12. Rötzer V, Hartlieb E, Vielmuth F, Gliem M, Spindler V, Waschke J. E-cadherin and Src associate with extradesmosomal Dsg3 and modulate desmosome assembly and adhesion. *Cell Mol Life Sci.* (2015) 72:4885–97. doi: 10.1007/s00018-015-1977-0
13. Tsang SM, Liu L, The MT, Wheeler A, Grose R, Hart IR, et al. Desmoglein 3, via an interaction with E-cadherin, is associated with activation of Src. *PLoS ONE.* (2010) 5:e14211. doi: 10.1371/journal.pone.0014211
14. Waschke J. Desmogleins as signaling hubs regulating cell cohesion and tissue/organ function in skin and heart—EFEM lecture 2018. *Ann Anat.* (2018). doi: 10.1016/j.aanat.2018.11.006. [Epub ahead of print].
15. Cirillo N, AlShwaimi E, McCullough M, Prime SS. Pemphigus vulgaris autoimmune globulin induces Src-dependent tyrosine-phosphorylation of plakophilin 3 and its detachment from desmoglein 3. *Autoimmunity.* (2014) 47:134–40. doi: 10.3109/08916934.2013.866100
16. Rötzer V, Breit A, Waschke J, Spindler V. Adducin is required for desmosomal cohesion in keratinocytes. *J Biol Chem.* (2014) 289:14925–40. doi: 10.1074/jbc.M113.527127
17. Wu H, Reynolds AB, Kanner SB, Vines RR, Parsons JT. Identification and characterization of a novel cytoskeleton-associated pp60src substrate. *Mol Cell Biol.* (1991) 11:5113–24. doi: 10.1128/MCB.11.10.5113
18. Tehrani S, Tomasevic N, Weed S, Sakowicz R, Cooper JA. Src phosphorylation of cortactin enhances actin assembly. *Proc Natl Acad Sci USA.* (2007) 104:11933–8. doi: 10.1073/pnas.0701077104
19. Lichti U, Anders J, Yuspa SH. Isolation and short-term culture of primary keratinocytes, hair follicle populations and dermal cells from newborn mice and keratinocytes from adult mice for *in vitro* analysis and for grafting to immunodeficient mice. *Nat Protoc.* (2008) 3:799–810. doi: 10.1038/nprot.2008.50
20. Kröger C, Loschke F, Schwarz N, Windoffer R, Leube RE, Magin TM. Keratins control intercellular adhesion involving PKC-alpha-mediated desmoplakin phosphorylation. *J Cell Biol.* (2013) 201:681–92. doi: 10.1083/jcb.201208162
21. Kumar V, Bouameur JE, Bär J, Rice RH, Hornig-Do HT, Roop DR, et al. A keratin scaffold regulates epidermal barrier formation, mitochondrial lipid composition, and activity. *J Cell Biol.* (2015) 211:1057–75. doi: 10.1083/jcb.201404147
22. Waschke J, Bruggeman P, Baumgartner W, Zillikens D, Drenckhahn D. Pemphigus foliaceus IgG causes dissociation of desmoglein 1-containing junctions without blocking desmoglein 1 transinteraction. *J Clin Invest.* (2005) 115:3157–65. doi: 10.1172/JCI23475
23. Spindler V, Rötzer V, Dehner C, Kempf B, Gliem M, Radeva M, et al. Peptide-mediated desmoglein 3 crosslinking prevents pemphigus vulgaris autoantibody-induced skin blistering. *J Clin Invest.* (2013) 123:800–11. doi: 10.1172/JCI60139
24. Maria Mulisch UW. *Romeis—Mikroskopische Technik.* Berlin Heidelberg: Springer-Verlag (2015).
25. Spindler V, Vielmuth F, Schmidt E, Rubenstein DS, Waschke J. Protective endogenous cyclic adenosine 5'-monophosphate signaling triggered by pemphigus autoantibodies. *J Immunol.* (2010) 185:6831–8. doi: 10.4049/jimmunol.1002675
26. Ishii K, Harada R, Matsuo I, Shirakata Y, Hashimoto K, Amagai M. *In vitro* keratinocyte dissociation assay for evaluation of the pathogenicity of anti-desmoglein 3 IgG autoantibodies in pemphigus vulgaris. *J Invest Dermatol.* (2005) 124:939–46. doi: 10.1111/j.0022-202X.2005.23714.x
27. Tsunoda K, Ota T, Aoki M, Yamada T, Nagai T, Nakagawa T, et al. Induction of pemphigus phenotype by a mouse monoclonal antibody against the amino-terminal adhesive interface of desmoglein 3. *J Immunol.* (2003) 170:2170–8. doi: 10.4049/jimmunol.170.4.2170
28. O'Keefe EJ, Briggaman RA, Herman B. Calcium-induced assembly of adherens junctions in keratinocytes. *J Cell Biol.* (1987) 105:807–17. doi: 10.1083/jcb.105.2.807
29. Hennings H, Holbrook KA. Calcium regulation of cell-cell contact and differentiation of epidermal cells in culture. *An ultrastructural study Exp Cell Res.* (1983) 143:127–42. doi: 10.1016/0014-4827(83)90115-5
30. Lewis JE, Jensen PJ, Wheelock MJ. Cadherin function is required for human keratinocytes to assemble desmosomes and stratify in response to calcium. *J Invest Dermatol.* (1994) 102:870–7. doi: 10.1111/1523-1747.ep12382690
31. Schnoor M, Stradal TE, Rottner K. Cortactin: cell functions of a multifaceted actin-binding protein. *Trends Cell Biol.* (2018) 28:79–98. doi: 10.1016/j.tcb.2017.10.009
32. Schnoor M, Lai FP, Zarbock A, Kläver R, Polaschegg C, Schulte D, et al. Cortactin deficiency is associated with reduced neutrophil recruitment but increased vascular permeability *in vivo*. *J Exp Med.* (2011) 208:1721–35. doi: 10.1084/jem.20101920
33. Egu DT, Walter E, Spindler V, Waschke J. Inhibition of p38MAPK signalling prevents epidermal blistering and alterations of desmosome structure induced by pemphigus autoantibodies in human epidermis. *Br J Dermatol.* (2017) 177:1612–8. doi: 10.1111/bjd.15721
34. Gil MP, Modol T, España A, López-Zabalza MJ. Inhibition of FAK prevents blister formation in the neonatal mouse model of pemphigus vulgaris. *Exp Dermatol.* (2012) 21:254–9. doi: 10.1111/j.1600-0625.2012.01441.x
35. España A, Mòdol T, Gil MP, López-Zabalza MJ. Neural nitric oxide synthase participates in pemphigus vulgaris acantholysis through upregulation of Rous sarcoma, mammalian target of rapamycin and focal adhesion kinase. *Exp Dermatol.* (2013) 22:125–30. doi: 10.1111/exd.12088
36. Sánchez-Carpintero I, España A, Pelacho B, López Moratalla N, Rubenstein DS, Diaz LA, et al. *In vivo* blockade of pemphigus vulgaris acantholysis by inhibition of intracellular signal transduction cascades. *Br J Dermatol.* (2004) 151:565–70. doi: 10.1111/j.1365-2133.2004.06147.x
37. Vielmuth F, Waschke J, Spindler V. Loss of desmoglein binding is not sufficient for keratinocyte dissociation in pemphigus. *J Invest Dermatol.* (2015) 135:3068–77. doi: 10.1038/jid.2015.324

38. Nekrasova O, Harmon RM, Broussard JA, Koetsier JL, Godsel LM, Fitz GN, et al. Desmosomal cadherin association with Tctex-1 and cortactin-Arp2/3 drives perijunctional actin polymerization to promote keratinocyte delamination. *Nat Commun.* (2018) 9:1053. doi: 10.1038/s41467-018-03414-6
39. Sokol E, Kramer D, Diercks GFH, Kuipers J, Jonkman MF, Pas HH, et al. Large-scale electron microscopy maps of patient skin and mucosa provide insight into pathogenesis of blistering diseases. *J Invest Dermatol.* (2015) 135:1763–70. doi: 10.1038/jid.2015.109
40. Getsios S, Simpson CL, Kojima S, Harmon R, Sheu LJ, Dusek RL, et al. Desmoglein 1-dependent suppression of EGFR signaling promotes epidermal differentiation and morphogenesis. *J Cell Biol.* (2009) 185:1243–58. doi: 10.1083/jcb.200809044

5

Bullous Pemphigoid IgG Induces Cell Dysfunction and Enhances the Motility of Epidermal Keratinocytes via Rac1/ Proteasome Activation

Duerna Tie[1], *Xia Da*[1], *Ken Natsuga*[2], *Nanako Yamada*[3], *Osamu Yamamoto*[3] *and Eishin Morita*[1*]

[1] *Department of Dermatology, Shimane University Faculty of Medicine, Izumo, Japan,* [2] *Department of Dermatology, Hokkaido University Graduate School of Medicine, Sapporo, Japan,* [3] *Division of Dermatology, Department of Medicine of Sensory and Motor Organs, Faculty of Medicine, Tottori University, Yonago, Japan*

Correspondence:
Eishin Morita
emorita@med.shimane-u.ac.jp

Bullous pemphigoid (BP) is an autoimmune disease characterized by the formation of blisters, in which autoantibodies mainly target type XVII collagen (ColXVII) expressed in basal keratinocytes. BP IgG is known to induce the internalization of ColXVII from the plasma membrane of keratinocytes through macropinocytosis. However, the cellular dynamics following ColXVII internalization have not been completely elucidated. BP IgG exerts a precise effect on cultured keratinocytes, and the morphological/functional changes in BP IgG-stimulated cells lead to the subepidermal blistering associated with BP pathogenesis. Based on the electron microscopy examination, BP IgG-stimulated cells exhibit alterations in the cell membrane structure and the accumulation of intracellular vesicles. These morphological changes in the BP IgG-stimulated cells are accompanied by dysfunctional mitochondria, increased production of reactive oxygen species, increased motility, and detachment. BP IgG triggers the cascade leading to metabolic impairments and stimulates cell migration in the treated keratinocytes. These cellular alterations are reversed by pharmacological inhibitors of Rac1 or the proteasome pathway, suggesting that Rac1 and proteasome activation are involved in the effects of BP IgG on cultured keratinocytes. Our study highlights the role of keratinocyte kinetics in the direct functions of IgG in patients with BP.

Keywords: bullous pemphigoid, keratinocyte, IgG, cell adhesion, cell migration

INTRODUCTION

Bullous pemphigoid (BP) is a skin-specific autoimmune disease characterized by subepidermal blisters (1–4). Systemic glucocorticoids and immunosuppressive agents are effective treatment options for BP (5, 6), but they increase the risk of lethal infections, particularly in elderly patients (7, 8). The autoimmune mechanisms involved in BP have been well-discussed based on clinical and experiential evidence (9, 10). IgG is the principal antibody involved, which recognizes the non-collagenous 16a domain (NC16a) of type XVII collagen (ColXVII, also known as BP180 or BPAg2) (9, 11–14).

ColXVII, a transmembrane protein, is located either at the core of the hemidesmosome in the skin (1) or in the hemidesmosome protein complexes of cultured keratinocytes (15, 16). ColXVII contains a long extracellular collagenous tail, which traverses the basement membrane zone (BMZ) (17), and serves as a signaling connector and/or a "mucilage" between the epidermis and the dermis (18–21). A genetic deficiency in ColXVII leads to junctional epidermolysis bullosa, resulting in the separation of the epidermis from the dermis (22, 23). Binding of the specific IgG to ColXVII is considered to contribute to intra-lamina lucida blistering in subjects with BP (24–26).

ColXVII-NC16a is a juxtamembrane region that plays a central role in the formation of the collagen-like-triple helix (27, 28). Moreover, IgG binding to ColXVII-NC16a is the most essential initial event in BP, and detection of the ColXVII-NC16a-specific IgG is important for diagnosing BP (10, 29, 30). The pathological progress of blistering after BP IgG binding to ColXVII-NC16a remains a debatable issue. Previously, complement activation was considered a major cause of blistering, because immunofluorescence studies of skin biopsies from patients with BP have shown that most patients with BP exhibit C3 deposition. Moreover, according to laboratory investigations, the binding of IgG to murine ColXVII triggers complement activation, mast cell degranulation, and neutrophil infiltration, suggesting that the formation of blistering lesions require both IgG and the recruitment and activation of complement (31–35). Recently, another BP pathomechanism has been advocated in which IgG exerts a direct effect on inducing blistering in patients with BP (36, 37). Evidence supporting these direct effects of BP IgG has been reported. Immunofluorescence studies have revealed that >10% BP cases are positive for BP IgG but negative for C3 deposition (31, 35). Based on the findings from some case reports, IgG staining shows an intercellular pattern in basal cells rather than a linear deposition along the BMZ (38). Clinical observations identified a non-inflammatory BP variant that is often associated with dipeptidyl peptidase-4 inhibitors application (39). BP IgG has been reported to directly induce blisters between the epidermis and the dermis without complement activation (40, 41), influence cell morphology (42), and "deplete" ColXVII in cell culture systems (37). The binding of BP IgG to ColXVII has also been reported to cause internalization of the immune complex by forming macropinosomes, resulting in decreased cell adhesion at the single cell level (43).

Although our understanding of the mechanism by which BP IgG induces blistering at the single-cell-level has improved, knowledge regarding macropinosome formation in the pathogenesis of BP is still lacking. A macropinosome is a large endocytic vacuole formed during macropinocytosis (44). Macropinosome formation acts as an entry site for intracellular pathogens (e.g., bacteria) that helps cells recognize the antigens/microbe-associated molecules (45, 46) and accumulate the metabolites required for proliferation (e.g., cancer cells) (47). However, hyperstimulation of macropinosomes leads to cell death (48, 49). Thus far, the changes in the morphology of keratinocytes during BP IgG-induced macropinosome formation are incompletely understood. We hypothesized that BP IgG contributes to the pathogenesis of BP by inducing keratinocyte dysfunction. The aim of this study was to clarify the morphological and functional changes in human keratinocytes incubated with BP IgG and the subsequent effects of inhibitors of macropinosome formation on these morphological and functional events.

MATERIALS AND METHODS

Cell Culture

Normal human epidermal keratinocytes (NHEKs) were obtained from the American Type Culture Collection (ATCC, Manassas, VA, USA) and cultured in serum-free media (with calcium chloride at a final concentration of 0.09 mM, Defined Keratinocyte SFM supplemented with growth factors, Gibco, Invitrogen Corporation, Carlsbad, CA, USA), 1% penicillin-streptomycin (Wako Pure Chemical Industries, Japan), and 25 ng/ml amphotericin B (Wako Pure Chemical Industries) at 37°C in a humidified atmosphere containing 5% CO_2. Cells were used after two to six passages in all experiments.

Antibody Purification

Plasma samples were obtained from three patients with BP (BP-1, BP-2, and BP-3), and eluents were obtained by a double filtration plasmapheresis treatment. BP IgGs fractions were isolated from plasma using a HiTrap Protein G HP column (GE Healthcare, Marlborough, MA, USA) with a fast protein liquid chromatography system (Amersham Biosciences, Marlborough, MA, USA), according to the manufacturer's protocol. The functions of BP IgGs were confirmed using indirect immunofluorescence staining of the salt-spilt human skin and a ColXVII-NC16a chemiluminescent enzyme immunoassay test (CLEIA, SRL Inc., Hachioji, Japan). Immunoblotting using the normal human epidermal extracts confirmed that the BP IgGs used in this study only reacted with ColXVII (180 kDa) (data not shown) and not with other antigens. The purified BP IgGs were concentrated through extensive washed with 0.9% NaCl and 50 K ultrafiltration (Millipore, Lexington, MA), and then filter-sterilized (pore size 0.22 μm; Millipore). The pooled IgGs from healthy people (normal IgG, Kenketsu Glovenin I, Nihon Pharmaceutical Co. Ltd., Tokyo, Japan) were dissolved in 0.9% NaCl to 50 mg/ml. Normal rabbit IgGs were purified using a Pierce classic IP kit (Thermo Fisher Scientific, MA, USA) with normal rabbit serum (ab7487, Abcam, Cambridge, UK). All IgGs

Abbreviations: BP, bullous pemphigoid; BMZ, basement membrane zone; BSA, bovine serum albumin; CLEIA, chemiluminescent enzyme immunoassay; ColXVII, type XVII collagen; DAPI, 4′, 6-diamidino-2-phenylindole; DCFHDA, 2′,7′-dichlorofluorescein diacetate; DMSO, dimethyl sulfoxide; DPBS, dulbecco's phosphate-buffered saline; FCCP, carbonyl cyanide-4-(trifluoromethoxy)phenylhydrazone; GTPases, guanosine triphosphate phosphohydrolases; h, hour; IgG, immunoglobulin G; MG132, carbobenzoxy-Leu-Leu-leucinal; min, minutes; NC16a, noncollagenous 16a domain; NHEKs, normal human epidermal keratinocytes; NSC23766, n6-[2-(4-diethylamino-1-methyl-butylamino)-6-methyl-pyrimidin-4-yl]-2-methyl-quinoline-4,6-diamine trihydrochloride; Rac1, ras-related C3 botulinum toxin substrate 1; ROS, reactive oxygen species; RT, room temperature; SEM, scanning electron microscope; TBHP, tert-butyl hydroperoxide; TEM, transmission electron microscope; QY-1, n-butyl glycidyl ether; $\Delta\Psi$m, mitochondria membrane potential.

protein concentrations were measured spectrophotometrically at 280 nm and samples were stored at −20°C.

This study was approved by the Ethics Committee of Shimane University and the Dean of the Faculty of Medicine (approval nos. 1746 and 2679).

Reagents

Carbobenzoxy-Leu-Leu-leucinal (MG132), cytochalasin D, and n6-[2-(4-diethylamino-1-methyl-butylamino)-6-methyl-pyrimidin-4-yl]-2-methyl-quinoline-4,6-diamine trihydrochloride (NSC23766) were purchased from Sigma (St. Louis, MO, USA). MG132 and cytochalasin D were dissolved in DMSO to generate 10 and 2 mM stock solutions, respectively. NSC23766 was dissolved in distilled water to generate a 10 mM stock solution. All inhibitor stock solutions were frozen at −20°C. For the application of inhibitors to cell cultures, all reagents were diluted in warm culture medium at the indicated concentrations. NHEKs were pretreated with cytochalasin D for 30 min, NSC23766 for 1 h, or MG132 for 0 h, and then IgGs were added prior to the analysis.

Flow Cytometry Analyses

Upon reaching ~60% confluence, NHEKs were treated with 2 mg/ml IgGs obtained from patients with BP (BP IgGs) or normal IgG. After 0, 0.25, 0.5, 1, 2, and 6 h incubations, the cells were washed with Dulbecco's phosphate-buffered saline (DPBS). Non-trypsin detached cells were immediately fixed with 4% paraformaldehyde and resuspended in DPBS. Cells were first incubated with a monoclonal rabbit IgG specific for human ColXVII-COOH (ColXVII IgG, ab184996, Abcam) and then incubated with anti-rabbit IgG-Alexa488 (ab150077, Abcam) to analyze the cell surface ColXVII expression. Cells were directly incubated with anti-human IgG-FITC (Dako, Copenhagen, Denmark) and examined using flow cytometry to determine the amount of IgG bound to the cell surface.

Immunostaining Assay

NHEKs were seeded on sterile glass coverslips at a density of 0.2 × 10^6 cells/ml, and after a 16 h incubation, NHEKs were pretreated with or without cytochalasin D, NSC23766, or MG132, and incubated with BP IgGs (2 mg/ml), normal IgG (2 mg/ml), or ColXVII IgG (12 μg/ml) for 0, 0.5, or 2 h. Afterwards, the cells were washed with DPBS, fixed with cold 4% (w/v) paraformaldehyde for 10 min, permeabilized and then blocked with 0.3 M (w/v) glycine/1% (w/v) BSA/10% (v/v) normal rabbit serum/0.1% (v/v) Tween-20 in DPBS for 1 h at room temperature (RT). NHEKs that had been treated with IgGs for 0 h were further incubated with BP IgGs (2 mg/ml) or normal IgG (2 mg/ml) for 1 h at RT or incubated with ColXVII IgG (12 μg/ml) overnight at 4°C. Cells were then washed three times with DPBS. All cells treated with IgGs were subsequently incubated with Alexa488- or FITC-conjugated secondary antibodies and rabbit or human IgG for 1 h at RT. The nuclei were stained with 4′, 6-diamidino-2-phenylindole (DAPI, Thermo Fisher Scientific). Cells on the coverslips were washed, mounted in mounting medium (Vector Laboratories, Burlingame, CA, USA), and viewed under a confocal scanning laser microscope (FV-100V, Olympus, Tokyo, Japan).

For the 3D reconstruction assay, a series of z-planes captured at 0.38 μm intervals were imaged with an Olympus FV-100V confocal microscope after staining. The 2D z-stack images from each channel were projected onto one 3D plane using the Olympus FV-100V software 3D view function. A red box indicated projected z-stack images, a yellow boxed region indicated one frame of a z-stack image, and a cut-off XZ or XY-section was shown in a yellow slice to better display the staining.

Quantification of the fluorescence intensity was performed using ICY software (icy.bioimageanalysis.org).

Cell Counting Assay

NHEKs were cultured in 96-well culture plates to 40–60% confluence in the presence or absence of cytochalasin D, NSC23766, or MG132. Cells were labeled with Hoechst 33342 (Thermo Fisher Scientific) and treated with BP IgGs (2 mg/ml), normal IgG (2 mg/ml), ColXVII IgG (12 μg/ml), or normal rabbit IgG (2 mg/ml). Live cell imaging was performed with an In Cell analyzer 2000 (GE Biosciences, Piscataway, NJ, USA) equipped with a ×20 objective. After a 6 h incubation with IgGs, the numbers of adherent cells in a ×20 area (0.57 mm^2) were automatically counted every hour with the In Cell Analyzer 1000 Workstation software (GE Biosciences) using the cell count analysis module.

Transmission Electron Microscopy (TEM) and Scanning Electron Microscopy (SEM)

NHEKs were incubated with BP IgGs (2 mg/ml) or normal IgG (2 mg/ml). Cells grown on four-well culture slides to 60% confluence were observed with TEM and the cells grown on 15 mm round cover-slips to 60% confluence were observed with SEM. For TEM, after the incubation with the indicated IgGs, cells were washed and immediately fixed with 2.5% (v/v) glutaraldehyde (Sigma) in 0.1 M cacodylate buffer (pH 7.4, Wako Pure Chemical Industries) for 2 h. Cells were then washed and postfixed with 1% (v/v) osmium tetroxide for 1 h and 1% (v/v) uranyl acetate for 1 h at 4°C in the dark. Dehydration was achieved in a graded series of ethanol solutions. Dehydrated cells were cleared in n-butyl glycidyl ether (QY-1), embedded in Epon (TAAB Epon 812 Resin, Berkshire, England), and cut into ultrathin sections at a thickness of 80 nm using an ultramicrotome. Sections were collected on a 300-mesh copper grid, and ultrathin sections were double stained with uranyl acetate and lead citrate. For SEM, after the incubation with the indicated IgGs, the debris were removed from the culture by gentle washes with sterile DPBS. Cells were fixed with 2.5% (v/v) glutaraldehyde for 2 h at 4°C and washed with a 0.1 M cacodylate buffer (pH 7.2) solution. Cells were postfixed with 1% (v/v) osmium tetroxide for 1 h at 4°C, stained with 1% (w/v) tannic acid for 1 h at 4°C in the dark, and then fixed with 1% (v/v) osmium tetroxide for 1 h at 4°C. Cells were subsequently dehydrated in an increasing gradient of ethanol solutions, critical point dried in liquid CO_2, mounted on aluminum stubs with the cell layer facing up, and then coated with gold. Cells were observed with a JSM-6510 scanning electron microscope (JEOL Co., Ltd., Tokyo, Japan) at a 10 kV accelerating voltage.

LysoTracker® Green DND-26 Staining Assay

NHEKs seeded on a 35 mm dish (Ibidi GmbH, Martinsried, Germany) at ~40% confluence were treated with BP IgGs (2 mg/ml) or normal IgG (2 mg/ml) for 2 h. Cells were stained with 50 nM Lysotracker® Green DND-26 (Thermo Fisher Scientific) for 15 min in the dark and the fluorescence of lysosomes was immediately detected using confocal microscopy (Olympus FV-1000). Images were quantified using CellProfiler image analysis software (cellprofiler.org) with the spot detection pipeline.

Analysis of Cell Morphology

NHEKs cultured in 96-well plate to 60% confluence were stained with 100 nM MitoTracker® Red CMXRos (Thermo Fisher Scientific) and 5 μg/ml Hoechst 33342. BP IgGs (2 mg/ml) or normal IgG (2 mg/ml) were then added to the culture, which was immediately imaged. Nuclear masks were generated from images of Hoechst 33342 staining at 0 and 2 h, and the found edge and overlay functions of ImageJ software were employed to identify enlarged cell nuclei. The cytoplasm was visualized by overlaying the images of MitoTracker® Red CMXRos staining with nuclear staining. The whole-cell area and the area of typical macropinosomes was determined in phase-contrast images, and the numbers of total observed cells and the cells that formed macropinosomes were counted using ImageJ software (imagej.nih.gov/ij/). For the cell size calculation, nuclear staining was used to mark each individual cell, and then phase-contrast images matched to nuclear channel images were employed to calculate the size of each cell using In Cell Analyzer 1000 Workstation software with the multitarget analysis module. The cell size was calculated from the sum of pixel areas for each cell based on the pixel sizes of the images (2.73 pixels/μm).

NHEKs were treated with BP-1 IgG (2 mg/ml) or normal IgG (2 mg/ml) and imaged to identify the rupture of the plasma membrane. Bright field images of cells were obtained at 10 min intervals up to 16 h. The found edge and overlay functions of ImageJ software were employed to analyze the images.

MitoTracker® Red CMXRos Staining Assay

NHEKs cultured in 96-well plates to 60% confluence were labeled with MitoTracker® Red CMXRos and Hoechst 33342 and treated with BP IgGs (2 mg/ml) or normal IgG (2 mg/ml) for 16 h to calculate the relative signal intensities and numbers of MitoTracker® Red CMXRos fluorescent dots per cell. Cells were fixed with cold 4% (w/v) paraformaldehyde for 10 min, and images of the cells were captured using an In Cell analyzer 2000 equipped with a ×20 objective (GE Biosciences). Images were quantified using CellProfiler image analysis software with the spot detection pipeline.

Cellular Reactive Oxygen Species (ROS) Assay

Intracellular ROS production in NHEKs was measured using the fluorescent dye 2′,7′-dichlorofluorescein diacetate (DCFHDA, Abcam) according to the manufacturer's instructions. Cells cultured in a 96-well plate to 60% confluence were incubated with DCFHDA for 45 min at 37°C in the dark, and fresh medium containing BP IgGs (2 mg/ml) or normal IgG (2 mg/ml) were added and cultured for 6 h at 37°C. The fluorescence intensity was determined using a fluorescence microplate reader (DTX880, Beckman Coulter, Brea, CA, USA). The relative ROS fluorescence intensity was calculated as follows: [T_{6h} (fluorescence intensity at 6 h)−T_{0h} (fluorescence intensity at 0 h)]/numbers of adherent cells measured by cell counting.

Mitochondrial Membrane Potential Assay

The mitochondrial membrane potential was measured using a JC-1 mitochondrial membrane potential assay kit (Mitosciences, Abcam) according to the manufacturer's instructions. NHEKs cultured in a 96-well culture plate to 60% confluence were stained with the JC-1 dye and incubated with BP IgGs (2 mg/ml) or normal IgG (2 mg/ml) for 20 h. The fluorescence intensity was analyzed using a fluorescence microplate reader (DTX880).

Analysis of C_{12}-Resazurin/SYTOX Green Staining

A C_{12}-resazurin/SYTOX green kit (Molecular Probes, Eugene, OR, USA) was used to visualize the cell viability according to the manufacturer's instructions. Briefly, NHEKs cultured to 60% confluence in T-25 flasks in the presence or absence of inhibitors were incubated with BP IgGs (2 mg/ml) or normal IgG (2 mg/ml) for 16 h. Cells were harvested with the TrypLE Express Enzyme (Gibco) and resuspended in 100 μl of DPBS containing 1 μM SYTOX green and 50 nM C_{12}-resazurin. After a 15 min incubation in the dark, 400 μL of DPBS were added. The cell suspension was mixed gently and then immediately subjected to flow cytometry analysis.

Cell Motility Assay

NHEKs were incubated in 96-well culture plates (Falcon) to ~60% confluence. Cells cultured in the presence or absence of inhibitors were labeled with Hoechst 33342, and then treated with BP IgGs (2 mg/ml) or normal IgG (2 mg/ml). Images of the cells were captured at 10 min intervals up to 6 h using an In Cell analyzer 2000 equipped with a ×20 objective (GE Biosciences). The motility of ~2,000 cells was analyzed using ImageJ software with WrMtrack plugins (www.phage.dk/plugins/wrmtrck.html). The Euclidean distance and velocity were calculated using the Chemotaxis and Migration Tool (Ibidi GmbH) and the mean square displacements were obtained using Motility Lab (www.motilitylab.net/).

Statistical Analysis

The results are presented either as the mean values ± standard errors of the means or mean values ± standard deviations (*SD*) from at least triplicate experiments. One-way or two-way ANOVA or Student's *t*-test was used to compare the means, and differences were deemed significant when the calculated *p*-value was < 0.05. All statistical analyses were performed with the R language (www.r-project.org).

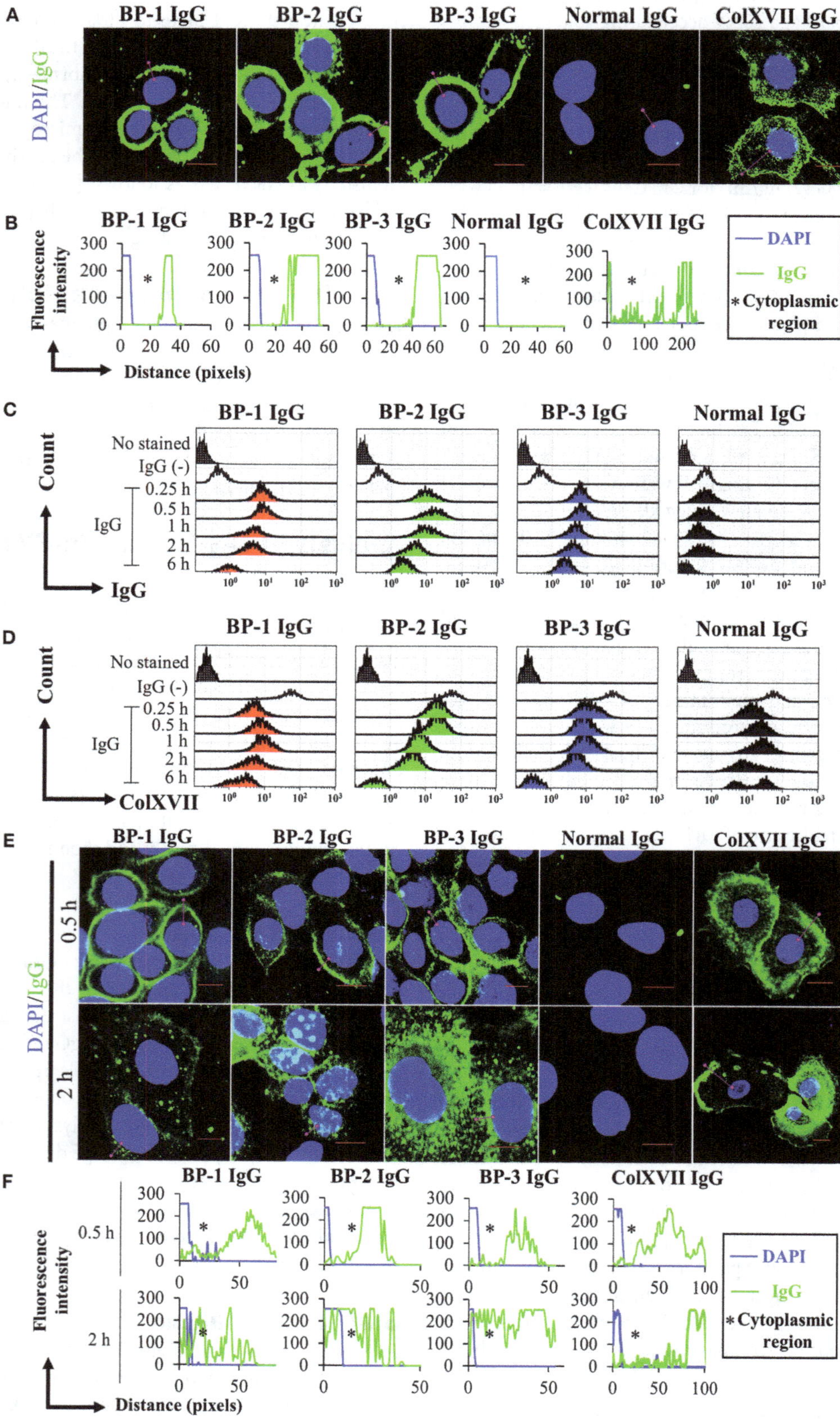

FIGURE 1 | Kinetics of the cell surface IgG binding and ColXVII expression. **(A)** Immunofluorescence staining for IgG bound to fixed NHEKs. NHEKs were fixed with paraformaldehyde and permeabilized. Cells were incubated with BP IgGs (BP-1, BP-2, or BP-3, 2 mg/ml), normal IgG (2 mg/ml), or rabbit anti-human

(Continued)

FIGURE 1 | ColXVII COOH IgG (ColXVII IgG, 12 μg/ml) and then subsequently stained with FITC- or Alexa Fluor 488-conjugated secondary antibodies (green). The nucleus was stained with DAPI (blue). Scale bar 10 μm. **(B)** Quantification of the fluorescence intensity of IgG bound to fixed NHEKs. Data were analyzed using ICY software. **(C)** Evaluation of the cell surface IgG binding using flow cytometry. NHEKs were cocultured with 2 mg/ml IgGs for the indicated times and then immediately fixed without permeabilization. The cells were directly incubated with anti-human IgG-FITC and were examined using flow cytometry. **(D)** Evaluation of the cell surface ColXVII expression using flow cytometry. NHEKs were cocultured with 2 mg/ml IgGs for the indicated times, and then immediately fixed without permeabilization. Then, cells were first incubated with an IgG specific for human ColXVII-COOH, and then incubated with Alexa Fluor 488-conjugated anti-IgG. Cells were examined using flow cytometry. **(E)** Fluorescence microscopy images of the binding of the indicated IgGs to NHEKs. NHEKs were incubated with BP IgGs (BP-1, BP-2, or BP-3, 2 mg/ml), normal IgG (2 mg/ml), or ColXVII IgG (12 μg/ml) for the indicated times. Then, the cells were fixed, permeabilized, subsequently stained with FITC- or Alexa Fluor 488-conjugated secondary antibodies (green). The nucleus was stained with DAPI (blue). Scale bar 10 μm. **(F)** Quantification of the fluorescence intensity of IgG bound to NHEKs. Data were analyzed using ICY software.

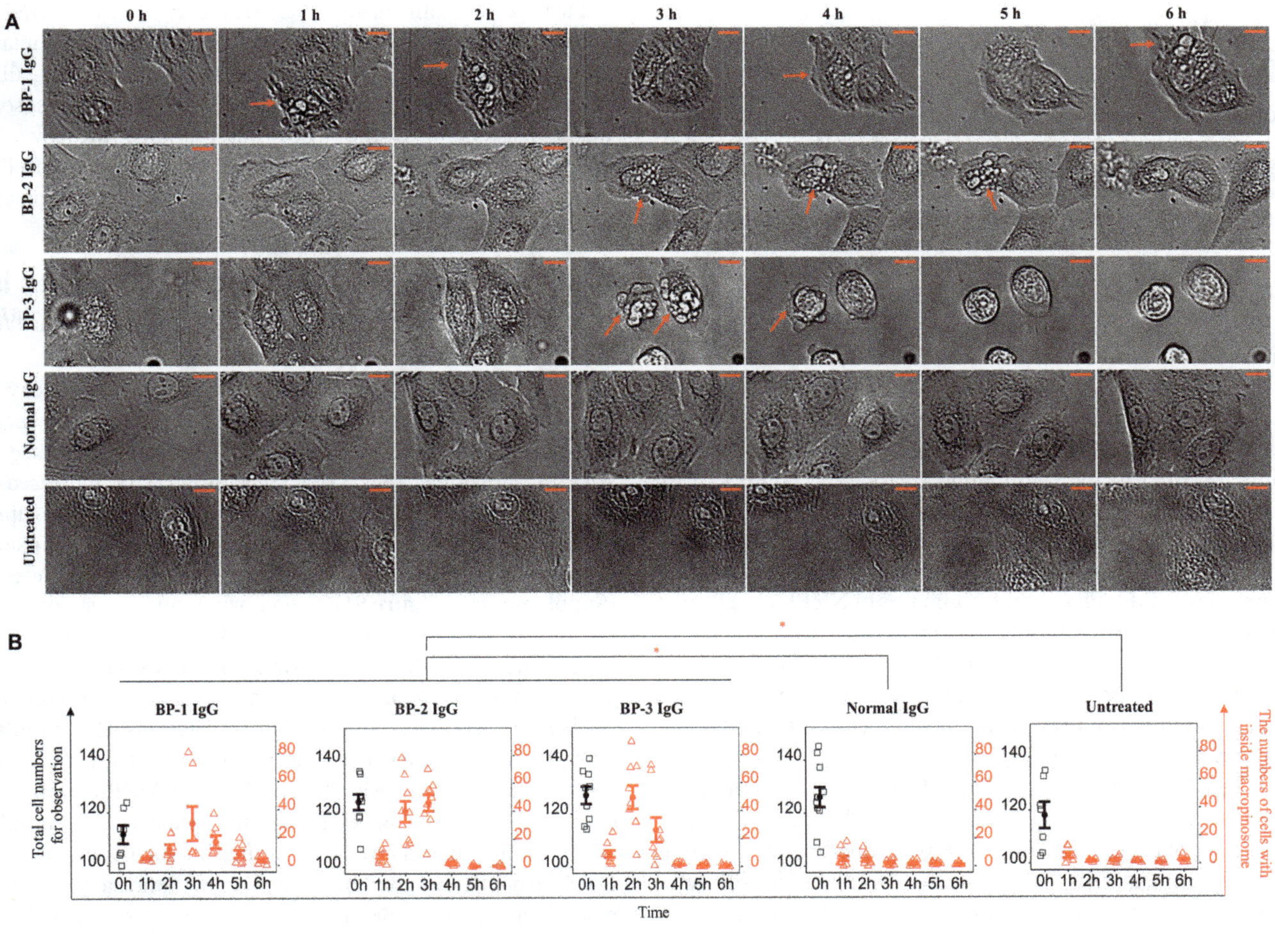

FIGURE 2 | Phase-contrast images of macropinosome formation in NHEKs treated with BP IgG. **(A)** Phase-contrast images were captured every 10 min after the addition of IgGs obtained from three patients with BP (BP-1, BP-2, and BP-3) or normal IgG to NHEKs and culture for up to 6 h. The figure shows images captured every 1 h. Cells with macropinosomes were indicated with arrows. Scale bar 10 μm. **(B)** The numbers of cells present during BP IgGs stimulation. Black: Total cell numbers observed at 0 h. Red: Numbers of cells containing macropinosomes at the indicated time points. Two-way ANOVA was used to analyze the significance of differences induced by BP IgGs. *p-value < 0.05.

RESULTS

Kinetics of the Cell Surface IgG Binding, ColXVII Expression, and the Numbers of Adherent NHEKs Treated With BP IgG

We performed immunostaining and analyzed the results with a confocal laser-scanning microscope and flow cytometry to obtain spatial and kinetic information about BP IgG binding and ColXVII expression in NHEKs treated with BP IgGs. BP IgGs binding to the NHEK surface were verified by positive immunostaining for FITC-labeled anti-human IgG, and ColXVII expression on the surface of NHEKs was verified using ColXVII IgG (**Figures 1A,B**). In the flow cytometry analysis, the cell surface IgG binding and ColXVII expression on the surface

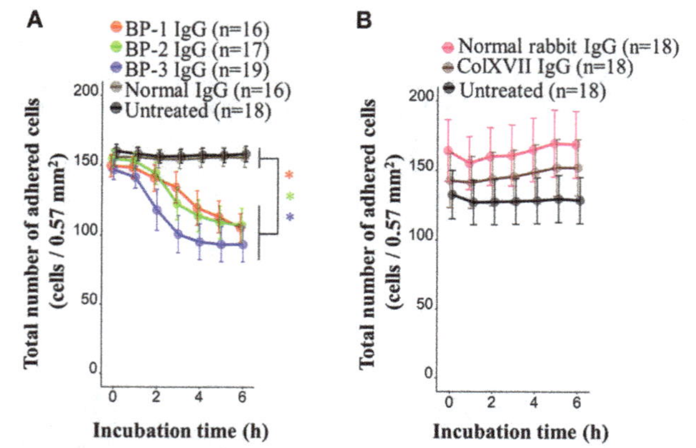

FIGURE 3 | Kinetics of the numbers of adherent NHEKs stimulated with BP IgG. Total numbers of adherent cells after stimulation with **(A)** BP IgGs, normal IgG, or **(B)** ColXVII IgG or normal rabbit IgG. The cell numbers were counted hourly in a ×20 area (0.57 mm^2) for up to 6 h. Two-way ANOVA was used to determine the significance of differences induced by BP IgGs. *p-value < 0.05.

of BP IgG-stimulated NHEKs decreased over time, whereas ColXVII expression and the binding of IgG to normal IgG-stimulated cells was not obviously altered (**Figures 1C,D**). Based on the confocal laser-scanning microscope observations, the cell surface localization of BP IgGs were visualized after a 0.5 h incubation, and most of the punctate IgGs staining were mainly localized in the cytoplasmic area at 2 h (**Figures 1E,F**). No significant IgG staining was observed when NHEKs were cocultured with normal IgG (**Figures 1A–E**). Immunostaining with ColXVII IgG did not show obvious internalization (**Figures 1A,B,E,F**). Phase-contrast images of NHEKs cocultured with BP IgGs displayed the BP IgG-induced formation of typical macropinosomes in NHEKs (**Figure 2A**), and compared to normal IgG- or untreated cells, BP IgG-stimulated cells exhibited a significant increase in the number of cells containing macropinosomes (**Figure 2B**).

BP IgG is known to cause the detachment of keratinocytes in 40% confluent cultures, although the adhesive function of ColXVII remains unclear (37). We performed a cell counting assay with living cells to determine the effect of BP IgGs on keratinocyte adhesion. BP IgGs significantly decreased the number of attached cells (reduced by ~40%) compared to the cells treated with normal IgG or untreated cells, and the effects were evident beginning 2 h after the incubation (**Figure 3A**). We also assessed the effect of IgG on detaching the COOH-termini of ColXVII (ColXVII IgG) and found that the addition of ColXVII IgG to the NHEKs did not obviously affect adhesion (**Figure 3B**).

BP IgG Treatment Alters the Morphology of NHEKs

We hypothesized that internalization of BP IgG-ColXVII complexes alters the properties and morphology of NHEKs. First, we used SEM to characterize the status of the plasma membrane after BP IgGs were added to the culture. Compared to the cells incubated with normal IgG and/or the untreated cells, the BP IgG-stimulated cells exhibited alterations in the cell membrane structure (indicated with arrows in **Figure 4**).

The TEM examination revealed larger vesicles with villi-like structures inside the cytoplasmic space in BP IgG-treated NHEKs. BP IgG-treated NHEKs displayed vacuolar structures containing myelin-like structures. BP IgG-stimulated cells accumulated lysosomes and/or autophagosomes (**Figures 5A,B**), whereas cell nuclei showed neither damage nor chromatin condensation (**Figure 5A**). Since lysosomes have been suggested to play important roles in cell death (50), we further characterized the involvement of lysosomes in the BP IgG-induced cell death using a LysoTracker® Green DND-26 uptake assay. The live cell imaging revealed the accumulation of lysosomes 2 h after BP IgGs were added to the culture (**Figure 5B**), and the intracellular distribution of lysosomes was consistent with the TEM observations. Moreover, BP IgG-stimulated cells contained a greater number intracellular LysoTracker® Green DND-26-labeled dots with high fluorescent intensity (**Figures 5C,D**).

Morphological and Functional Changes in the Mitochondria of NHEKs Incubated With BP IgG

We used time-lapse microscopy to analyze cell morphology and calculated the sizes of individual cells to determine whether the increased number of intracellular vesicles increased the sizes of individual cells. The sizes of NHEKs increased 1 h after adding BP IgGs to the culture, followed by the rupture of the cell membrane (**Supplementary Figure S1A**). The larger cell sizes reverted to the average size of normal cells after 3 h (**Supplementary Figure S1B**). Following nuclear staining and the capture of phase-contrast images, the sizes of NHEKs that had been incubated with BP IgGs for 2 h increased (**Figures 6A,B**). The TEM observations of mitochondria revealed numerous swollen mitochondria and a loss of cristae in cells stimulated with BP IgGs (**Figure 6C**). The mitochondrial functions were further analyzed with MitoTracker® Red CMXRos staining to observe the effect of BP IgGs, and the mitochondrial numbers and staining intensity were quantified in each individual cell. After 16 h, the number of stained mitochondria per cell did not differ between BP IgG-treated cells and normal IgG-treated or untreated cells (data not shown), whereas the staining intensity of mitochondria in BP IgG-treated cells decreased (**Figure 7A**).

ROS were generated 6 h after BP IgGs were added to the culture, whereas normal IgG did not increase ROS levels compared to untreated cells (**Figure 7B**). By performing JC-1 staining to analyze the mitochondrial membrane potential ($\Delta\Psi m$), JC-1 aggregates, a sign of intact mitochondria, were more abundant in the normal IgG-stimulated cells, and untreated cells. On the other hand, dysfunctional mitochondria with a dissipation of $\Delta\Psi m$, as evidenced by the increased number of JC-1 monomers, were pronounced in BP IgG-treated NHEKs at 20 h (**Figure 7C**).

The two-color fluorescence assay that distinguishes metabolically active cells was performed using SYTOX

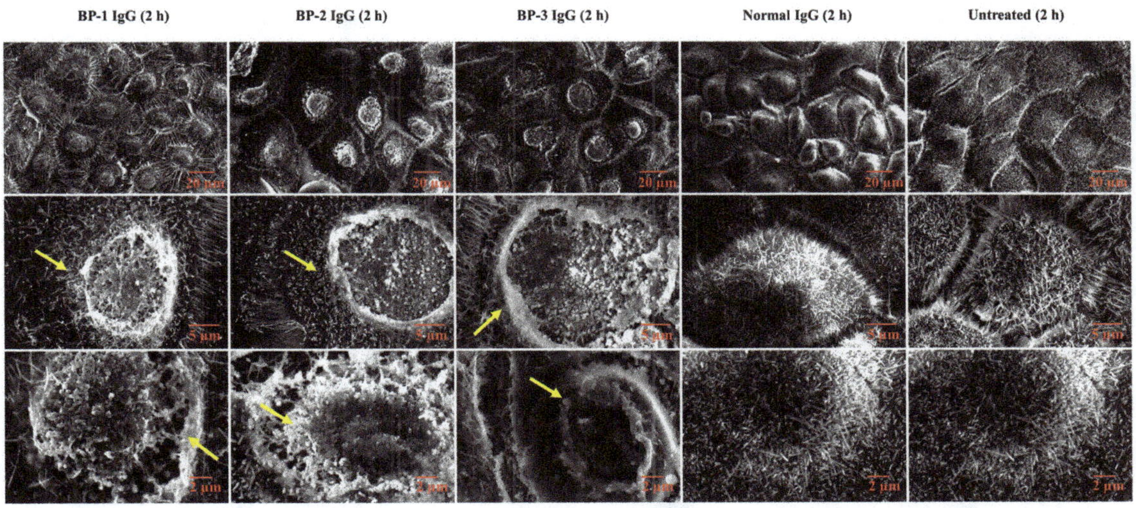

FIGURE 4 | SEM images of NHEKs stimulated with BP IgG. SEM images of NHEKs treated with BP IgGs (BP-1, BP-2, and BP-3) or normal IgG for 2 h. The lower magnification pictures show the connections of cells and filopodia. The higher magnification pictures show the cell surface and microvilli of individual cells. The alterations in the cell membrane structure are indicated with arrows.

green and C_{12}-resazurin dye. SYTOX green labels cells with compromised plasma membranes, and C_{12}-resazurin is used to assess mitochondrial metabolic activity. After a 2 h incubation with BP-1 IgG or normal IgG, the pattern of SYTOX green and C_{12}-resorufin staining did not differ between BP-1 IgG-, normal IgG-stimulated, or untreated NHEKs (data not shown). Therefore, we postulated that BP IgG-induced ColXVII internalization does not immediately induce a loss of metabolic activity in NHEKs. Since the dissipation of $\Delta\Psi m$ is usually regarded as a sign of decreased cell viability (51) and $\Delta\Psi m$ was not significantly decreased in NHEKs incubated with BP IgGs for up to 6 h (data not shown), we harvested the NHEKs that had been incubated with BP IgGs for 16 h and performed SYTOX green/C_{12}-resazurin staining. A greater percentage of BP IgG-stimulated cells was stained with SYTOX green and a relatively lower percentage was stained with C_{12}-resazurin than normal IgG-stimulated or untreated cells (**Figure 7D**), suggesting a decrease in the metabolic ability of BP IgG-treated cells. As DNA fragments were not found (data not shown) and chromatin condensation was not observed in our TEM images of BP IgG-stimulated cells (**Figure 5A**), we concluded that BP IgG did not induce apoptosis.

BP IgG Increased NHEK Motility

Next, we extended our observations to evaluate cell motility. According to the results of the electron microscopy analysis, BP-1 IgG-stimulated cells displayed longer lamellipodia (**Figure 4**), and the extension of lamellipodia is closely related to cell migration (52). Throughout the 6 h observation of live cells, BP IgG-treated cells showed increased cell motility compared with normal IgG-stimulated and untreated cells (**Figure 8**). Notably, both the migration distance (**Figures 8A,C**) and velocity (**Figure 8B**) increased.

Effects of cytochalasin D, NSC237766, and MG132 on the BP IgG-Induced Alterations in keratinocytes

The findings of BP IgG-induced cell dysfunction led us to investigate the pathway involved in the BP IgG-induced alterations. Three inhibitors that have been established as involved in the ColXVII internalization process were employed to further investigate the direct effect of BP IgGs on cell adhesion, metabolic activity, and motility.

Consistent with previous reports (43), application of cytochalasin D (inhibitor of the actin-cofilin interaction) inhibited the internalization of the BP IgG-ColXVII immune complex in BP IgG-stimulated NHEKs (**Figures 9A–C**). In the cell counting assay, the application of cytochalasin D did not exert a protective effect but instead increased the adhesion of NHEKs treated with BP IgGs (**Figure 10**). The cytochalasin D treatment did not completely relieve the BP IgG-induced loss of metabolic activity in NHEKs (**Figure 11**). In the motility assay, cytochalasin D significantly decreased the migration speed and distance of untreated NHEKs (**Figure 12A**), although it did not consistently exert the inhibitory effect on the NHEKs stimulated with BP IgGs (**Figures 12A,B**).

MG132 (inhibitor for proteasome) suppresses ColXVII depletion in both mouse and human keratinocytes stimulated with BP IgG (41). Thus, we hypothesized that the reduction in the adhesion of NHEKs treated with BP IgG is related to the depletion of ColXVII. MG132 did not prevent BP IgG-induced internalization (**Figures 9A–C**) or delay the BP IgG-induced decrease in cell number (**Figure 10**). However, MG132 protected NHEKs from the BP IgG-induced loss of

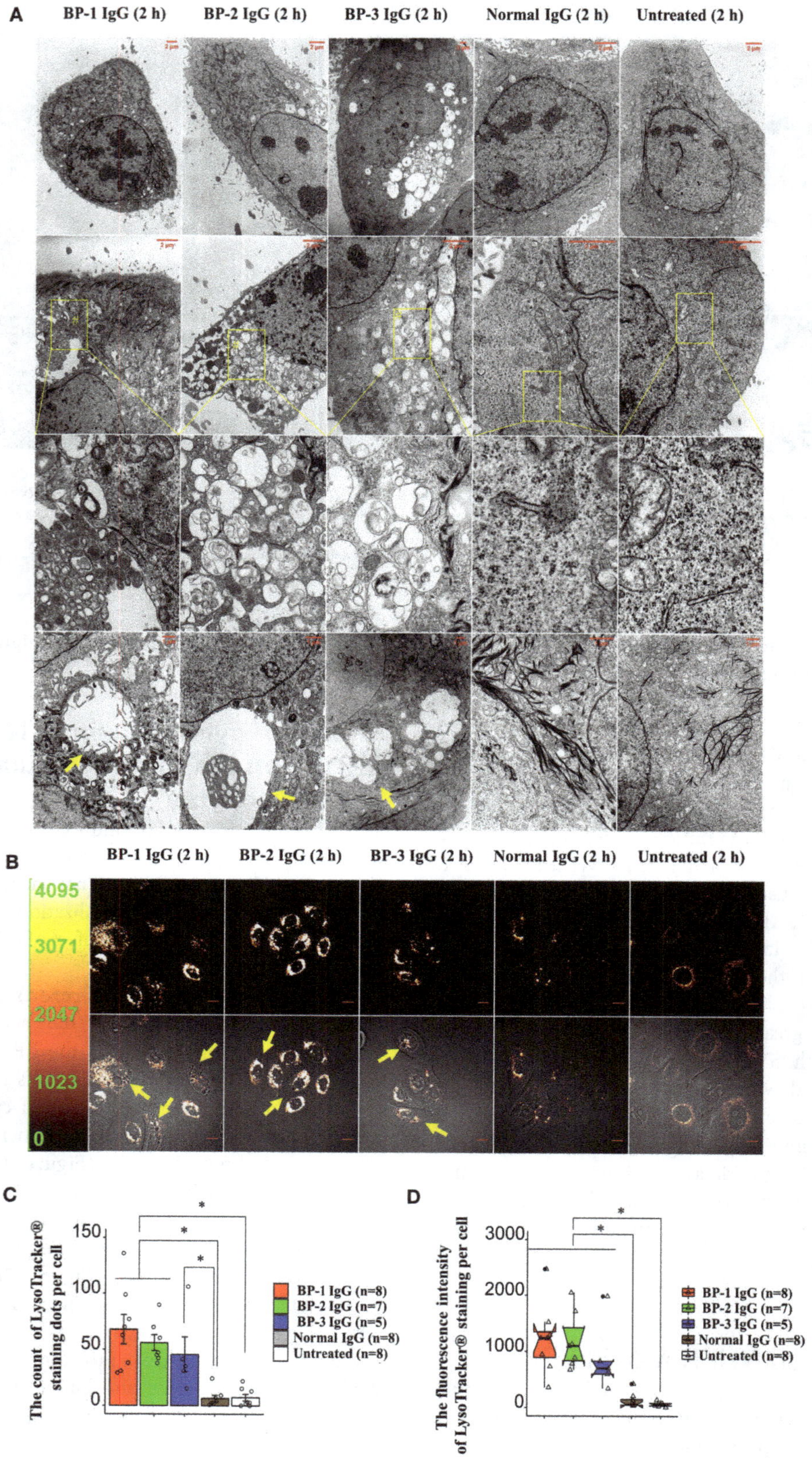

FIGURE 5 | Changes in the morphology of NHEKs stimulated with BP IgG. **(A)** TEM images of NHEKs stimulated with BP IgGs (BP-1, BP-2, and BP-3) or normal IgG for 2 h. Zoomed-out images labeled with the # symbol shows vacuolar structures containing myelin-like structures. Vacuolar structures are indicated with arrows.

(Continued)

FIGURE 5 | (B) The intracellular distribution of lysosomes in NHEKs stimulated with BP IgGs (BP-1, BP-2, and BP-3) or normal IgG. After a 2 h incubation with IgGs, cells were incubated with 50 nM LysoTracker® Green DND-26 for 15 min in dark, and live cells were imaged using confocal microscopy. Arrows indicate vesicles surrounded by lysosomes. Scale bar 10 μm. Y-axis in the left panel: fluorescence intensity. **(C)** Quantification of the fluorescently stained dots in cells. The LysoTracker® Green DND-26-stained dots in the cytoplasmic region of individual cells were counted using the CellProfiler image analysis software. One-way ANOVA was used for the statistical analysis. *p-value < 0.05. **(D)** Measurement of the fluorescence intensity per cell. The fluorescence intensity of LysoTracker® Green DND-26-stained cells was measured using CellProfiler image analysis software. One-way ANOVA was used for the statistical analysis. *p-value < 0.05.

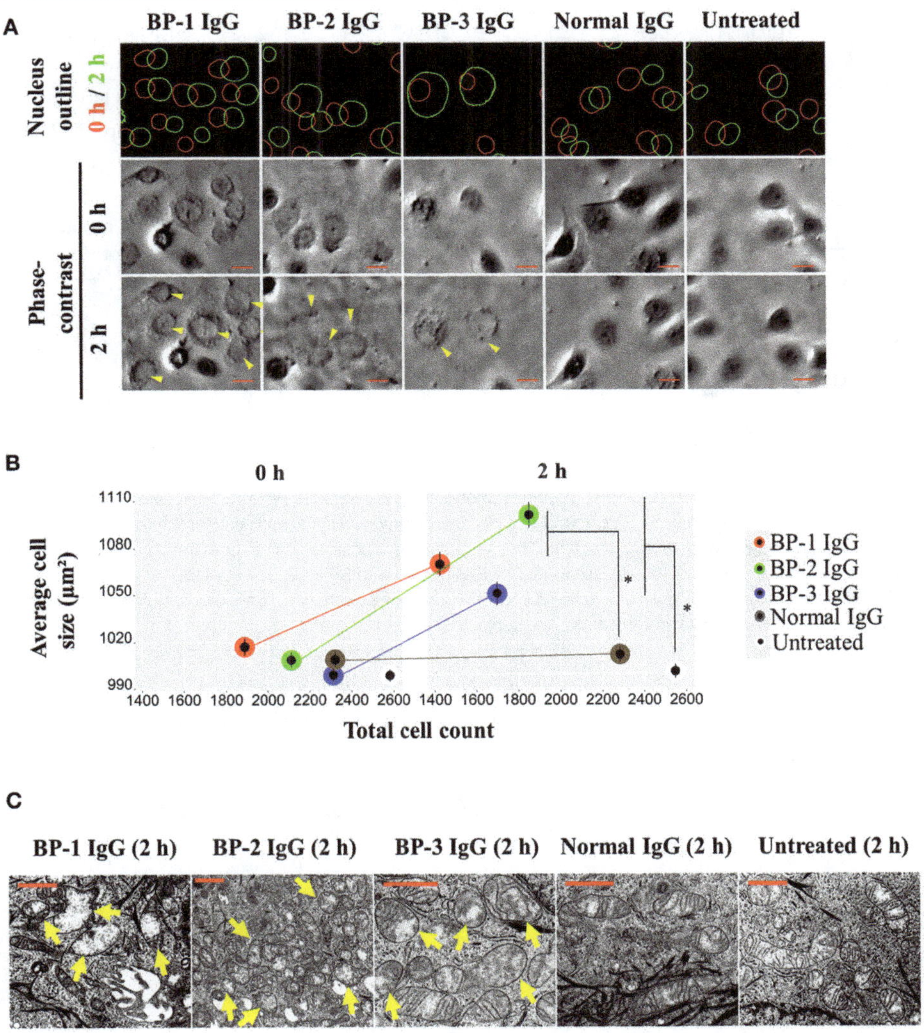

FIGURE 6 | Changes in the mitochondrial morphology in NHEKs treated with BP IgG. NHEKs were stained with Hoechst 33342 and then stimulated with BP IgGs (BP-1, BP-2, and BP-3) or normal IgG. **(A)** Nuclei were labeled at 0 h (red circle) and 2 h (green circle); the whole-cell area is shown with a phase-contrast image. Arrows indicate enlarged cells. Scale bar 20 μm. **(B)** Average cell sizes at 0 and 2 h were calculated from at least 1,500 individual cells per group. Two-way ANOVA was used for the statistical analysis. *p-value < 0.05. **(C)** TEM images of mitochondrial morphology in NHEKs that had been incubated with the indicated IgGs for 2 h. Damaged mitochondria are indicated with arrows. Scale bar 1 μm.

metabolic activity (**Figure 11**). These data support our hypothesis that the metabolic activity was associated with proteasome activation in NHEKs stimulated with BP IgGs. Additionally, MG132 slightly decreased the migration of BP IgG-treated cells (**Figures 12A,B**).

The formation of macropinosomes in epithelial cells as an early response to combat intracellular pathogens requires the activation of a Rho-GTPase such as Rac1 (46, 53). NSC23766 (a Rac1 inhibitor) suppresses the internalization of BP IgG-ColXVII immune complexes (54). In the immunostaining assay, we also confirmed that the inhibition of Rac1 activity prevented BP IgG-ColXVII internalization (**Figures 9A–C**). Surprisingly, the application of NSC23766 to the NHEKs treated with BP IgGs did not exert a protective effect on adhesion (**Figure 10**). As shown in **Figure 11**, the application of NSC23766 to the BP IgG-treated NHEKs prevented the loss of metabolic activity, but did not reduce the cell motility (**Figure 12**).

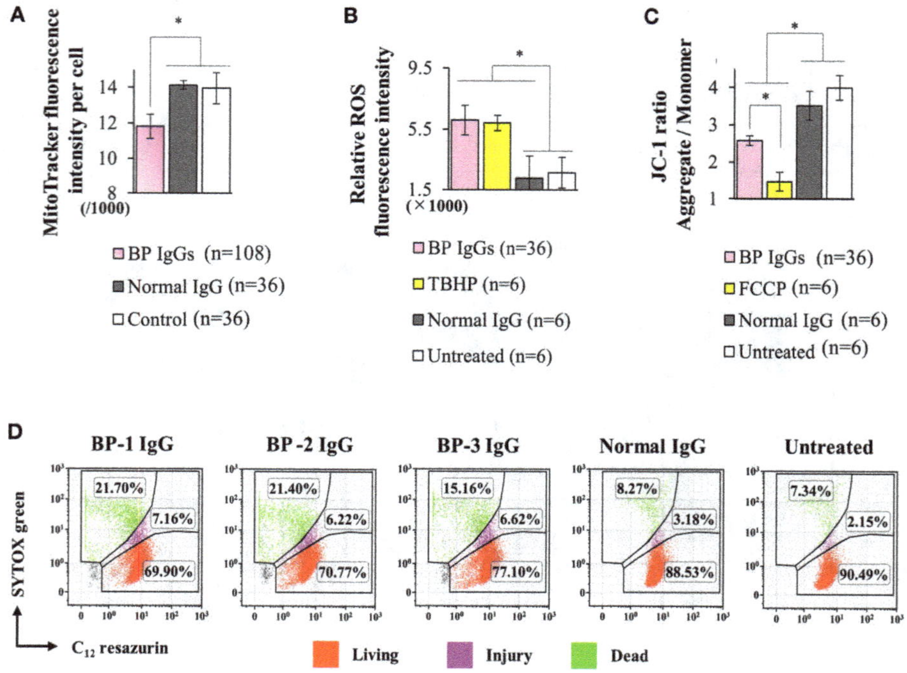

FIGURE 7 | Effects of BP IgG on mitochondrial function in NHEKs. **(A)** Mitochondrial staining intensities (MitoTracker® Red CMXRos) were evaluated in NHEKs incubated with a pool of BP IgGs (from BP-1, BP-2, and BP-3) or normal IgG for 16 h. One-way ANOVA was used for the statistical analysis. *p-value < 0.05. **(B)** ROS were detected in NHEKs stimulated with BP IgGs or normal IgG for 6 h. TBHP was used as a positive control. One-way ANOVA was used for the statistical analysis. *p-value < 0.05. **(C)** The mitochondrial membrane potential was assayed in NHEKs treated with BP IgGs or normal IgG for 20 h. FCCP was used as a positive control. One-way ANOVA was used for the statistical analysis. *p-value < 0.05. **(D)** NHEKs were collected after a 16 h incubation with the indicated IgGs, then stained with SYTOX green (stains dead cells) and C_{12}-resazurin (stains living cells), and subjected to flow cytometry.

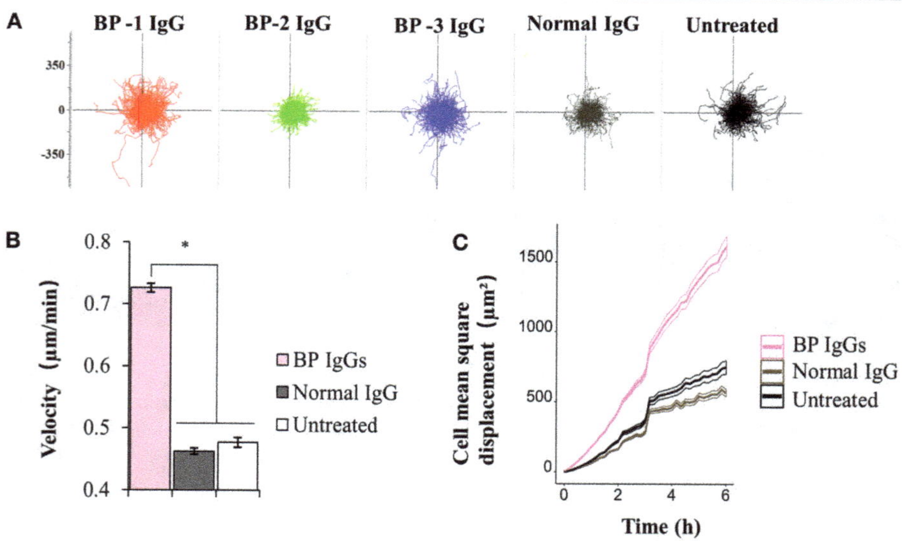

FIGURE 8 | Results of the cell motility assay using NHEKs stimulated with BP IgG. Hoechst 33342-labeled NHEKs were incubated with IgGs obtained from 3 patients with BP (BP-1, BP-2, and BP-3) or normal IgG, and imaged using time-lapse microscopy. Images were captured at 10 min intervals for up to 6 h. **(A)** Migration displacement maps were generated by centering the cell migration paths at a common starting point. Axes of vector diagrams = 500 μm. **(B)** Cell velocity of NHEKs treated with IgGs. One-way ANOVA was employed to determine the significance of differences induced by BP IgGs. *p-value < 0.05. **(C)** Mean square displacement of the NHEKs treated with IgGs.

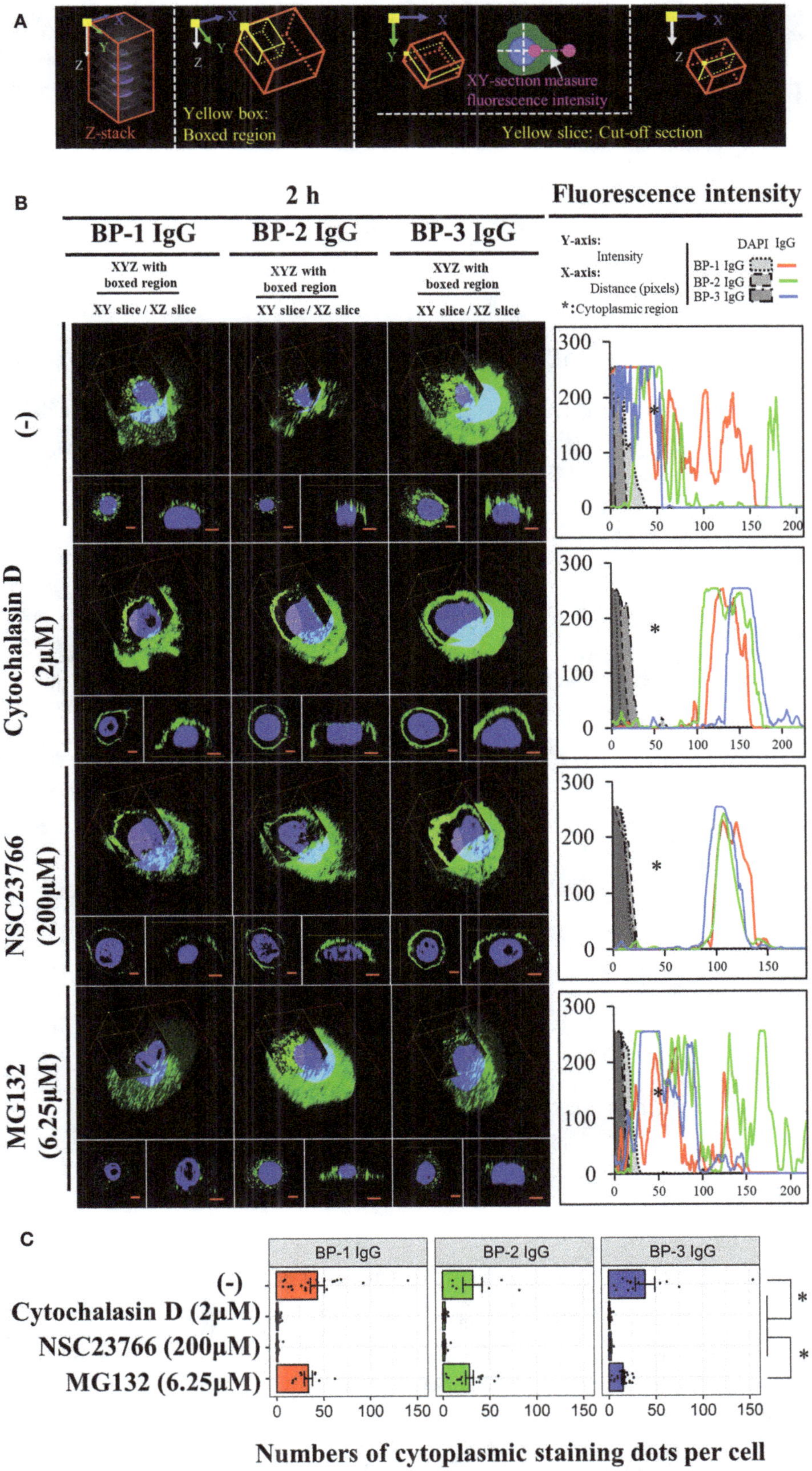

FIGURE 9 | Effects of cytochalasin D, NSC237766, and MG132 on the BP IgG-induced internalization. **(A)** Overview of the 3D reconstruction assay. The 3D reconstruction was performed as described in the methods. The boxed region indicates XYZ boxed area, XY slice indicates the horizontal slice and used to measure

(Continued)

FIGURE 9 | the fluorescence intensity, and XZ slice indicates the longitudinal slice. **(B)** Fluorescence microscopy images of the binding of the indicated IgGs to the NHEKs at 2 h. NHEKs were pretreated with cytochalasin D (2 μM) for 30 min, NSC23766 (200 μM) for 1 h, or MG132 (6.25 μM) for 0 h, and then 2 mg/ml BP IgGs (BP-1, BP-2, BP-3) or normal IgG were added to the cultured cells. The 3D reconstruction assay was applied to observe the changes. Scale bar 5 μm. **(C)** Quantification of the IgG-stained dots in cells. The anti-IgG-FITC-stained dots in the cytoplasmic region of individual cells were counted using the CellProfiler image analysis software. One-way ANOVA was used for the statistical analysis. *p-value < 0.05.

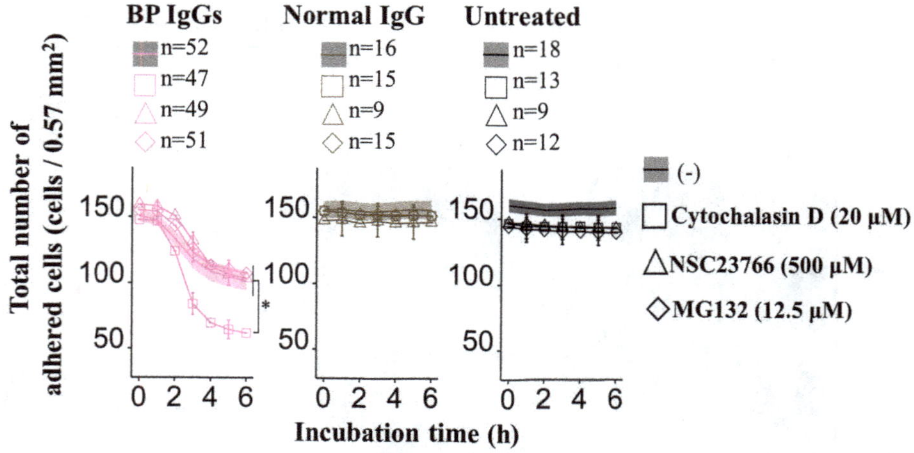

FIGURE 10 | Effects of cytochalasin D, NSC237766, and MG132 on the BP IgG-induced decrease in the number of adherent cells. NHEKs were pretreated with cytochalasin D (20 μM) for 30 min, NSC23766 (500 μM) for 1 h, or MG132 (12.5 μM) for 0 h, and then 2 mg/ml BP IgGs (BP-1, BP-2, and BP-3) or normal IgG were added to the cultured cells. Total numbers of adherent cells after the incubation with BP IgGs or normal IgG were counted every hour in a ×20 area (0.57 mm^2) for up to 6 h. One-way ANOVA was used for the statistical analysis. *p-value < 0.05.

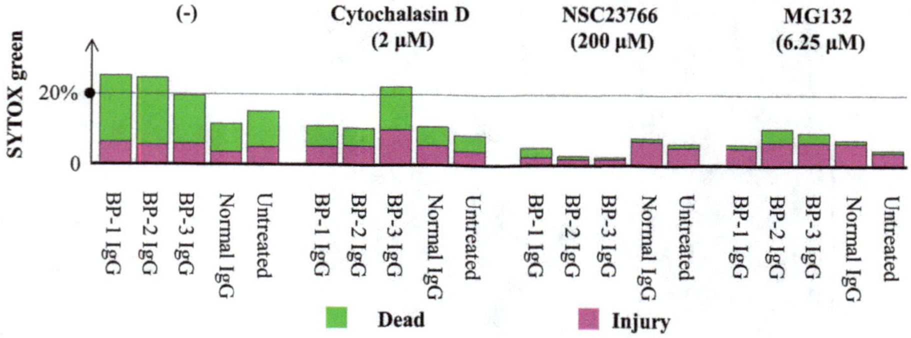

FIGURE 11 | Effects of cytochalasin D, NSC237766, and MG132 on the BP IgG-induced decrease in cellular metabolic activity. NHEKs were pretreated with cytochalasin D (2 μM) for 30 min, NSC23766 (200 μM) for 1 h, or MG132 (6.25 μM) for 0 h, and then 2 mg/ml BP IgGs (BP-1, BP-2, and BP-3) or normal IgG were added to the cultured cells for 16 h. Then, NHEKs were collected, stained with SYTOX green (stains dead cells) and C_{12}-resazurin (stains living cells), and analyzed using flow cytometry.

DISCUSSION

As shown in the present study, BP IgG directly induces NHEK dysfunction, as BP IgG stimulation increases SYTOX green staining, revealing structural disintegration of the plasma membrane, intercellular vesicle formation, and mitochondrial dysfunction, but not chromatin condensation. In addition, BP IgG induced cell dysfunction by activating Rac1 and the proteasome. Our findings support the hypothesis proposed by Ujiie et al. that BP IgG directly causes subepidermal bulla formation in patients with BP (41).

We considered two possible explanations for BP IgG-induced cell dysfunction: methuosis or oncosis. The well-known response of NHEKs to BP IgG stimulation is macropinosome formation (43, 54). In mammalian cells, hyperstimulation of macropinosomes is known to lead to methuosis, which is defined as the maturation of macropinosomes (48, 49). We first tested whether the BP IgG-induced accumulation of fluid-filled endocytic vesicles was catastrophic and ultimately merged with the lysosomes, as previously reported (55), to distinguish between these mechanisms. However, refuting our methuosis hypothesis, BP IgG-induced

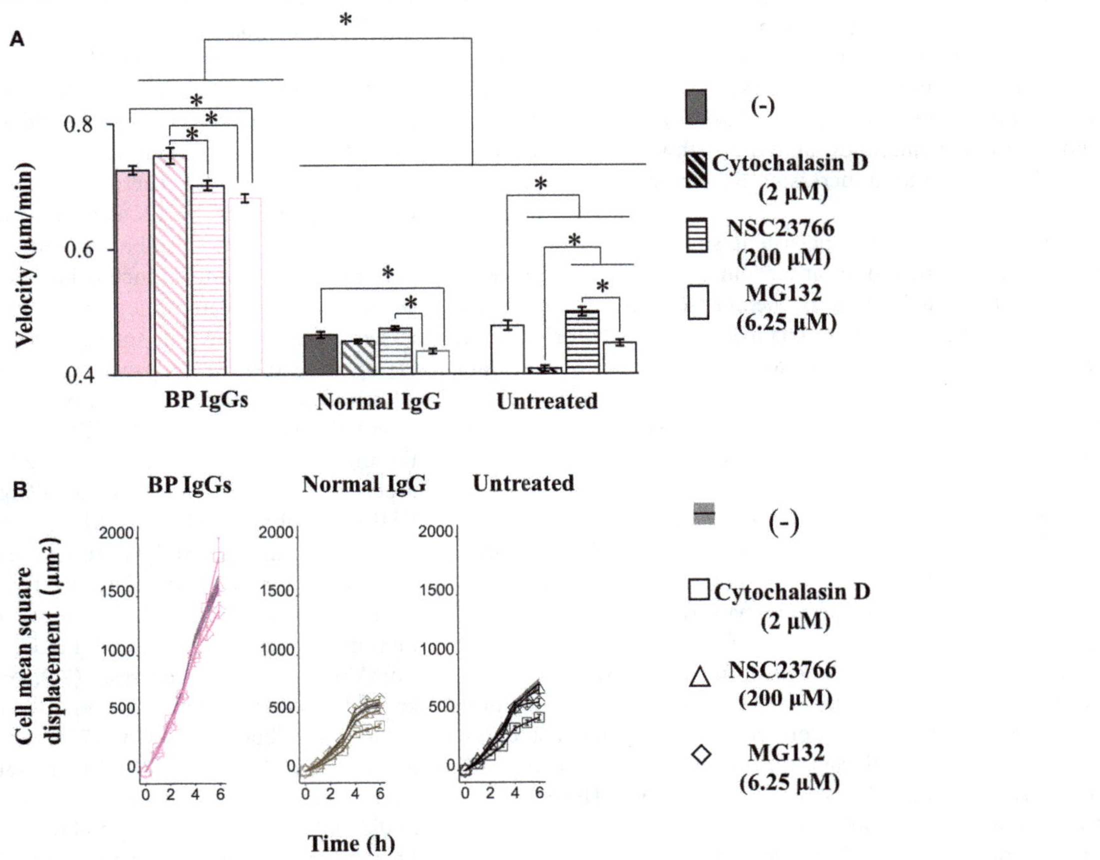

FIGURE 12 | Effects of cytochalasin D, NSC237766, and MG132 on the BP IgG-induced increase in cell motility. NHEKs were pretreated with cytochalasin D (2 μM) for 30 min, NSC23766 (200 μM) for 1 h, or MG132 (6.25 μM) for 0 h, and then 2 mg/ml BP IgGs (BP-1, BP-2, BP-3) or normal IgG were incubated with the cultured cells for 6 h. **(A)** Velocity of the NHEKs stimulated with IgGs. One-way ANOVA was used for the statistical analysis. *: p-value < 0.05. **(B)** Mean square displacement of the NHEKs stimulated with IgGs.

macropinosomes did not merge with lysosomes, excluding the possibility of methuosis. The alternative explanation is oncosis, a type of cell dysfunction caused by cell membrane damage characterized by cellular and/or organelle swelling (56). Our ultrastructural and morphological observations were consistent with these changes (**Figures 4, 5** and **Supplementary Figure S1**).

Importantly, our data provided evidence supporting the relationship between BP IgG-induced cell dysfunction and lysosome accumulation and mitochondria dysfunction (**Figures 5–7**). Cell membrane injury directly results in acute cell dysfunction, and the dying cells release endogenous alarm signals, which trigger the innate immune system and modulate inflammation through the lysosome-induced increase in the levels and excessive formation of ROS (50, 57). In contrast, the lysosomes mediate plasma membrane repair and control cellular dysfunction (50, 58). Mitochondrial dysfunction usually leads to mammalian cell death and influences the immune system to perceive/react to the dying cells (51, 59). Lysosome-mediated cellular dysfunction is characterized by simultaneous membrane damage and the proteolysis of a wide range of proteins (60). Lysotracker® Green DND-26, a marker of the lysosome membrane potential (60), helped identify BP IgG-treated cells with a higher lysosome membrane potential. Conceivably, the proteolytic enzymes released from lysosomes trigger a forward loop promoting lysosome rupture after a 2 h treatment with BP IgG. Moreover, the proteasome inhibitor MG132 efficiently blocks lysosome rupture (61) and has attracted considerable attention as an anti-BP agent (41). Therefore, MG132 likely exerted its protective effects on BP IgG-induced cell dysfunction in our study through its antilysosome/proteasome effects. Not surprisingly, several skin diseases are reported to be associated with alterations in mitochondria-related metabolic pathways (59). Consistent with the results of our ROS assay, the BP disease process was recently reported to be characterized by ROS production (62). We provided direct evidence that cell membrane fragility follows ROS production induced by BP IgG stimulation, which ultimately significantly increases cell membrane fragility, although we have not identified the molecular events underlying ROS production. The cell membrane is the site of activation of numerous signaling cascades that induce mitochondrial dysfunction. Interestingly, Rac1 is reported to be located both at the plasma membrane and mitochondrial membrane (63). The administration of NSC23766 decreases ROS production and promotes cell survival (64). Rac1 activation might serve as the initial step to "destroy" both the cell and mitochondrial membranes, and the pathways downstream of Rac1 also contribute to increasing ROS production to promote cellular dysfunction.

We conclude that the persistent stimulation with BP IgG induced the formation of macropinosomes in keratinocytes, resulting in a fragile plasma membrane, intercellular vesicle formation, lysosome accumulation, and ROS production, which ultimately contribute to mitochondrial dysfunction. The BP IgG-induced alterations in keratinocytes trigger the immune system to digest the basal keratinocytes, causing the formation of blisters on the skin along with BMZ.

Our study has limitations. For example, we had limited explanations for the association of BP IgG-induced keratinocyte alterations with blister formation. Similar to the results from a previous study of basal keratinocytes (*in vivo*) from patients with BP (65), intercellular vesicles filled with villi and swelled mitochondria were also observed in our TEM experiment. We first considered that the intercellular vesicles likely form in response to the maturation of macropinosomes, and the lysosome-mediated pathway contributes to vesicle expansion and exerts potential effects on skin blistering. However, the intracytoplasmic accumulation of lysosomes/autophagosomes are not observed in ultrastructural images *in vivo* (65–67). In addition, histopathology rarely reveals degenerated keratinocytes in patients with early-stage BP. We considered that the pattern of ColXVII expression differs between keratinocytes *in vivo* (hemidesmosome ColXVII) and *in vitro* (nonhemidesmosome ColXVII) (15, 16, 21); future studies should provide insights into the different changes in keratinocytes *in vitro* and *in vivo* during the BP IgG-induced blistering process.

We also describe the role of ColXVII in regulating cell adhesion and motility (**Figures 3**, **8**, **10**, **12**). The formation of the BP IgG-ColXVII complex has been shown to tear the weakened lamina lucida, leading to a specific split at the lamina lucida and induction of BMZ blistering (37). According to another report, ColXVII mediates the anchorage of basal keratinocytes by regulating cell motility (68). Thus, we speculate that the changes in the adhesion and motility of keratinocytes are involved in the pathogenesis of blistering in patients with BP. As shown in reports (69, 70), IgGs targeting proteins other than ColXVII-NC16a do not detach cells from culture dishes. Interestingly, an IgG targeting the C-terminus of ColXVII neither induced obvious IgG-ColXVII internalization nor had any significant effect on cell detachment. Together with the results of the *in vivo* study showing that IgGs targeting the ColXVII ectodomain fail to reproduce blistering in an animal model (71), the findings from previous studies and our data confirm the pathogenicity of the anti-ColXVII-NC16a antibodies in subjects with BP. Based on the existing literature, the reduction in the cell adhesion observed upon BP IgG stimulation can be accounted for by ColXVII internalization (43, 72). However, researchers have not clearly determined how ColXVII internalization might influence cell adhesion. In the present study, the BP IgG-induced cell detachment was not directly induced by macropinosome formation, because alterations in actin, the well-known and necessary molecule for macropinosome formation (73), did not completely prevent NHEK detachment. NHEKs disassembled their contacts with neighboring cells and detached from the culture dish following an incubation with BP IgG. Furthermore, epithelial cell "destabilization" has also been shown to require a step mediated by the proteasome (74). For this reason, we speculated and confirmed that the BP IgG-induced cell detachment was associated with proteasome activation, and the internalization of the IgG-ColXVII complex probably requires the initial event of proteasome activation. Another interesting aspect of this study was that the BP IgG treatment increased NHEK motility. Based on the BP IgG-induced cell detachment, we speculate that the BP IgG-induced alterations in cell motility are likely due to a decrease in the cell density. On the other hand, ColXVII has been shown to regulate keratinocyte motility, while changes in cell motility following the loss of ColXVII remain controversial (26). Studies using ColXVII-knockdown keratinocytes have reported that the loss of ColXVII reduces lamellipodial stability (75) and induces cell migration mediated by Rac1 (76, 77). Cell migration is associated with the remodeling of the actin cytoskeleton. However, cytochalasin D did not affect cell motility following the BP IgG treatment. This discrepancy might be explained by the binding of ColXVII to two different cytoskeleton systems in keratinocytes: actin-associated focal contacts and keratin-associated hemidesmosome compounds (15, 78, 79).

Our findings provide a better understanding of the direct effects of BP IgG on keratinocytes by increasing the fragility of the cell membrane, resulting in keratinocyte dysfunction, probably through oncosis. In addition, the BP IgG-induced cellular dysfunction was reversed by Rac1/proteasome inhibition. We believe that our identification of the Rac1/proteasome-mediated signaling pathway provides valuable new insights that have improved our understanding of the direct effects of BP IgG on keratinocytes.

AUTHOR CONTRIBUTIONS

DT designed the study and wrote the initial draft of the manuscript. XD contributed to data collection and interpretation, and critically reviewed the manuscript. KN contributed to data interpretation and critically reviewed the manuscript. NY and OY contributed to the electron microscopy experiments and data interpretation, and OY critically reviewed the manuscript. EM supervised the entire study, provided critical intellectual input, and approved the final version of the manuscript. All authors approved the final version of the manuscript and agree to be accountable for all aspects of the work and ensuring that questions related to the accuracy or integrity of any part of the work are appropriately investigated and resolved.

ACKNOWLEDGMENTS

We thank the staff of the Department of Dermatology, Faculty of Medicine, Shimane University for the support they provided during daily experiments. We would like to acknowledge the technical expertise of the Interdisciplinary Center for Science Research, Organization for Research and Academic Information, Shimane University.

REFERENCES

1. Giudice GJ, Emery DJ, Diaz LA. Cloning and primary structural analysis of the bullous pemphigoid autoantigen BP180. *J Invest Dermatol.* (1992) 99:243–50. doi: 10.1111/1523-1747.ep12616580
2. Liu Z. Immunopathology of bullous pemphigoid, an autoimmune and inflammatory skin blistering disease. *Keio J Med.* (2003) 52:128–33. doi: 10.2302/kjm.52.128
3. Iwata H, Ujiie H. Complement-independent blistering mechanisms in bullous pemphigoid. *Exp Dermatol.* (2017) 26:1235–9. doi: 10.1111/exd.13367
4. Ludwig RJ, Vanhoorelbeke K, Leypoldt F, Kaya Z, Bieber K, McLachlan SM, et al. Mechanisms of Autoantibody-Induced Pathology. *Front Immunol.* (2017) 8:603. doi: 10.3389/fimmu.2017.00603
5. Joly P, Roujeau J-C, Benichou J, Delaporte E, D'Incan M, Dreno B, et al. A comparison of two regimens of topical corticosteroids in the treatment of patients with bullous pemphigoid: a multicenter randomized study. *J Invest Dermatol.* (2009) 129:1681–7. doi: 10.1038/jid.2008.412
6. Kubin ME, Hellberg L, Palatsi R. Glucocorticoids: the mode of action in bullous pemphigoid. *Exp Dermatol.* (2017) 26:1253–60. doi: 10.1111/exd.13408
7. Moghadam-Kia S, Werth VP. Prevention and treatment of systemic glucocorticoid side effects. *Int J Dermatol.* (2010) 49:239–48. doi: 10.1111/j.1365-4632.2009.04322.x
8. Wojnarowska F, Kirtschig G, Highet AS, Venning VA, Khumalo NP. Guidelines for the management of bullous pemphigoid. *Br J Dermatol.* 147:214–21. doi: 10.1046/j.1365-2133.2002.04835.x
9. Liu Y, Li L, Xia Y. BP180 is critical in the autoimmunity of bullous pemphigoid. *Front Immunol.* (2017) 8:1752. doi: 10.3389/fimmu.2017.01752
10. Schmidt E, Zillikens D. Pemphigoid diseases. *Lancet* (2013) 381:320–32. doi: 10.1016/S0140-6736(12)61140-4
11. Iwasaki T, Olivry T, Lapiere JC, Chan LS, Peavey C, Liu YY, et al. Canine bullous pemphigoid (BP): identification of the 180-kd canine BP antigen by circulating autoantibodies. *Vet Pathol.* (1995) 32:387–93. doi: 10.1177/030098589503200407
12. Kobayashi M, Amagai M, Kuroda-Kinoshita K, Hashimoto T, Shirakata Y, Hashimoto K, et al. BP180 ELISA using bacterial recombinant NC16a protein as a diagnostic and monitoring tool for bullous pemphigoid. *J Dermatol Sci.* (2002) 30:224–32. doi: 10.1016/S0923-1811(02)00109-3
13. Haeberle S, Wei X, Bieber K, Goletz S, Ludwig RJ, Schmidt E, et al. Regulatory T-cell deficiency leads to pathogenic bullous pemphigoid antigen 230 autoantibody and autoimmune bullous disease. *J Allergy Clin Immunol.* (2018) 142:1831–42.e7. doi: 10.1016/j.jaci.2018.04.006
14. Muramatsu K, Ujiie H, Kobayashi I, Nishie W, Izumi K, Ito T, et al. Regulatory T-cell dysfunction induces autoantibodies to bullous pemphigoid antigens in mice and human subjects. *J Allergy Clin Immunol.* (2018) 142:1818–30.e6. doi: 10.1016/j.jaci.2018.03.014
15. Hiroyasu S, Colburn ZT, Jones JCR. A hemidesmosomal protein regulates actin dynamics and traction forces in motile keratinocytes. *FASEB J.* (2016) 30:2298–310. doi: 10.1096/fj.201500160R
16. Ozawa T, Tsuruta D, Jones JCR, Ishii M, Ikeda K, Harada T, et al. Dynamic relationship of focal contacts and hemidesmosome protein complexes in live cells. *J Invest Dermatol.* (2010) 130:1624–35. doi: 10.1038/jid.2009.439
17. Nonaka S, Ishiko A, Masunaga T, Nishikawa T, Akiyama M, Owaribe K, et al. The extracellular domain of BPAG2 has a loop structure in the carboxy terminal flexible tail *in vivo*. *J Invest Dermatol.* (2000) 115:889–92. doi: 10.1046/j.1523-1747.2000.00136.x
18. Hägg P, Väisänen T, Tuomisto A, Rehn M, Tu H, Huhtala P, et al. Type XIII collagen: a novel cell adhesion component present in a range of cell–matrix adhesions and in the intercalated discs between cardiac muscle cells. *Matrix Biol.* (2001) 19:727–42. doi: 10.1016/S0945-053X(00)00119-0
19. Nievers MG, Schaapveld RQJ, Sonnenberg A. Biology and function of hemidesmosomes. *Matrix Biol.* (1999) 18:5–17. doi: 10.1016/S0945-053X(98)00003-1
20. Nishimura M, Nishie W, Shirafuji Y, Shinkuma S, Natsuga K, Nakamura H, et al. Extracellular cleavage of collagen XVII is essential for correct cutaneous basement membrane formation. *Hum Mol Genet.* (2016) 25:328–39. doi: 10.1093/hmg/ddv478
21. Watanabe M, Natsuga K, Nishie W, Kobayashi Y, Donati G, Suzuki S, et al. Type XVII collagen coordinates proliferation in the interfollicular epidermis. *eLife* (2017) 6:26635. doi: 10.7554/eLife.26635
22. Jonkman MF, de Jong MC, Heeres K, Pas HH, van der Meer JB, Owaribe K, et al. 180-kD bullous pemphigoid antigen (BP180) is deficient in generalized atrophic benign epidermolysis bullosa. *J Clin Invest.* (1995) 95:1345–52. doi: 10.1172/JCI117785
23. Walko G, Castañón MJ, Wiche G. Molecular architecture and function of the hemidesmosome. *Cell Tissue Res.* (2015) 360:529–44. doi: 10.1007/s00441-015-2216-6
24. Yancey KB. The pathophysiology of autoimmune blistering diseases. *J Clin. Invest.* (2005) 115:825–8. doi: 10.1172/JCI200524855
25. Ujiie H, Shibaki A, Nishie W, Shimizu H. What's new in bullous pemphigoid. *J Dermatol.* (2010) 37:194–204. doi: 10.1111/j.1346-8138.2009.00792.x
26. Natsuga K, Watanabe M, Nishie W, Shimizu H. Life before and beyond blistering: the role of collagen XVII in epidermal physiology. *Exp Dermatol.* doi: 10.1111/exd.13550. [Epub ahead of print].
27. Franzke C-W, Bruckner P, Bruckner-Tuderman L. Collagenous transmembrane proteins: recent insights into biology and pathology. *J Biol Chem.* (2005) 280:4005–8. doi: 10.1074/jbc.R400034200
28. Nishie W, Jackow J, Hofmann SC, Franzke C-W, Bruckner-Tuderman L. Coiled coils ensure the physiological ectodomain shedding of collagen XVII. *J Biol Chem.* (2012) 287:29940–8. doi: 10.1074/jbc.M112.345454
29. Yasukochi A, Teye K, Ishii N, Hashimoto T. Clinical and immunological study of 332 Japanese patients tentatively diagnosed with anti-BP180-type mucous membrane pemphigoid: a novel BP180 C-terminal domain enzyme-linked immunoassay. *Acta Dermatol Venereol.* (2014) 96:762–7. doi: 10.2340/00015555-2407
30. van Beek N, Lüttmann N, Huebner F, Recke A, Karl I, Schulze FS, et al. Correlation of serum levels of IgE autoantibodies against BP180 with bullous pemphigoid disease activity. *JAMA Dermatol.* (2017) 153:30. doi: 10.1001/jamadermatol.2016.3357
31. Arbache ST, Nogueira TG, Delgado L, Miyamoto D, Aoki V. Immunofluorescence testing in the diagnosis of autoimmune blistering diseases: overview of 10-year experience. *An Bras Dermatol.* (2014) 89:885–9. doi: 10.1590/abd1806-4841.20143221
32. Giang J, Seelen MAJ, van Doorn MBA, Rissmann R, Prens EP, Damman J. Complement activation in inflammatory skin diseases. *Front Immunol.* (2018) 9:639. doi: 10.3389/fimmu.2018.00639

33. de Graauw E, Sitaru C, Horn M, Borradori L, Yousefi S, Simon H-U, et al. Evidence for a role of eosinophils in blister formation in bullous pemphigoid. *Allergy* (2017) 72:1105–13. doi: 10.1111/all.13131
34. Riani M, Le Jan S, Plée J, Durlach A, Le Naour R, Haegeman G, et al. Bullous pemphigoid outcome is associated with CXCL10-induced matrix metalloproteinase 9 secretion from monocytes and neutrophils but not lymphocytes. *J Allergy Clin Immunol.* (2017) 139:863–72.e3. doi: 10.1016/j.jaci.2016.08.012
35. Vassileva S. Immunofluorescence in dermatology. *Int J Dermatol.* (2007) 32:153–61. doi: 10.1111/j.1365-4362.1993.tb02785.x
36. Dainichi T, Chow Z, Kabashima K. IgG4, complement, and the mechanisms of blister formation in pemphigus and bullous pemphigoid. *J Dermatol Sci.* (2017) 88:265–70. doi: 10.1016/j.jdermsci.2017.07.012
37. Iwata H, Kamio N, Aoyama Y, Yamamoto Y, Hirako Y, Owaribe K, et al. IgG from patients with bullous pemphigoid depletes cultured keratinocytes of the 180-kDa bullous pemphigoid antigen (Type XVII Collagen) and weakens cell attachment. *J Invest Dermatol.* (2009) 129:919–26. doi: 10.1038/jid.2008.305
38. Imanishi A, Imanishi H, Hiroyasu S, Ozawa T, Koga H, Ishii N, et al. Anti-BP180-type mucous membrane pemphigoid immunoglobulin G shows heterogeneity of internalization of BP180/collagen XVII into keratinocyte cytoplasm. *Med Mol Morphol.* (2016) 49:89–97. doi: 10.1007/s00795-015-0128-x
39. Chijiwa C, Takeoka S, Kamata M, Tateishi M, Fukaya S, Hayashi K, et al. Decrease in eosinophils infiltrating into the skin of patients with dipeptidyl peptidase-4 inhibitor-related bullous pemphigoid. *J Dermatol.* (2018) 45:596–9. doi: 10.1111/1346-8138.14245
40. Natsuga K, Nishie W, Shinkuma S, Ujiie H, Nishimura M, Sawamura D, et al. Antibodies to pathogenic epitopes on type XVII collagen cause skin fragility in a complement-dependent and -independent manner. *J Immunol.* (2012) 188:5792–9. doi: 10.4049/jimmunol.1003402
41. Ujiie H, Sasaoka T, Izumi K, Nishie W, Shinkuma S, Natsuga K, et al. Bullous pemphigoid autoantibodies directly induce blister formation without complement activation. *J Immunol.* (2014) 193:4415–28. doi: 10.4049/jimmunol.1400095
42. Diaz LA, Marcelo CL. Pemphigoid and pemphigus antigens in cultured epidermal cells. *Br J Dermatol.* (1978) 98:631–7. doi: 10.1111/j.1365-2133.1978.tb03581.x
43. Hiroyasu S, Ozawa T, Kobayashi H, Ishii M, Aoyama Y, Kitajima Y, et al. Bullous pemphigoid IgG induces BP180 internalization via a macropinocytic pathway. *Am J Pathol.* (2013) 182:828–40. doi: 10.1016/j.ajpath.2012.11.029
44. Ha KD, Bidlingmaier SM, Liu B. Macropinocytosis exploitation by cancers and cancer therapeutics. *Front Physiol.* (2016) 7:381. doi: 10.3389/fphys.2016.00381
45. Norbury CC. Drinking a lot is good for dendritic cells. *Immunology* (2006) 117:443–51. doi: 10.1111/j.1365-2567.2006.02335.x
46. Weiner A, Mellouk N, Lopez-Montero N, Chang Y-Y, Souque C, Schmitt C, et al. Macropinosomes are key players in early shigella invasion and vacuolar escape in epithelial cells. *PLOS Pathog.* (2016) 12:e1005602. doi: 10.1371/journal.ppat.1005602
47. Kerr MC, Teasdale RD. Defining macropinocytosis. *Traffic* (2009) 10:364–71. doi: 10.1111/j.1600-0854.2009.00878.x
48. Maltese WA, Overmeyer JH. Methuosis. *Am J Pathol.* (2014) 184:1630–42. doi: 10.1016/j.ajpath.2014.02.028
49. Sun L, Li B, Su X, Chen G, Li Y, Yu L, et al. An ursolic acid derived small molecule triggers cancer cell death through hyperstimulation of macropinocytosis. *J Med Chem.* (2017) 60:6638–48. doi: 10.1021/acs.jmedchem.7b00592
50. Kroemer G, Jäättelä M. Lysosomes and autophagy in cell death control. *Nat Rev Cancer* (2005) 5:886–97. doi: 10.1038/nrc1738
51. Tait SWG, Green DR. Mitochondrial regulation of cell death. *Cold Spring Harb Perspect Biol.* (2013) 5:8706. doi: 10.1101/cshperspect.a008706
52. Ridley AJ. Rho GTPases and cell migration. *J Cell Sci.* (2001) 15:2713–22.
53. Egami Y. Molecular imaging analysis of Rab GTPases in the regulation of phagocytosis and macropinocytosis. *Anatom Sci Int.* (2016) 91:35–42. doi: 10.1007/s12565-015-0313-y
54. Iwata H, Kamaguchi M, Ujiie H, Nishimura M, Izumi K, Natsuga K, et al. Macropinocytosis of type XVII collagen induced by bullous pemphigoid IgG is regulated via protein kinase C. *Lab Invest.* (2016) 96:1301–10. doi: 10.1038/labinvest.2016.108
55. Dolat L, Spiliotis ET. Septins promote macropinosome maturation and traffic to the lysosome by facilitating membrane fusion. *J Cell Biol.* (2016) 214:517–27. doi: 10.1083/jcb.201603030
56. Weerasinghe P, Buja LM. Oncosis: an important non-apoptotic mode of cell death. *Exp Mol Pathol.* (2012) 93:302–8. doi: 10.1016/j.yexmp.2012.09.018
57. Mayer D, Armstrong D, Schultz G, Percival S, Malone M, Romanelli M, et al. Cell salvage in acute and chronic wounds: a potential treatment strategy. Experimental data and early clinical results. *J Wound Care* (2018) 27:594–605. doi: 10.12968/jowc.2018.27.9.594
58. Michelet X, Tuli A, Gan H, Geadas C, Sharma M, Remold HG, et al. Lysosome-mediated plasma membrane repair is dependent on the small GTPase Arl8b and determines cell death type in mycobacterium tuberculosis infection. *J Immunol.* (2018) 200:3160–9. doi: 10.4049/jimmunol.1700829
59. Feichtinger RG, Sperl W, Bauer JW, Kofler B. Mitochondrial dysfunction: a neglected component of skin diseases. *Exp Dermatol.* (2014) 23:607–14. doi: 10.1111/exd.12484
60. Jacobson LS, Lima H, Goldberg MF, Gocheva V, Tsiperson V, Sutterwala FS, et al. Cathepsin-mediated necrosis controls the adaptive immune response by Th2 (T helper type 2)-associated Adjuvants. *J Biol Chem.* (2013) 288:7481–91. doi: 10.1074/jbc.M112.400655
61. Brojatsch J, Lima H, Kar AK, Jacobson LS, Muehlbauer SM, Chandran K, et al. A proteolytic cascade controls lysosome rupture and necrotic cell death mediated by lysosome-destabilizing adjuvants. *PLoS ONE* (2014) 9:e95032. doi: 10.1371/journal.pone.0095032
62. de Graauw E, Sitaru C, Horn MP, Borradori L, Yousefi S, Simon D, et al. Monocytes enhance neutrophil-induced blister formation in an *ex vivo* model of bullous pemphigoid. *Allergy* (2018) 73:1119–30. doi: 10.1111/all.13376
63. Payapilly A, Malliri A. Compartmentalisation of RAC1 signalling. *Curr Opin Cell Biol.* (2018) 54:50–6. doi: 10.1016/j.ceb.2018.04.009
64. Kowluru RA, Kowluru A, Veluthakal R, Mohammad G, Syed I, Santos JM, et al. TIAM1-RAC1 signalling axis-mediated activation of NADPH oxidase-2 initiates mitochondrial damage in the development of diabetic retinopathy. *Diabetologia* (2014) 57:1047–56. doi: 10.1007/s00125-014-3194-z
65. Schaumburg-Lever G, Orfanos CE, Lever WP. Electron microscopic study of bullous pemphigoid. *Arch Dermatol.* (1972) 106:662–7.
66. Hashimoto K. Electron microscopy and histochemistry of pemphigus and pemphigoid. *Oral Surg Oral Med Oral Pathol.* (1972) 33:206–19. doi: 10.1016/0030-4220(72)90390-8
67. Rodrigo FG. Ultrastructural aspects of pemphigoid. *Br J Dermatol.* (2006) 88:143–9. doi: 10.1111/j.1365-2133.1973.tb07519.x
68. Tasanen K, Tunggal L, Chometon G, Bruckner-Tuderman L, Aumailley M. Keratinocytes from patients lacking collagen XVII display a migratory phenotype. *Am J Pathol.* (2004) 164:2027–38. doi: 10.1016/S0002-9440(10)63762-5
69. Wada M, Nishie W, Ujiie H, Izumi K, Iwata H, Natsuga K, et al. Epitope-dependent pathogenicity of antibodies targeting a major bullous pemphigoid autoantigen collagen XVII/BP180. *J Invest Dermatol.* (2016) 136:938–46. doi: 10.1016/j.jid.2015.11.030
70. Imafuku K, Iwata H, Kamaguchi M, Izumi K, Natsuga K, Ujiie H, et al. Autoantibodies of non-inflammatory bullous pemphigoid hardly deplete type XVII collagen of keratinocytes. *Exp Dermatol.* (2017) 26:1171–4. doi: 10.1111/exd.13331
71. Nishie W, Natsuga K, Iwata H, Izumi K, Ujiie H, Toyonaga E, et al. Context-dependent regulation of collagen XVII ectodomain shedding in skin. *Am J Pathol.* (2015) 185:1361–71. doi: 10.1016/j.ajpath.2015.01.012
72. Kitajima Y, Nojiri M, Yamada T, Hirako Y, Owaribe K. Internalization of the 180 kDa bullous pemphigoid antigen as immune complexes in basal keratinocytes: an important early event in blister formation in bullous pemphigoid. *Br J Dermatol.* (1998) 138:71–6.

73. Swanson JA. Shaping cups into phagosomes and macropinosomes. *Nat Rev Mol Cell Biol.* (2008) 9:639–49. doi: 10.1038/nrm2447
74. Tsukamoto T, Nigam SK. Cell-cell dissociation upon epithelial cell scattering requires a step mediated by the proteasome. *J Biol Chem.* (1999) 274:24579–84.
75. Hamill KJ, Hopkinson SB, Jonkman MF, Jones JCR. Type XVII collagen regulates lamellipod stability, cell motility, and signaling to Rac1 by targeting bullous pemphigoid antigen 1e to α6β4 integrin. *J Biol Chem.* (2011) 286:26768–80. doi: 10.1074/jbc.M110.203646
76. Pullar CE, Baier BS, Kariya Y, Russell AJ, Horst BAJ, Marinkovich MP, et al. β4 integrin and epidermal growth factor coordinately regulate electric field-mediated directional migration via Rac1. *Mol Biol Cell* (2006) 17:4925–35. doi: 10.1091/mbc.E06-05-0433
77. Maurer M, Altrichter S, Schmetzer O, Scheffel J, Church MK, Metz M. Immunoglobulin E-mediated autoimmunity. *Front Immunol.* (2018) 9:689. doi: 10.3389/fimmu.2018.00689
78. Kitajima Y. Cross-talk between hemidesmosomes and focal contacts: understanding subepidermal blistering diseases. *J Invest Dermatol.* (2010) 130:1493–6. doi: 10.1038/jid.2010.77
79. Seltmann K, Roth W, Kröger C, Loschke F, Lederer M, Hüttelmaier S, et al. Keratins mediate localization of hemidesmosomes and repress cell motility. *J Invest Dermatol.* (2013) 133:181–90. doi: 10.1038/jid.2012.256

6

Perspective From the 5th International Pemphigus and Pemphigoid Foundation Scientific Conference

Jinmin Lee[1], Victoria P. Werth[1,2], Russell P. Hall III[3], Rüdiger Eming[4], Janet A. Fairley[5], David C. Fajgenbaum[6], Karen E. Harman[7], Marcel F. Jonkman[8], Neil J. Korman[9], Ralf J. Ludwig[10], Dedee F. Murrell[11], Philippe Musette[12], Haley B. Naik[13], Christian D. Sadik[14], Jun Yamagami[15], Marc L. Yale[16] and Aimee S. Payne[1]*

[1] Department of Dermatology, University of Pennsylvania, Philadelphia, PA, United States, [2] Corporal Michael J. Crescenz VAMC, Philadelphia, PA, United States, [3] Department of Dermatology, Duke University, Durham, NC, United States, [4] Department of Dermatology and Allergology, Philipps-Universität Marburg, Marburg, Germany, [5] Department of Dermatology, University of Iowa, Iowa City, IA, United States, [6] Orphan Disease Center, Perelman School of Medicine, University of Pennsylvania, Philadelphia, PA, United States, [7] Centre of Evidence Based Dermatology, University of Nottingham, Nottingham, United Kingdom, [8] Department of Dermatology, University Medical Center Groningen, University of Groningen, Groningen, Netherlands, [9] Department of Dermatology, University Hospitals Cleveland Medical Center, Case Western Reserve University, Cleveland, OH, United States, [10] Department of Dermatology, Lübeck Institute of Experimental Dermatology, University of Lübeck, Lübeck, Germany, [11] Department of Dermatology, University of New South Wales, Sydney, NSW, Australia, [12] Department of Dermatology, Rouen University Hospital, Rouen, France, [13] Program for Clinical Research, Department of Dermatology, University of California, San Francisco, San Francisco, CA, United States, [14] Department of Dermatology, Allergy, and Venereology, University of Lübeck, Lübeck, Germany, [15] Department of Dermatology, Keio University, Tokyo, Japan, [16] International Pemphigus and Pemphigoid Foundation, Sacramento, CA, United States

***Correspondence:**
Aimee S. Payne
aimee.payne@uphs.upenn.edu

The 5th Scientific Conference of the International Pemphigus and Pemphigoid Foundation (IPPF), "Pemphigus and Pemphigoid: A New Era of Clinical and Translational Science" was held in Orlando, Florida, on May 15–16, 2018. Scientific sessions covered recent, ongoing, and future clinical trials in pemphigus and bullous pemphigoid, disease activity and quality of life instruments, and the IPPF Natural History Study. Furthermore, the meeting provided an opportunity to hear firsthand from patients, investigators, and industry about their experience enrolling for clinical trials.

Keywords: rituximab, Btk, FcRn, eotaxin, T-cell, fumarate, leukotriene, doxycycline

INTRODUCTION

Following successful meetings in Bethesda, Maryland, USA in 2001, 2005, and 2010, and Lübeck, Germany in 2017, the 5th International Pemphigus and Pemphigoid Foundation (IPPF) Scientific Conference was the first meeting to focus on clinical trials in pemphigus and pemphigoid and their methodologies. The meeting was organized by Drs. Aimee S. Payne, Victoria P. Werth, Russell P. Hall III, and IPPF Director Marc L. Yale and brought together over 175 researchers, clinicians, industry representatives, and patients representing 13 different countries to discuss the latest scientific and clinical data from technologies advancing to clinical trials in pemphigus and pemphigoid.

WHAT'S NEW IN PEMPHIGUS AND PEMPHIGOID CLINICAL TRIALS?

The first session of the meeting focused on results of ongoing and recently completed clinical trials in pemphigus, moderated by Drs. John Stanley (University of Pennsylvania, Philadelphia, PA, USA) and Ron Feldman (Emory University, Atlanta, GA, USA), as well as pemphigoid, moderated by Drs. David Woodley (University of Southern California, Los Angeles, CA, USA) and Enno Schmidt (University of Lübeck, Lübeck, Germany).

Pemphigus

B cells are major effector cells in autoimmunity, both through autoantibody production as well as cellular tolerance mechanisms. Dr. Philippe Musette (Rouen University Hospital, Rouen, France) spoke about major advances being made in refractory pemphigus patients by using B cell depleting therapies, in particular the anti-CD20 monoclonal antibody rituximab. A recent clinical trial (NCT00784589) supports rituximab usage as a first line therapy in pemphigus patients (1). Additionally, B cell depletion in patients represents an opportunity to better understand pemphigus pathophysiology and human B cell biology. Dr. Musette reported that rituximab induces a prolonged and continuous repopulation of naive B cells with a new repertoire after the initial B cell depletion, whereas the reappearance of memory B cells is markedly delayed (2). IL-10-producing regulatory B cells are also expanded and are capable of downregulating inflammation, making them potentially important for maintenance of tolerance. This delay of B cell maturation is associated with a blockage of the auto-reactive IgM to IgG class switching process. Thus, B cell depletion induces a two-step mechanism of immunosuppression in pemphigus by eliminating the autoreactive B cells involved in the production of pathogenic IgG+ autoantibodies and by promoting the appearance of regulatory B cells that can maintain long term immune tolerance.

Inhibition of Bruton's tyrosine kinase (BTK), a protein essential for B cell development, is an appealing therapeutic strategy for pemphigus based on the dual mechanism of action to block autoantibody production as well as to quickly dampen inflammation by inhibiting B cell activation. Dr. Dedee Murrell (University of New South Wales, Sydney, Australia) reported on an open label study of the oral BTK inhibitor, PRN1008 (NCT02704429), which was previously tested in healthy volunteers (3). In the current study, safety and efficacy was demonstrated in 21 pemphigus patients with mild to moderate disease (Pemphigus Disease Area Index score of 8–39), with a disease duration between 0 and 20 years. The primary endpoint of control of disease activity after 4 weeks treatment with PRN1008 was met in 61% of patients, who were concomitantly using a daily prednisone dose between 0 and 30 mg. PRN1008 will shortly commence a large, global, placebo-controlled, randomized phase 3 study in patients with pemphigus.

Inhibition of the neonatal Fc receptor (FcRn) can promote protection from autoimmunity by reducing serum antibody levels and blocking pro-inflammatory immune pathways. Recently, a humanized IgG4 monoclonal antibody was developed that specifically inhibits FcRn function (SYNT001) (4). This antibody has been evaluated in a phase 1b open label safety, tolerability, and activity study to treat subjects with pemphigus (NCT03075904). Dr. Russell Hall (Duke University, Durham, NC, USA) presented results of the phase 1b study showing that infusion of SYNT001 in human subjects resulted in a rapid lowering of circulating levels of IgG and was safe and well-tolerated. Subjects were found to have a mean total IgG reduction of 56% by Day 30, and 5 of 7 subjects showed reduction in disease activity by day 42 (5). Further studies are ongoing to evaluate the efficacy and safety of FcRn blockade in the treatment of pemphigus.

Pemphigoid

Dr. Karen Harman (University of Nottingham, Nottingham, UK) explained the characteristics of pragmatic and non-inferiority trials, illustrated by the BLISTER (bullous pemphigoid steroids and tetracyclines) study (ISRCTN13704604). A pragmatic trial is designed to reflect everyday clinical practice and represents the opposite end of the spectrum to an explanatory trial, performed under ideal conditions. The degree of pragmatism is measured over 9 domains using the PRECIS-2 tool. A non-inferiority trial is used to assess whether a test treatment is not clinically worse than standard care (control) by more than an acceptable predetermined margin (the non-inferiority margin) and comes from the concept of an acceptable alternative that may not be quite as effective standard care but may have other advantages such as cost, convenience or side-effects. The BLISTER study concluded that doxycycline is non-inferior to oral prednisolone for short-term disease control in bullous pemphigoid and significantly safer in the long-term (6).

Since bullous pemphigoid is characterized by a predominance of eosinophils both in the skin and in the blood, it is logical to target the eosinophil by treating with an antibody directed against eotaxin, a chemokine whose levels are elevated in the skin and blood of patients with BP. Dr. Neil Korman (Case Western Reserve University, Cleveland, OH, USA) discussed the results of a pilot phase 2a study of the safety and efficacy of bertilimumab, an anti-eotaxin-1 antibody, in the treatment of patients with bullous pemphigoid (NCT02226146). The results demonstrated that bertilimumab was safe and efficacious in the treatment of bullous pemphigoid. Despite only receiving three bertilimumab infusions and low doses of prednisone that were rapidly tapered, the nine subjects in this study showed rapid and durable improvement in disease activity with an 81% reduction in disease severity, along with a significant steroid-sparing effect. These promising preliminary findings should be followed up with larger controlled trial of longer duration.

Dr. Janet Fairley (University of Iowa, Iowa City, IA, USA) reviewed the current state of therapeutic clinical trials in bullous pemphigoid and studies of the mechanisms of lesion formation that could lead to new treatments. Currently there are no approved drugs for pemphigoid, and the advanced age of these patients and their co-morbidities have made clinical trials challenging. However, recently a number of new treatment options have been identified. Potential targets include complement, eosinophil chemotaxis and activation, polymorphonuclear cells, IgE and IgE receptors, IgG turnover, and cytokines. Several of these therapeutic strategies have shown promise in pre-clinical trials and case reports or case series. Larger controlled trials may lead to better treatments for pemphigoid patients.

CLINICAL TRIAL ENROLLMENT AND OUTCOMES

The second session of the meeting discussed data using disease-specific instruments that may help to determine clinical trial enrollment and outcomes, moderated by Drs. Katerina Patsatsi (Aristotle University School of Medicine, Thessaloniki, Greece) and Michael Hertl (Philipps-Universität Marburg, Marburg, Germany).

Dr. Jun Yamagami (Keio University, Tokyo, Japan) discussed a longitudinal study to quantify disease extent throughout the course of pemphigus and pemphigoid therapy, in order to better understand how the change in PDAI (Pemphigus Disease Area Index) or BPDAI (Bullous Pemphigoid Disease Area Index) score within the first 2 weeks from the initial treatment predicts whether the patient will require additional treatment. The study found significant change in the PDAI/BPDAI scores from baseline to 2 weeks between patients who needed additional treatment and those who did not, indicating that the ratio of PDAI/BPDAI scores could be useful as an objective parameter to determine the necessity of additional treatments.

Dr. Victoria Werth (University of Pennsylvania, Philadelphia, USA) discussed assessing the "quality" of quality of life surveys in autoimmune blistering disease. There are currently a number of skin-specific and one disease-specific autoimmune blistering disease quality of life instruments. A meta-analysis of health related quality of life in pemphigus identified at least 16 quality of life studies using 8 different instruments. It is important to determine which of the main instruments used capture the impact of disease on patients for both epidemiologic and therapeutic studies. This study sought to compare the change in three quality of life measures, including the autoimmune bullous diseases quality of life (ABQOL) questionnaire, the Dermatology Life Quality Index (DLQI), and the Skindex-29 (the latter of which has three subscores for symptoms, function, and emotion), with change in disease severity (measured in pemphigus with the Pemphigus Disease Area Index (PDAI) and Autoimmune Bullous Skin Disorder Intensity Score (ABSIS), and in bullous pemphigoid with the Bullous Pemphigoid Disease Area Index (BPDAI) and ABSIS) (7). Twenty three patients with mucosal involvement and 27 without mucosal involvement were enrolled and followed prospectively for a mean of 4.6 months. Sixty eight percent had pemphigus vulgaris, 12% had pemphigus foliaceus, and 20% had bullous pemphigoid. The Skindex-29 symptoms subscore correlated best with the change in disease severity ($r = 0.75$) relative to the ABQOL and DLQI ($r = 0.65$ and 0.68). The ABQOL had the best correlation with change in mucosal disease severity relative to Skindex-29 symptoms and DLQI ($r = 0.77$ vs. 0.66 and 0.56), and the Skindex-29 symptoms relative to ABQOL and DLQI had the best correlation with change in skin disease severity ($r = 0.81$ vs. 0.0.59 and 0.75). Overall the change in BPDAI and PDAI correlated more strongly with quality of life measurements than the ABSIS. Dr. Werth noted that the patients enrolled in the study had relatively mild disease, and higher correlations with the PDAI and BPDAI may reflect the ability to capture low disease activity accurately with these instruments.

PATIENT REPORTED OUTCOMES

The third session of the meeting focused on patient-reported outcomes, moderated by Drs. Meng Pan (Shanghai Jiao Tong University, Shanghai, China) and Animesh Sinha (University at Buffalo, Buffalo, NY, USA).

On behalf of the International Pemphigus and Pemphigoid Foundation (IPPF), Marc Yale (IPPF, Sacramento, CA, USA) summarized the Natural History Study being conducted by the IPPF. The IPPF Natural History Study is a new patient registry sponsored by the National Organization for Rare Disorders (NORD) and the US Food and Drug Administration (FDA). This online data system collects, stores, and retrieves patient data for analysis in research studies (https://pemphigus.iamrare.org/). The IPPF Natural History Study serves to provide a convenient online platform for patients or their legally authorized representative to report cases of pemphigus and pemphigoid, conduct a prospectively-planned natural history study that will result in the most comprehensive understanding of both diseases and their progression over time, and characterize and describe the pemphigus and pemphigoid population as a whole. In addition, it also serves to assist the pemphigus and pemphigoid community with the development of recommendations for standards of care, assist researchers studying the pathophysiology of pemphigus and pemphigoid, and support the design of clinical trials that explore new pemphigus and pemphigoid treatments. The IPPF Natural History Study is designed to help the medical and research community understand illness trends, treatment outcomes, disease burden, and some important demographic information about patient age and gender. With this vital information from large numbers of pemphigus and pemphigoid patients, the IPPF can better advocate for resources to improve patient support, education and outreach, as well as accelerate research.

Subsequently, Odette Miller (pemphigus patient, New Jersey, USA), Jeff Weisgerber (pemphigus patient, North Carolina, USA), Dr. Diana Chen (Genentech, South San Francisco, CA, USA), Ann Neale (Principia Biopharma, South San Francisco, CA, USA), and Dr. Donna Culton (University of North Carolina, Chapel Hill, NC, USA) led a panel discussion to allow patients who have participated in recent trials, as well as pharmaceuticals and investigators who have enrolled advanced phase clinical trials in pemphigus and pemphigoid to share their experiences.

COLLABORATIVE NETWORKS FOR RARE DISEASE RESEARCH

The co-founder of the Castleman Disease Collaborative Network, Dr. David Fajgenbaum (University of Pennsylvania, Philadelphia,

PA, USA) gave a keynote speech on the "collaborative network approach" that has helped to spearhead to accelerate research and drug discovery for Castleman disease (8). This information is significant because Castleman disease is one of the most common causes of paraneoplastic pemphigus, a highly deadly form of pemphigus. As rare diseases share many of the same hurdles in the way of drug discovery, there are great opportunities to leverage aspects of the collaborative network approach to make progress for pemphigus and other rare diseases.

CLINICAL TRIALS OF NOVEL CELLULAR THERAPIES FOR PEMPHIGUS

The fifth session of the meeting focused on future clinical trials in pemphigus, moderated by Drs. Annette Czernik (Icahn School of Medicine at Mount Sinai, New York, NY, USA) and Donna Culton (University of North Carolina, Chapel Hill, NC, USA).

In the pathogenesis of pemphigus, loss of immune tolerance to the major autoantigen desmoglein (Dsg) 3 is the key event leading to the production of Dsg-reactive autoantibodies. Dr. Rüdiger Eming (Philipps-Universität Marburg, Marburg, Germany) described strategies to restore immune tolerance to Dsg3 in the CD4+ T cell compartment by applying an HLA-transgenic mouse model of pemphigus. The study has shown that injecting animals with a set of immunodominant HLA-DRß1*04:02-binding Dsg3 peptides that are linked either to cellular carriers (splenocytes) or to defined particles (nanoparticles) prevents the induction of Dsg3-specific IgG antibodies upon Dsg3 immunization. Moreover, T cell reactivity to Dsg3 *in vitro* is markedly reduced in mice that previously received immunodominant Dsg3 peptides under tolerizing conditions. These results in the preclinical model provide the rationale for the development of a future phase I/II clinical trial to restore immune tolerance to Dsg3 in pemphigus vulgaris (PV) patients.

Adapted from a groundbreaking gene-engineered chimeric antigen receptor (CAR) T cell therapy that has led to long-lasting remissions of previously refractory B cell leukemia and lymphoma, Dsg3 chimeric autoantibody receptor T cell (DSG3-CAART) therapy has been shown to induce histologic and serologic remission of experimental pemphigus without detectable off-target toxicity in preclinical mouse models (9). Dr. Aimee Payne (University of Pennsylvania, Philadelphia, PA, USA) discussed strategies to move CAART technology forward to clinical trials in both mucosal PV, caused by antibodies to Dsg3, and in mucocutaneous PV, characterized by autoantibodies to Dsg3 and the homologous protein Dsg1. Dr. Payne reported that DSG1-CAART alone, and combined DSG1- and DSG3-CAART cells showed specific cytolysis of anti-DSG B cells, and no detectable toxicity to human skin xenografts *in vivo*. A first-in-human phase 1 clinical trial of DSG3-CAART in PV is planned to evaluate its safety and therapeutic potential.

Dr. Haley Naik (University of California San Francisco, San Francisco, CA, USA) reported on an autologous polyclonal regulatory T cell therapy as a strategy for limiting autoantibody production by augmenting immune regulation and re-establishing immune tolerance. A phase 1 open-label multicenter trial of autologous polyclonal regulatory T cells in patients with active pemphigus vulgaris and pemphigus foliaceus is being conducted toward this end (NCT03239470). In addition to clinical evaluation for safety, this study also aims to assess the presence and persistence of transferred regulatory T cells in blood and skin, alterations in the tissue immunologic milieu, and disease-specific and immunologic biomarkers in blood and skin. Safety and efficacy data generated from this study will lay the foundation for future studies using antigen-specific regulatory T cell therapy.

EMERGING THERAPIES IN CLINICAL DEVELOPMENT FOR PEMPHIGOID

The final invited speaker session covered future clinical trials in pemphigoid, moderated by Drs. Peter Marinkovich Stanford University, Stanford, CA, USA) and Soo-Chan Kim (Yonsei University, Seoul, Korea).

Dr. Marcel Jonkman (University of Groningen, Groningen, Netherlands) summarized an international survey on unmet needs in pemphigoid diseases to explore and prioritize unmet needs from the perspectives of patients, clinicians, and researchers. The priority need for patients is a quicker diagnosis, for clinicians labeling of new drugs, and for researchers more head-to-head randomized controlled trials. All surveyed groups agreed on a high need for improvement of current treatment options, and future research should focus on this unmet need.

Dr. Ralf Ludwig (University of Lübeck, Lübeck, Germany) reported on an upcoming clinical trial evaluating the safety and efficacy of dimethyl fumarate (DMF) in bullous pemphigoid, which will enroll the first patients this year in France, Germany, Poland and Turkey (DPem Trial). This trial was based on findings in preclinical animal models of epidermolysis bullosa acquisita (EBA) (10), where DMF reduced clinical disease severity in mice with already clinically manifest skin lesions. In addition to DMF, preclinical EBA models (11) have defined several new therapeutic targets, i.e., SYK (12, 13) and novel compounds (14).

Dr. Christian Sadik (University of Lübeck, Lübeck, Germany) presented the topic of the C5a-LTB_4 axis in bullous pemphigoid diseases (15). The eicosanoid leukotriene B_4 (LTB_4) and the complement factor C5, the precursor of the anaphylatoxin C5a, are both abundant in lesional skin of bullous pemphigoid patients, but their significance for the pathogenesis of bullous pemphigoid or other pemphigoid diseases is still largely elusive. In his talk, Dr. Christian Sadik demonstrated preclinical results from mouse models of pemphigoid diseases pointing at a critical role of LTB_4 in the recruitment of granulocytes to the dermal-epidermal junction (16). He discussed evidence that LTB_4 may closely interact with C5a in the regulation of skin inflammation and that hence, inhibiting these two factors individually or in parallel may be effective in the treatment of pemphigoid diseases.

CONCLUSIONS

The next decade offers exciting promise for an increasing number of clinical trials in pemphigus and pemphigoid as new preclinical programs advance to clinic and existing clinical stage companies apply their technologies to the treatment of pemphigus and pemphigoid. The patients, physicians, and researchers in the pemphigus and pemphigoid community remain committed to advocating for treatment options that improve the health and quality of life for pemphigus and pemphigoid patients.

AUTHOR CONTRIBUTIONS

JL wrote the first draft of the manuscript; VW, RH, RE, JF, DF, KH, MJ, NK, RL, DM, PM, HN, CS, JY, MY, and AP wrote sections of the manuscript. All authors contributed to manuscript revision, read and approved the submitted version.

ACKNOWLEDGMENTS

The conference was made possible by the sponsorship of Principia Biopharma, Syntimmune, Eli Lilly, Genentech, Immune Pharmaceuticals, argenx, and the EveryLife Foundation for Rare Diseases. We are indebted to Patrick Dunn, Nelly Filippov, Becky Strong, and Amethyst Yale at the IPPF for coordinating the conference.

REFERENCES

1. Joly P, Maho-Vaillant M, Prost-Squarcioni C, Hebert V, Houivet E, Calbo S, et al. French study group on autoimmune bullous skin, First-line rituximab combined with short-term prednisone versus prednisone alone for the treatment of pemphigus (Ritux 3): a prospective, multicentre, parallel-group, open-label randomised trial. *Lancet* (2017) 389:2031–40. doi: 10.1016/S0140-6736(17)30070-3
2. Colliou N, Picard D, Caillot F, Calbo S, Le CS, Lim A, et al. Long-term remissions of severe pemphigus after rituximab therapy are associated with prolonged failure of desmoglein B cell response. *Sci. Transl. Med.* (2013) 5:175ra30. doi: 10.1126/scitranslmed.3005166
3. Smith PF, Krishnarajah J, Nunn PA, Hill RJ, Karr D, Tam D, et al. A phase I trial of PRN1008, a novel reversible covalent inhibitor of Bruton's tyrosine kinase, in healthy volunteers. *Br J Clin Pharmacol.* (2017) 83:2367–76. doi: 10.1111/bcp.13351
4. Blumberg L, Humphries JE, Lasseter KC, Blumberg RS. SYNT001: a humanized IgG4 monoclonal antibody that disrupts the interaction of FcRn and IgG for the treatment of IgG-mediated autoimmune diseases. *Blood* (2017) 130:3483. Available online at: http://www.bloodjournal.org/content/130/Suppl_1/3483
5. Werth VP, Culton D, Blumberg L, Humphries J, Blumberg R, Hall R. FcRn blockade with SYNT001 for the treatment of pemphigus. *J Invest Dermatol.* (2018) 138:S92. doi: 10.1016/j.jid.2018.03.546
6. Williams HC, Wojnarowska F, Kirtschig G, Mason J, Godec TR, Schmidt E, et al. Doxycycline versus prednisolone as an initial treatment strategy for bullous pemphigoid: a pragmatic, non-inferiority, randomised controlled trial. *Lancet* (2017) 389:1630–8. doi: 10.1016/S0140-6736(17)30560-3
7. Kushner CJ, Pearson D, Tarazi M, Gaffney RG, Feng R, Payne AS, et al. Assessing the quality of quality of life measurement tools in autoimmune blistering disease. *J Invest Dermatol.* (2018) 138:S88. doi: 10.1016/j.jid.2018.03.523
8. Fajgenbaum DC, Ruth JR, Kelleher D, Rubenstein AH. The collaborative network approach: a new framework to accelerate Castleman's disease and other rare disease research. *Lancet Haematol.* (2016) 3:e150-2. doi: 10.1016/S2352-3026(16)00007-7
9. Ellebrecht CT, Bhoj VG, Nace A, Choi EJ, Mao X, Cho MJ, et al. Reengineering chimeric antigen receptor T cells for targeted therapy of autoimmune disease. *Science* (2016) 353:179–84. doi: 10.1126/science.aaf6756
10. Muller S, Behnen M, Bieber K, Moller S, Hellberg L, Witte M, et al. Dimethylfumarate impairs neutrophil functions. *J Invest Dermatol.* (2016) 136:117–26. doi: 10.1038/JID.2015.361
11. Bieber K, Koga H, Nishie W. *In vitro* and *in vivo* models to investigate the pathomechanisms and novel treatments for pemphigoid diseases. *Exp Dermatol.* (2017) 26:1163–70. doi: 10.1111/exd.13415
12. Samavedam UK, Mitschker N, Kasprick A, Bieber K, Schmidt E, Laskay T, et al. Whole-genome expression profiling in skin reveals SYK as a key regulator of inflammation in experimental epidermolysis bullosa acquisita. *Front Immunol.* (2018) 9:249. doi: 10.3389/fimmu.2018.00249
13. Nemeth T, Virtic O, Sitaru C, Mocsai A. The syk tyrosine kinase is required for skin inflammation in an *in vivo* mouse model of epidermolysis bullosa acquisita. *J Invest Dermatol.* (2017) 137:2131–9. doi: 10.1016/j.jid.2017.05.017
14. Koga H, Kasprick A, Lopez R, Auli M, Pont M, Godessart N, et al. Therapeutic effect of a novel phosphatidylinositol-3-kinase delta inhibitor in experimental epidermolysis bullosa acquisita. *Front Immunol.* (2018) 9:1558. doi: 10.3389/fimmu.2018.01558
15. Sadik CD, Miyabe Y, Sezin T, Luster AD. The critical role of C5a as an initiator of neutrophil-mediated autoimmune inflammation of the joint and skin. *Semin Immunol.* (2018) 37:21–9. doi: 10.1016/j.smim.2018.03.002
16. Sezin T, Krajewski M, Wutkowski A, Mousavi S, Chakievska L, Bieber K, et al. The leukotriene B4 and its receptor BLT1 act as critical drivers of neutrophil recruitment in murine bullous pemphigoid-like epidermolysis bullosa acquisita. *J Invest Dermatol.* (2017) 137:1104–13. doi: 10.1016/j.jid.2016.12.021

7

Immune Reaction to Type XVII Collagen Induces Intramolecular and Intermolecular Epitope Spreading in Experimental Bullous Pemphigoid Models

Hideyuki Ujiie, Norihiro Yoshimoto, Ken Natsuga, Ken Muramatsu, Hiroaki Iwata, Wataru Nishie and Hiroshi Shimizu*

Department of Dermatology, Hokkaido University Graduate School of Medicine, Sapporo, Japan

Correspondence:
Hideyuki Ujiie
h-ujiie@med.hokudai.ac.jp

Bullous pemphigoid (BP), the most common autoimmune blistering disease, is induced by autoantibodies to type XVII collagen (COL17). Previous studies demonstrated that COL17 harbors several epitopes targeted by autoreactive T and B cells and that the target epitopes change sequentially during the disease course. To elucidate the details of the humoral immune response to COL17, we used an active BP mouse model in which BP is induced by the adoptive transfer of spleen cells from wild-type mice immunized with human COL17-expressing skin grafting to immunodeficient COL17-humanized (Rag-$2^{-/-}$, mouse Col$17^{-/-}$, human COL17^{+}) mice. By immunoblot analysis, antibodies to the NC16A domain and other extracellular domains (ECDs) of COL17 were detected earlier than antibodies to intracellular domains (ICDs) in the active BP model. Time course analysis by enzyme-linked immunosorbent assay demonstrated a delayed peak of antibodies to ICD epitopes in active BP model. The blockade of CD40–CD40 ligand interaction soon after the adoptive transfer suppressed the production of antibodies to the non-collagenous 16A (NC16A) domain but not to an ICD epitope, suggesting the sequential activation from T and B cells against the ECD epitopes including the NC16A domain to those against ICD epitopes *in vivo*. Both wild-type mice immunized with a fragment of the NC16A domain and the recipients of those spleen cells produced IgG antibodies to ICD and ECD epitopes, showing intramolecular epitope spreading from the NC16A domain to other epitopes of COL17. Furthermore, we found that a portion of the active BP model mice show intermolecular epitope spreading from human COL17 to murine BP230. The appearance of antibodies to ICD epitopes of COL17 or of antibodies to murine BP230 did not correlate with the skin changes in the mice, suggesting that those antibodies have low pathogenicity. These results suggest that the immune response to the ECD epitopes of COL17, especially to the NC16*A* domain, triggers intramolecular, and intermolecular epitope spreading to ICD epitopes of COL17 and to murine BP230. These novel findings provide insight into the mechanism of epitope spreading in organ-specific, antibody-mediated autoimmune disorders.

Keywords: BP180, COL17, BP230, active mouse model, CD40 ligand, autoimmunity, autoantibody, NC16A domain

INTRODUCTION

Bullous pemphigoid (BP) is the most common autoimmune blistering disorder and is characterized by tense blisters with itchy urticarial plaques and erythema on the entire body. BP characteristically affects the elderly, and recent studies reported a trend of increased incidence of BP (1). BP is reported to be associated with increased risk for cardiovascular disease and neurological disease (2). Autoantibodies in BP react with two structural components of the dermal-epidermal junction (DEJ): type XVII collagen (COL17, also called BP180, or BPAG2) and BP230 (also called dystonin or BPAG1). The autoantibodies to COL17 are considered to trigger the inflammatory and non-inflammatory processes, resulting in the disruption of dermal-epidermal connection. COL17 is a hemidesmosomal transmembrane protein that spans the lamina lucida and projects into the lamina densa of the DEJ (3–10). The extracellular portion of COL17 contains 15 collagenous domains separated from one another by non-collagenous domains (4). The juxtamembranous extracellular non-collagenous 16A (NC16A) domain, located at the membrane-proximal region of COL17, is preferentially recognized by autoantibodies in BP patients (11, 12). Several studies have demonstrated that the serum levels of autoantibodies to the NC16A domain of COL17 are related to the disease activity of BP (13, 14). The passive transfer of IgG antibodies to the NC16A domain of human COL17 or its murine counterpart into neonatal mice directly demonstrates the *in vivo* pathogenicity of those antibodies (15, 16). Thus, the NC16A domain of COL17 contains the major pathogenic epitope for BP. In addition, it is well-known that the intracellular domain (ICD) and the extracellular domain (ECD) of COL17 are also targeted by autoantibodies of BP (17, 18). A previous study demonstrated that 47% of BP sera reacted to the C-terminal region of COL17 (19). Autoantibodies to the C-terminal region of COL17 are thought to be involved in mucous membrane pemphigoid (7). Furthermore, a recent study demonstrated that autoantibodies in BP patients which react to the full-length recombinant COL17 protein but not to the NC16A domain preferentially react to epitopes within the mid-portion of the ECD of COL17 (20).

BP230 is another autoantigen of BP and was originally identified as the major antigen of BP (21, 22). BP230 is a cytoplasmic component of hemidesmosomes that belongs to the plakin family; it promotes the linkage of keratin intermediate filaments to hemidesmosomes (23). More than 80% of BP sera show reactivity to BP230 (24, 25). It remains uncertain whether anti-BP230 autoantibodies directly contribute to blister formation or whether they are just by-products of epitope spreading associated with disease extension, although several studies have pointed to the pathogenicity of autoantibodies to BP230 (26–28).

Epitope spreading is a phenomenon in which the targets of T- and/or B-cell responses can extend from the initial dominant epitope to other epitopes on the same protein (intramolecular epitope spreading) or to other proteins in the same tissue (intermolecular epitope spreading) over time (29, 30). Intramolecular epitope spreading has been reported in several autoimmune disorders, such as multiple sclerosis (31) and myasthenia gravis (32). It is well-known that epitope spreading frequently occurs in BP. *In vivo* experiments using a human COL17-expressing skin-grafted BP mouse model showed that IgG antibodies to human COL17 initially react to the ECD epitopes and that, subsequently, the humoral immune responses target additional ECD and ICD epitopes (33). A prospective multicenter study demonstrated that 49% of 35 BP patients showed epitope spreading that preferentially occurred at an early stage of the disease and was associated with disease severity (34). Thus, epitope spreading has been shown in both experimental murine BP and human BP. However, many questions remain, such as whether the T- and B-cell interactions for different epitopes of COL17 occur at different times and whether an immune response to the NC16A domain of COL17 actually triggers intramolecular epitope spreading to other epitopes of COL17 and/or intermolecular epitope spreading to other hemidesmosomal antigens.

To address these issues, we utilized an active disease model for BP that we previously established (35). It is generated by the adoptive transfer of human COL17-immunized spleen cells into adult immunodeficient *Rag-2*$^{-/-}$/COL17-humanized (*COL17*$^{m-/-,h+}$) mice. This model continuously produces IgG antibodies to human COL17 in a CD4^{+} T-cell-dependent manner and reproduces the BP disease phenotype. By using this active BP model, the current study demonstrates that the production of antibodies to the ECD epitopes of COL17 precedes that to the ICD epitopes, especially to the inner portion of the ICD. The interference of T- and B-cell interaction by monoclonal antibody to the CD40 ligand (CD40L) shows that T- and B-cell interactions for ECD epitopes precede those to ICD epitopes of COL17 in an active BP model. Wild-type mice that were immunized with a fragment of the NC16A domain produced antibodies to ICD epitopes of COL17. Furthermore, the active BP model generates antibodies to murine BP230 as a result of intermolecular epitope spreading. These findings clarify the details of epitope spreading in BP.

MATERIALS AND METHODS

Mice

C57BL/6-background *Rag-2*$^{-/-}$ mice were received as a gift from the Central Institute for Experimental Animals (Kawasaki, Japan). We crossed *COL17*$^{m-/-,h+}$ (COL17-humanized) mice that we had previously generated (16) with *Rag-2*$^{-/-}$ mice to produce *Rag-2*$^{-/-}$/*COL17*$^{m-/-,h+}$ (Rag-2$^{-/-}$/COL17-humanized) mice.

Abbreviations: BP, bullous pemphigoid; COL17, type XVII collagen; NC16A, non-collagenous 16A; ICD, intracellular domain; ECD, extracellular domain; CD40L, CD40 ligand; IF, immunofluorescence; ELISA, enzyme-linked immunosorbent assay; NHS, normal human skin; skin-grafted wild-type mice, wild-type mice grafted with human COL17-expressing skin

Generation of Recombinant Proteins and Synthesized Peptides

Recombinant proteins covering all parts of human COL17 were generated in a previous study (36). Briefly, human ICD-1 (amino acids Met^1 to Ser^{204}), ICD-2 (Thr^{197} to Lys^{466}), NC16A (Glu^{490} to Arg^{566}), ECD-1 (Gly^{567} to Gly^{860}), ECD-2 (Leu^{853} to Gly^{1218}), and ECD-3 (Ser^{1211} to Pro^{1497}) were generated as GST-fusion proteins using the expression vector pGEX6P-1 (GE Healthcare) and the bacteria BL21 (GE Healthcare). These GST-fusion proteins were purified using GSTrap HP (GE Healthcare) according to the manufacturer's instructions. NC16A-R7 (Asp^{522} to Gln^{545}), 2 ICD peptides (ICD-149: Ala^{149} to Ser^{172}, ICD-320: Thr^{320} to Lys^{343}) and 3 ECD peptides (ECD-917: Lys^{917} to Ser^{940}, ECD-1084: Ser^{1084} to Pro^{1107}, ECD-1330: Ala^{1330} to Gly^{1353}) of human COL17 were chemically synthesized (Greiner Bio-One, Kremsmünster, Austria). The amino acid numbering system is based on the human COL17 sequence (NP_000494.3). Recombinant proteins covering all parts of murine BP230 were generated as previously reported (37). Briefly, total RNA of murine BP230 was extracted from murine keratinocytes, and cDNAs were synthesized by reverse transcription polymerase chain reaction. Plasmid vectors of 3 fragments of murine BP230 with His-tag at the C-terminus were designed. The 3 cDNA fragments were named BP230-1 (Met^1-Gly^{3264}), containing the N-terminal (plakin) domain; BP230-2 (Glu^{3223}-Pro^{5562}), containing the (coiled-coil) rod domain; and BP230-3 (Asp^{5533}-Gln^{7833}), containing the C-terminal (intermediate filament-binding) domain, according to GenBank (AF396877.1) and a previous report (38). These cDNAs were inserted into the pSeq Tag2/Hygro B vector (Thermo Fisher Scientific). Vectors were transfected into HEK293 cells with Lipofectamine 2000 (Thermo Fisher Scientific) for transient expression of BP230. Supernatants were collected and centrifuged for purification by using Amicon Ultra Centrifugal Filters (Merck Millipore, Darmstadt, Germany).

Generation of the Active BP Model

To make an active BP model, we first immunized wild-type mice with human COL17-expressing mouse skin graft according to the reported method (39). Briefly, full-thickness 1-cm^2 pieces of dorsal skin were removed from sacrificed COL17-humanized mice and grafted onto the backs of gender-matched, 6- to 8-week-old C57BL/6 wild-type mice. After the topical application of antibiotic ointment, the grafted site was covered with gauze and an elastic bandage for 14 days. Antibody production was confirmed at 5 weeks after skin grafting by immunofluorescence (IF) analysis, as described below. Spleen cells were isolated 5 weeks after the skin graft and pooled from several immunized wild-type mice, and 2.0×10^8 cells/mouse were adoptively transferred into *Rag-2*$^{-/-}$/COL17-humanized mice through a tail vain in 500 μL of PBS as previously reported (35). In some experiments, the wild-type mice were immunized at the hind footpad with 50 μg NC16A-R7 (fused with KLH) peptides emulsified in the adjuvant TiterMax Gold (TiterMax USA, Norcross, GA). The mice received an additional boost at the tail base 1 week after initial immunization. Negative controls were generated by immunization with phosphate-buffered saline (PBS) and TiterMax Gold. Spleen cells were isolated 5 weeks after immunization and pooled from several immunized wild-type mice, and 1.0×10^8 cells/mouse were transferred into *Rag-2*$^{-/-}$/COL17-humanized mice by retroorbital injection in 100 μL of PBS as previously described (40).

In vivo Anti-CD40L Antibody Treatment

Rag-2$^{-/-}$/COL17-humanized recipients that were adoptively transferred with immunized spleen cells were intraperitoneally injected with 1,000 μg hamster monoclonal antibody MR1 specific to mouse CD40L (Taconic Farms, Hudson, NY) at day 0 soon after the adoptive transfer of immunized splenocytes as previously reported (41). All of the treated mice were carefully observed for at least 10 weeks after adoptive transfer.

Evaluation of Recipient Mice

Weekly, the recipient mice were examined for general condition and for percentage of body surface area affected by cutaneous lesions (i.e., erythema, hair loss, blisters, erosions, and crusts). Serum samples were also obtained from recipient mice weekly and assayed by indirect IF microscopy and enzyme-linked immunosorbent assay (ELISA).

Indirect IF Study

Indirect IF using mice sera was performed on normal human skin (NHS) and wild-type mouse skin using standard protocols. We used 1:20 diluted mouse sera as the primary antibodies and 1:100 diluted FITC-conjugated antibodies to murine IgG (Jackson ImmunoResearch Laboratories, West Grove, PA) as the secondary antibodies.

Immunoblot Analysis

Immunoblotting of recombinant proteins covering human COL17 was performed as described previously (36). Briefly, each sample was solubilized in Laemmli's sample buffer and applied to SDS-polyacrylamide gels and then transferred to a nitrocellulose membrane. The membrane was blocked for 1 h at room temperature in 3% skimmed milk in TBS and then incubated with 1:20 diluted mouse serum samples overnight at 4°C. Bound antibodies were visualized using 1:500 diluted HRP-conjugated goat anti-rat IgG (Jackson ImmunoResearch). Color was developed with 4-chloro-1-naphthol in the presence of H_2O_2. For the detection of antibodies to murine BP230, recombinant murine BP230 proteins were used as a substrate. The membranes were incubated with 1:20 diluted mouse serum samples overnight at 4°C. Bound antibodies were visualized using 1:5,000 diluted HRP-conjugated goat anti-rat IgG (Jackson ImmunoResearch). As a positive control, 1:5,000 HRP-conjugated mouse anti-His-tag mAb-HRP-DirecT (MBL, Nagoya, Japan) was used. The blots were detected using the ECL Plus Detection Kit (GE Healthcare, Fairfield, CT).

ELISA

To determine the titer of antibodies to the NC16A domain of human COL17 in serum samples from the experimental mice, 96-well microtiter plates coated with recombinant NC16A protein purchased from MBL were incubated with diluted mouse sera for 1 h at room temperature. After being washed, bound antibodies were developed with 1:40,000-diluted, HRP-conjugated antibodies to mouse IgG (Jackson ImmunoResearch Laboratories), and the OD was read at 450 nm. The ELISA index value was defined by the following formula: index = (OD_{450} of tested serum—OD_{450} of negative control)/(OD_{450} of positive control—OD_{450} of negative control) ×100 (35). To examine the titers of antibodies to various regions of human COL17, synthesized peptides in 0.1 M sodium carbonate buffer (pH 9.5) were coated on F96 Maxisorp Nunc-Immuno plates (Thermo Scientific, Roskilde, Denmark) at 5 μg/ml and left overnight at 4°C. The plates were washed three times with PBS containing 0.05% Tween 20 and were blocked for 1 h at room temperature with ELISA assay diluent (BD Biosciences). They were incubated for 2 h at room temperature with 1:100-diluted mouse sera for NC16A-R7 or 1:25 for other peptides in assay diluent. The plates were washed four times and were incubated for 30 min at room temperature with 1:20,000-diluted HRP-conjugated antibodies to mouse IgG for NC16A-R7 or 1:10,000 for other peptides in an assay diluent. After four washings, the plates were displayed in a 1:1 mixture of substrate reagent A containing hydrogen peroxide and substrate reagent B containing tetramethylbenzidine (BD Biosciences) and were then stopped with 1 M phosphoric acid (BD Biosciences). The results were shown by OD at 450 nm. In some experiments, binding activities were calculated by the following formula: index value = (OD_{450} of tested serum—OD_{450} of negative control)/(OD_{450} of positive control—OD_{450} of negative control) ×100.

Statistical Analyses

Data were expressed as mean ± SEM. Statistical analyses were performed using GraphPad Prism (GraphPad Software, La Jolla, California, USA). The unpaired *t*-test with Welch's correction was used for comparisons of ELISA index in wild-type mice grafted with human COL17-expressing skin (skin-grafted wild-type mice). *P*-values of <0.05 were considered significant compared with the control.

RESULTS

Antibodies to the NC16A Domain of COL17 Decreased Earlier Than Those to the DEJ in the Active BP Model

First, we prepared the active BP mouse model by the adoptive transfer of spleen cells from a wild-type mouse that was immunized with human COL17-expressing skin grafting onto adult immunodeficient $Rag^{-/-}$/COL17-humanized mice (n = 4) (**Figure 1A**). Because human COL17-expressing skin contains full-length human COL17, the skin grafting theoretically induces polyclonal IgG antibodies to various regions of human COL17 in the skin-grafted wild-type mice as well as $Rag^{-/-}$/COL17-humanized recipient mice. As we previously reported (35), around day 7 after the adoptive transfer, the $Rag^{-/-}$/COL17-humanized recipients began to scratch their snouts, ears, and chests. Patchy hair loss with erythema started to develop on the neck and chest around 14 days after the adoptive transfer in the recipients. Ear swelling with crusts was also observed (**Figure 1B**). The dehaired patches gradually enlarged and spread to other regions on the trunk, face and extremities over the next 2–4 weeks, resulting in large areas of alopecia (**Figure 1B**). Dermal-epidermal separation with mild inflammatory cell infiltration was also seen in some of the ear samples at 5 weeks (**Figure 1B**). The affected body surface area plateaued 6 weeks after the transfer and remained high until 10 weeks after the transfer (**Figure 1C**).

Indirect IF examination using sera from the active BP model revealed that IgG bound to the DEJ of normal human skin. Time-course analysis revealed that IgG antibodies to the DEJ, which reflects the presence of antibodies to human COL17, became detectable in recipients' sera 1 week after the transfer. Although the titer gradually decreased after the peak, it remained high (> ×2,560) for 10 weeks (**Figure 1D**). We next examined the titer of antibodies to the NC16A domain of human COL17 by ELISA (MBL, Nagoya Japan). ELISA analysis revealed that antibodies to the NC16A domain of COL17 appeared in the recipients' sera as early as 1 week after the transfer. The antibody level peaked around day 9 after the transfer and then rapidly decreased, falling to a low level (<10% of the peak) at 6 weeks after the transfer (**Figure 1E**). These results demonstrate that the titers of total antibodies to human COL17 remained elevated for longer than did those to the NC16A domain, suggesting the presence of additional antibodies which are elevated in the late phase of the disease.

Antibodies to ECD and ICD Epitopes of COL17 Become Detectable at Different Times in the Active BP Model

To examine the presence of antibodies to various regions of human COL17 in the active BP model, we utilized 6 fragments of COL17 which were previously reported (**Figure 2A**) (36). By immunoblotting using those fragments from 4 active BP model mice, we analyzed the sera at days 8 and 56. All sera at day 8 strongly reacted to the NC16A domain and ECD fragments, but only one serum clearly reacted to ICD-2 and no serum bound to ICD-1 (**Figure 2B**). Interestingly, the reactivity of sera to NC16A, ECD-1, and ECD2 was apparently decreased at day 56, while the reactivity to ICD-2 was increased and ICD-1 was recognized by all sera (**Figure 2B**). The relative intensity of the reactivity is summarized in **Figure 2C**. To confirm these findings, we additionally analyzed sera from 4 active BP model mice at days 8, 35, and 56 after the adoptive transfer, and they showed a similar tendency (**Supplementary Figure 1**) Thus, antibodies to ECD epitopes of human COL17 are detectable from the early phase of the disease, whereas antibodies to ICD epitopes, especially to the inner portion of the ICD, were elevated in the late phase in the active BP model.

The Peak of Antibodies to an ICD Epitope of COL17 Lags That to the NC16A Domain and ECD Epitopes in the Active BP Model

To investigate the time course of antibodies to various epitopes of human COL17 in the active BP model, we newly generated

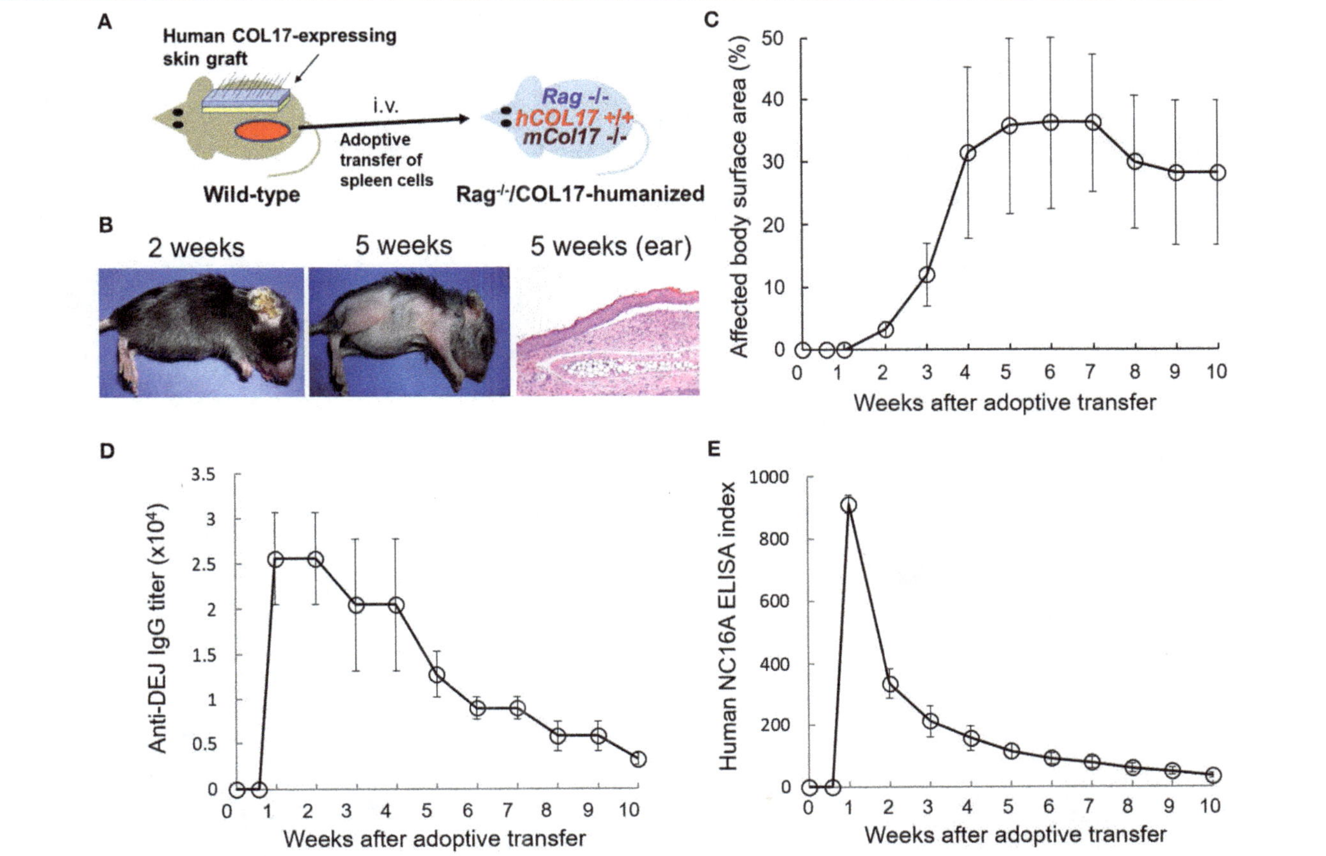

FIGURE 1 | Antibodies to the NC16A domain of COL17 decrease more rapidly than those to the dermal-epidermal junction (DEJ) in an active BP mouse model. **(A)** Schematic of the generation of an active BP mouse model. **(B)** Representative clinical presentations of the active BP model at 2 and 5 weeks after the adoptive transfer of immunized spleen cells and hematoxylin and eosin staining of the ear at 5 weeks (original magnification $\times 20$). **(C)** Time course of disease severities for the *Rag*$^{-/-}$/COL17-humanized recipients ($n = 4$). **(D)** Time course of titers of circulating IgG antibodies to the dermal-epidermal junction (DEJ) of the skin as determined by indirect IF using sera of an active BP model and normal human skin ($n = 4$). **(E)** Time course of the titers of circulating IgG antibodies to the NC16A domain as determined by ELISA ($n = 4$). Results are shown as mean $\pm$ SEM.

an ELISA using synthesized peptides of human COL17. As a fragment of the NC16A domain, we utilized the NC16A-R7 (Asp^{522} to Gln^{545}) peptide because we previously reported that IgG antibodies to R7, but not to other portions of the NC16A domain, are pathogenic *in vivo* (36). We also synthesized 2 ICD peptides (ICD-149: Ala^{149} to Ser^{172}, ICD-320: Thr^{320} to Lys^{343}) and 3 ECD peptides (ECD-917: Lys^{917} to Ser^{940}, ECD-1084: Ser^{1084} to Pro^{1107}, ECD-1330: Ala^{1330} to Gly^{1353}) with reference to previous studies (18, 33, 42) (**Figure 3A**). First, we measured the titers of antibodies in skin-grafted wild-type mice ($n = 16$) at 5 weeks after the skin grafting and compared them to those in untreated wild-type mice ($n = 8$) by ELISA. Although we expected the skin grafting to induce antibodies to every epitope of human COL17, it preferentially induced antibodies to NC16A-R7 but not to ICD-149 nor to ECD-1330 (**Figure 3B**). Next, we examined the titers of antibodies in the active BP model ($n = 6$). As expected, the titer of antibodies to NC16A-R7 peaked at day 9 and decreased rapidly thereafter (**Figure 3C**). The titers of antibodies to ECD-917, −1084 and −1330 also peaked at day 9 and then rapidly decreased, similar to the antibodies to NC16A-R7 (**Figure 3D**). The titer of antibodies to ICD-320 also peaked at day 9 and remained stable after the peak. Notably, the titer of antibodies to ICD-149 slowly increased and peaked at day 21 and then gradually decreased (**Figure 3D**). It should be noted that the titers of antibodies to NC16A-R7 were far higher than those to other epitopes of COL17, because 1:100 and 1:25 diluted sera were used to check the reactivity to NC16A-R7 and to other peptides, respectively. These results suggest that humoral immune response occurs preferentially to the NC16A domain in skin-grafted wild-type mice and then spreads to other epitopes of COL17 in the active BP model in which the response to ECD epitopes precedes that to ICD epitopes.

Blockade of CD40–CD40 Ligand Interaction at Day 0 Preferentially Suppresses the Production of Antibodies to the NC16A Domain but not to Other Epitopes of COL17

To further investigate the timing of T- and B-cell responses to various epitopes of COL17 in an active BP model, we interfered with the interaction between T and B cells by administrating

A

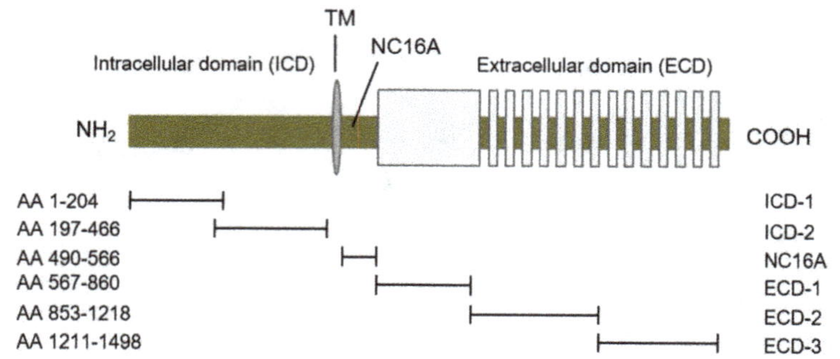

B

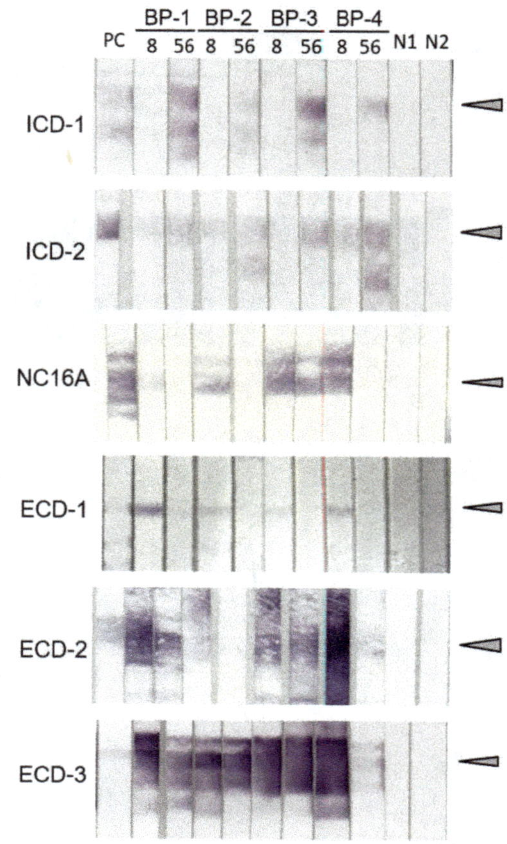

C

		ICD-1	ICD-2	NC16A	ECD-1	ECD-2	ECD-3
BP-1	D7		±	+	+	++	+++
BP-2	D7		±	++	±	+	++
BP-3	D8			+++	±	+	++
BP-4	D8		+	+++	+	+++	+++
BP-1	D56	++	+			+	++
BP-2	D56	+	+				++
BP-3	D56	++	++	++		+	+++
BP-4	D56	+	++			±	±

-	±	+	++	+++

FIGURE 2 | Antibodies to ICD epitopes of COL17 become detectable later than those to ECD epitopes by immunoblotting in an active BP model. **(A)** Schematic of human COL17 and recombinant proteins. TM, transmembrane domain; NH_2, N-terminus; COOH, C-terminus; AA, amino acid. **(B)** Reactivity of sera from active BP model mice ($n = 4$, days 8 and 56) to fragments of COL17 as measured by immunoblotting. PC; positive control (BP patient serum), 8, day 8; 56, day 56; BP-1-4, active BP model mice #1-4, respectively; N1, negative control-1 (wild-type serum); N2, negative control-2 (normal human serum). Arrowheads indicate positive levels. **(C)** Relative intensities of reactivity as measured by immunoblotting. –, negative; ±, faint; +, weakly positive; ++, positive; + + +, strongly positive.

monoclonal antibodies to CD40 ligand (CD40L) at day 0 of the adoptive transfer ($n = 4$) and compared the titers of antibodies in untreated active BP model ($n = 9$) (**Figure 4A**). As we previously reported (41), a single dose of antibodies to CD40L at day 0 strongly suppressed the production of antibodies to the NC16A domain (**Figure 4B**). Antibodies to ECD epitopes of COL17 (ECD-917 and 1330) were not suppressed by the treatment (**Figures 4D,E**). Interestingly, the peak of antibodies to ICD-149 was increased and prolonged by the treatment compared to the untreated active BP model (**Figure 4C**). These results suggest that T- and B-cell interaction for the ECD epitopes occurs very soon after adoptive transfer, whereas the interaction regarding ICD epitopes occurs late, so it is unaffected by the early treatment of antibodies to CD40L.

Immunization With NC16A-R7 Induces Antibodies to ICD and ECD Epitopes of COL17 *in vivo*

Because COL17-humanized skin contains full-length human COL17, skin grafting can activate lymphocytes to multiple epitopes of COL17 in wild-type mice. To simply analyze epitope spreading from the NC16A domain to other domains of COL17, we immunized wild-type mice with NC16A-R7 peptides fused with KLH twice at days 0 and 7 (**Figure 5A**). The immunized mice started to produce antibodies to NC16A-R7 within 1 week. However, interestingly, the mice also produced antibodies to ICD-149, which were detected from 2 weeks after the immunization and which gradually increased (**Figure 5B**). Meanwhile, the titers of antibodies to ECD-1330 were very low. Indirect IF study demonstrated that NC16A-R7-immunized wild-type sera reacted to the DEJ of normal human skin (NHS) (positive/total = 5/5). Additionally, they reacted to the surface of basal keratinocytes in wild-type mouse skin (positive/total = 4/5) (**Figure 5C**), suggesting the presence of antibodies that recognize murine COL17 and/or other keratinocyte antigens. We transferred the spleen cells to *Rag-2*$^{-/-}$/COL17-humanized mice at 5 weeks after immunization ($n = 8$) (**Figure 5A**). As a control, spleen cells obtained from untreated wild-type mice were transferred to *Rag-2*$^{-/-}$/COL17-humanized recipients ($n = 8$). As expected, the recipients receiving NC16A-R7-immunized

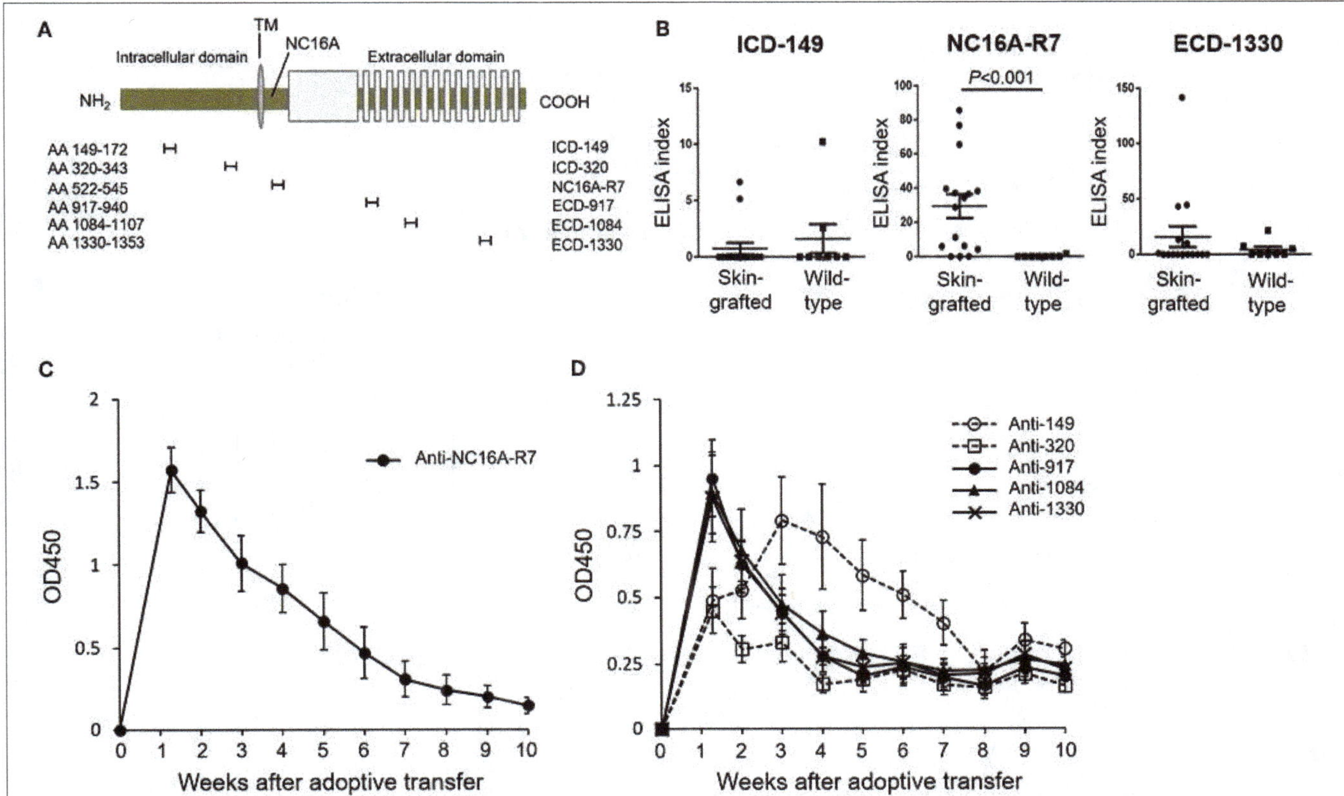

FIGURE 3 | The peak of antibodies to ICD-149 lags that of antibodies to the NC16A domain and ECD epitopes by ELISA in an active BP model. **(A)** Schematic of human COL17 and synthesized peptides. TM, transmembrane domain; NH_2, N-terminus; COOH, C-terminus; AA, amino acid. **(B)** ELISA index of skin-grafted wild-type sera (day 35, $n = 16$) and untreated wild-type sera ($n = 8$) measured by ELISA. Sera were diluted to 1:100 for NC16A-R7 and 1:25 for ICD-149 and ECD-1330. **(C)** Time course of titers of circulating IgG antibodies to NC16A-R7 as determined by ELISA ($n = 6$). **(D)** Time course of titers of circulating IgG antibodies to ICD-149, ICD-320, ECD-917, ECD-1084 and ECD-1330 as determined by ELISA ($n = 6$, respectively). Results are shown as mean ± SEM.

spleen cells developed antibodies to NC16A-R7 shortly after adoptive transfer, and then the titer gradually decreased (**Figure 5D**). Additionally, antibodies to ICD-149 and ECD-1330 became detectable 2 weeks after transfer and then slowly increased. These results indicate that the re-activation of T and B cells to ICD-149 occurs later than that to NC16A-R7 in the recipients. All the recipients developed faint or no skin changes that accounted for <2% of skin surface area, suggesting that the immune response in the recipients is unrelated to the inflammation of the skin. Notably, the recipients of spleen cells from the untreated wild-type mice produced low titers of antibodies to ICD and ECD epitopes but not to the NC16A domain at a late phase (**Figure 5E**), suggesting that a small number of naïve T and B cells from untreated wild-type mice can weakly react to ICD and ECD epitopes of human COL17 in the recipients.

A Portion of the Active BP Model Mice Produce a Low Titer of Antibodies to Murine BP230

Next, we examined whether intermolecular epitope spreading occurs in an active BP model. First, we performed indirect IF analysis using sera from an active BP model and NHS containing human COL17, and COL17-deficient mouse skin lacking both murine and human COL17. As expected, sera from the active BP model strongly reacted to the DEJ of NHS; furthermore, they showed weak reactivity around the basal keratinocytes in COL17-deficient mouse skin (**Figure 6A**), suggesting the presence of antibodies to the antigens on basal keratinocytes other than COL17. Then, we focused on BP230, another major autoantigen of BP, and examined the presence of antibodies to murine BP230 by using recombinant proteins. Recombinant murine BP230 proteins were prepared as 3 fragments; the N-terminus domain (referred to as BP230-1), the rod domain (BP230-2) and the C-terminus domain (BP230-3) (37) (**Figure 6B**). The sizes were confirmed by Western blotting using anti-His-tag antibody (**Figure 6C**). We examined sera from skin-grafted wild-type mice at day 35 ($n = 8$), and they showed no reactivity (data not shown). We then examined sera from the active BP model at days 8, 21 and 84 ($n = 8$). No reactivity was observed in sera at day 8 (data not shown) nor at day 84 (**Figure 6D**), but interestingly, 4 sera at day 21 weakly reacted to BP230-1 (**Figure 6D**). No reactivity was observed on BP230-2 or BP230-3 fragments. There was no correlation between the appearance of antibodies to BP230-1 and disease severity (data not shown). Thus, the humoral immune response that started from COL17 extended to BP230 *in vivo*.

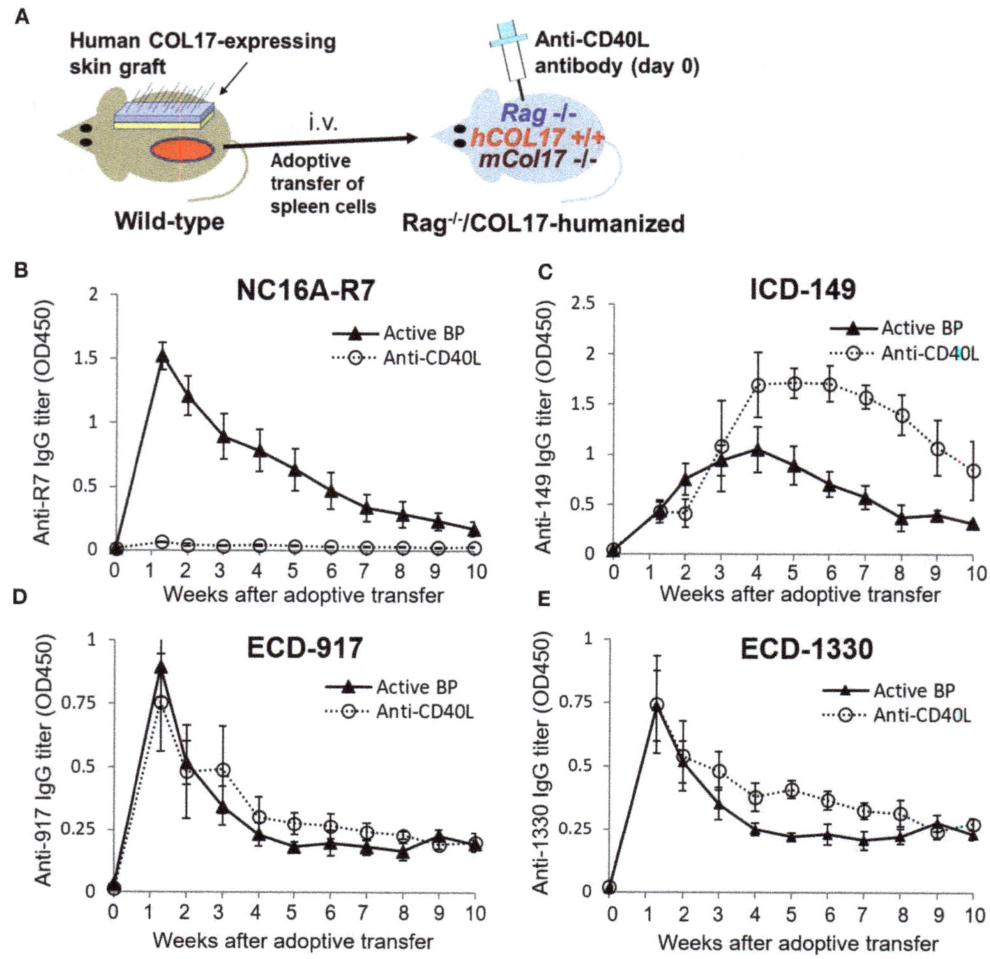

FIGURE 4 | Blockade of CD40–CD40 ligand interaction preferentially decreases antibodies to the NC16A domain but not to other epitopes of COL17. **(A)** Schematic of treatment of the active BP model with antibodies to murine CD40 ligand (CD40L). **(B–E)** Time course of titers of circulating IgG antibodies to NC16A-R7 **(B)**, ICD-149 **(C)**, ECD-917 **(D)**, and ECD-1330 **(E)** in an anti-CD40L antibody-treated active BP model ($n = 4$) and in an untreated active BP model ($n = 9$) as determined by ELISA. Results are shown as mean ± SEM.

DISCUSSION

This study has shown that intramolecular epitope spreading within COL17 and intermolecular epitope spreading from COL17 to BP230 occurs in experimental BP mouse models (**Figure 7**). Although the titer of antibodies to the NC16A domain drops rapidly (**Figure 1E**), the active BP model maintains a similar clinical disease severity for a long period (**Figure 1C**) in association with the clear deposition of IgG at the DEJ of lesional skin, even 35 days after the adoptive transfer of spleen cells as we previously reported (43). We had also noticed the discrepancy in time-course between the titer of antibodies to the DEJ as measured by indirect IF and that to the NC16A domain as measured by ELISA. In this study, we showed that this discrepancy is due to the delayed increase of antibodies to ICD epitopes of COL17. This is consistent with a previous study using a human COL17-expressing skin-grafted mouse model (33). In that study, antibodies to ICD epitopes emerged mostly later than 40 days after skin grafting, which is also consistent with our results in which antibodies to ICD-149 were not detected at day 35 in skin-grafted wild-type mice (**Figure 3B**). As reasons for the delayed increase of antibodies to ICD epitopes in the active BP model, we consider two possibilities. First, intramolecular epitope spreading from the NC16A domain to ICD epitopes occurs shortly after adoptive transfer. Second, ICD epitope-reactive T and B cells were already activated in skin-grafted wild-type mice as a result of intramolecular epitope spreading, and when these cells were transferred into $Rag^{-/-}$/COL17-humanized recipients, they encountered ICD antigens probably a little bit later than ECD antigens *in vivo*, resulting in the delayed peak of antibodies to ICD epitopes.

Unexpectedly, wild-type mice immunized with NC16A-R7 produced antibodies to ICD-149 (**Figure 5B**). We speculate that NC16A-R7-reactive T and B cells also recognized a corresponding site of murine COL17, which induced

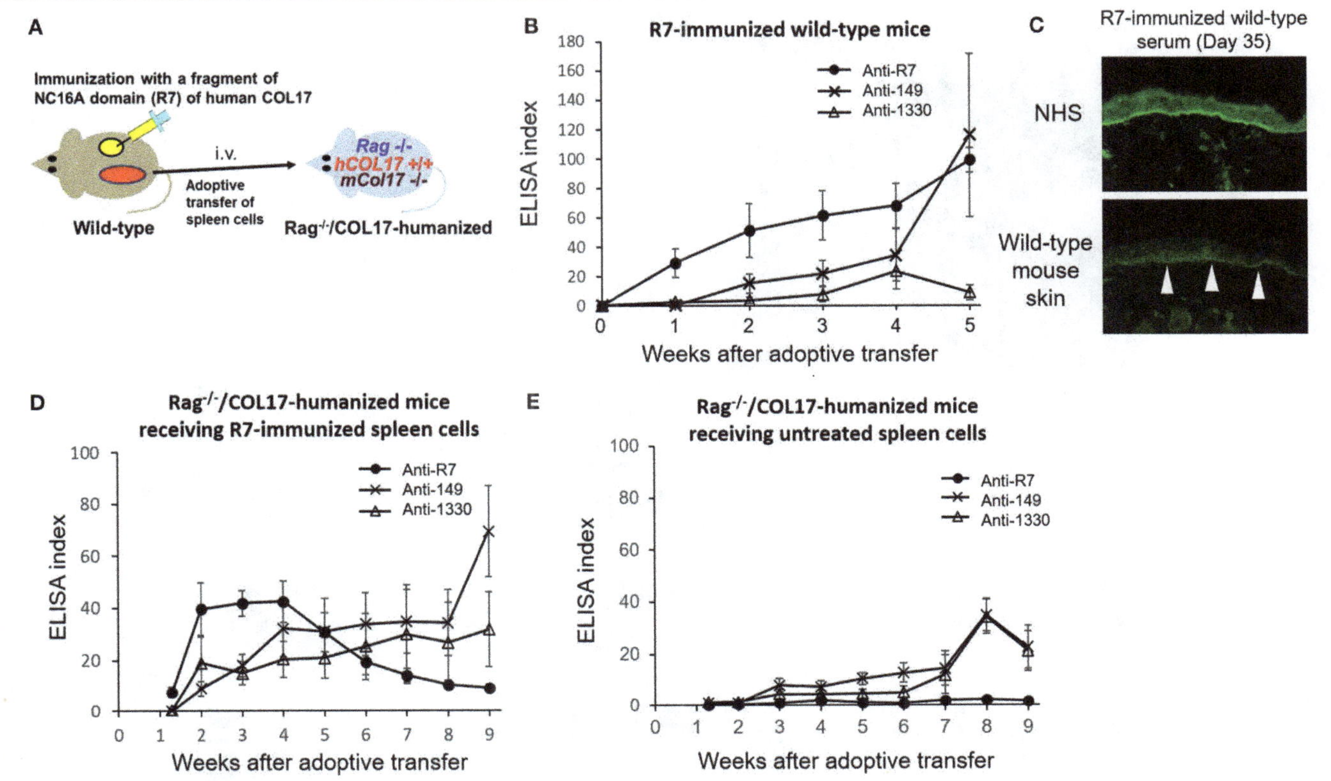

FIGURE 5 | The immune response to the NC16A domain spreads to ICD and ECD epitopes of COL17 *in vivo*. **(A)** Schematic of the immunization of wild-type mice with NC16A-R7 and the adoptive transfer of spleen cells to make the active BP model. **(B)** Time course of titers of circulating IgG antibodies to NC16A-R7, ICD-149, and ECD-1330 in NC16A-R7-immunized wild-type mice ($n = 5$) as determined by ELISA. **(C)** Representative images of IgG deposition in indirect IF study using normal human skin (NHS) and wild-type mouse skin as substrates and 1:20 diluted sera from NC16A-R7-immunized wild-type mice at day 35 as primary antibodies. Arrowheads indicate IgG deposition around the basal keratinocytes. **(D,E)** Time course of titers of circulating IgG antibodies to NC16A-R7, ICD-149, and ECD-1330 in *Rag*$^{-/-}$/COL17-humanized mice that received spleen cells from NC16A-R7-immunized mice ($n = 8$) **(D)** and in those that received spleen cells from untreated wild-type mice ($n = 8$) **(E)** as determined by ELISA. Results are shown as mean ± SEM.

intramolecular epitope spreading to other epitopes of murine COL17 in wild-type mice. Although the homology of the amino acid sequence of NC17A-R7 (human COL17) and the corresponding site of murine COL17 is 54.1%, that of ICD-149 (human COL17) and the corresponding site of murine COL17 is 95.8%. The positive reactivity of NC16A-R7-immunized sera at day 35 to mouse skin shown in **Figure 5C** supports our hypothesis. Thus, intramolecular epitope spreading from the NC16A domain to ICD epitopes occurs in NC16A-immunized wild-type mice.

Two major mechanisms are considered to be behind the epitope spreading phenomenon: an "independent" or "dependent" of a physical association of antigens (30, 44). The former involves the development of secondary epitopes due to the release of antigens or the disclosure of parts of antigens during a chronic inflammatory or autoimmune response. The latter is independent of inflammatory processes. T cells specific for one epitope of an antigen can activate B cells that are specific for other antigens of the same multi-antigen complex, resulting in the generation of autoantibodies to antigens that are not initially targeted by the immune response (45). In this study, we demonstrated epitope spreading from the NC16A domain to other epitopes of COL17 in NC16A-R7-immunized wild-type mice, even though the mice developed no skin changes. This suggests that intramolecular epitope spreading within COL17 can occur under a mechanism that is "dependent" on a physical association of antigens.

We can estimate the timing of COL17-reactive T-cell activation more easily in the active BP mouse model than in the skin-grafted BP model, because in the former model, it starts soon after the adoptive transfer of spleen cells. By utilizing this advantage, we previously demonstrated that the activation of anti-human COL17 NC16A IgG-producing B cells via CD40–CD40L interaction is completed within 5 days after the transfer of spleen cells (41). The study also showed that antibodies to the DEJ were restored long after the single administration of antibodies to CD40L at day 0 and that the restored antibodies do not react to the NC16A domain. The results in **Figure 4** suggest that the restored antibodies are mainly specific for ICD epitopes of COL17 and that the interaction between T and B cells regarding ICD epitopes may arise slightly bit later than that to the NC16A domain after the adoptive transfer of spleen cells. We previously reported that the blockade of CD40L at

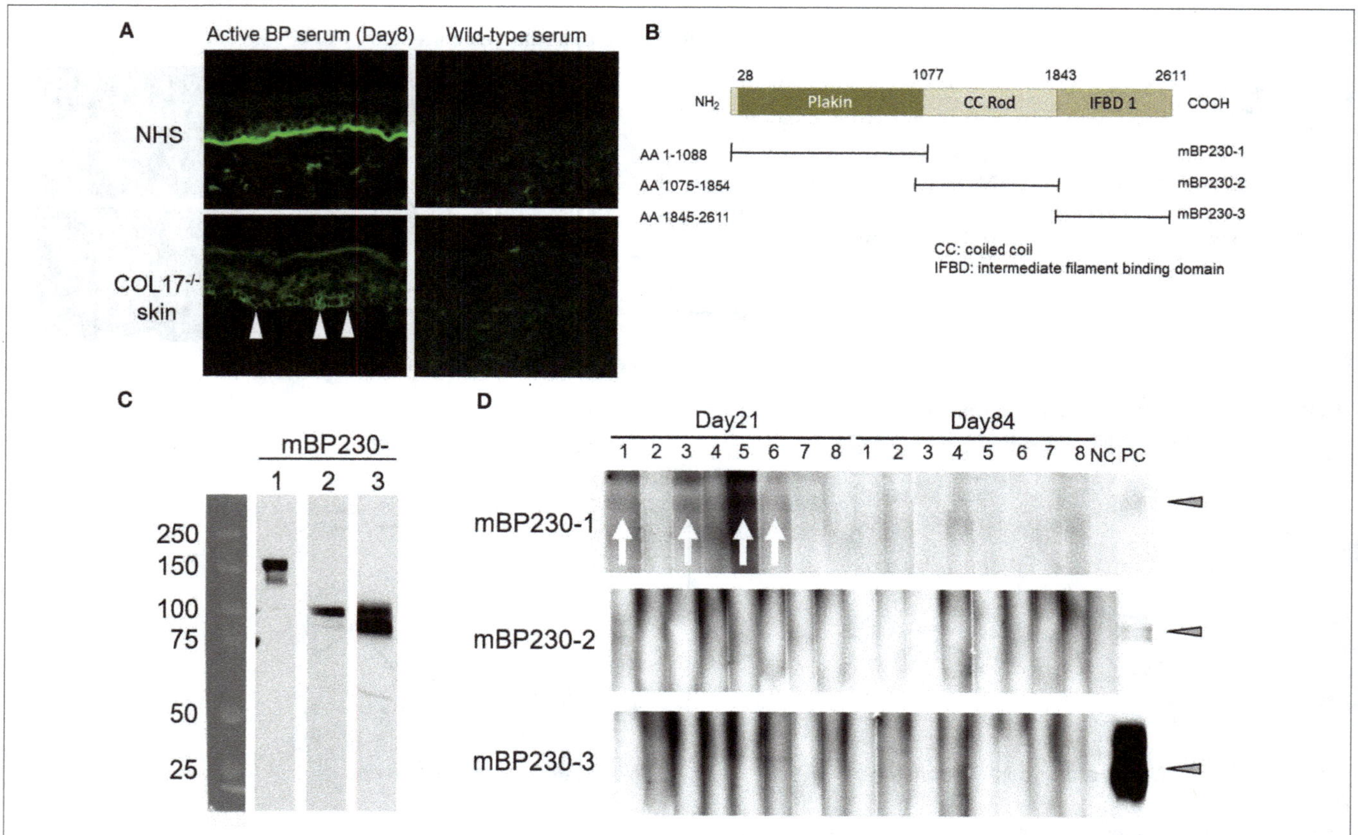

FIGURE 6 | Antibodies to murine BP230 are detected in a portion of the active BP model mice. **(A)** Representative images of IgG deposition in indirect IF study using normal human skin (NHS) and murine COL17$^{-/-}$ mouse skin as substrates and 1:20 diluted sera from an active BP model at day 35 and from wild-type mice as primary antibodies. Arrowheads indicate IgG deposition around the basal keratinocytes. **(B)** Schematic of murine BP230 and recombinant proteins. NH_2, N-terminus; COOH, C-terminus; AA, amino acid; mBP230, murine BP230. **(C)** The sizes of recombinant proteins were confirmed by immunoblotting using anti-His-tag antibody. **(D)** Reactivity of sera from the active BP model ($n = 8$, days 21 and 84) to fragments of murine BP230 was measured by immunoblotting. NC, negative control (wild-type serum); PC, positive control (anti-His-tag antibody). Arrowheads indicate a positive level. Arrows indicate a positive band.

day 13, 16, and 19 after the adoptive transfer did not suppress antibodies to the NC16A domain (examined by ELISA), nor did it suppress antibodies to the DEJ (examined by indirect IF) (41). This strongly suggests that the delayed blockade of CD40-CD40L interaction does not suppress the production of antibodies to ICD epitopes and that the CD40-CD40L interaction between T and B cells regarding ICD epitopes was completed within 13 days after the adoptive transfer. The reason for the discrepancy between the results for NC16A-R7 and those for other ECDs in **Figure 4** is unclear. As mentioned above, the reactivity of antibodies to NC16A-R7 is far stronger than those to ECD-917 and ECD-1330 in the untreated active BP model. This would be due to the high antigenicity of the NC16A domain of COL17 as reported previously (36, 46). It is commonly known that CD40L is transiently expressed on the surface of activated CD4$^+$ T cells (47). Given the above, we consider that a treatment of CD40L-blocking antibody preferentially affects the highly activated T cells reacting to the NC16A domain rather than those reacting to the other ECD epitopes. Further investigations are required to confirm this.

This study also showed intermolecular epitope spreading from COL17 to BP230 in an active BP model. As mentioned above, intermolecular epitope spreading commonly occurs among different antigens of a single molecular complex or among antigens that colocalize to the same site (30). Both COL17 and BP230 are hemidesmosomal proteins, and they directly interact with each other at their N-termini (48). Di Zenzo et al. examined IgG reactivity to COL17 and BP230 during the course of the disease in 35 BP cases and detected epitope spreading in 17 cases (49%). Notably, 3 of those 17 cases showed intermolecular epitope spreading from COL17 to BP230, but the reactivity to BP230 never preceded that to COL17 (34). We demonstrated the reactivity of active BP mouse sera to murine BP230, but it was very weak, as shown in **Figure 6D**. This weak reactivity may be due to the strong self-tolerance in the wild-type mouse, a source of transferred spleen cells in the active BP model, because murine BP230 is originally expressed in wild-type mice. This hypothesis is supported by our recent finding that regulatory T cells, a main player in peripheral tolerance, play a crucial role in maintaining self-tolerance to murine BP230 in mice (37).

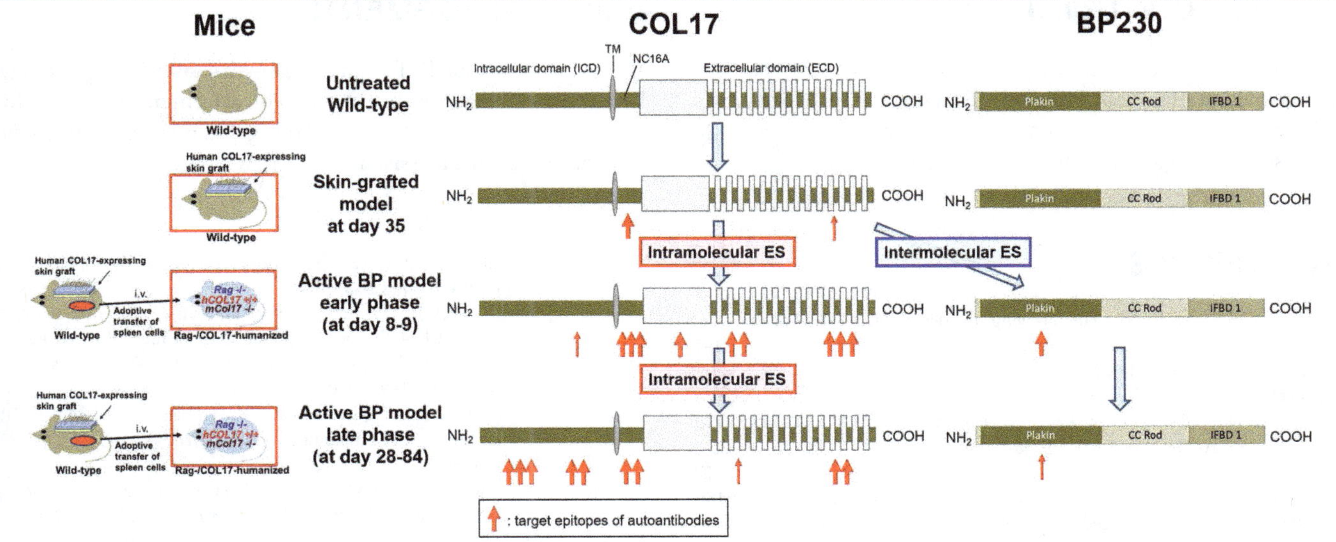

FIGURE 7 | Epitope spreading in the skin-grafted mouse model and in the active BP model. A schematic of COL17 and BP230. In the skin-grafted mouse model, antibodies mainly react to the NC16A domain and weakly react to ECD epitopes of COL17. After the adoptive transfer of immunized spleen cells, intramolecular epitope spreading to ECD epitopes and to the outer portion of the ICD as well as intermolecular epitope spreading to BP230 occur, followed by intramolecular epitope spreading to the inner portion of the ICD. ES: epitope spreading.

There are several limitations to this study. First, the synthesized peptides that were used for the ELISA account for only a small portion of human COL17. The titers of antibodies to ICD-1 (recombinant protein of 204 amino acids) were higher at day 56 than at day 8, as shown in **Figure 2C**, whereas the titers of antibodies to ICD-149 (synthesized peptides of 24 amino acids) were higher at day 8 than at day 56, as shown in **Figure 3D**. These results suggest that active BP mouse sera contain antibodies to ICD-1 epitopes (Met^1 to Ser^{204}) other than ICD-149 (Ala^{149} to Ser^{172}). Second, a correlation between disease severity and epitope spreading remains unclear. As mentioned above, previous studies demonstrated that the disease severities of BP are associated with the appearance of antibodies to ICD epitopes in both mouse models and human patients (33, 34). Meanwhile the appearance of antibodies to BP230-1 or BP230 was not related to the disease severity of the active BP model in this study, which is probably due to the low titers of those antibodies. Third, we have not examined intramolecular epitope spreading that starts from ICD or ECD epitopes other than the NC16A domain. We recently reported 3 cases of dipeptidyl peptidase-4 inhibitor-associated BP in which autoantibodies to the NC16A domain were initially undetectable but became positive during the course of BP (49). To investigate this phenomenon, we immunized wild-type mice with recombinant proteins of ICD or ECD shown in **Figure 2A** and adoptively transferred the spleen cells to $Rag^{-/-}$/COL17-humanized mice. However, the titers of antibodies to COL17 were very low in all the immunized mice and the recipient mice (data not shown). This is probably due to the lower antigenicity of those proteins compared to that of the NC16A domain. Fourth, we have not examined intermolecular epitope spreading to hemidesmosomal proteins such as plectin, integrin α6, integrin β4, or laminin 332, which were reported to interact directly with COL17 (50–54), although those molecules become targets of autoantibodies less frequently than COL17 and BP230 do. We should also confirm whether the interaction between human COL17 and murine hemidesmosomal proteins in COL17-humanized mice is normal. To overcome these limitations, further investigations are necessary.

In conclusion, the immune reaction to human COL17 that starts from ECD epitopes, especially those of the NC16A domain, was found to spread over time to ICD epitopes and to murine BP230 in an experimental BP model. The timing of the interaction between COL17-reactive T and B cells differs *in vivo*, and it is dependent on the target epitope. These novel findings elucidate certain details of epitope spreading in BP and give us a hint for new therapeutic strategies for BP that involve the regulation of this phenomenon.

ETHICS STATEMENT

This study was carried out in accordance with the recommendations of the local ethics committee and the Institutional Review Board of Hokkaido University, with written informed consent obtained from all subjects in accordance with the Declaration of Helsinki. All animal procedures were conducted according to guidelines provided by the Hokkaido University Institutional Animal Care and Use Committee under an approved protocol.

AUTHOR CONTRIBUTIONS

HU and NY performed the experiments. KN, KM, HI, and WN provided materials. HU and HS designed the experiments. HU wrote the manuscript, and all the coauthors reviewed the manuscript and gave final approval of the submission.

ACKNOWLEDGMENTS

We thank Professor K. B. Yancey (Department of Dermatology, University of Texas Southwestern Medical Center, Dallas, TX) for providing human COL17 cDNA transgenic mice and Ms. Keiko Abe for her technical assistance.

REFERENCES

1. Kridin K, Ludwig RJ. The growing incidence of bullous pemphigoid: overview and potential explanations. *Front Med.* (2018) 5:1–7. doi: 10.3389/fmed.2018.00220
2. Bech R, Kibsgaard L, Vestergaard C. Comorbidities and treatment strategies in bullous pemphigoid: an appraisal of the existing litterature. *Front Med.* (2018) 5:238. doi: 10.3389/fmed.2018.00238
3. Diaz LA, Ratrie H, Saunders WS, Futamura S, Squiquera HL, Anhalt GJ, Giudice GJ. Isolation of a human epidermal cDNA corresponding to the 180-kD autoantigen recognized by bullous pemphigoid and herpes gestationis sera. Immunolocalization of this protein to the hemidesmosome. *J Clin Invest.* (1990) 86:1088–94. doi: 10.1172/JCI114812
4. Giudice GJ, Emery DJ, Diaz LA. Cloning and primary structural analysis of the bullous pemphigoid autoantigen BP180. *J Invest Dermatol.* (1992) 99:243–50. doi: 10.1111/1523-1747.ep12616580
5. Hopkinson SB, Riddelle KS, Jones JC. Cytoplasmic domain of the 180-kD bullous pemphigoid antigen, a hemidesmosomal component: molecular and cell biologic characterization. *J Invest Dermatol.* (1992) 99:264–70. doi: 10.1111/1523-1747.ep12616615
6. Ishiko A, Shimizu H, Kikuchi A, Ebihara T, Hashimoto T, Nishikawa T. Human autoantibodies against the 230-kD bullous pemphigoid antigen (BPAG1) bind only to the intracellular domain of the hemidesmosome, whereas those against the 180-kD bullous pemphigoid antigen (BPAG2) bind along the plasma membrane of the hemidesmosome. *J Clin Invest.* (1993) 91:1608–15. doi: 10.1172/JCI116368
7. Bédane C, McMillan JR, Balding SD, Bernard P, Prost C, Bonnetblanc JM, Diaz LA, Eady RA, Giudice GJ. Bullous pemphigoid and cicatricial pemphigoid autoantibodies react with ultrastructurally separable epitopes on the BP180 ectodomain: evidence that BP180 spans the lamina lucida. *J Invest Dermatol.* (1997) 108:901–7. doi: 10.1111/1523-1747.ep12292701
8. Liu Y, Li L, Xia Y. BP180 is critical in the autoimmunity of bullous pemphigoid. *Front Immunol.* (2017) 8:1–15. doi: 10.3389/fimmu.2017.01752
9. Goletz S, Zillikens D, Schmidt E. Structural proteins of the dermal-epidermal junction targeted by autoantibodies in pemphigoid diseases. *Exp Dermatol.* (2017) 26:1154–62. doi: 10.1111/exd.13446
10. Ludwig RJ, Vanhoorelbeke K, Leypoldt F, Kaya Z, Bieber K, McLachlan SM, et al. Mechanisms of autoantibody-induced pathology. *Front Immunol.* (2017) 8:603. doi: 10.3389/fimmu.2017.00603
11. Matsumura K, Amagai M, Nishikawa T, Hashimoto T. The majority of bullous pemphigoid and herpes gestationis serum samples react with the NC16a domain of the 180-kDa bullous pemphigoid antigen. *Arch Dermatol Res.* (1996) 288:507–9. doi: 10.1007/BF02505245
12. Zillikens D, Rose PA, Balding SD, Liu Z, Olague-Marchan M, Diaz LA, Giudice GJ. Tight clustering of extracellular BP180 epitopes recognized by bullous pemphigoid autoantibodies. *J Invest Dermatol.* (1997) 109:573–9. doi: 10.1111/1523-1747.ep12337492
13. Tsuji-Abe Y, Akiyama M, Yamanaka Y, Kikuchi T, Sato-Matsumura KC, Shimizu H. Correlation of clinical severity and ELISA indices for the NC16A domain of BP180 measured using BP180 ELISA kit in bullous pemphigoid. *J Dermatol Sci.* (2005) 37:145–9. doi: 10.1016/j.jdermsci.2004.10.007
14. Döpp R, Schmidt E, Chimanovitch I, Leverkus M, Bröcker E-B, Zillikens D. IgG4 and IgE are the major immunoglobulins targeting the NC16A domain of BP180 in bullous pemphigoid: Serum levels of these immunoglobulins reflect disease activity. *J Am Acad Dermatol.* (2000) 42:577–83. doi: 10.1067/mjd.2000.103986
15. Liu Z, Diaz LA, Troy JL, Taylor AF, Emery DJ, Fairley JA, Giudice GJ. A passive transfer model of the organ-specific autoimmune disease, bullous pemphigoid, using antibodies generated against the hemidesmosomal antigen, BP180. *J Clin Invest.* (1993) 92:2480–8. doi: 10.1172/JCI116856
16. Nishie W, Sawamura D, Goto M, Ito K, Shibaki A, McMillan JR, et al. Humanization of autoantigen. *Nat Med.* (2007) 13:378–83. doi: 10.1038/nm1496
17. Nie Z, Hashimoto T. IgA antibodies of cicatricial pemphigoid sera specifically react with C- terminus of BP180. *J Invest Dermatol.* (1999) 112:254–5. doi: 10.1046/j.1523-1747.1999.00501.x
18. Di Zenzo G, Grosso F, Terracina M, Mariotti F, De Pità O, Owaribe K, et al. Characterization of the anti-BP180 autoantibody reactivity profile and epitope mapping in bullous pemphigoid patients. *J Invest Dermatol.* (2004) 122:103–10. doi: 10.1046/j.0022-202X.2003.22126.x
19. Hofmann SC, Thoma-Uszynski S, Hunziker T, Bernard P, Koebnick C, Stauber A, et al. Severity and phenotype of bullous pemphigoid relate to autoantibody profile against the NH2- and COOH-terminal regions of the BP180 ectodomain. *J Invest Dermatol.* (2002) 119:1065–73. doi: 10.1046/j.1523-1747.2002.19529.x
20. Izumi K, Nishie W, Mai Y, Wada M, Natsuga K, Ujiie H, et al. Autoantibody profile differentiates between inflammatory and noninflammatory bullous pemphigoid. *J Invest Dermatol.* (2016) 136:2201–10. doi: 10.1016/j.jid.2016.06.622
21. Stanley JR, Hawley-Nelson P, Yuspa SH, Shevach EM, Katz SI. Characterization of bullous pemphigoid antigen: a unique basement membrane protein of stratified squamous epithelia. *Cell.* (1981) 24:897–903. doi: 10.1016/0092-8674(81)90115-X
22. Stanley JR, Tanaka T, Mueller S, Klaus-Kovtun V, Roop D. Isolation of complementary DNA for bullous pemphigoid antigen by use of patients' autoantibodies. *J Clin Invest.* (1988) 82:1864–70. doi: 10.1172/JCI113803
23. Guo L, Degenstein L, Dowling J, Yu QC, Wollmann R, Perman B, Fuchs E. Gene targeting of BPAG1: abnormalities in mechanical strength and cell migration in stratified epithelia and neurologic degeneration. *Cell.* (1995) 81:233–43. doi: 10.1016/0092-8674(95)90333-X
24. Skaria M, Jaunin F, Hunziker T, Riou S, Schumann H, Bruckner-Tuderman L, et al. IgG autoantibodies from bullous pemphigoid patients recognize multiple antigenic reactive sites located predominantly within the B and C subdomains of the COOH-terminus of BP230. *J Invest Dermatol.* (2000) 114:998–1004. doi: 10.1046/j.1523-1747.2000.00893.x
25. Thoma-Uszynski S, Uter W, Schwietzke S, Hofmann SC, Hunziker T, Bernard P, et al. BP230- and BP180-specific auto-antibodies in bullous pemphigoid. *J Invest Dermatol.* (2004) 122:1413–22. doi: 10.1111/j.0022-202X.2004.22603.x
26. Hall RP, Murray JC, McCord MM, Rico MJ, Streilein RD. Rabbits immunized with a peptide encoded for by the 230-kD bullous pemphigoid antigen cDNA develop an enhanced inflammatory response to UVB irradiation: a potential animal model for bullous pemphigoid. *J Invest Dermatol.* (1993) 101:9–14. doi: 10.1111/1523-1747.ep12358276
27. Kiss M, Husz S, Jánossy T, Marczinovits I, Molnár J, Korom I, Dobozy A. Experimental bullous pemphigoid generated in mice with an antigenic epitope of the human hemidesmosomal protein BP230. *J Autoimmun.* (2005) 24:1–10. doi: 10.1016/j.jaut.2004.09.007
28. Haeberle S, Wei X, Bieber K, Goletz S, Ludwig RJ, Schmidt E, et al. Regulatory T-cell deficiency leads to pathogenic bullous pemphigoid antigen

230 autoantibody and autoimmune bullous disease. *J Allergy Clin Immunol.* (2018) 142:1831–42.e7. doi: 10.1016/j.jaci.2018.04.006
29. Chan LS, Vanderlugt CJ, Hashimoto T, Nishikawa T, Zone JJ, Black MM, et al. Epitope spreading: lessons from autoimmune skin diseases. *J Invest Dermatol.* (1998) 110:103–9. doi: 10.1046/j.1523-1747.1998.00107.x
30. Didona D, Di Zenzo G. Humoral epitope spreading in autoimmune bullous diseases. *Front Immunol.* (2018) 9:1–27. doi: 10.3389/fimmu.2018.00779
31. Tuohy VK, Yu M, Yin L, Kawczak JA, Philip Kinkel R. Spontaneous regression of primary autoreactivity during chronic progression of experimental autoimmune encephalomyelitis and multiple sclerosis. *J Exp Med.* (1999) 189:1033–42. doi: 10.1007/s12264-013-1313-3
32. Huijbers MG, Vink A-FD, Niks EH, Westhuis RH, van Zwet EW, de Meel RH, et al. Longitudinal epitope mapping in MuSK myasthenia gravis: implications for disease severity. *J Neuroimmunol.* (2016) 291:82–8. doi: 10.1016/j.jneuroim.2015.12.016
33. Di Zenzo G, Calabresi V, Olasz EB, Zambruno G, Yancey KB. Sequential intramolecular epitope spreading of humoral responses to human BPAG2 in a transgenic model. *J Invest Dermatol.* (2010) 130:1040–7. doi: 10.1038/jid.2009.309
34. Di Zenzo G, Thoma-Uszynski S, Calabresi V, Fontao L, Hofmann SC, Lacour JP, et al. Demonstration of epitope-spreading phenomena in bullous pemphigoid: Results of a prospective multicenter study. *J Invest Dermatol.* (2011) 131:2271–80. doi: 10.1038/jid.2011.180
35. Ujiie H, Shibaki A, Nishie W, Sawamura D, Wang G, Tateishi Y, et al. A novel active mouse model for bullous pemphigoid targeting humanized pathogenic antigen. *J Immunol.* (2010) 184:2166–74. doi: 10.4049/jimmunol.0903101
36. Natsuga K, Nishie W, Shinkuma S, Ujiie H, Nishimura M, Sawamura D, et al. Antibodies to pathogenic epitopes on type XVII collagen cause skin fragility in a complement-dependent and -independent manner. *J Immunol.* (2012) 188:5792–9. doi: 10.4049/jimmunol.1003402
37. Muramatsu K, Ujiie H, Kobayashi I, Nishie W, Izumi K, Ito T, et al. Regulatory T-cell dysfunction induces autoantibodies to bullous pemphigoid antigens in mice and human subjects. *J Allergy Clin Immunol.* (2018) 142:1818–30.e6. doi: 10.1016/j.jaci.2018.03.014
38. Leung CL, Zheng M, Prater SM, Liem RKH. The BPAG1 locus: Alternative splicing produces multiple isoforms with distinct cytoskeletal linker domains, including predominant isoforms in neurons and muscles. *J Cell Biol.* (2001) 154:691–7. doi: 10.1083/jcb.200012098
39. Olasz EB, Roh J, Yee CL, Arita K, Akiyama M, Shimizu H, Vogel JC, Yancey KB. Human bullous pemphigoid antigen 2 transgenic skin elicits specific IgG in wild-type mice. *J Invest Dermatol.* (2007) 127:2807–17. doi: 10.1038/sj.jid.5700970
40. Ujiie H, Shevach EM. γδ T Cells Protect the liver and lungs of mice from autoimmunity induced by scurfy lymphocytes. *J Immunol.* (2016) 196:1517–28. doi: 10.4049/jimmunol.1501774
41. Ujiie H, Shibaki A, Nishie W, Shinkuma S, Moriuchi R, Qiao H, Shimizu H. Noncollagenous 16A domain of type XVII collagen-reactive CD4 + T cells play a pivotal role in the development of active disease in experimental bullous pemphigoid model. *Clin Immunol.* (2012) 142:167–75. doi: 10.1016/j.clim.2011.10.002
42. Mariotti F, Grosso F, Terracina M, Ruffelli M, Cordiali-Fei P, Sera F, et al. Development of a novel ELISA system for detection of anti-BP180 IgG and characterization of autoantibody profile in bullous pemphigoid patients. *Br J Dermatol.* (2004) 151:1004–10. doi: 10.1111/j.1365-2133.2004.06245.x
43. Sasaoka T, Ujiie H, Nishie W, Iwata H, Ishikawa M, Higashino H, et al. Intravenous IgG reduces pathogenic autoantibodies, serum IL-6 levels, and disease severity in experimental bullous pemphigoid models. *J Invest Dermatol.* (2018) 138:1260–7. doi: 10.1016/j.jid.2018.01.005
44. McCluskey J, Farris AD, Keech CL, Purcell AW, Rischmueller M, Kinoshita G, et al. Determinant spreading: lessons from animal models and human disease. *Immunol Rev.* (1998) 164:209–29. doi: 10.1111/j.1600-065X.1998.tb01222.x
45. Cornaby C, Gibbons L, Mayhew V, Sloan CS, Welling A, Poole BD. B cell epitope spreading: mechanisms and contribution to autoimmune diseases. *Immunol Lett.* (2015) 163:56–68. doi: 10.1016/j.imlet.2014.11.001
46. Giudice GJ, Emery DJ, Zelickson BD, Anhalt GJ, Liu Z, Diaz LA. Bullous pemphigoid and herpes gestationis autoantibodies recognize a common non-collagenous site on the BP180 ectodomain. *J Immunol.* (1993) 151:5742–50. doi: 10.1016/0923-1811(93)90940-q
47. Foy T, Aruffo A, Janet E, Noelle R. Immune regulation by CD40 and its ligand GP39. *Annu Rev Immunol.* (1996) 14:591–617. doi: 10.1146/annurev.immunol.14.1.591
48. Hopkinson SB Jones JC. The N terminus of the transmembrane protein BP180 interacts with the N-terminal domain of BP230, thereby mediating keratin cytoskeleton anchorage to the cell surface at the site of the hemidesmosome. *Mol Biol Cell.* (2000) 11:277–86. doi: 10.1091/mbc.11.1.277
49. Mai Y, Nishie W, Izumi K, Yoshimoto N, Morita Y, Watanabe M, et al. Detection of anti-BP180 NC16A autoantibodies after the onset of dipeptidyl peptidase-IV inhibitor-associated bullous pemphigoid: a report of three patients. *Br J Dermatol.* (2018) 179:790–1. doi: 10.1111/bjd.16656
50. Natsuga K, Nishie W, Nishimura M, Shinkuma S, Watanabe M, Izumi K, et al. Loss of interaction between plectin and type XVII collagen results in epidermolysis bullosa simplex. *Hum Mutat.* (2017) 38:1666–70. doi: 10.1002/humu.23344
51. Hopkinson SB, Findlay K, deHart GW, Jones JC. Interaction of BP180 (type XVII collagen) and alpha6 integrin is necessary for stabilization of hemidesmosome structure. *J Invest Dermatol.* (1998) 111:1015–22. doi: 10.1046/j.1523-1747.1998.00452.x
52. Koster J, Geerts D, Favre B, Borradori L, Sonnenberg A. Analysis of the interactions between BP180, BP230, plectin and the integrin alpha6beta4 important for hemidesmosome assembly. *J Cell Sci.* (2003) 116:387–99. doi: 10.1242/jcs.00241
53. Schaapveld RQ, Borradori L, Geerts D, van Leusden MR, Kuikman I, Nievers MG, et al. Hemidesmosome formation is initiated by the beta4 integrin subunit, requires complex formation of beta4 and HD1/plectin, and involves a direct interaction between beta4 and the bullous pemphigoid antigen 180. *J Cell Biol.* (1998) 142:271–84. doi: 10.1083/jcb.142.1.271
54. Nishimura M, Nishie W, Shirafuji Y, Shinkuma S, Natsuga K, Nakamura H, et al. Extracellular cleavage of collagen XVII is essential for correct cutaneous basement membrane formation. *Hum Mol Genet.* (2016) 25:328–39. doi: 10.1093/hmg/ddv478

8

Thymoma-Associated Paraneoplastic Autoimmune Multiorgan Syndrome—From Pemphigus to Lichenoid Dermatitis

Farzan Solimani[1], Roberto Maglie[1], Robert Pollmann[1], Thomas Schmidt[1], Ansgar Schmidt[2], Norito Ishii[3], Björn Tackenberg[4], Andreas Kirschbaum[5], Dario Didona[1], Julia Pickert[1], Rüdiger Eming[1], Takashi Hashimoto[5,6] and Michael Hertl[1]*

[1] *Department of Dermatology and Allergology, Philipps-University, Marburg, Germany,* [2] *Institute of Pathology, Philipps-University, Marburg, Germany,* [3] *Department of Dermatology, Kurume University School of Medicine, and Kurume University Institute of Cutaneous Cell Biology, Kurume, Japan,* [4] *Department of Neuroimmunology, Philipps-University, Marburg, Germany,* [5] *Department of Surgery, Philipps-University, Marburg, Germany,* [6] *Osaka City University Graduate School of Medicine, Osaka, Japan*

***Correspondence:**
Farzan Solimani
farzan.solimani@charite.de

Introduction: Paraneoplastic autoimmune multi-organ syndrome (PAMS) is a rare clinical condition characterized by variable and heterogeneous clinical phenotypes in the presence of neoplasias which largely depend on the activation of humoral and cellular immune responses. Clinically, these patients present with a spectrum of antibody-driven pemphigus-like lesions to graft-vs.-host-disease-like exanthemas with a lichenoid inflammatory infiltrate in the skin. PAMS is occasionally associated with thymoma, in which altered immune surveillance eventually leads to multiorgan autoimmunity which often includes variable cutaneous symptoms. This disorder is associated with a profound disturbance of peripheral immune tolerance against human autoantigens.

Objectives: We here present a patient with relapsing thymoma who developed PAMS with several cutaneous and extracutaneous autoimmune disorders.

Materials: Peripheral blood mononuclear cells (PBMC), sera, and lesional skin biopsies were obtained at different clinical disease stages. Peripheral T cell subsets were characterized phenotypically and the cytokine profile of the peripheral blood T cellular response against distinct epidermal and dermal autoantigens of the skin was analyzed by ELISpot assay. Serological screening was performed by ELISA and immunoblot analysis. Skin biopsies were subjected to immunohistochemical analysis of distinct T cell subsets. Thymoma tissue was analyzed for the presence of T regulatory cells and compared with adult thymus and indolent thymoma.

Results and Conclusions: In the present case, thymoma was the cause of the observed multi-organ autoimmune syndromes as its recurrence and surgical removal was associated with the relapse and regression of the cutaneous symptoms, respectively. Initially, the patient presented with two autoimmune disorders with Th2/Th1 imbalance, myasthenia gravis (MG) and pemphigus foliaceus (PF), which regressed upon immunosuppressive treatment. Months later, the patient developed a lichenoid exanthema with a Th1-dominated skin infiltrate. Further clinical evaluation revealed the recurrence of the thymoma and the lichenoid exanthema gradually regressed upon thymectomy. Our contention that T cell recognition against distinct cutaneous autoantigens, such as desmoglein 1 (Dsg1), shifted from a Th2 to a Th1-dominated immune response could not be fully substantiated as the patient was on a stringent immunosuppressive treatment regimen. We could only observe a decrease of the initially present serum IgG autoantibodies against Dsg1. Phenotypic analysis of the associated thymoma showed a lower number of T regulatory cells compared to adult thymus and indolent thymoma, suggesting that impaired thymus-derived immune surveillance had a direct impact on the outcome of the observed cutaneous autoimmune disorders.

Keywords: ***Pemphigus foliaceous*****, autoimmunity, thymoma auto-immunity, PAMS, myasthenia (myasthenia gravis—MG), GVHD-like disease**

BACKGROUND

PAMS is an extremely rare clinical syndrome which arises in patients with lymphoproliferative or solid tumors, like thymomas (1, 2). It is increasingly debated whether PAMS and paraneoplastic pemphigus (PNP) should be considered as one entity, since, in both cases, production of IgG autoantibodies against desmosomal adhesions molecules, such as Dsgl and/or Dsg3, are related to an altered immune surveillance induced by the underlying neoplasia (3–5). In contrast to pemphigus vulgaris (PV) or PF, two well-characterized autoimmune bullous disorders of the skin associated with IgG autoantibodies against Dsg3 and Dsgl, respectively, PAMS is characterized by a wide clinical heterogeneity (6), ranging from classic pemphigus-like muco-cutaneous lesions with erosions, and blisters to lichenoid, graft vs. host disease (GVHD)-like, bullous pemphigoid (BP)-like, and erythema multiforme like-skin lesions (1). As in PNP, mortality of PAMS is high and largely dependent on the underlying malignancy or opportunistic infections (6, 7). As previously reported, PAMS may be associated with thymoma, a neoplasm which arises from epithelial cells of the thymus and accounts for ~50% of all mediastinal tumors (8–15).

Thymomas are often asymptomatic and are sometimes detected by chance by routine radiographic examinations (16). Nonetheless, given the central role of the thymus in adaptive immune regulation, ensuring T-cell tolerance against self-antigens and preventing the maturation of self-reactive T-cells, it is not surprising that thymomas can frequently lead to autoimmune syndromes (7, 17). Approximately 50% of the patients with thymomas experience associated autoimmune diseases, including MG, pure red cell aplasia, systemic lupus erythematosus, and Goodpasture's syndrome (17, 18). Cutaneous disorders associated with thymomas are widely heterogeneous and include pemphigus, BP, lichen planus (LP), vitiligo, alopecia areata, and lupus erythematosus (17).

CASE PRESENTATION

A 51 year old Caucasian woman presented with a diffuse skin rash associated with abdominal pain and diarrhea with a 2 weeks duration. Her past medical history was remarkable for a B2-type thymoma which was diagnosed about 7 years earlier. The patient underwent complete surgical resection of the tumor and then received adjuvant radiotherapy (50.4 Gy). Few months after surgical removal of the thymoma, the patient developed diffuse muscle weakness and was diagnosed with MG. She was started on azathioprine and pyridostigmine resulting in a good clinical control of her symptoms. Physical examination revealed erythematous plaques with shallow erosions and overwhelming yellow-to-brown crusts, involving the trunk, mainly back, upper and, to lesser extent, lower limbs, dorsal aspect of hands, face, and scalp (**Figure 1A**). There was no mucosal involvement. The results of the routine laboratory investigations were unremarkable except for elevated serum concentrations of the transaminases, GOT and GPT.

Initially, after surgical removal of the thymoma, direct immunofluorescence (DIF) from perilesional biopsy of the scaly erythematous skin rash revealed deposits of both IgG and C3 on the surface of epidermal keratinocytes (**Figures 2A,C**). Another DIF which was taken later at the time of GVHD-like dermatitis revealed instead linear deposits of IgG and C3 along the dermal-epidermal basement membrane zone (BMZ) (**Figures 2B,C**). Indirect immunofluorescence (IIF) on normal human skin, 1M NaCl-split human skin and monkey esophagus showed neither IgG autoantibodies to either the surface of epithelial cells nor on the dermal-epidermal BMZ (not shown). In addition, IIF on rat bladder was negative on transitional epithelia (not shown). Of note, the patient had IgG autoantibodies against Dsgl (719 relative units (RU)/ml, cutoff $<$ 20 RE/ml) and desmocollin 1 (Dscl) (0.448 OD, cutoff $<$ 0.200 OD) by ELISA and IgG autoantibodies against laminin 332 by immunoblot analysis (**Table 1**).

Based on clinical, histologic, and immunologic findings, the diagnosis of PF with additional anti-BMZ IgG reactivity was established. As there was neither evidence for IgG antibodies against desmosomal plaque proteins nor the 170 kDa alpha2-macroglobulin-like protein-1, the diagnosis of PNP was abandoned.

The patient initially received a cycle of intravenous immunoglobulins (IVIg) at 2 g/kg/cycle, followed by infusions of rituximab 2 × 1 g two weeks apart (19, 20). The patient's skin erosions improved significantly and fully regressed eventually, in association with the decrease of anti-Dsgl serum IgG antibodies.

Several months later, she developed diffuse erythroderma (**Figure 1B**). Erythematous targetoid plaques, resembling

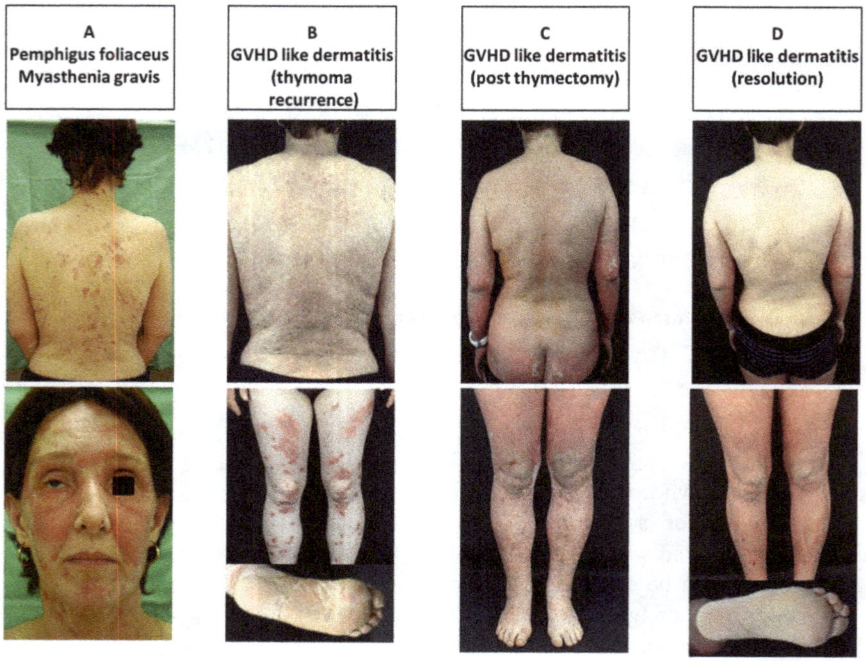

FIGURE 1 | (A–D) Clinical manifestations of the patient during clinical observational period. **(A)** Initially pemphigus foliaceus with involvement of the seborrheic skin areas and ptosis in myasthenia gravis, **(B)** lichenoid eruption at the time of thymoma recurrence, **(C)** erythroderma with lichenoid eruption right after thymectomy, and **(D)** resolution of the lichenoid eruption.

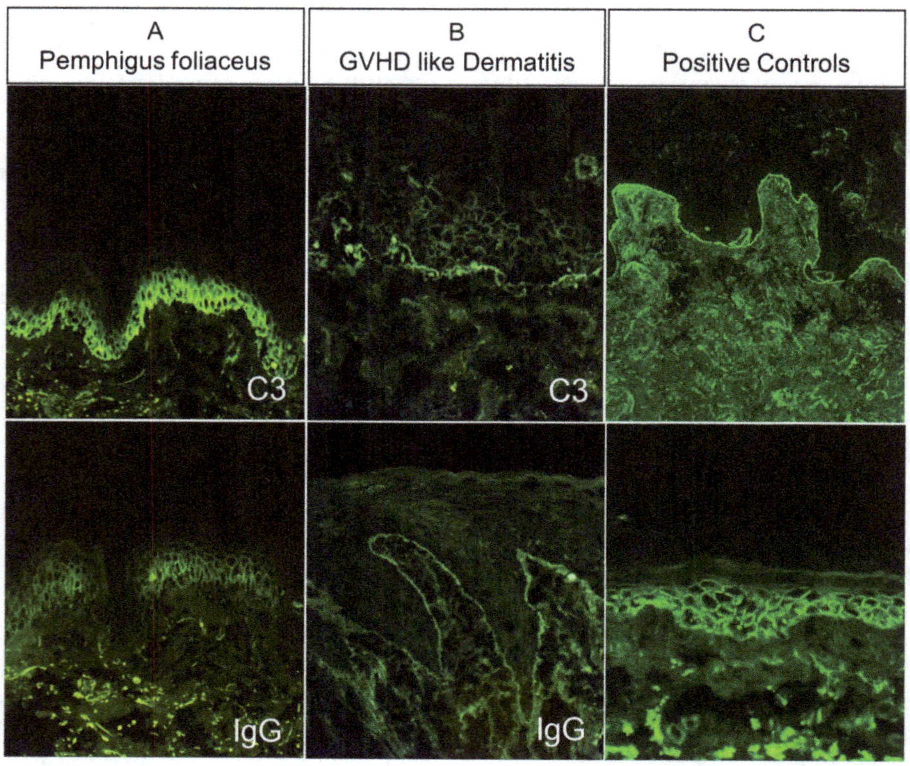

FIGURE 2 | Immune serological characteristics of the patient, **(A)** direct immunofluorescence (DIF) at time of pemphigus foliaceus, which showed IgG and C3 deposits at the surface of epidermal keratinocytes and **(B)** DIF at time of GVHD-like dermatitis which showed IgG C3 deposits along the BMZ. **(C)** positive DIF controls of perilesional BP skin, showing linear deposition of IgG along the BMZ (above), and positive DIF from perilesional PV skin presenting deposits at the surface of epidermal keratinocytes.

TABLE 1 | Autoantibody profile of the studied patient with thymoma-associated paraneoplastic autoimmune multiorgan syndrome.

Antigens	pemphigus foliaceus + myasthenia gravis	Thymoma reoccurrence	After thymectomy	Immunoassay
Dsg1	719 RE/ml (Cutoff < 20 RU/ml)	71 RU/ml	6 RU/ml	ELISA
Dsg3	0 (Cutoff < 20 RU/ml)	0	0	ELISA
Desmocollin 1	0.448 OD (Cutoff < 0.200 OD)	nd	nd	ELISA
Plakins	–	–	–	Immunoblot
BP180	0 (Cutoff < 20 RU/ml)	0	0	ELISA
BP230	0 (Cutoff < 20 RU/ml)	0	0	ELISA
Laminin γ-1	–	–	–	Immunoblot
Laminin 332	+	+	+	Immunoblot
Human type VII collagen	0 (Cutoff < 6 RU/ml)	0	0	ELISA
Skeletal muscle (titin)	++	+	–	BIOCHIP MOSAIC
Parotid gland	–	nd	nd	BIOCHIP MOSAIC
Stomach and bowels	–	nd	nd	BIOCHIP MOSAIC
Granulocytes, eosinophils, platelets, lymphocytes	–	nd	nd	BIOCHIP MOSAIC
Spinal cord, cerebrum, nerves, and cerebellum	–	nd	nd	BIOCHIP MOSAIC
HEP-2 cells	–	nd	nd	BIOCHIP MOSAIC
Liver, kidney, heart	–	nd	nd	BIOCHIP MOSAIC

nd, not determined; OD, optical densitiy; RU, relative units.

erythema multiforme (EM), and hyperkeratotic plaques appeared at her lower limbs and soles, respectively (**Figure 1B**). A skin biopsy from the erythrodermic skin revealed liquefactive degeneration and apoptotic keratinocytes and a band-like lymphocytic infiltrate along the BMZ (**Figure 3A**). These cutaneous symptoms were associated with persistent diarrhea and elevated liver enzymes and were thus considered as thymoma-associated GVHD-like disease. A chest X-ray and magnetic resonance imaging revealed a large mass in the left anterior mediastinum which was diagnosed by histopathology as a recurrent type-B2 thymoma. Prior to surgical removal, the patient received a cycle of intravenous cyclophosphamide (1,300 mg total dose) and IVIg (2 g/kg given on three consecutive days). After tumor resection, erythroderma with multiform lesions gradually regressed (**Figure 1C**) and eventually disappeared (**Figure 1D**). Of note, MG significantly improved and anti-Dsg1 serum IgG antibodies were no longer detectable (**Table 1**). A third skin biopsy revealed findings consistent with GVHD-like erythroderma (**Figure 3A**). Despite the clinical response, the patient eventually died because of an opportunistic bacterial infection leading to fulminant sepsis.

LABORATORY INVESTIGATIONS

Autoantibody Profile in the Patient With Thymoma-Associated Autoimmune Syndrome

The patient's serum IgG antibodies were reactive with Dsg1 and Dsc1 by ELISA and laminin 332 by immunoblot analysis (**Table 1**). Immunoblot analysis with epidermal extracts failed to identify IgG against plakins including periplakin and envoplakin (**Table 1**). Autoantibody profiling against various tissues showed the presence of IgG antibodies against muscle tissue (anti-titin IgG antibodies) which is characteristic for MG (**Table 1**) (21). More detailed information regarding the IgG autoantibody profile is given in the **Supplementary Material**. For information regarding detection of autoantibodies against laminin-γ1 please see (22).

Immunohistochemical Analysis of the T Cell Infiltrate in Skin Lesions and Thymoma Tissue

Skin samples taken from PF lesions, pre- and post-thymectomy GVHD-like skin lesions were further analyzed

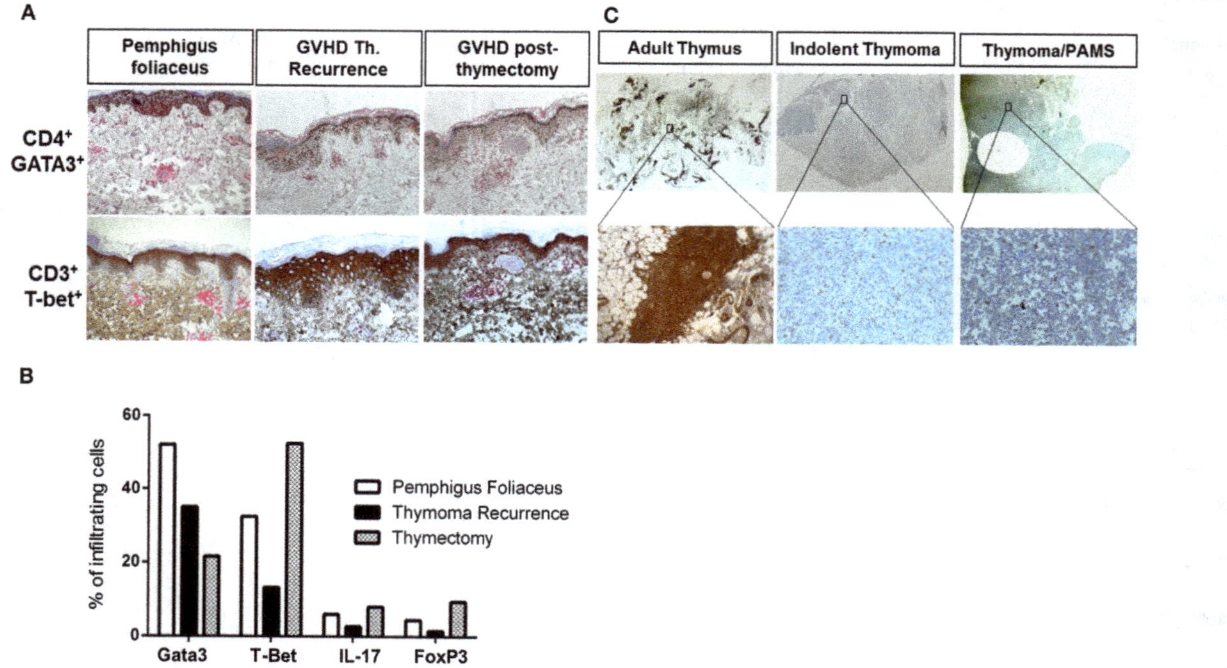

FIGURE 3 | (A) Immunohistochemical analysis of T cell subsets in pemphigus foliaceus (PF) and lichenoid skin lesions during the observational period. **(A)** CD3^{+}/Tbet^{+} and CD4^{+}/GATA3^{+} T cell skin infiltrate in PF, the lichenoid eruption at thymoma recurrence, and after thymectomy. **(B)** Percentage of CD4^{+}/GATA3^{+}, T-Bet+, IL17A^{+}, and FoxP3^{+} T cells in PF skin lesions, at thymoma recurrence and after thymectomy, **(C)** expression pattern of FoxP3+ T cells in adult thymus, indolent thymoma, and in PAMS-associated thymoma (present case).

by immunohistochemistry as recently described (23) (more detailed information is given in the **Supplementary Materials**). PF skin lesions showed more CD4^{+}GATA-3^{+} Th2 cells than CD3^{+}T-Bet^{+} compared to the Th1-dominated GVHD-like skin lesions which inversely showed a stronger presence of CD3^{+}T-Bet^{+} Th1 cells than CD4^{+}GATA-3^{+} Th2 cells (**Figures 3A,B**). The numbers of IL-17^{+} T cells and of FoxP3^{+} Treg cells were not different between PF and GVHD-like skin lesions (**Figure 3B**). Moreover, the number of FoxP3^{+} Treg cells in the patient's thymoma at the time of recurrence was significantly lower compared to adult persistent thymus and indolent thymoma without associated autoimmune syndromes (**Figure 3C**).

Peripheral Blood T Cell Response Against Cutaneous Autoantigen

By ELISpot assay, the peripheral blood T cell response of the patient against different cutaneous autoantigens, i.e., Dsg1, Dsg3, BP180, and BP230, was studied at different time points as recently described (21) (more detailed information is given in the **Supplementary Materials**).

Tetanus toxoid served as a control protein. Due to the strong immunosuppressive therapy, it was impossible to systematically study peripheral blood T cell responses against distinct cutaneous autoantigens (**Supplementary Figure 1**). Except for the initial treatment phase of PF with rituximab, Th1 and Th2 responses against the recall antigen, i.e., tetanus toxoid, were visible. After thymectomy, distinct Th1 and Th2 responses against Dsg3 and BP180 became apparent.

DISCUSSION

The association of thymoma, MG and PF is uncommon and is only rarely described in the literature (12). PF, MG, and thymoma can manifest as part of multiple autoimmune syndrome type 1, which consists of at least three autoimmune diseases including polymyositis, autoimmune thyroid disease, and giant cell myocarditis (18, 24). There have been sporadic cases of co-existing MG and PF which were not linked to thymoma (7, 8, 25). The etiopathogenesis of the simultaneous occurrence of MG, PF, and thymoma is only poorly understood. It has been proposed that a defective negative selection of autoreactive T-cells in neoplastic thymus leads to a loss of tolerance associated with autoantibody production against epithelial cells in Hassall's corpuscles and myeloid cells. These autoantibodies may then cross-react with homologous antigens of the epidermis and striate muscle, respectively (12). This contention is supported by the finding that the number of FoxP3^{+} Treg cells in thymomas is inversely correlated with the occurrence of associated autoimmune disorders, i.e., impaired Treg cell function favors the onset of autoimmune disorders (26, 27).

Tsuchisaka et al. reported on a patient with PF associated with thymoma which expressed higher levels of Dsg3, Dsc2, Dsc3, and autoimmune regulator (AIRE) but not Dsg1 compared to normal adult thymus, indolent thymomas, and thymic carcinoma. These findings suggest that lack of AIRE-induced expression of Dsg1 lead to an autoimmune response against this epidermal adhesion protein (28).

Our patient was diagnosed with PF based on the characteristic skin lesions and presence of anti-Dsg1 IgG antibodies. In addition, serum IgG against Dsc1 was also initially detected, and was likely linked to impaired desmosomal function (29). The patient did not fulfill all the criteria for PNP based on; (i) a lack of mucosal involvement, (ii) negative IIF on urinary bladder, and (iii) the absence of serum IgG antibodies against plakins, which are major autoantigens of PNP (6, 30).

Anti-laminin 332 antibodies are pathogenic autoantibodies in anti-laminin 332 mucous membrane pemphigoid, a distinct subepidermal autoimmune bullous disorder showing predominant mucosal lesions. However, the pathogenic role of anti-laminin 332 antibodies detected in the present case is unclear, as the patient neither presented subepithelial blisters on the skin nor on the mucous membranes. Due to the profound impaired immunological tolerance status, the presence of IgG autoantibodies against laminin 332 is likely the consequence of epitope spreading (31).

Although considered as a separate entity based on its characteristic spectrum of pathology, there is not a clear-cut distinction between thymoma associated multiorgan autoimmunity (TAMA) and PAMS. Accordingly, (i) thymomas are the second most frequent neoplasms associated with PAMS, following Castleman's disease (2); (ii) among the various cutaneous presentations, which also include pemphigus-like, BP-like or multiforme lesions, several cases of PAMS resembling cutaneous GVHD have been reported (2); (iii) involvement of liver and colon in PAMS has been also reported (2). As for thymoma, both PAMS and TAMA are thought to occur as a result of incomplete deletion of self-reactive T cells in the tumors (32). A decreased number of Treg cells in neoplastic thymus is believed to be also involved (33). In line with previous studies, we also observed a reduction of Treg cells in our patient's thymoma compared to adult thymus and indolent thymoma. The observed clinical spectrum, ranging from pemphigus-like to lichenoid lesions, likely depends on the T-cellular profile of the cutaneous immune response, either humoral (Th2), and later T cell-mediated (Th1).

IgG antibodies against envoplakin and periplakin are characteristic serological markers of PAMS, while anti-Dsg1 and anti-Dsg3 IgG antibodies are rarely seen (34–36). Conversely, anti-Dsc1-3 IgG antibodies are seen in almost 60% of PAMS cases, as the presence of anti-Dsc1 IgG in the present case. Although unusual, the detection of initial epidermal cell surface staining and, at a later time point, linear staining at the BMZ is a classic feature of PAMS. The presence of both patterns has been considered as a criteria for the diagnosis of PAMS (2, 37), while systematic studies on the prevalence of IgG antibodies against epidermal or BMZ antigens in TAMA are lacking. In addition, one case of cutaneous thymoma associated GVHD-like erythroderma was reported to show IgG deposits on the surface of epidermal keratinocytes by DIF (38).

In our case, even though IIF failed to show the presence of IgG autoantibodies against epidermal keratinocytes, DIF taken from perilesional skin at two different clinical stages showed initially the presence of IgG and C3 deposits on the surface of epidermal keratinocytes (**Figure 2A**) and, later on, the presence of linear IgG and C3 deposits at the BMZ (**Figure 2B**), which was supported by the detection of anti-Dsg1, anti-Dsc1, and anti-laminin 332 IgG antibodies. It could be argued that Dsg1, Dsc1, and/or laminin 332 function as antigenic targets and triggers for the activation of autoreactive T cells driving GVHD-like erythroderma (39). This contention is supported by a recent study of our group which suggested that lichenoid dermatoses such as LP harbor a T-cellular response against epidermal (Dsg3) or BMZ (BP180) autoantigens commonly associated with autoimmune blistering diseases (23). As recently suggested by Amber, it should be discussed if PNP should be classified as a subtype of PV or if PNP is just a variant of PAMS, a large group of clinically variable disorders which are all linked the occurrence of various neoplasias. We also tend to believe that PNP, as TAMA, should be considered as a variant of PAMS, but this requires a broader consensus (3). In conclusion, the present study proposes an immunologic conversion from an initial Th2-driven to a Th1-type dominated cutaneous immune response triggered by the recurrence of the thymoma (**Figures 1, 3A**). This shift to a Th1 response was paralleled by the complete resolution of the initial Th2 driven autoimmune disorders, PF and MG (**Figure 1**), and by the disappearance of serum anti-Dsg1/Dsc1 IgG antibodies (**Table 1**).

Of note, a study by Fujisao and Tsuda (40) described a patient with thymoma-associated pure red aplasia in which thymectomy resulted in an increased ratio of peripheral blood Th1/Th2 cells leading to significant amelioration of anemia (40). In 2015, Garrwan et al. reported on a patient with thymoma and associated proteinuria due to minimal change glomerulonephritis, in which antitumoral therapy with belinostat, cisplatin, doxorubicin, and cyclophosphamide resulted in a complete resolution of the tumor, reduction of proteinuria and increase in the Th1/Th2 ratio (41). Further accumulation of cases is required to better understand how thymectomy modulates thymoma-associated autoimmune syndromes via specific T-cell signatures and impacts on the course of these associated paraneoplastic syndromes.

ETHICS STATEMENT

In accordance with the declaration of Helsinki, written consent for the publication of this case report, and the accompanying images was obtained from the patient.

AUTHOR CONTRIBUTIONS

FS, RM, RP, and TS wrote the manuscript, performed the experiments, analyzed data, and designed figures. RE and MH designed and supervised the study. TH and NI provided help for extensive serological diagnostic. BT, AK, DD, and JP helped during clinical follow-ups and helped during manuscripts writing. RP, TS, RE, MH, and TH revised the study. All authors revised and finally approved the study.

REFERENCES

1. Nguyen VT, Ndoye A, Bassler KD, Shultz LD, Shields MC, Ruben BS, et al. Classification, clinical manifestations, and immunopathological mechanisms of the epithelial variant of paraneoplastic autoimmune multiorgan syndrome: a reappraisal of paraneoplastic pemphigus. *Arch Dermatol.* (2001) 137:193–206.
2. Czernik A, Camilleri M, Pittelkow MR, Grando SA. Paraneoplastic autoimmune multiorgan syndrome: 20 years after. *Int J Dermatol.* (2011) 50:905–14. doi: 10.1111/j.1365-4632.2011.04868.x
3. Amber KT. Paraneoplastic autoimmune multi-organ syndrome is a distinct entity from traditional pemphigus subtypes. *Nat Rev Dis Primers.* (2018) 4:18012. doi: 10.1038/nrdp.2018.12
4. Payne AS, Kasperkiewicz M, Ellebrecht CT, Takahashi H, Yamagami J, Zillikens D, et al. Correction: paraneoplastic autoimmune multiorgan syndrome and paraneoplastic pemphigus describe the same spectrum of disease pathology. *Nat Rev Dis Primers.* (2018) 4:18032. doi: 10.1038/nrdp.2018.32
5. Hashimoto T. Production of numerous autoantibodies in paraneoplastic pemphigus. *Br J Dermatol.* (2015) 172:849–50. doi: 10.1111/bjd.13648
6. Kasperkiewicz M, Ellebrecht CT, Takahashi H, Yamagami J, Zillikens D, Payne AS, et al. Pemphigus. *Nat Rev Dis Primers.* (2017) 3:17026. doi: 10.1038/nrdp.2017.27
7. Holbro A, Jauch A, Lardinois D, Tzankov A, Dirnhofer S, Hess C. High prevalence of infections and autoimmunity in patients with thymoma. *Hum Immunol.* (2012) 73:287–90. doi: 10.1016/j.humimm.2011.12.022
8. Huh WK, Tada J, Fujimoto W, Toi Y, Arakawa K, Arata J, et al. Thyroid gland tumour, pemphigus foliaceus and myasthenia gravis in the daughter of a woman with myasthenia gravis. *Clin Exp Dermatol.* (2001) 26:504–6. doi: 10.1046/j.1365-2230.2001.00877.x
9. Nakayama M, Itoh M, Kikuchi S, Tanito K, Nakagawa H. Thymoma-associated cutaneous graft-versus-host-like disease possibly treated with Narrow-band UVB phototherapy. *Eur J Dermatol.* (2016) 26:208–9. doi: 10.1684/ejd.2015.2716
10. Qiao J, Zhou G, Ding Y, Zhu D, Fang H. Multiple paraneoplastic syndromes: myasthenia gravis, vitiligo, alopecia areata, and oral lichen planus associated with thymoma. *J Neurol Sci.* (2011) 308:177–9. doi: 10.1016/j.jns.2011.05.038
11. Slavik T, Potgieter FM, Brittain D. Thymoma-associated multiorgan autoimmunity with exclusive gastrointestinal tract involvement: case report and review of the literature. *Virchows Arch.* (2018) 473:121–5. doi: 10.1007/s00428-018-2304-6
12. Takeshita K, Amano M, Shimizu T, Oyamada Y, Abiko T, Kobayashi K, et al. Thymoma with pemphigus foliaceus. *Internal Med.* (2000) 39:742–7. doi: 10.2169/internalmedicine.39.742
13. Wadhera A, Maverakis E, Mitsiades N, Lara PN, Fung MA, Lynch PJ. Thymoma-associated multiorgan autoimmunity: a graft-versus-host-like disease. *J Am Acad Dermatol.* (2007) 57:683–9. doi: 10.1016/j.jaad.2007.02.027
14. Winkler DT, Strnad P, Meier ML, Roten S, Went P, Lyrer P, et al. Myasthenia gravis, paraneoplastic pemphigus and thymoma, a rare triade. *J Neurol.* (2007) 254:1601–3. doi: 10.1007/s00415-007-0588-6
15. Yamawake N, Koyo T, Kakuta T, Kurisu H, Iida Y, Sekine M, et al. [A case of pemphigus vulgaris with thymoma]. *Nihon Naika Gakkai Zasshi.* (1988) 77:22–5. doi: 10.2169/naika.77.22
16. Kondo K, Yoshizawa K, Tsuyuguchi M, Kimura S, Sumitomo M, Morita J, et al. WHO histologic classification is a prognostic indicator in thymoma. *Ann Thorac Surg.* (2004) 77:1183–8. doi: 10.1016/j.athoracsur.2003.07.042
17. Bernard C, Frih H, Pasquet F, Kerever S, Jamilloux Y, Tronc F, et al. Thymoma associated with autoimmune diseases: 85 cases and literature review. *Autoimmun Rev.* (2016) 15:82–92. doi: 10.1016/j.autrev.2015.09.005
18. Humbert P, Dupond JL. The multiple autoimmune syndromes (MAS). *Br J Dermatol.* (1997) 136:468–9. doi: 10.1111/j.1365-2133.1997.tb14972.x
19. Amber KT, Maglie R, Solimani F, Eming R, Hertl M. Targeted therapies for autoimmune bullous diseases: current status. *Drugs.* (2018) 78:1527–48. doi: 10.1007/s40265-018-0976-5
20. Maglie R, Didona D, Eming R, Hertl M. Pemphigus: current and future therapeutic strategies. *Front Immunol.* (2019) 10:1418. doi: 10.3389/fimmu.2019.01418
21. Yamamoto AM, Gajdos P, Eymard B, Tranchant C, Warter JM, Gomez L, et al. Anti-titin antibodies in myasthenia gravis: tight association with thymoma and heterogeneity of nonthymoma patients. *Arch Neurol.* (2001) 58:885–90. doi: 10.1001/archneur.58.6.885
22. Solimani F, Pollmann R, Ishii N, Eming R, Hashimoto T, Schmidt T, et al. Diagnosis of anti-laminin gamma-1 pemphigoid by immunoblot analysis. *J Eur Acad Dermatol Venereol.* (2018) 33:735–41. doi: 10.1111/jdv.15170
23. Schmidt T, Solimani F, Pollmann R, Stein R, Schmidt A, Stulberg I, et al. TH1/TH17 cell recognition of desmoglein 3 and bullous pemphigoid antigen 180 in patients with lichen planus. *J Allergy Clin Immunol.* (2018) 142:669–72 e7. doi: 10.1016/j.jaci.2018.02.044
24. Seiffert-Sinha K, Khan S, Attwood K, Gerlach JA, Sinha AA. Anti-thyroid peroxidase reactivity is heightened in pemphigus vulgaris and is driven by human leukocyte antigen status and the absence of desmoglein reactivity. *Front Immunol.* (2018) 9:625. doi: 10.3389/fimmu.2018.00625
25. Kim HT, Kim SH, Kim JH, Kim MH, Lee CW. Coexistence of myasthenia gravis and pemphigus foliaceus. *J Korean Med Sci.* (1995) 10:298–302. doi: 10.3346/jkms.1995.10.4.298
26. Liu Y, Zhang H, Zhang P, Meng F, Chen Y, Wang Y, et al. Autoimmune regulator expression in thymomas with or without autoimmune disease. *Immunol Lett.* (2014) 161:50–6. doi: 10.1016/j.imlet.2014.04.008
27. Bieber K, Sun S, Witte M, Kasprick A, Beltsiou F, Behnen M, et al. Regulatory T cells suppress inflammation and blistering in pemphigoid diseases. *Front Immunol.* (2017) 8:1628. doi: 10.3389/fimmu.2017.01628
28. Tsuchisaka A, Kaneko S, Imaoka K, Ota M, Kishimoto K, Tomaru U, et al. Presence of autoimmune regulator and absence of desmoglein 1 in a thymoma in a patient with pemphigus foliaceus. *Br J Dermatol.* (2015) 173:268–71. doi: 10.1111/bjd.13617
29. Didier K, Bolko L, Giusti D, Toquet S, Robbins A, Antonicelli F, et al. Autoantibodies associated with connective tissue diseases: what meaning for clinicians? *Front Immunol.* (2018) 9:541. doi: 10.3389/fimmu.2018.00541
30. Witte M, Zillikens D, Schmidt E. Diagnosis of autoimmune blistering diseases. *Front Med.* (2018) 5:296. doi: 10.3389/fmed.2018.00296
31. Didona D, Di Zenzo G. Humoral epitope spreading in autoimmune bullous diseases. *Front Immunol.* (2018) 9:779. doi: 10.3389/fimmu.2018.00779
32. Liu ZH, Xu JZ, Shen H. Fetal sequential multiorgan autoimmunity associated with recurrent post thymectomy thymoma. *Autoimmun Rev.* (2017) 16:1090–1. doi: 10.1016/j.autrev.2017.08.003
33. Hanafusa T, Azukizawa H, Kitaba S, Murota H, Umegaki N, Terao M, et al. Diminished regulatory T cells in cutaneous lesions of thymoma-associated multi-organ autoimmunity: a newly described paraneoplastic autoimmune disorder with fatal clinical course. *Clin Exp Immunol.* (2011) 166:164–70. doi: 10.1111/j.1365-2249.2011.04472.x
34. Inaoki M, Kodera M, Fujimoto A, Nousari HC, Anhalt GJ, Takehara K. Paraneoplastic pemphigus without antidesmoglein 3 or antidesmoglein 1 autoantibodies. *Br J Dermatol.* (2001) 144:610–3. doi: 10.1046/j.1365-2133.2001.04095.x
35. Joly P, Richard C, Gilbert D, Courville P, Chosidow O, Roujeau JC, et al. Sensitivity and specificity of clinical, histologic, and immunologic features in the diagnosis of paraneoplastic pemphigus. *J Am Acad Dermatol.* (2000) 43:619–26. doi: 10.1067/mjd.2000.107488
36. Ohyama M, Amagai M, Hashimoto T, Nousari HC, Anhalt GJ, Nishikawa T. Clinical phenotype and anti-desmoglein autoantibody profile in paraneoplastic pemphigus. *J Am Acad Dermatol.* (2001) 44:593–8. doi: 10.1067/mjd.2001.112222
37. Amber KT, Valdebran M, Grando SA. Non-desmoglein antibodies in patients with pemphigus vulgaris. *Front Immunol.* (2018) 9:1190. doi: 10.3389/fimmu.2018.01190
38. Yatsuzuka K, Tohyama M, Oda F, Hashimoto T, Sayama K. Case of thymoma-associated cutaneous graft-versus-host disease-like disease successfully

improved by narrowband ultraviolet B phototherapy. *J Dermatol.* (2018) 45:479–82. doi: 10.1111/1346-8138.14176

39. Ludwig RJ, Vanhoorelbeke K, Leypoldt F, Kaya Z, Bieber K, McLachlan SM, et al. Mechanisms of autoantibody-induced pathology. *Front Immunol.* (2017) 8:603. doi: 10.3389/fimmu.2017.00603
40. Fujisao S, Tsuda H. Th1/Th2 balance alteration in the clinical course of a patient with pure red cell aplasia and thymoma. *Br J Haematol.* (1998) 103:308–10. doi: 10.1046/j.1365-2141.1998.01011.x
41. Gharwan H, Tomita Y, Lee MJ, Thomas A, Berman A, Giaccone G, et al. Alterations of immune cell subsets in relapsed, thymoma-associated minimal change disease: a case report. *Oncol Lett.* (2015) 10:1155–8. doi: 10.3892/ol.2015.3325

9

Identification of a Novel Non-Desmoglein Autoantigen in Pemphigus Vulgaris

Giulia Di Lullo[1], *Valentina Calabresi*[2], *Feliciana Mariotti*[2], *Giovanna Zambruno*[3], *Antonio Lanzavecchia*[4] *and Giovanni Di Zenzo*[2*]

[1] *Tumor Immunology Unit, Division of Immunology, Transplantation and Infectious Diseases, Istituto di Ricovero e Cura a Carattere Scientifico (IRCCS) San Raffaele Scientific Institute, Milan, Italy,* [2] *Laboratory of Molecular and Cell Biology, IDI-IRCCS, Rome, Italy,* [3] *Genetic and Rare Diseases Research Division, Bambino Gesù Children's Hospital, IRCCS, Rome, Italy,* [4] *Institute for Research in Biomedicine, Università della Svizzera italiana, Bellinzona, Switzerland*

Correspondence:
Giovanni Di Zenzo
g.dizenzo@idi.it

Pemphigus vulgaris (PV) is an autoimmune bullous disease of the skin and mucous membranes characterized by the presence of circulating and tissue-bound autoantibodies against keratinocyte cell surface antigens, specifically desmoglein (Dsg) 1 and 3. The pathogenic role of anti-Dsg antibodies is well-established, while the mechanism of blister formation is only partly defined. We have applied a previously developed method for the efficient immortalization of IgG+ memory B cells to identify novel target antigens in PV. A human monoclonal antibody reactive with a hitherto unreported non-Dsg antigen was isolated. Immunoprecipitation and immunoblotting studies with keratinocyte extracts indicated α-catenin as the putative antigen, then confirmed by immunoblotting on the recombinant protein. Four of ten PV sera reacted with recombinant α-catenin. Although the isolated human monoclonal antibody was *per se* unable to dissociate keratinocyte monolayers and also to synergize with a pathogenic antibody *in vitro,* further studies are warranted to assess its possible *in vivo* contribution in the multifactorial pathogenesis and heterogeneous manifestations of PV disease.

Keywords: pemphigus vulgaris, non-desmoglein autoantigens, autoantibodies, memory B cells, α-catenin, skin, mucous membranes

INTRODUCTION

Pemphigus vulgaris (PV) is a rare but highly disabling and, if untreated, almost always fatal immunobullous disease of the skin and mucous membranes. PV is characterized histologically by loss of cell-cell adhesion between suprabasal keratinocytes, leading to acantholysis, and immunopathologically by the presence of circulating and tissue-bound autoantibodies (autoAbs) against keratinocyte cell surface antigens, specifically desmoglein (Dsg) 1 and 3. PV is considered as a paradigmatic organ-specific autoimmune disease in view of (i) present knowledge of disease autoantigens and pathogenesis and (ii) reproducibility of major clinical and pathogenic features in animal models (1). The existence of both pathogenic and non-pathogenic anti-Dsg autoAbs has recently been underscored by isolation of human monoclonal antibodies (hMabs) from pemphigus patients. Anti-Dsg hMabs characterization has shown that their pathogenic potential primarily depends on the targeted epitopes (1). We have been interested in characterizing the repertoire of naturally occurring autoreactive epithelium-specific memory B cells in pemphigus vulgaris patients. In a first work, we focused on autoantibodies targeting Dsg3 (2). However, (i) the lack of tight correlation between anti-Dsg autoAb titers and disease activity in some patients and (ii) the significant degree of disease heterogeneity point at the importance of non-Dsg autoAbs, that have been progressively, even though not exhaustively, described (3, 4). In fact, besides Dsg3 and Dsg1, other non-desmoglein autoAbs, either pathogenic or non-pathogenic, have been identified in pemphigus patients. AutoAbs endowed with an acantholytic potential target desmocollin 3, α-acetylcholine receptor, pemphaxin, and keratinocyte mitochondria (5–8). On the other hand, the pathogenic role of autoAbs recognizing other autoantigens, such as ATP2C1, desmocollin 1, BP230, periplakin, E-cadherin, desmoglein 4, desmoplakin 1, and desmoplakin 2, remains to be demonstrated (9). In line with this interest, our current work aimed to identify autoAbs targeting non-Dsg membrane-bound or membrane-associated intracellular antigens.

In the present study, we report on the characterization of a hMab isolated from a PV patient and directed to a novel non-Dsg antigen. The hMab reacts with α-catenin that is recognized by almost half of PV sera analyzed.

MATERIALS AND METHODS

Patients, Sera and Isolation of hMabs From a PV Patient

Peripheral blood was obtained from 2 patients (PVC and PVF) suffering from active mucocutaneous PV. The patients showed typical clinical, histological, and immunopathological features and had high-titer anti-Dsg circulating autoantibodies (PVC: Dsg3, 127 U/ml, Dsg1, 90 U/ml; PVF: Dsg3, 191 U/ml, Dsg1, 170 U/ml), as assessed by ELISA kits based on ectodomain of Dsg1 and Dsg3 (MBL, Nagoya, Japan). hMabs were isolated by a highly-efficient protocol for the immortalization of IgG+ memory B cell with Epstein Barr virus (EBV) in the presence of a Toll-like receptor agonist, as previously described (2). In detail, IgG+ memory B cells were isolated from cryopreserved peripheral blood mononuclear cells using anti-CD22 microbeads (Miltenyi Biotec, Bo, Italy) followed by depletion of cells carrying IgM, IgD, and IgA by cell sorting. Multiple replicate microcultures of 10–30 IgG+ memory B cells/well (for a total of 2 to 8 × 10^4 purified cells) were infected with EBV and CpG as previously described (10). Culture supernatants were tested for binding to Dsg1- and Dsg3-coated ELISA plates and for binding to HaCaT keratinocyte cell line monolayers (both on live cells and on fixed and permeabilized cells) by immunofluorescence (IF) assay using an automated fluorescence microscope (Pathway 855, BD). The specificity of positive polyclonal cultures was further assessed by IF on primary human keratinocytes. Positive reactivities were confirmed by the propagation of oligoclonal cultures. Positive cultures were cloned by limiting dilution and expanded; antibodies were purified using protein G columns. Serum samples were collected from 10 PV and 16 bullous pemphigoid (BP) patients and 10 healthy donors. This study was carried out in conformity with the Helsinki guidelines and with approval of the IDI-IRCCS Ethics Committee. All the biological samples were obtained after patient's informed consent.

Immunofluorescence Analyses

IF studies were performed according to the procedure described in Di Zenzo et al. with minor modifications (2). Briefly, supernatants from immortalized human memory B cells were screened on monolayers of live and fixed/permeabilized HaCaT cells. After washing with phosphate-buffered saline, cells were stained with Alexa Fluor 488–conjugated goat anti-human IgG (Invitrogen, Carlsbad, CA, USA). The isolated monoclonal antibodies were further tested on permeabilized HaCaT cells and on primary keratinocytes. Non-keratinocyte cell lines, i.e., MRC9, Hela, and SKMEL cells, were used as controls for IF analyses on cell monolayers. Human antibodies of irrelevant specificity were used as negative controls. Serial images of stained keratinocyte monolayers were acquired by the BD Pathway 855 automated fluorescence microscope. Staining was also performed on cryo sections of normal human skin, guinea pig and monkey esophagus and revealed with fluorescein isothiocyanate-conjugated anti-human IgG antibody (Agilent DAKO, Santa Clara, CA, USA).

Immunoprecipitation and Immunoblotting Analyses

Immunoprecipitation (IP) of ^{35}S-labeled keratinocyte extracts by hMab PVF144 was carried out as previously described (11). The precipitated proteins, separated on sodium dodecyl sulfate-polyacrylamide gel electrophoresis on 6% gels under reducing conditions, were detected by autoradiography. Immunoblotting (IB) experiments on keratinocyte extracts were performed as previously reported using both horseradish peroxidase (HRP)-conjugated and alkaline phosphatase-conjugated secondary antibodies (12). Bands were quantified using ImageJ Software (National Institutes of Health, Bethesda, MD, USA) and their intensities were normalized respect to the positive control signal obtained by anti-α-catenin antibody. The cut-off value was set as the medium value +2 standard deviations obtained measuring signals obtained with healthy donors. Commercial primary antibodies were purchased from Progen Biotechnik GmbH (Heidelberg, Germany) (anti-desmocollin 2), BD Biosciences (San Jose, CA, USA; anti-α-catenin), and Santa Cruz Biotechnology, Inc (Dallas, TX, USA; anti-γ-catenin, anti-β-catenin, anti-p120, and anti-E-cadherin). Recombinant tagged human α1-catenin was purchased from Abcam (Cambridge, UK). To rule out that PV sera were mainly reacting against the fused glutathione S-transferase (GST) moiety of the α-catenin recombinant protein, IB experiments by using commercial tagged protein and equimolar GST were performed (data not shown).

Enzyme Linked ImmunoSorbent Assay (ELISA)

Briefly, recombinant Dsg1 and Dsg3 ectodomains were produced in baculovirus and used for coating of ELISA plates. The plates were, then, blocked with 1% bovine serum albumin and incubated with antibodies followed by HRP-conjugated anti-human IgG (Jackson ImmunoResearch, Baltimore, PA, USA) (2).

Keratinocyte Dissociation Assay

The assay was performed as previously reported (13). Briefly, primary human keratinocyte cells were seeded onto 12-well plates and 24 h post-confluence treated with monoclonal antibodies.

After adding exfoliative toxin A to cleave Dsgl protein, the cell monolayers were detached with dispase I (Merck, KGaA, Darmstadt, Germany) and subjected to mechanical stress by pipetting. The monolayer fragments, fixed by adding a 3% formaldehyde solution, were subsequently stained using crystal violet. To investigate a possible synergistic effect PVF144 was applied to the monolayer together with a pathogenic antibody (PVB28) (2) at optimal (4 μg/ml) and suboptimal concentrations (1 μg/ml and 0.25 μg/ml; **Figure 4**) and a non-pathogenic antibody (2, PVB28 in a germline version that is not able to dissociate the keratinocyte monolayer; data not shown).

RESULTS

Isolation of hMabs Specific for Non-Dsg Epithelial Antigens in Pemphigus Patients

In order to identify hMabs targeting non-Dsg membrane-bound or membrane-associated intracellular antigens, we took advantage of the same strategy by which we had previously isolated and finely characterized several Dsg-reactive PV patient-derived monoclonal autoantibodies (2). In detail, peripheral blood samples were collected from 2 patients with mucocutaneous PV: one with long-lasting steroid-resistant disease (PVC) and the other prior to treatment initiation (PVF). IgG+ memory B cells were isolated by magnetic and fluorescence-activated cell sorting, seeded in 96-well microplates, and immortalized with EBV in the presence of irradiated mononuclear cells and oligodeoxynucleotides containing CpG motifs, as previously described (10). The reactivity of antibodies secreted in the supernatants of growing polyclonal cultures was screened by IF staining both on live and on fixed and permeabilized cells from the human keratinocyte HaCaT cell line. The polyclonal antibodies produced by the vast majority of isolated cultures bound to surface antigens on the keratinocyte membrane and were reactive with Dsgl and/or Dsg3 ectodomains by ELISA, as previously reported (2, and data not shown). Besides such prevalent pattern of reactivity, supernatants of rare cultures from both patients showed a distinctive membrane-associated fishnet reactivity, detected only on permeabilized keratinocytes, and were negative in ELISA on Dsgl and Dsg3 ectodomains. The human Mabs PVF144 (IgG1-isotype), PVC6 (IgG1-isotype), and PVC33 (isotype IgG3-isotype) were cloned by limiting dilution and showed the same IF pattern as the original polyclonal cultures also on permeabilized HaCaT keratinocytes (**Figure 1A**), suggesting their specificity for a membrane-associated intracellular (i.e., non-exposed) autoantigen. In addition, they showed an intercellular staining pattern by IF on human skin, guinea pig, and monkey esophagus (**Figures 1B–D**), very similar to IF staining pattern of anti-Dsg3 antibodies (2, and data not shown). Supernatants from the selected clones were tested on non-keratinocyte cell lines, i.e., MRC-9 (fibroblast), SKMEL (melanoma), and Hela (epithelial) cells: they failed to stain both live and permeabilized cells, apart from a reactivity on permeabilized Hela cells (data not shown), hinting at a specificity for membrane-associated intracellular antigens expressed on keratinocytes and other epithelial cells.

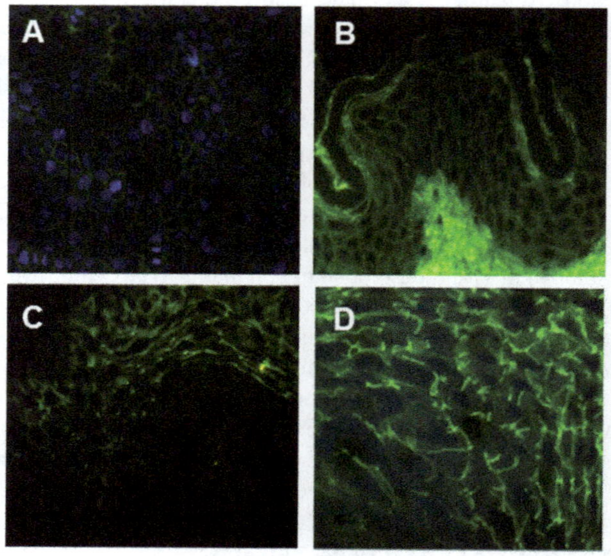

FIGURE 1 | Intercellular staining pattern of hMab PVF144. PVF144 binds a membrane associated epithelial antigen showing a typical intercellular staining pattern on permeabilized HaCaT keratinocytes (nuclear counterstain is obtained with DAPI) (20X) **(A)**, human skin (40X) **(B)** guinea pig (40X) **(C)**, and monkey esophagus (40X) **(D)**.

Identification of the Intracellular Epithelial Target Antigen of hMab PVF144

IP studies with the 3 selected clones on radiolabelled keratinocyte extracts to identify the target antigen showed reactivity to a 100 kDa antigen for PVF144 (**Figure 2A**) and to 190–210 kDa antigens for PVC6 and PVC33, respectively (data not shown). As the IP results from the latter two clones pointed at members of the plakin-family as candidate target antigens and autoreactivity of PV sera to plakin family members has been already documented (14, 15), we chose to further characterize PVF144 with the aim to identify a possible novel membrane-associated PV autoantigen. Subsequent IB experiments using commercial antibodies reacting with keratinocyte membrane-associated proteins with a molecular weight of ~100 kDa (desmocollin 2–115 kDa; α-catenin-102 kDa; E-cadherin-120 kDa; β-catenin-92 kDa; γ-catenin-83 kDa; P120-catenin 80–100 kDa) indicated α-catenin as the putative antigen (**Figure 2B**). Sequential IP and IB experiments further supported α-catenin as the target antigen of PVF144. Specifically, a protein immunoprecipitated from keratinocyte extracts with PVF144 was recognized by a commercial anti-α-catenin antibody, and an anti-α-catenin antibody was in turn able to immunoprecipitate a protein recognized by PVF144 in IB (**Figure 2C**). Finally, IB experiments with the recombinant tagged protein unequivocally confirmed the specific binding of PVF144 to α-catenin (**Figure 2D**).

α-Catenin Is Recognized by PV Patient Sera

To determine whether autoAbs of the same specificity as PVF144 were present in the sera of PV patients, we performed IB experiments with 10 PV sera on recombinant tagged α-catenin

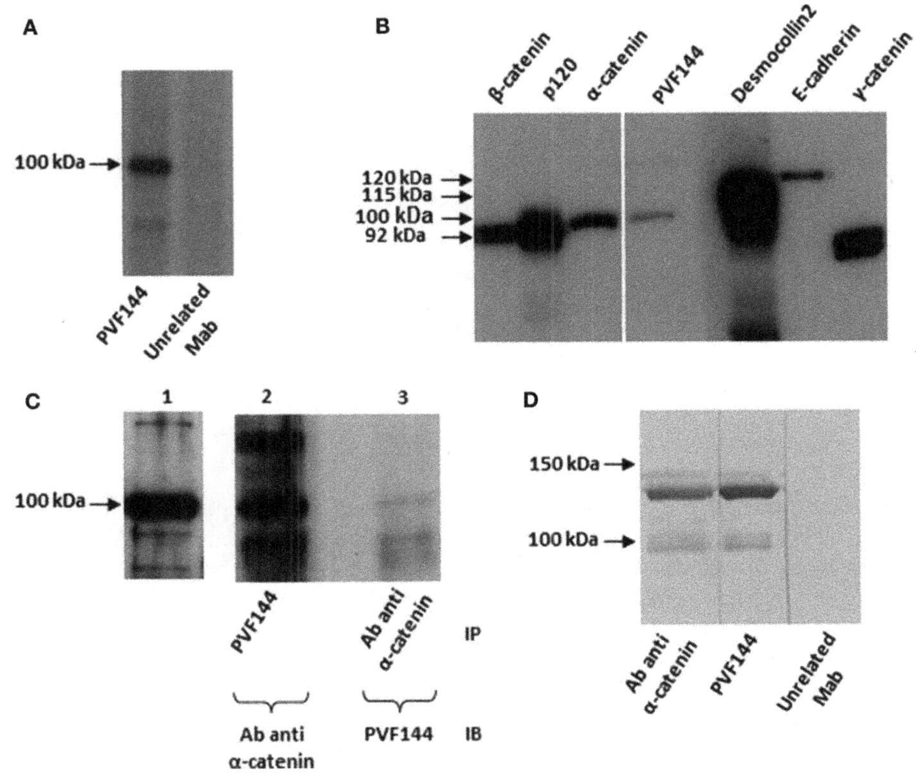

FIGURE 2 | PVF144 binds a membrane-associated epithelial antigen: α-catenin. PVF144 immunoprecipitates (IP) an unknown antigen of 100 kDa from radiolabeled normal human keratinocyte extracts **(A)**. Immunoblotting (IB) experiments on keratinocyte extracts by using PVF144 and commercial antibodies suggest that α-catenin could be the putative antigen of 100 kDa: PVF144 and a monoclonal murine anti-α-catenin antibody (Ab) react with a keratinocyte antigen of similar molecular weight (100 kDa) **(B)**. Anti-α-catenin commercial antibody reacts to α-catenin from keratinocyte extracts by IB (lane 1); PVF144 immunoprecipitates α-catenin recognized by the commercial anti-α-catenin antibody by IB (lane 2) and, viceversa, anti-α-catenin antibody immunoprecipitates α-catenin recognized by PVF144 by IB (lane 3). The faint reactivity observed in lane 3 could be related to the epitope recognized **(C)**. IB performed with a recombinant GST-tagged human α-catenin (120 kDa) confirms that the target of PVF144 is α-catenin. The lower bands are likely degradation products **(D)**.

(**Figure 3**). Four out of 10 PV patients (40%) showed the same reactivity of PVF144 to α-catenin, whereas the other PV sera and 10 normal human control sera showed only a faint signal, indicating that this autoreactivity was well-represented in PV patients, even though not shared by all patients. In order to evaluate whether this reactivity is disease-specific, 16 BP patient sera were analyzed on recombinant α-catenin by IB. Only one of 16 BP (7 representative BP sera shown and other 9 not shown) reacted to α-catenin (**Supplementary Figure 1**) underlining the specificity of this autoantigen. The weak signals found in the other remaining PV, PB, and healthy donor sera might be ascribed to reactivity to the tag protein (GST).

PVF144 Is Not Able to Dissociate a Keratinocyte Monolayer and to Synergize With a Human Pathogenic Antibody

The presence of anti-α-catenin autoAbs in several PV sera raised the question as to their pathogenic potential. Previous studies showed the ability of intact autoAbs to enter the cytosol or nucleus of living cells (16, 17). More recently, Marchenko et al. reported that PV autoAbs could penetrate keratinocytes and react with intracellular mitochondrial proteins (8). These findings suggested that a hMab to an intracellular antigen could exert its pathogenic ability on live keratinocytes. Thus, an *in vitro* dissociation assay was used to evaluate the pathogenic activity of the hMab PVF144. This approach allows to measure the ability of a specific antibody or a mixture of antibodies, such as a serum, to fragment a monolayer of primary human keratinocytes seeded to confluence. The keratinocyte monolayers, incubated for 24 h with PVF144, remained intact, similarly to monolayers incubated with an unrelated hMab used as negative control (**Figure 4**). As expected, human (PVB28) and murine (AK23) pathogenic anti-Dsg3 antibodies were able to dissociate the monolayers (2, 18) (**Figure 4**). In addition, PVF144 failed to synergize with a pathogenic antibody (**Figure 4**). These findings exclude a primary pathogenic function of anti-α-catenin autoAbs in PV, nevertheless a potential secondary role in the immunobiology of the disease cannot be excluded and warrants future studies.

DISCUSSION

In the present work we went forward in the characterization of the diverse targets of epithelium-specific autoreactive B cells from PV patients. To this purpose, we took advantage of the

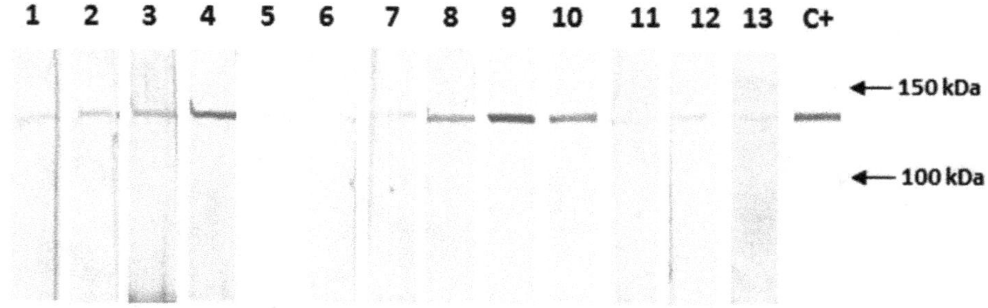

FIGURE 3 | Almost half of PV sera specifically react with recombinant α-catenin. Immunoblotting with sera obtained from 10 pemphigus vulgaris (PV) patients shows that 4 of 10 sera (4, 8, 9, 10) react with the novel epithelial antigen, while 3 healthy donor sera (11, 12, 13), representative of 10 sera analyzed, show only a background signal. The positive control (C+) is the commercial anti-α-catenin antibody. The background signal, could be also due to reactivity to the tag protein (GST). Quantification and normalization of bands using ImageJ analysis (data not shown) have confirmed the reported results (see Materials and Methods section).

high-efficiency immortalization protocol of IgG+ memory B cells we had previously developed (10) and applied to isolate and molecularly characterize a number of anti-Dsg3 hMabs (2). Our present focus was to detect plasma-membrane-associated antigens, either expressed on the cell surface or intracellularly, therefore we chose to screen the isolated polyclonal cultures on both live and permeabilized keratinocytes. Our choice was based on the hypothesis that antigens associated to the cell membrane, even those with intracellular localization, could have a higher chance to contribute to pemphigus pathogenesis, which is due to the loss of cell-cell adhesion.

As expected, the vast majority of cultures resulted specific for Dsg1 and/or Dsg3, further confirming the major role of these antigens in pemphigus pathogenesis. Among polyclonal cultures that reacted only with permeabilized keratinocytes, we selected and cloned those giving a membrane-associated fishnet-like staining pattern on stratified epithelia. Among the cloned cultures, we further characterized clone PVF144 and demonstrated by IF, IP and IB studies that α-catenin is its target. α-catenin is a component of adherens junctions (AJs), i.e., cell-cell anchoring structures that, together with desmosomes, allow keratinocytes to adhere to one another and maintain epithelial integrity. α-catenin binds to β-catenin in AJs and is required for their formation and maintenance (19, 20). In addition, α-catenin was reported to be necessary for the organization of desmosomes in epithelial cells (21).

A previous study reported a reactivity of pemphigus sera to another AJ component, i.e., E-cadherin (22). Likewise, we showed that anti-α-catenin autoreactivity was: (i) well-represented in PV patient sera, as α-catenin was recognized by almost half of the PV sera tested; (ii) more frequently associated with pemphigus than with other autoimmune bullous diseases, as α-catenin was very rarely recognized by the BP sera analyzed.

Then, considering that previous studies demonstrated the ability of intact autoAbs to enter living cells (8, 16, 17), we addressed the potential pathogenicity of α-catenin-specific Mab PVF144 by evaluating its acantholytic activity in an *in vitro* keratinocyte dissociation assay. In this regard, several observations suggest that AJs, and in particular E-cadherin, may be involved in pemphigus pathogenesis (23, 24). Of note, with the exception of anti-desmocollin 3 autoAbs, all known non-Dsg-reactive autoAbs with reported pathogenicity do not possess acantholytic potential on their own but may act synergistically with anti-Dsg antibodies (1, 25, 26). Accordingly, Marchenko et al. described a pathogenic role for intracellular anti-mitochondrial autoAbs, even though not on their own (8). In our hands, the anti-α-catenin Mab PVF144 was not able to dissociate the keratinocyte monolayer either alone or in combination with a suboptimal dose of a pathogenic anti-Dsg3 antibody. Nevertheless, we cannot exclude that regions of α-catenin different from that recognized by PVF144 could be recognized by PV sera and contribute to acantholysis. In addition, a possible role of anti-α-catenin hMabs as co-factors in disease initiation or maintenance could not be exhaustively addressed by our approach. In previous studies, several antibodies against intracellular antigens have been considered as triggers for autoimmunity. Mabs specific for the cytoplasmic precursor form of Dsg1 (preDsg1) have been cloned from pemphigus patients and from healthy individuals (25, 26). Yamagami et al. postulated that the presence of anti-preDsg1 B cells is involved in the initiation of the autoimmune response in pemphigus patients. In particular, in the context of tissue damage they could present peptides which are part of mature Dsg1 (i.e., the extracellular autoantigen recognized by most pathogenetic autoAbs) derived from the processing of preDsg1. This intramolecular epitope spreading phenomenon could lead to the production of pathogenic autoAbs targeting mature Dsg1 and to the initiation of disease pathogenesis (27, 28). Moreover, natural autoAbs (NAAs), i.e., antibodies to intracellular autoantigens that naturally occur in the healthy population and are *per se* unable to cause immune phatology, have been theorized as cofactors in the onset of autoimmunity, possibly by participating in the mechanisms of chronic tissue injury at the basis of intermolecular epitope spreading (29–31).

In conclusion, while our previous study (2) demonstrated that pathogenic PV antibodies primarily target the Dsg-3 cis-interface, thus leading to desmosome disruption, our current results reveal novel antibodies targeting intracellular keratinocyte proteins. We are tempted to speculate that the cellular damage

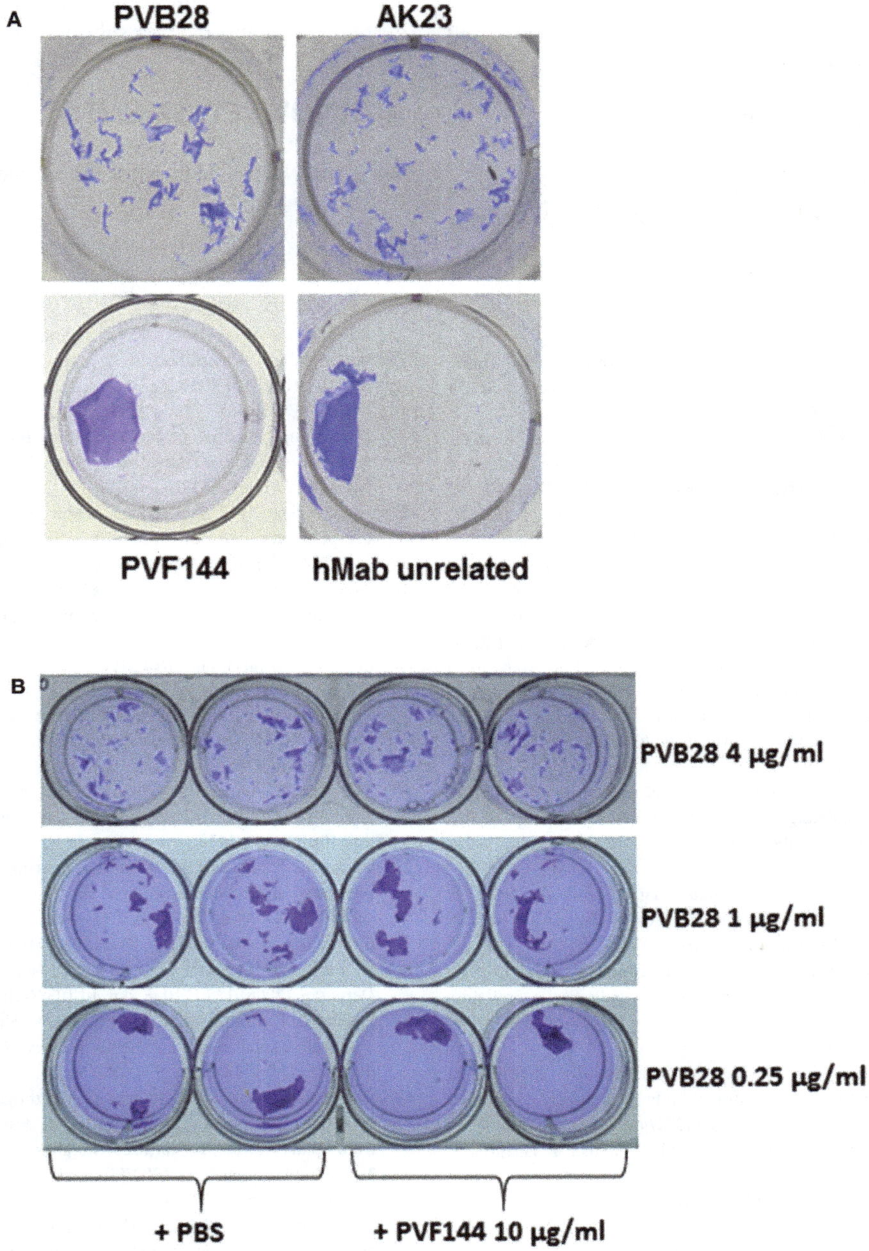

FIGURE 4 | PVF144 is not able to dissociate a keratinocyte monolayer even in the presence of suboptimal concentrations of PVB28. A representative keratinocyte dissociation experiment. Primary human keratinocytes, seeded to confluence, were incubated with PVF144, an unrelated human Mab (negative control) and, as positive controls, the human pathogenic Mab PVB28 (7) and the murine pathogenic Mab AK23 (14), both Dsg3-specific **(A)**. To investigate synergistic potential of cloned antibody we have employed PVF144 (10 μg/ml) together with optimal (4 μg/ml) and suboptimal concentrations (1 μg/ml and 0.25 μg/ml) of the pathogenic anti-Dsg3 antibody PVB28 without obtaining any difference in ability of PVB28, with or without PVF144, to dissociate the keratinocyte monolayer **(B)**.

induced by pathogenic anti-Dsg antibodies may trigger an intermolecular epitope-spreading phenomenon resulting in an antibody response against intracellular antigens, among which α-catenin. Further studies are needed: (i) to evaluate whether PVF144 may act synergistically with anti-Dsg antibodies using more informative approaches, such as *in vitro* organ culture or *in vivo* models; (ii) to assess the possible role of anti-α-catenin autoAbs in pemphigus initiation and evolution *in vivo*; and (iii) to characterize this novel antigen as a possible target of epitope spreading phenomena in PV.

ETHICS STATEMENT

This study was carried out in accordance with the recommendations of Helsinki guidelines, IDI-IRCCS Ethics

Committee. The protocol was approved by the IDI-IRCCS Ethics Committee. All subjects gave written informed consent in accordance with the Declaration of Helsinki.

AUTHOR CONTRIBUTIONS

GDZ and GDL have written the manuscript. GDZ, GZ, and AL have designed the study. GDZ, GDL, VC, and FM performed the experiments. All the authors have revised the manuscript and given the final approval for submission.

ACKNOWLEDGMENTS

We thank Naomi De Luca for the excellent technical assistance.

REFERENCES

1. Di Zenzo G, Amber KT, Sayar BS, Müller EJ, Borradori L. Immune response in pemphigus and beyond: progresses and emerging concepts. *Semin Immunopathol.* (2016) 38:57–74. doi: 10.1007/s00281-015-0541-1
2. Di Zenzo G, Di Lullo G, Corti D, Calabresi V, Sinistro A, Vanzetta F, et al. Pemphigus autoantibodies generated through somatic mutations target the desmoglein-3 cis-interface. *J Clin Invest.* (2012) 122:3781–90. doi: 10.1172/JCI64413
3. Amber KT, Valdebran M, Grando SA. Non-desmoglein antibodies in patients with pemphigus vulgaris. *Front Immunol.* (2018) 9:1190. doi: 10.3389/fimmu.2018.01190
4. Sinha AA, Sajda T. The evolving story of autoantibodies in pemphigus vulgaris: development of the "super compensation hypothesis". *Front Med.* (2018) 5:218. doi: 10.3389/fmed.2018.00218
5. Rafei D, Muller R, Ishii N, Llamazares M, Hashimoto T, Hertl M, et al. IgG autoantidodies against desmocollin 3 in pemphigus sera induce loss of keratinocyte adhesion. *Am J Pathol.* (2011) 178:718–23. doi: 10.1016/j.ajpath.2010.10.016
6. Nguyen VT, Ndoye A, Grando SA. Novel human alpha9 acetylcholine receptor regulating keratinocyte adhesion is targeted by pemphigus vulgaris autoimmunity. *Am J Pathol.* (2000) 157:1377–91. doi: 10.1016/S0002-9440(10)64651-2
7. Nguyen VT, Ndoye A, Grando SA. Pemphigus vulgaris antibody identifies pemphaxin. A novel keratinocyte annexinlike molecule binding acetylcholine. *J Biol Chem.* (2000) 275:29466–76. doi: 10.1074/jbc.M003174200
8. Marchenko S, Chernyavsky AI, Arredondo J, Gindi V, Grando SA. Antimitochondrial autoantidodies in pemphigus vulgaris: a missing link in disease pathophysiology. *J Biol Chem.* (2010) 285:3695–704. doi: 10.1074/jbc.M109.081570
9. Kalantari-Dehaghi M, Anhalt GJ, Camilleri MJ, Chernyavsky AI, Chun S, Felgner PL, et al. Pemphigus vulgaris autoantibody profiling by proteomic technique. *PLoS ONE.* (2013) 8:e57587. doi: 10.1371/journal.pone.0057587
10. Traggiai E, Becker S, Subbarao K, Kolesnikova L, Uematsu Y, Gismondo MR, et al. An efficient method to make human monoclonal antibodies from memory B cells: potent neutralization of SARS coronavirus. *Nat Med.* (2004) 10:871–5. doi: 10.1038/nm1080
11. Di Zenzo G, El Hachem M, Diociaiuti A, Boldrini R, Calabresi V, Cianfarani F, et al. A truncating mutation in the laminin-332α chain highlights the role of the LG45 proteolytic domain in regulating keratinocyte adhesion and migration. *Br J Dermatol.* (2014) 170:1056–64. doi: 10.1111/bjd.12816
12. Cozzani E, Di Zenzo G, Calabresi V, Carrozzo M, Burlando M, Longanesi L et al. Autoantibody profile of a cohort of 78 italian patients with mucous membrane pemphigoid: correlation between reactivity profile and clinical involvement. *Acta Derm Venereol.* (2016) 96:768–73. doi: 10.2340/00015555-2311
13. Ishii K, Harada R, Matsuo I, Shirakata Y, Hashimoto K, Amagai M. *In vitro* keratinocyte dissociation assay for evaluation of the pathogenicity of anti-desmoglein 3 IgG autoantidodies in pemphigus vulgaris. *J Invest Dermatol.* (2005) 124:939–46. doi: 10.1111/j.0022-202X.2005.23714.x
14. Kiyokawa C, Ruhrberg C, Nie Z, Karashima T, Mori O, Nishikawa T, et al. Envoplakin and periplakin are components of the paraneoplastic pemphigus antigen complex. *J Invest Dermatol.* (1998) 111:1236–8. doi: 10.1046/j.1523-1747.1998.00449.x
15. Mimouni D, Foedinger D, Kouba DJ, Orlow SJ, Rappersberger K, Sciubba JJ, et al. Mucosal dominant pemphigus vulgaris with anti-desmoplakin autoantibodies. *J Am Acad Dermatol.* (2004) 51:62–7. doi: 10.1016/j.jaad.2003.11.051
16. Golan TD, Sigal D, Sabo E, Shemuel Z, Guedj D, Weinberger A. The penetrating potential of autoantibodies into live cells *in vitro* coincides with the *in vivo* staining of epidermal nuclei. *Lupus.* (1997) 6:18–26. doi: 10.1177/096120339700600103
17. Alascón-Segovia D. Proceedings of the second international conference on the penetration of autoantibodies into living cells. *J Autoimmun.* (1998) 11:509–10. doi: 10.1006/jaut.1998.0238
18. Tsunoda K, Ota T, Aoki M, Yamada T, Nagaim T, Nakagawa T, et al. Induction of pemphigus phenotype by a mouse monoclonal antibody against the amino-terminal adhesive interface of desmoglein 3. *J Immunol.* (2003) 170:2170–8. doi: 10.4049/jimmunol.170.4.2170
19. Hirano S, Kimoto N, Shimoyama Y, Hirohashi S, Takeichi M. Identification of a neural alpha-catenin as a key regulator of cadherin function and multicellular organization. *Cell.* (1992) 70:293–301. doi: 10.1016/0092-8674(92)90103-J
20. Kobielak A, Fuchs E. Alpha-catenin: at the junction of intercellular adhesion and actin dynamics. *Nat Rev Mol Cell Biol.* (2004) 5:614–25. doi: 10.1038/nrm1433
21. Taniguchi T, Miyazaki M, Miyashita Y, Arima T, Ozawa M. Identification of regions of alpha-catenin required for desmosome organization in epithelial cells. *Int J Mol Med.* (2005) 16:1003–8. doi: 10.3892/ijmm.16.6.1003
22. Evangelista F, Dasher DA, Diaz LA, Prisayanh PS, Li N. E-cadherin is an additional immunological target for pemphigus autoantibodies. *J Invest Dermatol.* (2008) 128:1710–8. doi: 10.1038/sj.jid.5701260
23. Furukawa F, Takigawa M, Matsuyoshi N, Shirahama S, Wakita H, Fujita M, et al. Cadherins in cutaneous biology. *J Dermatol.* (1994) 21:802–13. doi: 10.1111/j.1346-8138.1994.tb03294.x
24. Aoyama Y, Owada MK, Kitajima Y. A pathogenic autoantibody, pemphigus vulgaris-IgG, induces phosphorylation of desmoglein 3, and its dissociation from plakoglobin in cultured keratinocytes. *Eur J Immunol.* (1999) 29:2233–40. doi: 10.1002/(SICI)1521-4141(199907)29:07<2233::AID-IMMU2233>3.0.CO;2-4
25. Chernyavsky A, Webber RJ, Grando SA, Wang PH. Critical role of the neonatal Fc receptor (FcRn) in the pathogenic action of antimitochondrial autoantibodies synergizing with anti-desmoglein autoantibodies in pemphigus vulgaris. *J Biol Chem.* (2015) 290:23826–37. doi: 10.1074/jbc.M115.668061
26. Chernyavsky A, Amber KT, Agnoletti AF, Wang C, Grando SA. Synergy among non-desmoglein antibodies contributes to the immunopathology of desmoglein antibody-negative pemphigus vulgaris. *J Biol Chem.* (2019) 294:4520–8. doi: 10.1074/jbc.RA118.006743
27. Ishii K, Lin C, Siegel DL, Stanley JR. Isolation of pathogenic monoclonal anti-desmoglein 1 human antibodies by phage display of pemphigus foliaceus autoantidodies. *J Invest Dermatol.* (2008) 128:939–48. doi: 10.1038/sj.jid.5701132
28. Yamagami J, Kacir S, Ishii K, Payne AS, Siegel DL, Stanley JR. Antibodies to the desmoglein 1 precursor proprotein but not to the mature cell surface protein cloned from individuals without pemphigus. *J Immunol.* (2009) 183:5615–21. doi: 10.4049/jimmunol.0901691

29. Didona D, Di Zenzo G. Humoral epitope spreading in autoimmune bullous diseases. *Front Immunol.* (2018) 9:779. doi: 10.3389/fimmu.2018.00779

30. Goodnow CC, Sprent J, Fazekas de St. Groth B, Vinuesa CG. Cellular and genetic mechanisms of self tolerance and autoimmunity. *Nature.* (2005) 435:590–7. doi: 10.1038/nature03724

31. Wardemann H, Yurasov S, Schaefer A, Young JW, Meffre E, Nussenzweig MC. Predominant autoantibody production by early human B cell precursors. *Science.* (2003) 301:1374–7. doi: 10.1126/science.1086907

10

NET Formation in Bullous Pemphigoid Patients with Relapse is Modulated by IL-17 and IL-23 Interplay

Delphine Giusti [1,2†], Estela Bini [1†], Christine Terryn [3], Kevin Didier [1], Sébastien Le Jan [1], Grégory Gatouillat [1,2], Anne Durlach [4], Stéphane Nesmond [1], Celine Muller [1], Philippe Bernard [1,5], Frank Antonicelli [1,6‡] and Bach Nga Pham [1,2‡]*

[1] Laboratory of Dermatology, Faculty of Medicine of Reims, University of Champagne-Ardenne, Reims, France, [2] Laboratory of Immunology, Reims University Hospital, University of Champagne-Ardenne, Reims, France, [3] PICT Platform, University of Reims Champagne-Ardenne, Reims, France, [4] Laboratory of Pathology, Reims University Hospital, Reims, France, [5] Department of Dermatology, Reims University Hospital, University of Champagne-Ardenne, Reims, France, [6] Department of Biological Sciences, Immunology, UFR Odontology, University of Reims Champagne-Ardenne, Reims, France

***Correspondence:**
Delphine Giusti
dgiusti@chu-reims.fr

† These authors have contributed equally to this work

‡ These authors have contributed equally to this work

Background: DNA extracellular traps (ETs), released by neutrophils (NETs), or eosinophils (EETs), play a pathogenic role in several autoimmune disorders. However, to date, NETs have never been investigated in bullous pemphigoid (BP) with respect to clinical and immunological activities, both at baseline and at time of relapse which have been characterized with specific IL-17 and IL-23 patterns.

Objective: We sought to assess whether ETs were associated with BP as well as the relative contribution of IL-17 axis cytokines to NET induction.

Methods: Skin biopsy specimens were obtained from 11 patients with BP. Immuno-detection of neutrophils and eosinophils combined to DNA staining allowed us to investigate the *in-situ* presence of NETs and EETs using confocal scanning microscopy. NETs release was evaluated *ex vivo* by stimulating polymorphonuclear cells from BP patients with BP biological fluids in presence of IL-17A and IL-23 or of glucocorticoids.

Results: At baseline, ETs were observed in BP lesions at the site of dermal-epidermal cleavage. Despite an important infiltrate of eosinophils, ETs were essentially associated with neutrophils *in situ* and were not related to BP clinical activity at diagnosis. *In situ* observation of NETs was associated in 6 among 8 patients with serum capacity of NET induction. Notably both blister fluid and sera from BP patients at diagnosis and at time of relapse could induce NET formation *ex vivo*. In contrast, a longitudinal investigation showed a decrease of NET formation with time of treatment in patients undergoing remission. Mimicking relapse, complementation of sera from BP patients with ongoing remission with either IL-17A or IL-23 increased NET formation. Conversely, IL-17A inhibited NET formation induced by serum from BP patients with relapse supplemented or not with IL-23. Finally, glucocorticoids also inhibited NET formation *ex vivo* in BP.

Conclusion: NET formation is an associated phenomenon with BP. Furthermore, we showed that IL-23 favored NET formation, whereas the effects of IL-17A are environment dependent. Indeed, IL-17A displayed a protective effect on NET formation when associated with IL-23, showing for the first-time differential effects of these two cytokines in BP.

Keywords: neutrophil extracellular traps, eosinophil extracellular traps, cytokine, autoimmunity, inflammation, bullous pemphigoid

INTRODUCTION

Bullous pemphigoid (BP) is an invalidating autoimmune subepidermal blistering disease affecting preferentially the elderly. Eosinophils and neutrophils are the most represented cells in the skin inflammatory infiltrate of BP patients (1). Both cells have the capacity to form DNA traps (2–5) which play a pathogenic role in several autoimmune diseases (6, 7). The participation of eosinophil DNA extracellular traps (EET)s to blister formation has recently been reported in BP (7, 8). In contrast, neutrophil extracellular trap (NET) presence has not been demonstrated yet. Additionally, DNA trap formation has never been investigated in BP with respect to the clinical features of the disease i.e., activity and outcome. Also, the relationship between NET formation and the autoimmune or inflammatory responses, which characterize BP development, needs to be clarified.

Neutrophils and eosinophils are both involved in BP pathological process (8–13). Neutrophils play a crucial role in most BP experimental models to induce dermal-epidermal separation (10, 14–16). The cooperation with monocytic cell-line and the stimulation by CXCL-10, IL-17, or IL-23, lead neutrophils to release metalloproteinase MMP-9 and neutrophil elastase, which are responsible for dermal-epidermal junction (DEJ) disruption and BP180 cleavage (17–22). Besides, eosinophils are the predominant cells in the human BP inflammatory infiltrate (1). The activated eosinophils release a potent army of cytokines (9, 11) and granule proteins such as Eosinophil Cationic Protein (ECP), which serum concentrations parallel BP activity (23). The actions of both granulocytes converge to MMP-9 production, which suppresses the neutrophil elastase natural inhibitor, and thus contributes to dermal-epidermal splitting (24).

Stimuli inducing NETs release are numerous and highly variable. For instances auto-antibodies (AAb)s, as well as cytokines, appear to be able to induce this phenomenon (5, 6, 25). Indeed, AAbs from patients with rheumatoid arthritis and IL-17 were recently shown to induce NET formation in an *ex vivo* model of rheumatoid arthritis (25). In BP, the pathogenic role of anti-BP180 antibodies has been illustrated by both *in vitro* and *in vivo* studies, and their serum concentrations at diagnosis have been correlated with disease activity (14, 26–30). Cytokines also play a key role in BP pathogeny (17–19, 31–34). In previous studies, we showed that IL-17 levels were elevated in blister fluids, linked to a local production by neutrophils and mastocytes (17), and a relationship between IL-17 axis cytokines and BP outcome (18). More precisely, we evidenced an increased serum level of IL-23 or a high sustained serum level of IL-17 despite treatment in BP patient who later relapsed (18). Moreover, these inflammatory mediators are involved in BP pathophysiological process, as they enhance MMP-9 production by innate immune cells from patients (17, 18).

In the present study, we investigated DNA extracellular traps in BP with respect to clinical and immunological characteristics of the disease. Therefore, the aim of this study was to determine whether NETs or EETs or even both were associated with BP at tissue level, and to investigate IL-17 and IL-23 influence on NET formation *ex vivo*.

MATERIALS AND METHODS

Patients

This prospective, observational, and translational study was conducted in our tertiary Referral Center for Autoimmune Bullous Diseases at the Reims University Hospital. Consecutive patients with newly diagnosed BP were included in this prospective study. Diagnosis of BP was made when the following criteria were met: presence of at least 3 out of 4 established clinical criteria by Vaillant et al in combination with positive direct immunofluorescence findings (30). Routine skin biopsy specimens of 11 BP patients were provided by the Pathology Department of the Reims University Hospital to perform *in situ* analysis. *Ex-vivo* assays were performed with sera from these 11 patients collected at time of diagnosis (at the same time as the biopsy) and with biological samples [sera and polymorphonuclear cells (PMN)] collected at time of diagnosis and around 150 and 360 days after, from 17 other consecutive BP patients. Sera were also collected at time of relapse in patients who underwent relapse despite treatment. PMNs used for *ex vivo* experiments were freshly isolated PMNs from patients with BP collected at any time point (between D1 and D360 after diagnosis) throughout the course of the study. Seven sera and PMN from healthy controls were provided by French Blood Agency and volunteers (mean age 66.4 years).

In situ Analysis of NETs/EETs

Immunofluorescence and confocal analysis of NETs and EETs were performed on paraformaldehyde-fixed and paraffin-embedded skin biopsy specimens from 11 BP patients. DNA staining along with neutrophils and eosinophils immunostaining was performed as follow on tissues. Four consecutive deparaffanized sections were used by patient, using a distinct eosinophil marker on each. After 15 min heat retrieval in sodium citrate buffer pH6, the sections were then blocked with PBS-BSA 3% for 30 min at room temperature. Then, simultaneous staining was performed for 30 min at room temperature with mouse anti-human myeloperoxidase (1:150; *R&D Systems, Minneapolis, USA)* for neutrophil staining and another primary antibody (Ab) for eosinophil staining: either rabbit anti-human IL-5Rα (1:150; *Proteintech, Chicago, USA*), or rabbit anti-human MBP, EDN, or ECP (1:150; *Novus Biologicals, Littleton, USA*). This was followed by 30 min of incubation at room temperature with matched secondary Abs: chicken anti-rabbit IgG Alexa Fluor 488 and chicken anti-mouse IgG Alexa Fluor 594 (Invitrogen). Sytox Orange Nucleic Acid Stain (5 μM) *(Molecular Probes, Invitrogen, Carlsbad, USA)* was finally used to stain DNA prior to mounting slides with Dako® fluorescent mounting medium. The presence of NETs *in situ* was confirmed by an immunostaining performed with a rabbit polyclonal Ab to Histone H3 (1:100 overnight; *Abcam, Cambridge, UK)* revealed by a secondary chicken anti-rabbit Ab Alexa Fluor 594 (1:200. *Invitrogen, Carlsbad, USA*) and a mouse monoclonal Ab to human myeloperoxydase coupled to a FITC fluorochrome *(1:100; Abcam, Cambridge, UK).*

Extracellular DNA filaments associated to both eosinophils and neutrophils were investigated by 2 independent investigators using 3-dimensional imaging by confocal scanning microscope LSM 710 NLO Zeiss (Zeiss SAS, Germany). Image analysis was performed by using ZEISS ZEN software (Zeiss SAS, Germany) and IMARIS Software (Bitplane, Switzerland). ETs were identified as shapes of DNA extruding from cell and stained by nucleic acid probe SYTOX orange. NETs were defined as extracellular DNA filaments stained by Sytox Orange extruding from cells labeled by MPO Ab, while cell MBP, EDN, ECP or IL-5R labeling characterized EETs.

To qualify eosinophil and neutrophil cell infiltrate, hematoxylin-eosin coloration of serial sections was performed for these 11 biopsy specimens. A rating from 0 to + + + was assigned by two operators to eosinophil and neutrophil infiltrates in the papillary dermis and in the blister cavity to allow a comparative semi-quantification of these cells.

Ex vivo Analysis of NET Formation

Peripheral PMNs cells were obtained by density-gradient centrifugation from 25 mL heparinized-treated whole blood (Granulosep, Eurobio-Abcys). NET generation was performed following the protocol proposed by Brinkmann et al. (35) with the difference that SYTOX Orange was used to stain extracellular DNA. 2.10^5 PMNs were incubated with either 5% blister fluids or 5% sera from BP patients, following preliminary optimization assays (**Supplementary Figure S1**). To investigate their potential influence on NET formation, recombinant IL-17A and IL-23 were added to cell culture medium at concentrations close to those determined in the sera of BP patients (1.2 ng/mL) (18). To assess the effects of treatment on NET induction by BP sera, methylprednisolone MP (10 μM), and Compound A (10 μM) were added to the cell culture medium in presence of BP sera. Each condition was tested with biological fluids from at least 3 different subjects (patients or controls).

NETs were visualized using an inverted epifluorescence microscope (AxioObserver Z1: Zeiss, Germany; camera Cool Snap HQ2: Roper Scientific, France). For each slide, a mosaic of 4 × 4 consecutive images was taken (scale image: 0.625 μm/pixel, driven by Metamorph Software (Roper scientific, Evry, France), which represents an area of around 2 mm^2 per coverslips. Fluorescence signal was collected with bandpass 545/25 excitation filter and bandpass 605/70 emission filter. For each acquisition, fluorescence, and transmitted images were taken.

To assess NETs formation, the area occupied by the DNA filaments was determined using a dedicated home-made macro based on "skeletonize function" and the "analyse particle" tool running under IMAGE J® software (ImageJ, U. S. National Institutes of Health, Bethesda, USA.). Briefly, we skeletonized the fluorescent images, setting 40 pixels as the minimal resolution, and transformed these images into drawings of DNA filaments, which were measured and processed by the "Analyze particles" tool (**Supplementary Figure S1**). Area of each filament was measured, and the mean was calculated, making the conversion from pixels to μm (1pixel = 0.625 μm). The total number of cells was counted using the counter cell tool of Image J® software on the transmitted image acquired simultaneously with fluorescent image. Thus, this method allowed measuring the total number of PMNs, and the total area of NETs. Results were expressed in mean area of NETs per PMN (as proposed by Rebernick et al. (36). As variations were observed when using PMNs from different subjects, results were also expressed in ratio between mean area of NETs per cell for condition X and mean area of NETs per cell for the reference condition with the same PMNs.

Statistical Analysis

As the distribution of the variables could not be assumed to be normal, comparisons between two groups were performed using the Wilcoxon matched pairs signed rank test for paired data and the Mann-Whitney test for unpaired data. When more of two matched groups were compared, Friedman test was performed. Ratio paired t-test was used to compare NETs induction by sera with and without treatment (by cytokines, methylprednisolone or compound A). Statistical difference was considered significant if p-value was 0.05 or less.

RESULTS

DNA Extracellular Traps Mainly Originated From Neutrophils *in situ*

To investigate the presence of either NETs or EETs or even both in BP at site of lesion, immune-detection of neutrophils and eosinophils along with DNA staining was performed on paraffin-embedded skin biopsy specimens from 11 BP patients. The mean age of the 11 newly diagnosed BP patients (6 female (54.5%) and 5 males (45.5%), sex ratio F/M: 1.2) was of 78.9 years. At baseline, the clinical BP activity was assessed by the Bullous Pemphigoid Disease Assessment Index (BPDAI) score and by the number of new daily blisters. The BPDAI median value was of 53 [23–90], and 9 (81.8%) BP patients presented with a severe disease characterized by more than 10 blisters a day. Finally, 5 (45.5%) BP patients experienced a relapse despite treatment during the first year of follow up (**Table 1**).

Extracellular DNA filaments were identified *in situ* in 8 out of the 11 (73%) BP patients (**Figures 1A–C**). NETs were observed on lesional skin biopsy specimen, in the papillary dermis at the edge of the dermal-epidermal separation (**Figures 1A–G**). A 3-dimensional reconstruction picture corresponding to **Figure 1E** allowed defining NETs as shapes of DNA extruding from neutrophils stained by MPO (**Supplementary Video S1; Figure 1F**). EETs were only observed in one patient despite a higher number of eosinophils than neutrophils in BP lesional skin, corroborated by both HES staining and immunofluorescence using specific eosinophils markers including MBP, EDN, ECP, or IL-5Rα (**Figure 1H; Table 2**). DNA extracellular trap was observed neither in blister cavity nor in perilesional dermis, despite the presence of numerous inflammatory cells. Besides, in those 8 BP patients, NETs were absent from skin biopsy specimens performed at distance of the lesions (data not shown). Also, no DNA traps were evidenced in 4 plastic surgical normal skin specimens (mean age of controls 66.5 years) (data not shown).

In situ occurrence of NETs appeared to be independent of the disease activity at time of diagnosis. Indeed, patients in whom NETs were seen, showed miscellaneous BPDAI scores with values ranged from 23 to 90 and a median of 50.5 (**Tables 1, 3**). Furthermore, these 8 BP patients were evenly distributed according to the BPDAI score, as 3 patients displayed a BPDAI score superior to 56, 2 with a BPDAI close to mean value between 48 and 53, and 3 with a BPDAI inferior to 36. Also, NETs were observed in both patients with a multibullous BP (displaying more than 10 new blisters per day and up to 120 new daily blisters), and in those with a limited disease (down to only one blister per day). Likewise, the presence of NETs was not associated with BP relapse, as among the 8 BP patients displaying NETs at baseline, 4 later underwent a relapse and 4 remained on remission over the one-year of clinical follow-up (**Table 1**).

Both Neutrophils and Biological Fluids From Patients With BP Were Required for NET Formation

To further investigate the factors involved in NET formation associated with BP, we established an *ex vivo* NET generation model with peripheral blood PMNs from patients with BP stimulated with blister fluid collected at time of diagnosis (**Figure 2A**). Similar NET formation level was observed when PMNs from BP patients were stimulated with BP serum (**Figures 2B–D**, p =0.25, Wilcoxon matched pairs test). Besides, immunostaining of myeloperoxydase and citrullinated histones allowed to confirm that neutrophils were the source of the observed NETs in this *ex vivo* model (**Figure 2C**). The induction of NETs by blister fluids was independent from BPDAI score at diagnosis and from BP 180 Ab levels in blister fluids (**Figures 2E,F**). We then investigated the capacity of the sera from the 11 BP patients for whom *in situ* exploration of NETs was performed, to induce NET formation. Among the 8 patients previously identified with NETs *in situ*, 6 showed capacity of NET induction compared with 1 patient among the 3 for whom *in-situ* assessment was negative (**Table 1**).

In contrast, the capability of sera from healthy donors to induce NET formation by PMN from BP patients was significantly lower than sera from BP patients (0.15 vs. 0.74 μm^2/cell, p = 0.0006 Mann-Whitney test) (**Figures 2G,H**). To investigate whether circulating PMNs from BP patients were primed to release NETs, we assessed the ability of PMNs isolated from healthy donor peripheral blood to generate NETs upon BP serum stimulation. As showed in **Figure 2I**, NET quantification remained low in those conditions. Also, when PMNs from healthy donors were stimulated with heterologous sera from healthy donors, NET area remained low (**Figure 2J**).

BP Serum Capacity to Induce NET Formation Decreased in BP Patients With Ongoing Remission

Then, we evaluated the ability of BP sera collected during patient's follow up to induce NET release. Compared with baseline values, NET formation was gradually reduced with time of treatment as illustrated by *ex vivo* experiments conducted with sera collected at day150 and day 360 (0.18, 0.13, and 0.06 μm^2/cell, p = 0.0001Friedman test) (**Figures 3A–C,E**). Conversely, NET levels remained as elevated as with BP serum at diagnosis when NET generation was performed with the BP sera collected at time of relapse from the same patients (0.13 at baseline vs. 0.15 μm^2/cell at time of relapse, p = 0.68 Wilcoxon matched pairs test) (**Figures 3D,F**).

IL-17 and IL-23 Display Differential Effects on NET Formation

As we previously reported that IL-17 and IL-23 remained elevated or even increased in the sera of patients at risk of relapse (18), we further investigated whether these cytokines participated to NET induction in BP. In this line, we complemented BP sera collected after 150 days from patients with ongoing remission with either IL-17A or IL-23 or even both. Both IL-17A and IL-23 independently enhanced NET formation with an even greater effect under IL-23 stimulation (1.9-fold increase with IL-17, p = 0.029, and 10-fold increase with IL-23 with respect to the stimulation with D150 sera alone, p = 0.04 ratio paired t-test, **Figures 4A–D,F,G**). We then assessed the combined effects of both cytokines, IL-17A and IL-23 on NET generation. The high NET formation level induced by addition of IL-23 was reduced when IL-17A was added to the cell culture medium (**Figures 4E,H**).

To further investigate the potential lowering effects of IL-17A on IL-23-induced NETs release, we added IL-17A to the potent NET inducer sera collected at the time of relapse. Supporting the above-mentioned observation, IL-17A addition (alone or combined with IL-23) significantly decreased the area occupied by NETs with respect to the area obtained with the serum of BP patients collected at time of relapse (0.09, and 0.17 vs. 0.45

TABLE 1 | Individual characteristics of BP patients.

Patient	NETs		Baseline						Follow-up						
			Age at diagnosis	Sex	Nb blisters/ day	BPDAI	Serum antibodies		Relapse	Day 150			Day 360		
	Presence *in situ*	*Ex vivo* NET induction (mean area of NET µm²/cell)					Anti-BP180 (U/mL)	Anti-BP230 (U/mL)		BPDAI	Anti-BP180 (U/mL)	Anti-BP230 (U/mL)	BPDAI	Anti-BP180 (U/mL)	Anti-BP230 (U/mL)
1	+	**1.141**	84	F	120	**90***	**150**	**94**	+	34	**59**	**30**	7	**52**	**71**
2	+	**2.02**	95	F	30	**65***	**64**	**83**	+	**59***	**47**	7	10	**81**	**32**
3	+	0.285	81	F	73	**65***	**81**	**64**	–	7	**22**	**14**	7	**10**	**9**
4	+	0.130	58	F	26	53	**56**	1	+	32	**74**	5	D	D	D
5	+	**0.471**	75	M	10	48	**116**	5	–	2	9	5	0	0	0
6	+	**0.501**	87	M	15	36	1	1	–	2	7	5	0	7	7
7	+	**0.798**	78	M	10	23	1	2	+	0	2	4	4	0	0
8	+	**0.503**	81	M	1#	23	9	**20**	–	1	7	**10**	1	7	20
9	–	0.382	79	M	20	**73***	**68**	**35**	+	31	**41**	**21**	6	8	5
10	–	0.433	90	F	10	**56***	**79**	3	–	5	**38**	3	10	**21**	5
11	–	**0.636**	60	F	5#	30	**26**	1	–	6	**16**	0	23	**11**	5

**Severe disease according to BPDAI ≥56;*
#patients with moderate disease defined by a number of new daily blisters <10; Relapse was defined as the reappearance of at least 3 new daily blisters in between one-year follow-up. Bold characters: out of normal range values i.e., NET area per PMN >0.445 µm²/PMN, which is the mean value obtained by stimulation of the same PMNs with healthy sera + 2SD; Anti-BP180 Ab >9 U/ml, Anti-BP230 Ab >7 U/ml. BPDAI, bullous pemphigoid disease area index, Nb number.

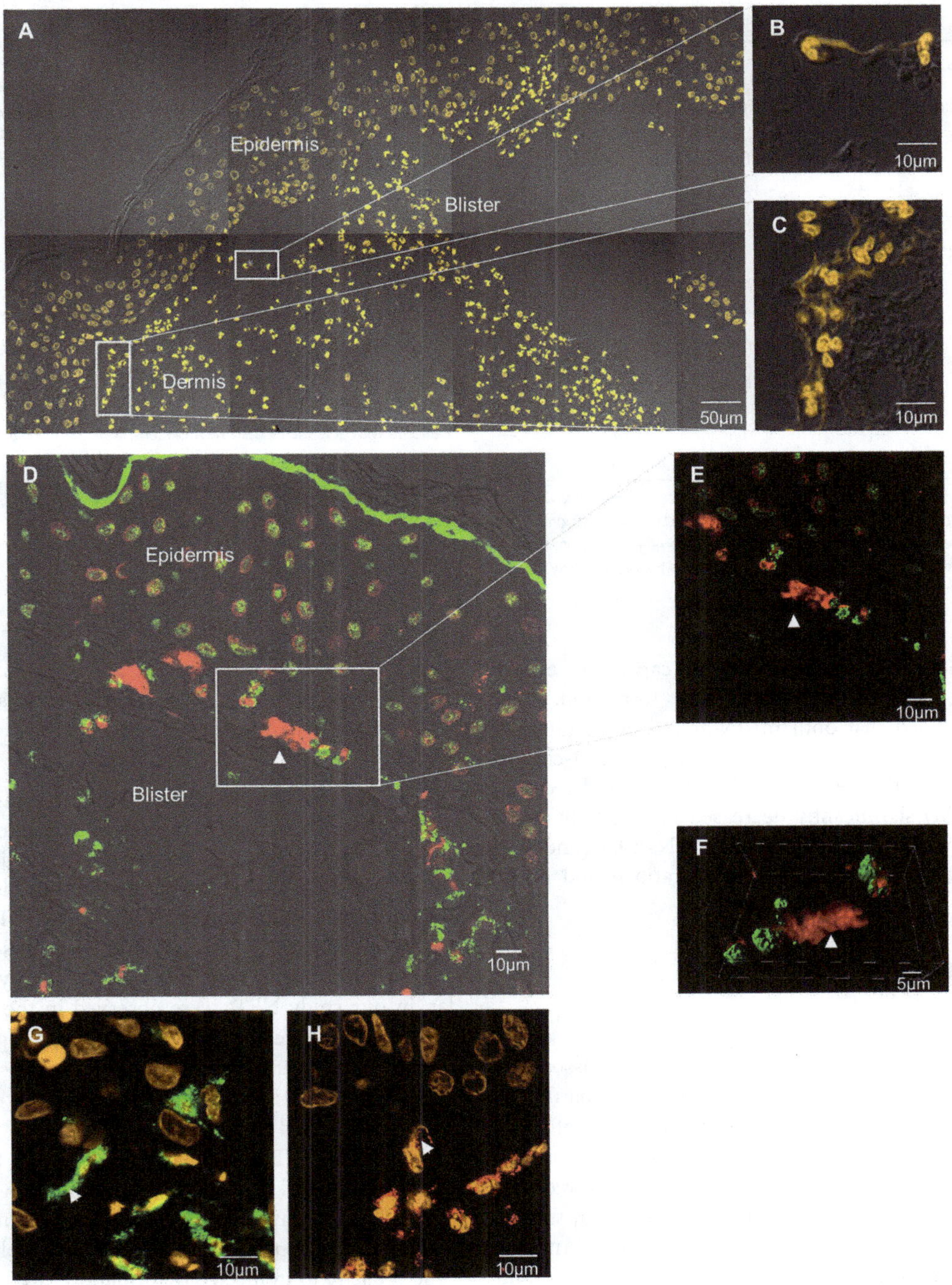

FIGURE 1 | *In situ* exploration of DNA traps in BP. DNA extracellular traps are located at the edge of the DEJ splitting, in the papillary dermis of BP patient skin. Skin biopsy specimen stained by SYTOX Orange nucleic acid probe **(A–C)**. Neutrophil extracellular trap stained by anti-histone H3 Ab *(red)* and anti-myeloperoxidase Ab *(green)* **(D–F)**. 3-dimensional reconstruction imaging by confocal microscopy and IMARIS® software of this NET **(F)**. Magnification 80x, numerical aperture of 1, z-stack with 0.67µm step-size. Neutrophil extracellular trap stained by Sytox orange and anti-myeloperoxidase *(green)* **(G)**. Eosinophil extracellular trap stained by Sytox orange and anti-eosinophil-derived-neurotoxin Ab *(red)* **(H)**.

μm^2/cell, $p = 0.05$ and $p = 0.02$, respectively, ratio paired t-test) (**Figures 5A–C,E,F**). In contrast, supplementation of these sera collected at time of relapse with IL-23, did not affect their capacity to induce NET formation (0.48 vs. 0.45 μm^2/cell, $p = 0.89$ ratio paired t-test) (**Figures 5D,G**).

NET Formation Is Inhibited by Methylprednisolone and by Compound A

Having demonstrated that the capacity of BP sera to induce NET release progressively decreased in BP patients with ongoing remission upon treatment, we then wondered whether

TABLE 2 | Inflammatory cell infiltrate in BP skin according to the presence of NETs forming cells *in situ*.

Patient	Blister cavity		Papillary dermis		NETS
	Eosinophils	Neutrophils	Eosinophils	Neutrophils	
1	+	0/+	0/+	0/+	+
2	+ + +	+	++/+ + +	+/++	+
3	++	+ + +	0/+	0/+	+
4	++/+ + +	++	++/+ + +	++	+
5	+ + +	++	++	+	+
6	+ + +	0/+	+ + +	+	+
7	+ + +	++	++/+ + +	+	+
8	+	+	0/+	0/+	+
9	+ + +	+ /++	+ + +	+	–
10	+ + +	+/++	++	0/+	–
11	++	+ + +	+	+	–

Quality of cell infiltrate assessed independently by two operators on Hematoxylin-eosin stained sections with respect to the presence of NETs determined by immunofluorescence on a serial section of the same skin biopsy. A rating from 0 to + + + was assigned to eosinophil and neutrophil infiltrates in the papillary dermis and in the blister cavity to allow a comparative semi-quantification of these cells. (n = 11).

TABLE 3 | Clinical and biological characteristics of BP patients according to the *in-situ* observation of NETs.

	"NETs positive" patients	"NETs negative" patients
CLINICAL CHARACTERISTICS		
Number of patients, *n*	8	3
Age (y); sex ratio F/M	79.9y; 1	76.3y; 2
BPDAI total score, mean ± SD	50.3 ± 23	53 ± 21.6
Total skin activity, mean ± SD	49.9 ± 23	50.6 ± 23.6
Blisters/Erosions, mean ± SD	32.2 ± 16.7	41.7 ± 13.8
Erythema/urticaria, mean ± SD	17.6 ± 9.6	9 ± 14.7
Patients with severe disease according BPDAI,[a] *n*	3/8	2/3
Patients with at least 10 daily new blisters, *n*	7/8	2/3
Relapse[b]	4/8	1/3
BIOLOGICAL CHARACTERISTICS		
Positive serum anti-BP180 NC16A IgG, *n*	5/8	3/3
Mean anti BP180 NC16A IgG, U/ml	93.4	57.7
Positive serum anti-BP230 IgG, *n*	4/8	1/3

[a]*Severe disease was defined by BPDAI ≥56.*
[b]*Relapse was defined as the reappearance of at least 3 new daily blisters in between one-year follow-up. No statistically significant difference was observed using Mann Whitney test. n, effective, y, years. BPDAI, bullous pemphigoid disease area index.*

corticosteroid therapy also reduced the capability of BP sera collected at baseline to induce NET formation. NET quantification revealed that both methylprednisolone (10 μM) and compound A (also named 2-(4-acetoxyphenyl)-2-chloro-N-ethyl ammonium chloride, a natural glucocorticoid receptor ligand (37), 10 μM) significantly decreased the capacity of BP serum to induce NET formation by BP PMNs (0.05 and 0.04 vs. 0.14 μm^2/cell, $p = 0.04$ and $p = 0.01$, ratio paired t-test) (**Figure 6**).

DISCUSSION

NET formation has recently been reported in several autoimmune diseases as a phenomenon potentially associated to tissue damage and/or loss of tolerance mechanisms (6). In this study, we brought *in situ* evidence of the presence of NETs in BP at the extremity of the blister where dermis separates from epidermis. Using an *ex vivo* model, we also showed that both BP neutrophils and biological fluids (blister fluid, serum) from BP patients were required for NET formation. Analysis of NET presence at tissue level with respect to BP clinical and to immunological data revealed that NET formation was not associated with specific characteristics of the disease at baseline. However, a longitudinal analysis of NET formation using our *ex vivo* model discriminated sera from BP patients with ongoing remission under treatment from those collected at time of relapse. Based on our previous studies (17, 18), we identified IL-23 as a potent NETs enhancer in BP. In contrast, we evidenced in BP a protective role of IL-17A despite the presence of potent inducers such as IL-23 or relapse sera, demonstrating for the first time in BP antagonist functions for these 2 cytokines.

To the best of our knowledge, we here evidenced for the first time the presence *in situ* of NETs in BP. Actually, NETs were observed in 8 out of 11 patients with BP at baseline. In contrast, EETs were present only in 1 case despite the use of 4 different markers on 4 sequential sections for eosinophil immunostaining. The absence of EETs could not be explained by the quality of the inflammatory infiltrate, as eosinophils were the most represented immune cells where NETs were detected. It is possible that EETs formation rather occurs in the skin of BP patients with tissue eosinophilia as previously described (7). So far, in our study NETs were observed in the skin biopsy from BP patients whatever disease activity, although the quantity of NETs observed remained low in all cases. Thus, our observations suggest that NET formation is a common but quantitatively rare process associated with BP.

Noticeably, NETs localized precisely at the very edge of dermal-epidermal separation. NET formation could be dictated by skin microenvironment. Furthermore, most patients for whom *in situ* exploration was positive, displayed at the same time capacity to induce NET formation *ex vivo* when BP PMNs were cultured in presence of their sera. Actually, we showed that both body fluid and PMNs from BP patients were required for NET formation. Such specific NET localization at the extremity of blister where the epidermis separates from the dermis could be related to a role of NETs in blister formation as it was demonstrated using an *ex vivo* model that degradation of DNA filaments inhibited DEJ splitting (8).

Although immunoglobulins have been associated with NET formation (38–42), such process could not be foreseen in BP. Indeed, no correlation could be drawn between NETs' presence *in situ* or NET formation *ex vivo* and serum or blister fluids levels of anti-BP180 AAb. Besides, the fact that NETs were observed in most skin biopsy specimen independently of disease

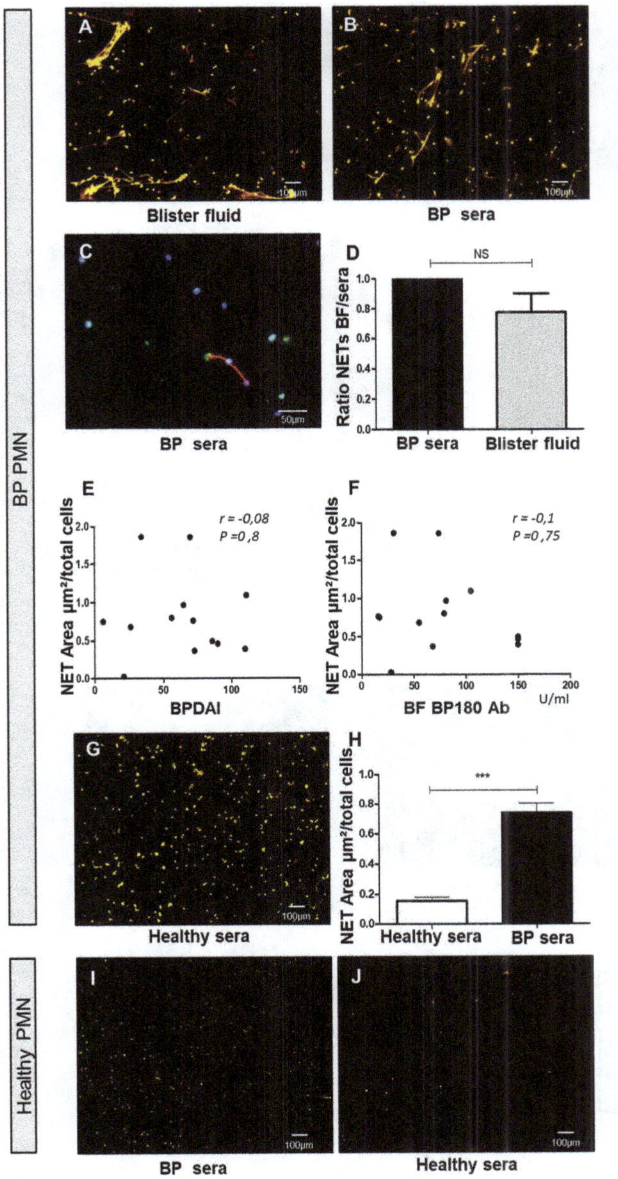

FIGURE 2 | Blister fluids and BP sera induce NET formation by BP PMN but not by control PMN. *Ex vivo* stimulation of BP PMNs with BP blister fluids (BF) **(A)**, and BP sera **(B,C)** stained by Sytox orange **(A,B)** or anti-Histone H3 and anti-MPO Ab **(C)**. NET area induced by BP sera vs. BF from the same patients on heterologous BP PMNs **(D)** ($n = 3$); results expressed in ratio of NET area induced by BF to NET area induced by serum of the same patient, results represent mean ± SEM, NS, non-significant. Correlation of NET area induced by heterologous BF with BPDAI **(E)** and BF concentration of BP180 Ab **(F)**. Stimulation of BP PMN with healthy control sera **(G)** and comparison with NET area induced by BP sera **(H)** ($n = 7$), $^{***}p < 0.001$, results represent mean ± SEM. Stimulation of PMNs from healthy controls by BP sera **(I)**, or heterologous healthy sera **(J)**. Magnification 20x. BPDAI, Bullous Pemphigoid Disease Area Index; BF BP180 Ab, concentrations of anti-BP180 antibodies in blister fluids.

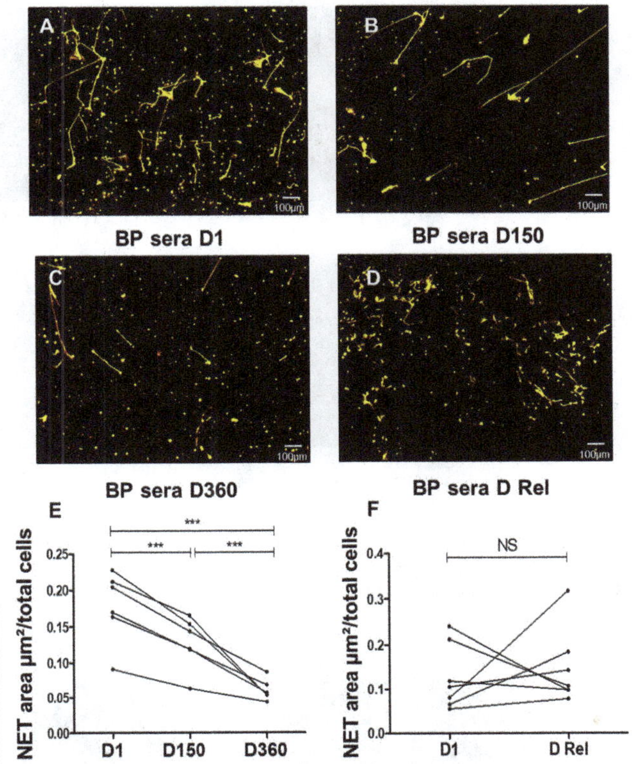

FIGURE 3 | NETs are induced more efficiently by BP sera at diagnosis and at time of relapse. *Ex vivo* stimulation of BP PMNs with heterologous BP sera collected: at baseline **(A)**, around 150 days after diagnosis in patients with controlled disease **(B)**, around 360 days after diagnosis in patients undergoing remission **(C)**, or at time of relapse in patients undergoing relapse **(D)**. Magnification 20x. NET area measured for each condition: stimulation of BP PMNs with BP sera collected Baseline (D1) vs matched sera collected at Day 150 and Day 360 **(E)** ($n = 6$), $^{***}p < 0.0001$. NET area measured after stimulation of BP PMNs with BP sera collected at baseline (D1) vs. matched sera collected at time of relapse (D Rel) from the same patients **(F)** ($n = 7$), NS: non-significant.

activity, suggests that NET inducers may be present in all body fluids from BP patients at baseline. Indeed, sera from BP patients in clinical remission were less efficient to induce NET formation. Altogether, this suggests that NET induction is rather associated with inflammatory mediators than with the autoimmune response in BP. In this setting, it was shown that inflammatory molecules such as cytokines and complement components were potent inducers of DNA traps (5, 6, 43–45).

Neutrophils' priming is a required step for NET formation in BP. In BP skin environment, the presence of cytokines able to activate innate cells such as neutrophils, eosinophils and monocytes has already been largely described (17–19, 31). Such inflammatory response may be responsible for neutrophils' priming and explain why NET formation level remained low in neutrophils from healthy donors even when stimulated with BP serum. Accordingly, it has been shown that neutrophils from normal individuals released NETs upon IL-17A stimulation only after having been primed by TNF-α (25). In BP, the importance of neutrophils was also highlighted by the capacity of both classical corticoids and Compound A to inhibit NET generation induced by serum collected at baseline. However, further studies are required to determine the cytokines involved in neutrophils sensitization to NET formation in BP.

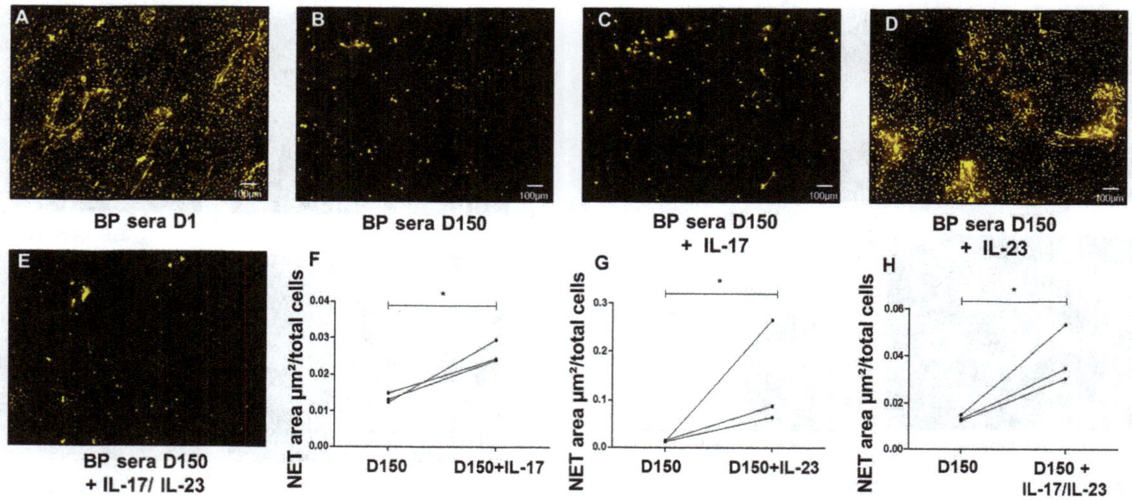

FIGURE 4 | IL23 is critical to NETs formation. *Ex-vivo* stimulation of BP PMNs with BP sera collected at baseline **(A)**, around 150 days after diagnosis in patients with controlled disease **(B)**, and day 150 sera added with either IL-17A **(C)**, IL-23 **(D)**, or both IL-17A and IL-23 **(E)** (1.2 ng/mL for both cytokines). Comparison of NET area measured when cytokines IL-17A, IL-23, or both were added to day 150-serum with NET area induced by day 150- serum alone **(F–H)** ($n = 3$), * $p<0.05$.

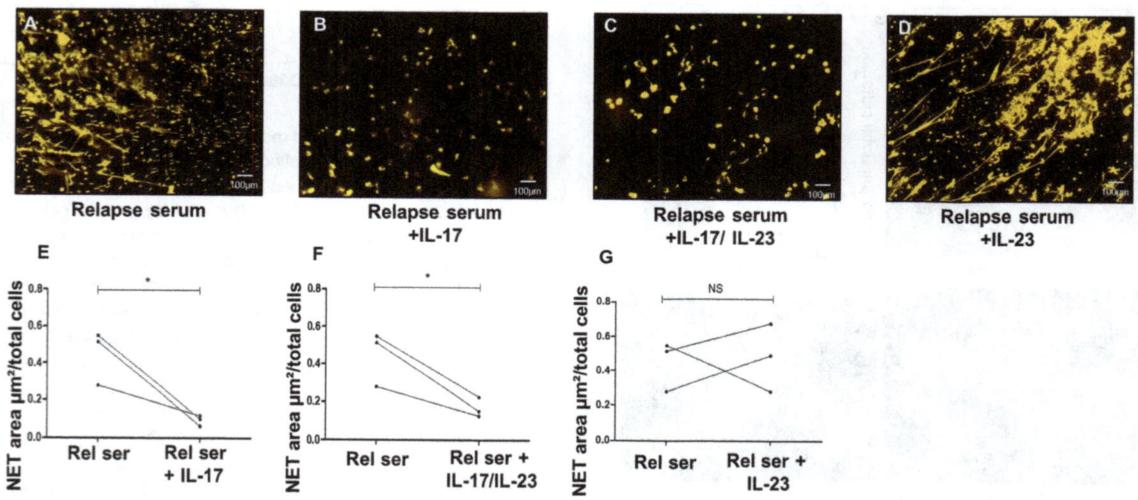

FIGURE 5 | IL-17A inhibits NET formation by BP sera at time of relapse. *Ex vivo* stimulation of BP PMNs with BP sera collected at time of relapse alone **(A)**, or in presence of either IL-17 **(B)**, or both IL-17 and IL-23 **(C)**, or IL-23 **(D)**. Comparison of NET area measured when cytokines were added to serum collected at time of relapse with NET level generated in presence of this relapse serum (Rel Ser) alone **(E–G)** ($n = 3$), *$p<0.05$.

Serum from BP patients with relapse holds on high level of NET formation. This suggests that NETs' triggers remained present in the serum of those patients even under therapy. In this line, we previously reported that the concentration of IL-17 and IL-23 remained elevated or even increased in the sera of BP patients at risk of relapse (18). Noteworthy, using our *ex vivo* model, we demonstrated that IL-23, and to a lesser extent IL-17A, could enhance NET formation in BP neutrophils. While IL-17 is known to potently recruit neutrophils, a role and the mechanisms associated with this cytokine in the induction of NET have still not been fully elucidated. Activation of p38-Mitogen-activated protein kinase (p38 MAPK) and Nuclear Factor Kappa B (NF-κB) pathways by IL-17A (46–49) may explain this property, as both are involved in NET formation (50–52), and p38 MAPK pathway mediates IL-17 induced ROS production (46). To our knowledge, the role of IL-23 in NET generation had not been evaluated yet. Neutrophils constitutively express low amount of IL-23R, which are up-regulated upon activation (53).Three activation cascades may be activated following IL-23 transduction signal among which the above-mentioned p38 MAPK and NF-κB pathways but also the mammalian target of rapamycin (mTOR) pathway which play a pivotal role in NET formation and may explain the higher capacity of IL-23 to induce NET formation in BP (50, 51, 53, 54). In this line, no correlation could be drawn between

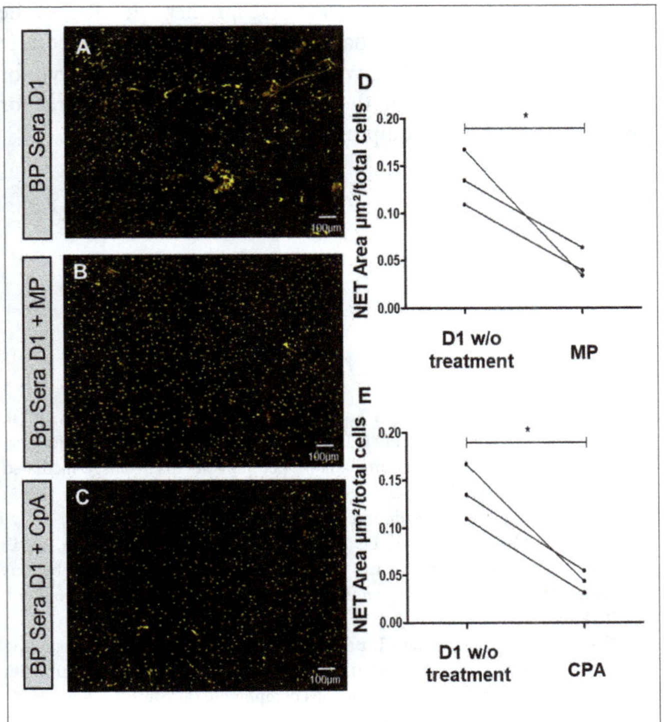

FIGURE 6 | NET formation is inhibited by methylprednisolone or Compound A. *Ex vivo* stimulation of BP PMNs with BP sera collected at diagnosis (D1) alone **(A)**, or in presence of either methylprednisolone **(B)**, or compound A **(C)**. Comparison of NET area measured when treatments were added to baseline serum with NET formation by this baseline serum without treatment **(D,E)** ($n = 3$). $^{*}p < 0.05$, mean ± SEM are represented. MP, Methylprednisolone; CpA, Compound A; w/o, without.

IL-17 or IL-23 blister fluids concentrations and NET formation ($r = -0.5$, $p = 0.14$, and $r = -0.71$, $p = 0.06$ respectively), suggesting that IL-17A and IL-23 were not the only triggers of NET formation in BP. Observed effects of these cytokines may also result from synergic actions of several cytokines and further studies are needed to understand mechanisms of NET induction in BP.

This study is the first to our knowledge to demonstrate tendentious functions of IL-17A with respect to IL-23 presence. Indeed, we observed a protective effect of IL-17A supplementation on NET formation induced either by IL-23 itself or by sera from BP patients with relapse, highlighting the role of disease specific microenvironment in cytokine's function. In the same line, blocking IL-17 signaling in inflammatory bowel diseases resulted in an increased expression of pro-inflammatory chemokines and cytokines (55, 56). Some molecules have recently been described in such regulation mechanisms. Suppressor of cytokine signaling 3 (SOCS3) is therefore known to inhibit Janus kinase 2 activity, thereby decreasing IL-23 induced effects (57–59). Yet, SOCS3 expression has recently been correlated with severity of inflammation, expression of proinflammatory cytokines, and activation of p38 MAPK pathway (60). SOCS3 expression is also induced by IL-17 family cytokines (61, 62). Then, although this has to be proven, we hypothesized that in BP IL-17A attenuates IL-23 induced NET formation by inducing SOCS3 expression as previously demonstrated in the airway epithelium (62). Such effects could explain the limited quantity of NETs observed in the skin of BP patients. Furthermore, our present results demonstrate that, in the future, patients with bullous pemphigoid could be further divided into subgroups according to the biomarkers expressed to identify an adequate candidate for biotherapy maintenance in relay of corticosteroid in patients at risk of relapse.

NETs are involved in loss of tolerance mechanisms in several autoimmune diseases (6). In BP, NETs release could participate to both autoimmune and inflammatory responses. Auto-antigens may be present at the surface of NETs, which prolongs their exposition, subsequently favoring an autoimmune response (63, 64). In this line, NET formation is associated with production of reactive oxygen species, and granule enzymes cover the DNA filaments (2, 6, 65). Several studies showed the involvement of NETs in tissue damage (66, 67). Brinkmann et al. reported the association of NETs with various proteases such as neutrophil elastase (5). Yet, neutrophil elastase has largely been implicated in BP pathological processes, as well as matrix metalloproteinase MMP-9 (14, 68). Thus, although NET formation does not directly correlate with BP activity, we showed in this study that NET formation depends on the presence of inflammatory cytokines, and therefore that the inflammatory response associated with BP may participate to BP antigen immunogenicity or to the perpetuation of the disease. Subsequently, our results showing NETs at the dermal-epidermal splitting area, along with the serum capacity to induce NETs at the same time, really advocate for a role of neutrophil in extracellular DNA release, although NET implication in BP still needs to be further demonstrated. Based on the literature, we hypothesize that NET-associated mechanisms may be involved in BP180 antigen immunogenicity, and further in epitope spreading in BP.

ETHICS STATEMENT

The investigation was conducted under the approval of the Ethic Committee of the University Hospital of Reims (CNIL authorization DR-2013-320), and all of the subjects gave their informed and written consent before participating in the study in accordance with the Helsinki Declaration.

AUTHOR CONTRIBUTIONS

PB, FA, and BP conceived the study. DG, EB, SL, GG, PB, FA, and BN contributed to the study design and data analysis. AD, CM, PB, and FA contributed to the clinical and histological metadata collection. DG, EB, CT, KD, SL, SN, CM, and BP contributed to the sample processing. CT conceived the macro allowing *ex vivo* NET quantification. DG, EB, and SL performed the statistical analyses. DG, PB, FA, and BP wrote the manuscript and all authors reviewed and approved the manuscript.

ACKNOWLEDGMENTS

This study was supported by research grants from the French Department of Health's Project Hospitalier de Recherche Clinique (PHRC) Interrégional 2012 and the Association pour la Recherche en Dermatologie. We also thank Christine Terryn for technical assistance during the study and the PICT platform for providing microscopy equipments.

REFERENCES

1. Dubertret L, Bertaux B, Fosse M, Touraine R. Cellular events leading to blister formation in bullous pemphigoid. *Br J Dermatol.* (1980) 103:615–24. doi: 10.1111/j.1365-2133.1980.tb01683.x
2. Jorch SK, Kubes P. An emerging role for neutrophil extracellular traps in noninfectious disease. *Nat Med.* (2017) 23:279–87. doi: 10.1038/nm.4294
3. Ueki S, Tokunaga T, Fujieda S, Honda K, Hirokawa M, Spencer LA, et al. Eosinophil ETosis and DNA traps: a new look at eosinophilic inflammation. *Curr Allergy Asthma Rep.* (2016) 16:54. doi: 10.1007/s11882-016-0634-5
4. Yousefi S, Simon D, Simon H-U. Eosinophil extracellular DNA traps: molecular mechanisms and potential roles in disease. *Curr Opin Immunol.* (2012) 24:736–9. doi: 10.1016/j.coi.2012.08.010
5. Brinkmann V, Reichard U, Goosmann C, Fauler B, Uhlemann Y, Weiss DS, et al. Neutrophil extracellular traps kill bacteria. *Science.* (2004) 303:1532–5. doi: 10.1126/science.1092385
6. Lee KH, Kronbichler A, Park DD-Y, Park Y, Moon H, Kim H, et al. Neutrophil extracellular traps (NETs) in autoimmune diseases: a comprehensive review. *Autoimmun Rev.* (2017) 16:1160–73. doi: 10.1016/j.autrev.2017.09.012
7. Simon D, Hoesli S, Roth N, Staedler S, Yousefi S, Simon H-U. Eosinophil extracellular DNA traps in skin diseases. *J Allergy Clin Immunol.* (2011) 127:194–9. doi: 10.1016/j.jaci.2010.11.002
8. de Graauw E, Sitaru C, Horn M, Borradori L, Yousefi S, Simon H-U, et al. Evidence for a role of eosinophils in blister formation in bullous pemphigoid. *Allergy.* (2017) 72:1105–13. doi: 10.1111/all.13131
9. Amber KT, Valdebran M, Kridin K, Grando SA. The role of eosinophils in bullous pemphigoid: a developing model of eosinophil pathogenicity in mucocutaneous disease. *Front Med.* (2018) 5:201. doi: 10.3389/fmed.2018.00201
10. Liu Z, Giudice GJ, Zhou X, Swartz SJ, Troy JL, Fairley JA, et al. A major role for neutrophils in experimental bullous pemphigoid. *J Clin Invest.* (1997) 100:1256–63. doi: 10.1172/JCI119639
11. Simon D, Borradori L, Simon H-U. Eosinophils as putative therapeutic targets in bullous pemphigoid. *Exp Dermatol.* (2017) 26:1187–92. doi: 10.1111/exd.13416
12. Hellberg L, Samavedam UKSRL, Holdorf K, Hänsel M, Recke A, Beckmann T, et al. Methylprednisolone blocks autoantibody-induced tissue damage in experimental models of bullous pemphigoid and epidermolysis bullosa acquisita through inhibition of neutrophil activation. *J Invest Dermatol.* (2013) 133:2390–9. doi: 10.1038/jid.2013.91
13. Fang H, Zhang Y, Li N, Wang G, Liu Z. The autoimmune skin disease bullous pemphigoid: the role of mast cells in autoantibody-induced tissue injury. *Front Immunol.* (2018) 9:407. doi: 10.3389/fimmu.2018.00407
14. Bieber K, Koga H, Nishie W. *In vitro* and *in vivo* models to investigate the pathomechanisms and novel treatments for pemphigoid diseases. *Exp Dermatol.* (2017) 26:1163–70. doi: 10.1111/exd.13415
15. Leighty L, Li N, Diaz LA, Liu Z. Experimental models for the autoimmune and inflammatory blistering disease, Bullous pemphigoid. *Arch Dermatol Res.* (2007) 299:417–22. doi: 10.1007/s00403-007-0790-5
16. Chen R, Fairley JA, Zhao M-L, Giudice GJ, Zillikens D, Diaz LA, et al. Macrophages, but not T and B lymphocytes, are critical for subepidermal blister formation in experimental bullous pemphigoid: macrophage-mediated neutrophil infiltration depends on mast cell activation. *J Immunol.* (2002) 169:3987–92. doi: 10.4049/jimmunol.169.7.3987
17. Le Jan S, Plée J, Vallerand D, Dupont A, Delanez E, Durlach A, et al. Innate immune cell-produced IL-17 sustains inflammation in bullous pemphigoid. *J Invest Dermatol.* (2014) 134:2908–17. doi: 10.1038/jid.2014.263
18. Plée J, Le Jan S, Giustiniani J, Barbe C, Joly P, Bedane C, et al. Integrating longitudinal serum IL-17 and IL-23 follow-up, along with autoantibodies variation, contributes to predict bullous pemphigoid outcome. *Sci Rep.* (2015) 5:18001. doi: 10.1038/srep18001
19. Riani M, Le Jan S, Plée J, Durlach A, Le Naour R, Haegeman G, et al. Bullous pemphigoid outcome is associated with CXCL10-induced matrix metalloproteinase 9 secretion from monocytes and neutrophils but not lymphocytes. *J Allergy Clin Immunol.* (2016) 139:863–72.e3. doi: 10.1016/j.jaci.2016.08.012
20. de Graauw E, Sitaru C, Horn MP, Borradori L, Yousefi S, Simon D, et al. Monocytes enhance neutrophil-induced blister formation in an *ex vivo* model of bullous pemphigoid. *Allergy.* (2018) 73:1119–30. doi: 10.1111/all.13376
21. Lin L, Betsuyaku T, Heimbach L, Li N, Rubenstein D, Shapiro SD, et al. Neutrophil elastase cleaves the murine hemidesmosomal protein BP180/type XVII collagen and generates degradation products that modulate experimental bullous pemphigoid. *Matrix Biol.* (2012) 31:38–44. doi: 10.1016/j.matbio.2011.09.003
22. Verraes S, Hornebeck W, Polette M, Borradori L, Bernard P. Respective contribution of neutrophil elastase and matrix metalloproteinase 9 in the degradation of BP180 (type XVII collagen) in human bullous pemphigoid. *J Invest Dermatol.* (2001) 117:1091–6. doi: 10.1046/j.0022-202x.2001.01521.x
23. Giusti D, Gatouillat G, Le Jan S, Plée J, Bernard P, Antonicelli F, et al. Eosinophil Cationic Protein (ECP), a predictive marker of bullous pemphigoid severity and outcome. *Sci Rep.* (2017) 7:4833. doi: 10.1038/s41598-017-04687-5
24. Liu Z, Li N, Diaz LA, Shipley M, Senior RM, Werb Z. Synergy between a plasminogen cascade and MMP-9 in autoimmune disease. *J Clin Invest.* (2005) 115:879–87. doi: 10.1172/JCI23977
25. Khandpur R, Carmona-Rivera C, Vivekanandan-Giri A, Gizinski A, Yalavarthi S, Knight JS, et al. NETs are a source of citrullinated autoantigens and stimulate inflammatory responses in rheumatoid arthritis. *Sci Transl Med.* (2013) 5:178ra40. doi: 10.1126/scitranslmed.3005580
26. Gammon WR, Merritt CC, Lewis DM, Sams WM, Carlo JR, Wheeler CE. An *in vitro* model of immune complex-mediated basement membrane zone separation caused by pemphigoid antibodies, leukocytes, and complement. *J Invest Dermatol.* (1982) 78:285–90. doi: 10.1111/1523-1747.ep12507222
27. Liu Z, Diaz LA, Troy JL, Taylor AF, Emery DJ, Fairley JA, et al. A passive transfer model of the organ-specific autoimmune disease, bullous pemphigoid, using antibodies generated against the hemidesmosomal antigen, BP180. *J Clin Invest.* (1993) 92:2480–8. doi: 10.1172/JCI116856

28. Sitaru C, Dähnrich C, Probst C, Komorowski L, Blöcker I, Schmidt E, et al. Enzyme-linked immunosorbent assay using multimers of the 16th non-collagenous domain of the BP180 antigen for sensitive and specific detection of pemphigoid autoantibodies. *Exp Dermatol.* (2007) 16:770–7. doi: 10.1111/j.1600-0625.2007.00592.x
29. Charneux J, Lorin J, Vitry F, Antonicelli F, Reguiai Z, Barbe C, et al. Usefulness of BP230 and BP180-NC16a enzyme-linked immunosorbent assays in the initial diagnosis of bullous pemphigoid: a retrospective study of 138 patients. *Arch Dermatol.* (2011) 147:286–91. doi: 10.1001/archdermatol.2011.23
30. Bernard P, Antonicelli F. Bullous pemphigoid: a review of its diagnosis, associations and treatment. *Am J Clin Dermatol.* (2017) 18:513–28. doi: 10.1007/s40257-017-0264-2
31. Giusti D, Le Jan S, Gatouillat G, Bernard P, Pham BN, Antonicelli F. Biomarkers related to bullous pemphigoid activity and outcome. *Exp Dermatol.* (2017) 26:1240–7. doi: 10.1111/exd.13459
32. Chakievska L, Holtsche MM, Künstner A, Goletz S, Petersen B-S, Thaci D, et al. IL-17A is functionally relevant and a potential therapeutic target in bullous pemphigoid. *J Autoimmun.* (2018) 96:104–12. doi: 10.1016/j.jaut.2018.09.003
33. D'Auria L, Cordiali Fei P, Ameglio F. Cytokines and bullous pemphigoid. *Eur Cytokine Netw.* (1999) 10:123–34.
34. Ameglio F, D'auria L, Bonifati C, Ferraro C, Mastroianni A, Giacalone B. Cytokine pattern in blister fluid and serum of patients with bullous pemphigoid: relationships with disease intensity. *Br J Dermatol.* (1998) 138:611–4.
35. Brinkmann V, Laube B, Abed UA, Goosmann C, Zychlinsky A. Neutrophil extracellular traps: how to generate and visualize them. *J Vis Exp.* (2010) 24:1724. doi: 10.3791/1724
36. Rebernick R, Fahmy L, Glover C, Bawadekar M, Shim D, Holmes CL, et al. DNA area and NETosis Analysis (DANA): a high-throughput method to quantify neutrophil extracellular traps in fluorescent microscope images. *Biol Proced Online.* (2018) 20:7. doi: 10.1186/s12575-018-0072-y
37. Lesovaya E, Yemelyanov A, Swart AC, Swart P, Haegeman G, Budunova I. Discovery of Compound A – a selective activator of the glucocorticoid receptor with anti-inflammatory and anti-cancer activity. *Oncotarget.* (2015) 6:30730–44. doi: 10.18632/oncotarget.5078
38. Alemán OR, Mora N, Cortes-Vieyra R, Uribe-Querol E, Rosales C. Differential use of human neutrophil Fcγ receptors for inducing neutrophil extracellular trap formation. *J Immunol Res.* (2016) 2016:2908034. doi: 10.1155/2016/2908034
39. Behnen M, Leschczyk C, Möller S, Batel T, Klinger M, Solbach W, et al. Immobilized immune complexes induce neutrophil extracellular trap release by human neutrophil granulocytes via FcγRIIIB and Mac-1. *J Immunol Baltim Md.* (2014) 193:1954–65. doi: 10.4049/jimmunol.1400478
40. Alemán OR, Mora N, Cortes-Vieyra R, Uribe-Querol E, Rosales C. Transforming growth factor-β-activated kinase 1 is required for human FcγRIIIb-induced neutrophil extracellular trap formation. *Front Immunol.* (2016) 7:277. doi: 10.3389/fimmu.2016.00277
41. Rosales C. Fcγ receptor heterogeneity in leukocyte functional responses. *Front Immunol.* (2017) 8:280. doi: 10.3389/fimmu.2017.00280
42. Bieber K, Sun S, Witte M, Kasprick A, Beltsiou F, Behnen M, et al. Regulatory T cells suppress inflammation and blistering in pemphigoid diseases. *Front Immunol.* (2017) 8:1628. doi: 10.3389/fimmu.2017.01628
43. Palmer LJ, Damgaard C, Holmstrup P, Nielsen CH. Influence of complement on neutrophil extracellular trap release induced by bacteria. *J Periodontal Res.* (2016) 51:70–6. doi: 10.1111/jre.12284
44. Yousefi S, Mihalache C, Kozlowski E, Schmid I, Simon HU. Viable neutrophils release mitochondrial DNA to form neutrophil extracellular traps. *Cell Death Differ.* (2009) 16:1438–44. doi: 10.1038/cdd.2009.96
45. Yipp BG, Petri B, Salina D, Jenne CN, Scott BNV, Zbytnuik LD, et al. Infection-induced NETosis is a dynamic process involving neutrophil multitasking *in vivo*. *Nat Med.* (2012) 18:1386–93. doi: 10.1038/nm.2847
46. Pietrowski E, Bender B, Huppert J, White R, Luhmann HJ, Kuhlmann CRW. Pro-inflammatory effects of interleukin-17A on vascular smooth muscle cells involve NAD(P)H- oxidase derived reactive oxygen species. *J Vasc Res.* (2011) 48:52–8. doi: 10.1159/000317400
47. Tokuda H, Kanno Y, Ishisaki A, Takenaka M, Harada A, Kozawa O. Interleukin (IL)-17 enhances tumor necrosis factor-alpha-stimulated IL-6 synthesis via p38 mitogen-activated protein kinase in osteoblasts. *J Cell Biochem.* (2004) 91:1053–61. doi: 10.1002/jcb.20004
48. Laan M, Lötvall J, Chung KF, Lindén A. IL-17-induced cytokine release in human bronchial epithelial cells *in vitro*: role of mitogen-activated protein (MAP) kinases. *Br J Pharmacol.* (2001) 133:200–6. doi: 10.1038/sj.bjp.0704063
49. Gaffen SL. Structure and signalling in the IL-17 receptor superfamily. *Nat Rev Immunol.* (2009) 9:556. doi: 10.1038/nri2586
50. Tatsiy O, McDonald PP. Physiological stimuli induce PAD4-dependent, ROS-independent NETosis, with early and late events controlled by discrete signaling pathways. *Front Immunol.* (2018) 9:2036. doi: 10.3389/fimmu.2018.02036
51. Lapponi MJ, Carestia A, Landoni VI, Rivadeneyra L, Etulain J, Negrotto S, et al. Regulation of neutrophil extracellular trap formation by anti-inflammatory drugs. *J Pharmacol Exp Ther.* (2013) 345:430–7. doi: 10.1124/jpet.112.202879
52. Nel JG, Theron AJ, Pool R, Durandt C, Tintinger GR, Anderson R. Neutrophil extracellular traps and their role in health and disease. *South Afr J Sci.* (2016) 112:w14352. doi: 10.4414/smw.2016.14352
53. Chen F, Cao A, Yao S, Evans-Marin HL, Liu H, Wu W, et al. mTOR Mediates IL-23 induction of neutrophil IL-17 and IL-22 production. *J Immunol.* (2016) 196:4390–9. doi: 10.4049/jimmunol.1501541
54. Itakura A, McCarty OJT. Pivotal role for the mTOR pathway in the formation of neutrophil extracellular traps via regulation of autophagy. *Am J Physiol - Cell Physiol.* (2013) 305:C348–54. doi: 10.1152/ajpcell.00108.2013
55. Maxwell JR, Zhang Y, Brown WA, Smith CL, Byrne FR, Fiorino M, et al. Differential roles for interleukin-23 and interleukin-17 in intestinal immunoregulation. *Immunity.* (2015) 43:739–50. doi: 10.1016/j.immuni.2015.08.019
56. Song X, Dai D, He X, Zhu S, Yao Y, Gao H, et al. Growth factor FGF2 cooperates with interleukin-17 to repair intestinal epithelial damage. *Immunity.* (2015) 43:488–501. doi: 10.1016/j.immuni.2015.06.024
57. Babon JJ, Kershaw NJ, Murphy JM, Varghese LN, Laktyushin A, Young SN. Suppression of cytokine signaling by SOCS3: characterization of the mode of inhibition and the basis of its specificity. *Immunity.* (2012) 36:239–50. doi: 10.1016/j.immuni.2011.12.015
58. Chen Z, Laurence A, Kanno Y, Pacher-Zavisin M, Zhu BM, Tato C. Selective regulatory function of Socs3 in the formation of IL-17-secreting T cells. *Proc Natl Acad Sci USA.* (2006) 103:8137–42. doi: 10.1073/pnas.0600666103
59. Carow B, Rottenberg ME. SOCS3, a major regulator of infection and inflammation. *Front Immunol.* (2014) 5:58. doi: 10.3389/fimmu.2014.00058
60. Chaves de Souza JA, Nogueira AVB, Chaves de Souza PP, Kim YJ, Silva Lobo C, Pimentel Lopes de Oliveira GJ, et al. SOCS3 expression correlates with severity of inflammation, expression of proinflammatory cytokines, and activation of STAT3 and p38 MAPK in LPS-induced inflammation *in vivo*. *Mediators Inflamm.* (2013) 2013:650812. doi: 10.1155/2013/650812
61. Caruso R, Stolfi C, Sarra M, Rizzo A, Fantini MC, Pallone F, et al. Inhibition of monocyte-derived inflammatory cytokines by IL-25 occurs via p38 Map kinase-dependent induction of Socs-3. *Blood.* (2009) 113:3512–9. doi: 10.1182/blood-2008-08-172767
62. Niwa M, Fujisawa T, Mori K, Yamanaka K, Yasui H, Suzuki Y, et al. IL-17A Attenuates IFN-λ expression by inducing suppressor of cytokine signaling expression in airway epithelium. *J Immunol.* (2018) 201:2392–402. doi: 10.4049/jimmunol.1800147
63. Bruschi M, Petretto A, Bertelli R, Galetti M, Bonanni A, Pratesi F, et al. Post-translational modified proteins are biomarkers of autoimmune-processes: NETosis and the inflammatory–autoimmunity connection. *Clin Chim Acta.* (2017) 464:12–16. doi: 10.1016/j.cca.2016.11.006
64. Bruschi M, Petretto A, Vaglio A, Santucci L, Candiano G, Ghiggeri GM. Annexin A1 and autoimmunity: from basic science to clinical applications. *Int J Mol Sci.* (2018) 19:E1348. doi: 10.3390/ijms19051348
65. Thieblemont N, Wright HL, Edwards SW, Witko-Sarsat V. Human neutrophils in auto-immunity. *Semin Immunol.* (2016) 28:159–73. doi: 10.1016/j.smim.2016.03.004
66. Kolaczkowska E, Jenne CN, Surewaard BGJ, Thanabalasuriar A, Lee W-Y, Sanz M-J, et al. Molecular mechanisms of NET formation and degradation revealed by intravital imaging in the liver vasculature. *Nat Commun.* (2015) 6:6673. doi: 10.1038/ncomms7673

11

ST18 Enhances PV-IgG-Induced Loss of Keratinocyte Cohesion in Parallel to Increased ERK Activation

Mariya Y. Radeva [1†], Elias Walter [1†], Ramona Alexandra Stach [2], Amir S. Yazdi [2,3], Nicolas Schlegel [4], Ofer Sarig [5], Eli Sprecher [5,6] and Jens Waschke [1]*

[1] Department I, Institute of Anatomy and Cell Biology, Ludwig-Maximilians-Universität (LMU) Munich, Munich, Germany, [2] Department of Dermatology, University Medical Center Tübingen, Eberhard Karls University, Tübingen, Germany, [3] Department of Dermatology, RWTH Aachen, Aachen, Germany, [4] Department of General, Visceral, Vascular and Paediatric Surgery, Julius-Maximilians-Universität, Würzburg, Germany, [5] Department of Dermatology, Tel-Aviv Sourasky Medical Center, Tel-Aviv, Israel, [6] Department of Human Molecular Genetics and Biochemistry, Sackler Faculty of Medicine, Tel-Aviv University, Tel-Aviv, Israel

***Correspondence:**
Jens Waschke
jens.waschke@med.uni-muenchen.de

[†] These authors have contributed equally to this work

Pemphigus is an autoimmune blistering disease targeting the desmosomal proteins desmoglein (Dsg) 1 and Dsg3. Recently, a genetic variant of the Suppression of tumorigenicity 18 (ST18) promoter was reported to cause ST18 up-regulation, associated with pemphigus vulgaris (PV)-IgG-mediated increase in cytokine secretion and more prominent loss of keratinocyte cohesion. Here we tested the effects of PV-IgG and the pathogenic pemphigus mouse anti-Dsg3 antibody AK23 on cytokine secretion and ERK activity in human keratinocytes dependent on ST18 expression. Without ST18 overexpression, both PV-IgG and AK23 induced loss of keratinocyte cohesion which was accompanied by prominent fragmentation of Dsg3 immunostaining along cell borders. In contrast, release of pro-inflammatory cytokines such as IL-1α, IL-6, TNFα, and IFN-γ was not altered significantly in both HaCaT and primary NHEK cells. These experiments indicate that cytokine expression is not strictly required for loss of keratinocyte cohesion. Upon ST18 overexpression, fragmentation of cell monolayers increased significantly in response to autoantibody incubation. Furthermore, production of IL-1α and IL-6 was enhanced in some experiments but not in others whereas release of TNF-α dropped significantly upon PV-IgG application in both EV- and ST18-transfected HaCaT cells. Additionally, in NHEK, application of PV-IgG but not of AK23 significantly increased ERK activity. In contrast, ST18 overexpression in HaCaT cells augmented ERK activation in response to both c-IgG and AK23 but not PV-IgG. Because inhibition of ERK by U0126 abolished PV-IgG- and AK23-induced loss of cell cohesion in ST18-expressing cells, we conclude that autoantibody-induced ERK activation was relevant in this scenario. In summary, similar to the situation in PV patients carrying ST18 polymorphism, overexpression of ST18 enhanced keratinocyte susceptibility to autoantibody-induced loss of cell adhesion, which may be caused in part by enhanced ERK signaling.

Keywords: pemphigus, desmosome, desmoglein, ST18, ERK, cytokines

INTRODUCTION

Pemphigus vulgaris (PV) is a potentially fatal autoimmune disease of the skin and the mucous membranes. The skin disorder is manifested by mucocutaneous blister formation caused by loss of keratinocytes intercellular cell adhesion, which is primarily promoted by IgG autoantibodies directed against desmosomal adhesion molecules such as desmoglein (Dsg) 1 and Dsg 3 (1). However, autoantibodies targeting desmocollin (Dsc) 3, which are rarely present in cases when antibodies against Dsg3 are missing, were also shown to be pathogenic (2–4). These desmosomal cadherins are transmembrane proteins forming the adhesive core of desmosomes, a special intercellular junction maintaining the mechanical integrity of tissues and bearing tension primarily if exposed to high levels of mechanical stress such as in the epidermis (5). With their cytoplasmic tail, via Plakoglobin (PG), and Desmoplakin (DP), the cadherins are linked to the intermediate filament skeleton, another structural unit providing mechanical strength to cells (6, 7). Besides their mechanical functions, desmosomes serve as signaling hubs coordinating tissue-specific functions with intercellular adhesion, which is required for instance during wound healing (8).

In response to binding of pemphigus autoantibodies to the keratinocyte surface, Dsg3-mediated homophilic interaction is impaired and desmosomal proteins are depleted from the membrane leading to keratin retraction and Dsg internalization (9–12). These structural alterations are induced by various PV-mediated outside-in intracellular signaling events such as p38 mitogen-activated protein kinase (p38MAPK) (13–15) and extracellular-signal regulated kinase (ERK) (16, 17). Signaling mechanisms have been shown to be important for loss of cell adhesion (17) and the importance of several signaling mechanisms is highlighted by the protective effects of pharmacological inhibitors *in vivo*, *in vitro*, or *ex vivo* (18–20).

Despite all efforts, the etiology of the disease is still not completely understood. Interestingly studies reporting ethnic susceptibility and familial occurrence of the PV- skin disorder provided evidence for a genetic predisposition to PV (21–25). In this respect, most of the reports provided data for PV associated genes belonging to a human leukocyte antigen (HLA) locus. Few studies, however, described PV genetic association of non-HLA genes (25). Amongst the latter is suppression of tumorigenicity 18 (ST18), the product of which functions as a transcription factor and thereby controls the mRNA levels of numerous proappoptotic and pro-inflammatory genes (26), participating in regulation of processes with potential relevance for loss of cell adhesion in PV (27, 28). Recently, a genetic variant located within the ST18 promoter was reported to cause ST18 up-regulation, associated with PV-IgG-mediated increase in cytokine secretion and more prominent loss of keratinocytes cohesion (29). In line with this, single nucleotide polymorphisms (SNP) identified in the ST18 gene were proposed to predispose to PV in a population-specific manner. SNPs promoted augmentation in ST18 expression was shown to be associated with more severe disease manifestation, indicative for the direct role of ST18 in PV pathogenesis (30, 31).

In the present study we investigated in both HaCaT and normal human epidermal keratinocytes (NHEK) the release of key pro-inflammatory molecules such as IL-1α, IL-6, TNF-α, and IFN-γ upon PV-IgG treatment. Additionally, the effect of ST18 overexpression on cytokine release but also on the modulation of pemphigus-associated ERK signaling was evaluated since both events would render keratinocytes more susceptible to PV-IgG-induced loss of keratinocyte adhesion.

MATERIALS AND METHODS

Cell Culture, Isolation of Human Primary Keratinocytes

For all experiments, primary normal human epithelial keratinocytes (NHEK) and HaCaT, a spontaneously immortalized human skin keratinocyte cell line were used. HaCaT cells were maintained in Dulbecco's Modified Eagle Medium (DMEM), (Life Technologies; Carlsbad; CA; USA) supplemented with 10% FCS (Biochrom, Berlin, Germany), 50 U/ml penicillin and 50 U/ml streptomycin, both antibiotics were purchased from AppliChem, Darmstadt, Germany.

NHEK were generated at Universitäts-Hautklinik Tübingen. The procedure was approved by the medical ethical committee of the Eberhard Karls University Tübingen (ethical approval: 547/2011BO2). Briefly, the cells were isolated from juvenile foreskin derived from patients, who have given written informed consent. The skin was divided into epidermis and dermis by using 50 mg/ml Dispase II (Roche; Basel, Switzerland). Epidermal cells were then separated from each other by using a trypsin-EDTA solution (Merck, Darmstadt, Germany) and afterwards cultivated in CnT-07 medium (CELLnTEC Advanced Cell Systems AG, Switzerland) containing 10 μg/ml gentamycin and 0.25 μg/ml amphotericin B. The cells were cultured in low calcium conditions (0.06 mM Ca^{2+}). 24 h prior treatment, cell differentiation was induced by increasing the Ca^{2+} concentration to 1.8 mM. All experiments were conducted on NHEK cells between passages 3 to 8.

Both cell lines were grown in a humidified atmosphere containing 5% CO_2 at 37°C. After cells reached confluency the medium was changed and 24 h later cell monolayers were treated accordingly.

Constructs and Transfection

The human ST18 construct (pCMV6-ST18-Myc/DDK) was generated by inserting the translated region of a human ST18 cDNA into the pCMV6-Entry target vector (Origene Technologies Company, Rockville, MD, USA). The latter was used also for a control transfection.

ST18 overexpression was accomplished by transient transfection with a plasmid DNA into HaCaT cells at 80% confluence using Turbofect transfection reagent (Fermentas, ThermoFisher Scientific). 24 h after transfection, medium was changed and cell monolayers were further exposed to treatment with various IgG fractions.

RNA Isolation, Complementary DNA (cDNA) Preparation, and PCR Performance

To confirm sufficient transfection efficiency with ST18 construct, PCR was performed with cDNA transcribed from an equal amount of total RNA. The latter was isolated by using RNeasy Plus mini kit (Qiagen, Venlo, Netherlands). cDNA was synthesized through the usage of SuperScript II reverse transcriptase kit (Invitrogen, ThermoFisher Scientific). All preparations were carried out according to manufacturer's instructions.

The transfection efficiency of each experiment requesting ST18 overexpression was tested by PCR using following primer pair:

hST18-164bp-Fw CACTAATCCAGGAGCTCAGTGTTG
hST18-164bp-Rev CCTGTCACTGCGGTCTTCTTG

To validate the PCR assay, positive (pCMV-ST18-Myc/DDK vector) and negative (instead of cDNA, H_2O was used as a template) controls were used. An empty negative control reflects the lack of contaminations, whereas manifestation of amplicon with correct size in the positive control guarantees accurate PCR conditions.

PCR was carried out as follows: 95°C for 3 min, followed by 22 cycles at 95°C for 30 s, 60°C for 30 s and 72°C for 30 s, the final extension was at 72°C for 5 min. Then, the PCR products were visualized by gel electrophoresis.

Dispase-Based Keratinocytes Dissociation Assay

Keratinocytes were seeded in 24-well plates and grown to confluency. NHEK cells were subsequently differentiated for 24 h by increasing the Ca^{2+}-concentration to 1.8 mM. HaCaT monolayers were transiently transfected either with control or pCMV-ST18-Myc/DDK vector 24 h prior to experimental procedure. Monolayers treated with PBS (Vehicle) or control IgG (c-IgG) for 24 h were considered as controls. Experimental conditions were treated with AK23 or different PV-IgG in a similar fashion.

The loss of cell cohesion was tested by dispase-based dissociation assay. The latter was performed as described elsewhere (32, 33). Briefly, after treatment, cell monolayers were washed with pre-warmed Hank's Balanced Salt Solution (HBSS) and subsequently released from the well-bottom by incubation with 2.4 U/ml Dispase II (Sigma-Aldrich) dissolved in HBSS for 20 min at 37°C. Next, the protease solution was substituted by HBSS and each condition was treated additionally for 10 min with thiazolyl blue tetrazolium bromide (MTT) (Sigma-Aldrich) at a final concentration of 10 μM to better visualize the monolayer sheets. The integrity of a single intact monolayer was compromised by applying controlled shear stress through pipetting the monolayers with an electrical 1 ml pipette. Resulting fragments were counted under a binocular microscope (Leica, Mannheim, Germany) as their number is an inverse measure of intercellular adhesion. Higher number of fragments correspond to stronger loss of intercellular adhesion. A Canon EOS 750D camera was used to record the dissociation experiments. Each experiment was repeated 6 to 10 times.

Analysis of the Cytokine Secretion

Simultaneous quantitative cytokine measurements were accomplished by high-throughput bead-based multiplex assays. A Milliplex kit (HCYTOMAG-60K, Merck KGaA, Darmstadt, Germany), precustomized for cytokines of interest, i.e., IL-1α, IL-6, IFN-γ, TNF-α, was used. Along with the serial standards, each sample was analyzed in duplicate or triplicate following the manufacturer's instructions. Collection of the data was achieved by using Luminex LX100/200 system (Luminex Corporation, Austin, Texas). Data analysis was performed using MILLIPLEX® Analyst 5.1.Software (Merck KGaA, Darmstadt, Germany). To estimate the cytokine concentration (expressed in pg/ml), standard curves derived from known reference concentrations supplied by the manufacturing company were utilized.

Immunostaining

Human keratinocytes (HaCaT and NHEK) were grown to confluence on glass coverslips. Twenty four hours prior treatment, the medium was changed and in the case of NHEK cells, the Ca^{2+} concentration was increased to 1.8 mM in order to induce cell differentiation. After 24 h of incubation at 37°C with different IgG fractions the culture medium was removed, cell monolayers were washed with PBS and subsequently fixed (with 2% paraformaldehyde (PFA) for 10 min) and permeabilized (with 0,1% Triton-X-100 for 5 min). To prevent unspecific binding the intact monolayers were blocked with a mix of 1% normal goat serum and 3% bovine serum albumin solved in PBS for at least 30 min at room temperature (RT). Consequent overnight incubation at 4°C with primary rabbit anti-Dsg3 antibody (Biozol Diagnostica Vertrieb GmbH, Germany) was performed. After washing with PBS, the cell monolayers were incubated with Cy3- conjugated secondary goat-anti-rabbit antibody (Dianova, Hamburg, Germany) for an hour at RT. After rinsing the monolayers with PBS and H_2O the cells were mounted on a glass slide with N-propyl gallate, an anti-fade reagent, which is used to reduce photobleaching of the fluorescent probes. Images were collected with 63xNA1.4 PL APO objective using a Leica SP5 confocal microscope.

PV Sera and Purification

Patient blood sera were obtained from the Department of Dermatology and Allergology, Philipps-Universität Marburg, Marburg, Germany. Prior serum collection, all patients gave their written informed consent. For disease determination, clinical and histological studies were carried out and the antibody scores for aDsg1 and 3 were obtained during disease diagnosis. Control serum was donated from healthy volunteers. Before experimental usage, patient sera were purified by column affinity chromatography as described elsewhere (34). Briefly, Protein-A Agarose (ThermoFisher, Waltham, USA) was washed with PBS. Subsequently, beads were incubated with patient sera for 2 h at room temperature on a rotator, which enables IgG binding to the beads. After washing the beads with PBS, IgGs were detached from the Agarose by using sodium citrate (20 mM, pH 2.4) followed up by neutralization with sodium carbonate. Next, a filter unit (Amicon Ultra−4, 100 k; Merck Millipore, Darmstadt, Germany) was used to wash the resulting salts out of the IgG fractions by centrifugation at 19,000 g for 20 min. As a final step the IgGs were resuspended in PBS. Protein amount of purified IgG fractions was determined by Bicinchoninic acid kit (BCA) (Thermo Fisher Scientific, Schwerte, Germany) and used for further experiments at a dilution of 1:50.

The monoclonal antibody AK23 reacting to Dsg3 was purchased from Biozol (Eching, Germany).

Triton X-100 Protein Fractionation, Electrophoresis, Western Blotting, and Tested Antibodies

Signaling pathway modulation was examined in either non-transfected or transfected keratinocytes exposed to different IgGs or AK23 for a time period of 30 min. After the incubation was accomplished, cell monolayers were washed with ice cold PBS. As next, extraction buffer (0.5% Triton X-100, 50 mmol/L MES, 25 mmol/L EGTA, 5 mmol/L $MgCl_2$) containing 0.1% of Leupeptin, Pepstatin and Aprotinin as well as 1% PMSF was applied for 15 min, on ice, under moderate shaking. Lysates were collected by scraping. In order to achieve successful fractionation of the cytoskeletal bound insoluble from the soluble fraction, a centrifugation step at 19,000 g for 10 min at 4°C was performed. Resulting supernatants defined the cytosolic pools. The obtained pellet, representing the cytoskeletal bound fraction, was further washed with Triton extraction buffer, centrifuged for 10 min and consequently re-suspended in SDS-buffer (25 mmol/l HEPES, 2 mmol/l EDTA, 25 mmol/l NaF, and 1% SDS, pH 7,4, complete Protease Inhibitor Cocktail). After sonication, protein concentration of both fractions was determined by Pierce BCA Protein Assay Kit (Thermo Fisher Scientific, Schwerte, Germany), following the manufacturer's instructions. Equal amounts of samples were mixed with Laemmli buffer and consequently subjected to Western blotting as described elsewhere (17).

Following primary antibodies were incubated overnight at 4°C in 5% bovine serum albumin (BSA) in Tris-buffered-saline (TBS) with 0.05% tween (TSB-T): p-ERK (Cell Signaling Technologies, Cambridge, United Kingdom), p44/42 MAPK pAB (Erkl/2) (Cell Signaling Technologies), GAPDH mAB (Santa Cruz), Desmoplakin I/II pAB (H-300) (Santa Cruz). Following peroxidase coupled secondary antibodies were used for 1 h at room temperature in TBS-T: HRP-coupled goat anti-mouse, a HRP-coupled goat anti-rabbit (Dianova, Hamburg, Germany). Afterwards antibodies were visualized by chemiluminescence with ECL reaction (GE Healthcare, Munich, Germany).

Data Analysis and Statistic

One-way ANOVA followed by Bonferroni correction (GraphPad Software, La Jolla, CA) was used to assess the differences among three or more treatments in dispase-based assay. To determine the cell response to different treatments in cells transfected with EV and ST18- vector either two-way ANOVA followed by Sidak's multiple comparisons test or multiple t-tests corrected by Holm-Sidak's method were applied as indicated. Each data point represents one single experiment. Data are presented as mean ± SEM. P-values less or equal to 0.05 assume significant differences between analyzed groups.

RESULTS

Pathogenicity of Pemphigus Autoantibodies on Human Keratinocytes

The pathogenic effect of IgG fractions derived either from an active pemphigus mouse model (AK23, a monoclonal autoantibody targeting Dsg3, (35)) or from pemphigus patients (PV-IgG) was evaluated by dispase-based dissociation assay in cultured immortalized HaCaT and primary normal human epidermal keratinocytes (NHEK) (**Figure 1A**). In contrast to control conditions, in which confluent monolayer exposed to PBS (vehicle) or control IgG (c-IgG) obtained from healthy volunteers remained intact, application of both AK23 and PV-IgG (PV-1 and PV-2) for 24 h induced loss of cell adhesion.

In HaCaT cell monolayers, the effect of pathogenic IgG-fractions on desmosomes was visualized by Dsg3 immunostaining. In all controls (vehicle and c-IgG), linearly organized Dsg3 staining at cell borders was observed. In contrast, 24 h incubation with autoantibodies induced fragmentation of the Dsg3 staining pattern along the borders (**Figure 1B**). Under the same conditions, NHEKs exhibited changes similar to those observed in HaCaT cells (**Supplementary Figure 1**).

ST18 Overexpression Promotes PV-IgG-Mediated Loss of Keratinocyte Cohesion

Recently, it has been reported that a PV-associated SNP leads to a significant increase in the expression of ST18 gene. As a consequence, in NHEK cells PV-IgG caused loss of keratinocyte adhesion as well as the release of key inflammatory molecules (29). In order to validate the effect of ST18 overexpression in human HaCaT keratinocytes, cells were transiently transfected with either empty vector (EV) or with ST18 expression vector. Consequently, the intact monolayers were exposed to control or pemphigus autoantibodies. Twenty four hours later, dispase-based dissociation assay was performed. Upon ST18 overexpression, the fragmentation of cell monolayers increased significantly in response to PV-IgG and AK23 incubation (**Figures 2A,B**). For each single experiment, sufficient transfection efficiency was confirmed by PCR analysis (**Figure 2C**).

Effect of Pemphigus Autoantibodies and ST18 Overexpression on Cytokine Release

Besides preserving the structure of the skin by forming strong intercellular junctions and thus functioning as a physical barrier, keratinocytes also mediate inflammation by synthesizing and secreting various cytokines in response to physical or chemical damage, inflammatory signals or UV radiation (36–38). Therefore, in the present study, the pattern of cytokines expressed by non-transfected or transiently transfected human keratinocytes exposed to either c-IgG or pathogenic IgG was further analyzed.

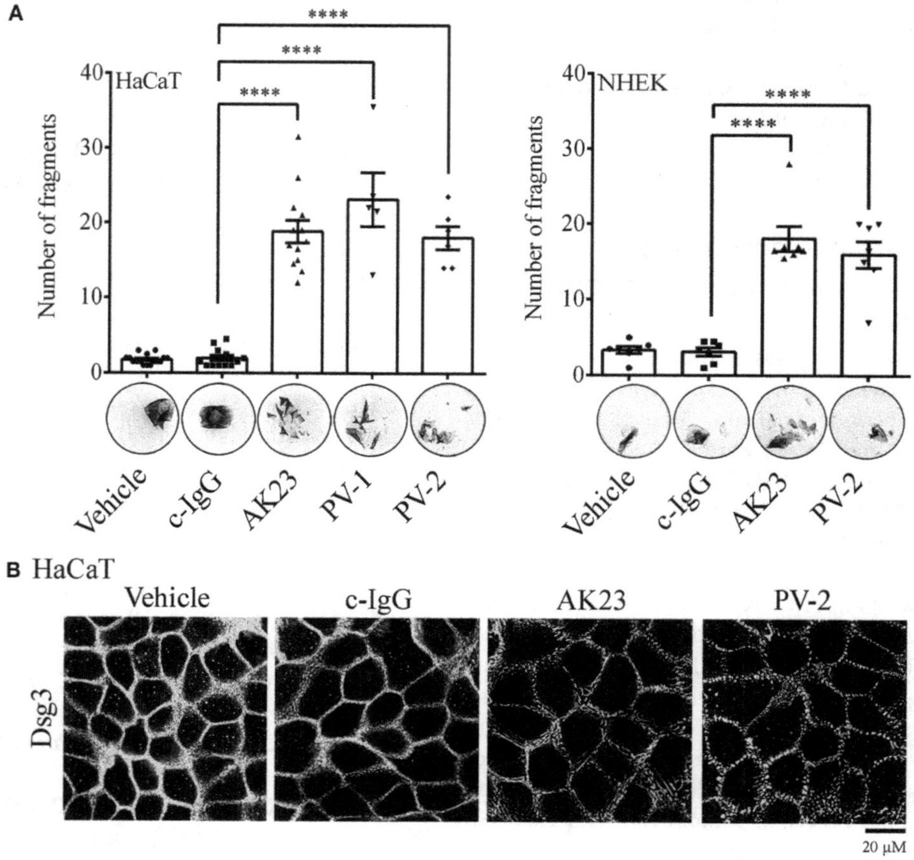

FIGURE 1 | Pemphigus autoantibody application induces loss of keratinocyte cohesion and fragmentation of Dsg3 immunostaining. **(A)** Dispase-based dissociation assay in human HaCaT and NHEK keratinocytes after treatment with pemphigus autoantibodies. Besides PBS-treated monolayers (Vehicle), cells exposed to c-IgG were also used as a control. Representative images of cell sheets pre-stained with MTT and subjected to defined mechanical stress ($n \geq 6$, One-way ANOVA, $^{****}p \leq 0.0001$ vs. c-IgG). **(B)** Dsg3 immunostaining in response to pathogenic autoantibodies (PV-IgG and monoclonal autoantibody AK23, targeting Dsg3). Representative images of $n \geq 4$ (Scale bar: 20 μm).

Twenty four hours after reaching confluency HaCaT and NHEK cells were exposed to pathogenic IgG for another 24 h. Respective controls (PBS or c-IgG treated) were run in parallel. After the incubation was completed, supernatants were collected and simultaneously assessed for multiple cytokines by Luminex assay. Cytokine secretion of IL-1α, IL-6, TNF-α, and IFN-γ in both HaCaT and primary NHEK cells was not affected significantly (**Figures 3A,B**). In case of IFN-γ, independent on the treatment, cytokine release in HaCaT was either not altered, similar as in NHEK cells, or often under the detection limit (**Supplementary Figures 2A,B**). The latter observation was in line with a recent study in PV-patients, where the serum levels of IFN-γ were undetectable (39). Taken together, these data demonstrate that at least *in vitro*, cytokine release is not strictly required for loss of keratinocyte cohesion.

It was reported that ST18 overexpression in NHEKs results in a PV-IgG-mediated release of key inflammatory cytokines (29). In order to validate the effect of ST18 overexpression in human HaCaT keratinocytes, cells were transiently transfected with either EV or ST18- expression vector. For the recent study, experiments were carried out in HaCaT keratinocytes since the transfection efficiency in NHEK was not consistent. The intact monolayers were consequently exposed to IgG fractions. Supernatants were collected and secretion profiles of IL-1α, IL-6, TNF-α, and IFN-γ were analyzed by Luminex assay. ST18 overexpression induced no significant increase in the secretion of any cytokine analyzed (**Figure 3C**). However, IL-1α and IL-6 levels were augmented in some experiments, but not in others. When compared to c-IgG treatment, the release of TNF-α was even reduced significantly upon PV-IgG application in both EV and ST18 transfected monolayers. Secretion of IFN-γ was either undetectable or not affected by ST18 overexpression (**Supplementary Figure 2C**).

Modulation of ERK Signaling Upon Treatment With PV-IgG Fractions and ST18 Overexpression

Several signaling pathways, including ERK signaling, have been implicated in the pathogenesis of pemphigus (16, 17). In order to evaluate ERK activity upon pemphigus autoantibody treatment, 24 h after differentiation with 1.8 mM Ca^{2+}, confluent NHEK

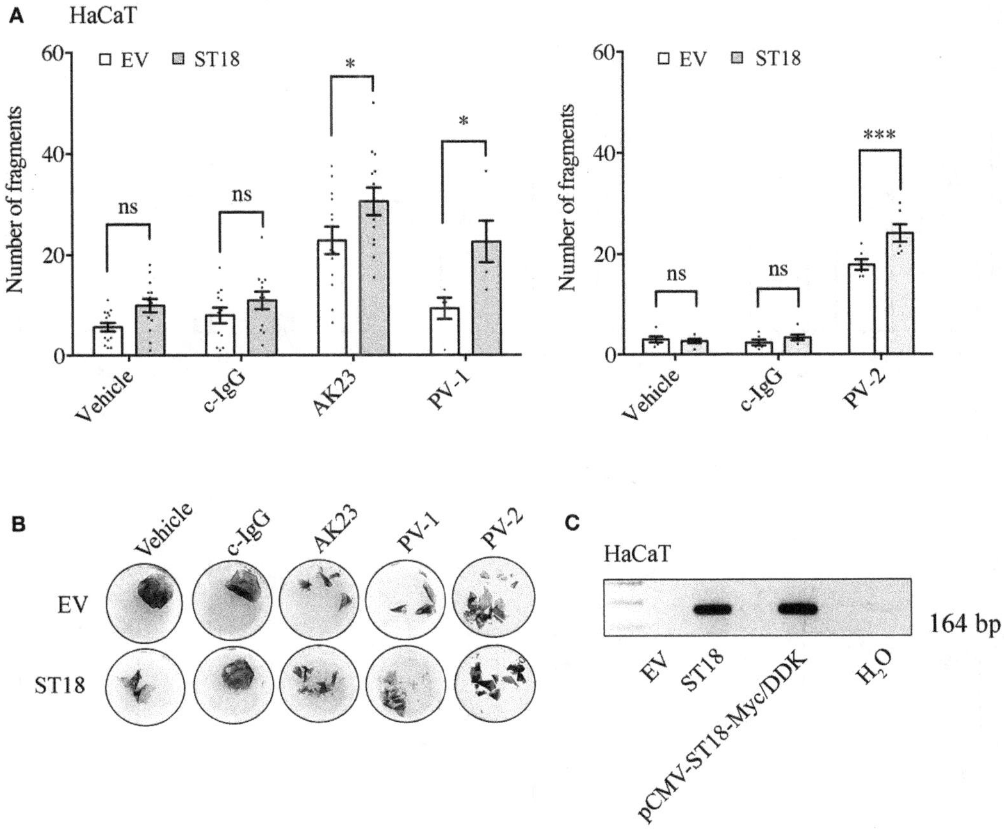

FIGURE 2 | ST18 enhances AK23- and PV-IgG-mediated loss of cohesion in cultured keratinocyte monolayers. **(A)** Dispase-based dissociation assay in HaCaT cells transiently transfected with a control empty (EV) or a ST18-expression vector and exposed to either c-IgG, AK23, or PV-IgG fractions ($n \geq 0.05$, two-way ANOVA, $^*p \leq 0.05$ and $^{***}p \leq 0.001$ vs. respective monolayers transfected with EV). **(B)** Representative images of keratinocyte monolayers pre-stained with 10 μM MTT for better visualization of the fragments. **(C)** PCR analysis validating sufficient transfection efficiency was performed for each single experiment. Positive (pCMV-ST18-Myc/DDK vector) and negative (H_2O) controls were run in parallel.

monolayers were incubated with different control or pathogenic IgGs for 30 min. ERK phosphorylation was investigated by triton fractionation and subsequent western blot analysis. The bands of phosphorylated and total ERK were densitometrically quantified and ERK activity was expressed as a ratio of phosphorylated-ERK to non-phosphorylated total ERK. Analysis revealed that compared to c-IgG, treatment with PV-2 IgG but not with AK23 induced significant activation of ERK (**Figure 4A**).

To evaluate the effect of ST18 overexpression on ERK signaling, 24 h after transfection HaCaT cells were incubated for 30 min with different IgGs (**Figure 4B**). Overexpression of ST18 resulted in significantly increased activity of ERK after c-IgG and AK23 treatment. Prominent but not significant elevation of ERK activity was observed in response to PV-2 application. Thus, we hypothesize that activation of ERK signaling is required to induce significant loss of cell cohesion as a result of ST18 overexpression. In order to test this hypothesis, inhibition of ERK activation by U0126, a widely used MEK inhibitor (40, 41), was performed in dispase assays using cell monolayers transiently transfected with either EV or ST18. Twenty four hours after transfection HaCaT cells were treated with 5 μM U0126 for an hour followed by incubation with either c-IgG, PV-IgG, or AK23 for another 2 h. Inhibition of ERK activation completely abolished autoantibody-induced loss of cell adhesion in ST18 transfected monolayers (**Figure 4C**).

Next, to test whether overexpression of ST18 modulates baseline adhesion via ERK, dispase-based dissociation assays were performed in vehicle or U0126-treated HaCaT keratinocytes transiently transfected with either EV or ST18 expression vector. Analysis revealed that neither in EV- nor in ST18- transfected cells adhesion was affected by ERK inhibition (**Figure 4D**). This indicates that an additional factor such as PV-IgG is required to facilitate ST18/ERK-mediated loss of adhesion.

DISCUSSIONS

Autoantibodies targeting Dsg1 and Dsg3 are pathogenic and cause blister formation by inducing structural desmosomal changes in the skin of PV patients (42). However, the mechanisms underlying disease development and the factors enhancing its manifestation have not yet been fully elucidated. Secondary

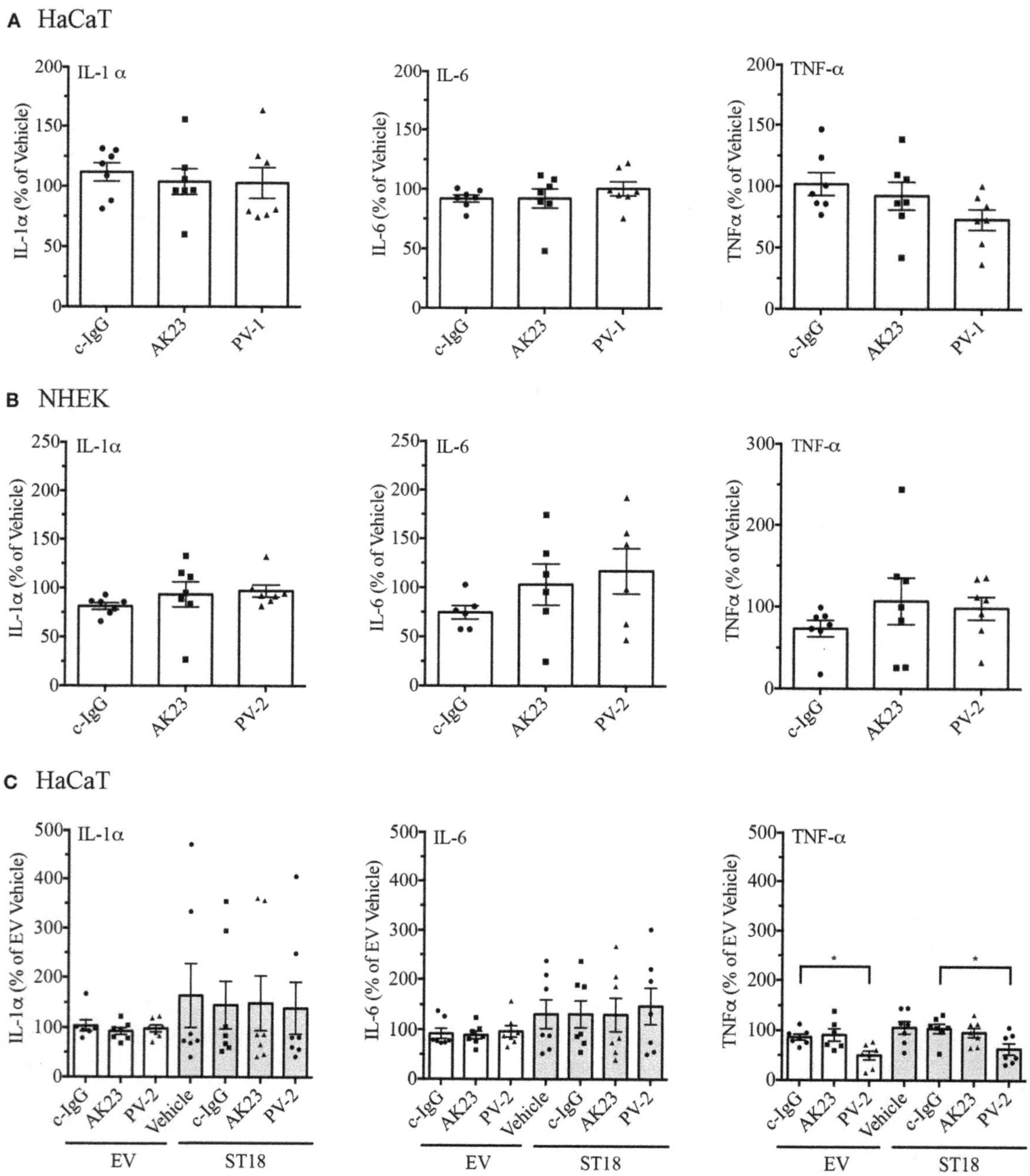

FIGURE 3 | Release of pro-inflammatory cytokines in response to pemphigus autoantibodies and ST18 overexpression. The content of cytokines in supernatants collected from cell monolayers, which were either treated with controls (Vehicle, c-IgG), AK23 or PV-IgGs, was evaluated in both HaCaT **(A)** and NHEK **(B)** cells. **(C)** Cytokine release by HaCaT cells transiently transfected with either EV or ST18 expression vectors and exposed to PV-IgG or AK23 was determined. All data are presented as percent of Vehicle ($n \geq 6$, two-way ANOVA; $^{*}p \leq 0.05$ vs. respective c-IgG).

factors promoting severity of the disease include non-Dsg antibodies (43) as well as genetic alterations such as recently reported ST18 SNPs (29–31) and may also entail keratinocyte-derived cytokine release.

Here, we investigate the effect of ST18 overexpression and cytokine secretion on PV-IgG mediated loss of adhesion. We observed that in both HaCaT and NHEK the release of key pro-inflammatory molecules such as IL-1α, IL-6, TNF-α, and IFN-γ is not strictly required for PV-IgG-induced loss of cell cohesion. However, ST18 overexpression did not only modulate cytokine release in some of the experiments but also altered ERK activity.

Pemphigus, as an autoimmune disease, depends highly on the activity of T-cells, the differentiation of which is regulated by autocrine cytokine signaling and is modulated by paracrine cytokine secretion from other cell type such as keratinocytes (44, 45). In skin, the production and secretion of cytokines has been

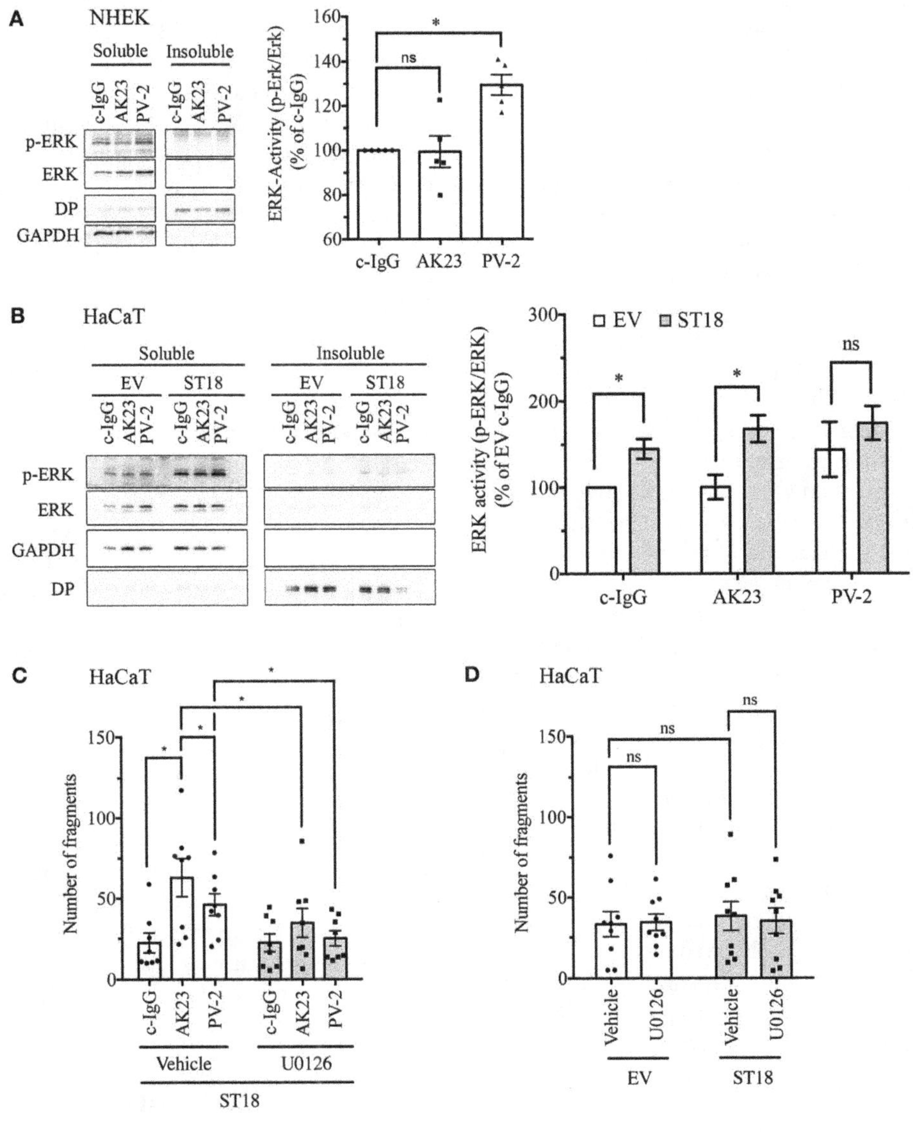

FIGURE 4 | Modulation of ERK signaling after incubation with pemphigus autoantibodies and ST18 overexpression. Twenty four hours after differentiation, NHEK cells were exposed for 30 min to different IgG fractions. Triton X-100-soluble (cytosolic) and Triton X-100-insoluble (representing cytoskeletal- bound) fractions were generated and further analyzed by Western blot. **(A)** Representative blot of ERK phosphorylation in response to IgG for each Triton X-100 fraction produced. GAPDH was used as a cytosolic marker, while Desmoplakin (DP) served as a cytoskeletal-bound marker. Densitometric quantification of ERK activity ($n = 5$, One-Way ANOVA, $^{*}p < 0.05$ vs. c-IgG). **(B)** Triton X-100 fractionation of HaCaT cells transfected with EV or ST18 vector and treated with IgG fractions for 30 min. Representative western blots showing total and phosphorylated ERK with respective markers for protein fractionation. Densitometric analysis of ERK activity within the soluble fraction using ImageJ software ($n = 7$, multiple T-tests, $^{*}p < 0.05$). **(C)** In HaCaT cells, 24 h after ST18 transfection an U0126 was applied for an hour followed by 2 h incubation with different IgG fractions, as indicated. Dispase-based assay evaluating the effect of ST18 mediated ERK activation in cell monolayers treated with autoantibody fractions. **(D)** Impact of U0126-mediated ERK inhibition on baseline cell adhesion in EV- and ST18-transfected monolayers assessed by dispase-based dissociation assays ($n \geq 8$, two-way ANOVA, $^{*}p < 0.05$).

recognized long ago and therefore intensely studied (46). These pro-inflammatory cytokines can also modulate keratinocyte behavior and could therefore be relevant for blister formation in pemphigus (47, 48).

Most studies on PV and cytokine release, however, are conflicting and report patient serum cytokine levels, which are most likely derived from T-cell signaling (49–52). Only few studies include cytokine assessment of blister fluid and only single reports evaluate production and secretion of cytokines *in vitro* (53). In the latter, polyclonal IgG fractions containing a plethora of antibodies, which could also include non-Dsg antibodies, were used (53). Therefore, in the present study, in addition to patient-derived PV-IgG the ability of a specific aDsg3 antibody, i.e., AK23, to induce cytokine secretion in keratinocytes was investigated. Both, AK23 and PV-IgG did not provoke significant cytokine secretion in HaCaT and NHEK cells (**Figures 3A,B**) but were efficient to impair keratinocyte adhesion. Therefore, secretion of keratinocyte-derived cytokines seems not to be primarily important for induction of loss of cell adhesion. Other antibodies such as mitochondrial antibodies or soluble FAS-ligand might change cytokine secretion profiles and thereby augment the disease as a secondary factor (54, 55).

Studies available on the transcription factor ST18 are limited. However, one of the first reports validated ST18 as a suppressor of tumor growth in breast cancer cell lines (56). Additionally, in fibroblasts, ST18 was reported to promote the expression of pro-inflammatory and pro-apoptotic genes, including cytokines (26). Furthermore, a relationship between a ST18 polymorphism and PV has now been shown to be relevant for Israelian, Egyptian (30) as well as Iranian (31) but not German (30) or Chinese (57) populations. In this respect, it was reported that increased loss of adhesion was associated with cytokine secretion in primary NHEK cells after introduction of ST18 expression vector and incubation with PV-IgG (29). Similarly, in HaCaT cells, we also detected decrease of cell adhesion upon simultaneous ST18 overexpression and pathogenic autoantibody treatment. However, we found elevated cytokine secretion in some but not all experiments following ST18 overexpression independently of IgG treatment. The discrepancy between both studies could possibly be based on the usage of different cell lines since in the study of Vodo et al. (29) NHEK cells were used whereas our experiments were performed with HaCaT cells. Nevertheless, these results indicate that mechanisms independent of cytokine secretion may also contribute to ST18-induced enhancement of adhesion loss.

Activation of several signaling pathways regulates desmosome stability and is involved in pemphigus skin blistering (58, 59). We focused on ERK because it was observed previously that this pathway is activated only when antibodies against Dsg1, which are known to be primarily important for epidermal blistering in pemphigus, were present in autoantibody fractions (1, 16, 17, 60). Similarly to ST18, ERK modulation also was shown to be associated with cytokine signaling (61–65) and could thereby link desmosome destabilization and ST18 expression. Here we show, that expression of ST18 induced significant ERK activation after c-IgG and AK23 treatment, which led to the hypothesis that ST18 promoted increase in disease severity is mediated by ERK activation independent of IgG treatment. In order to validate this hypothesis, ERK activation was inhibited by U0126. The mediator abolished loss of cell cohesion in monolayers transfected with ST18 and incubated with pemphigus antibodies indicating that ST18-mediated loss of adhesion is at least in part induced by ERK signaling pathway modulation.

Mechanisms underlying loss of cell adhesion in response to AK23 or PV-IgG may differ as the latter contain antibodies against Dsg1 and possibly against various other antigens (43). Moreover, it has been shown that in contrast to antibodies targeting Dsg3 such as AK23, which are capable to prevent homophilic interactions between Dsg3 molecules (66), antibodies targeting Dsg1 were not observed to inhibit Dsg1 interactions (34).

We previously reported that ERK was not activated by AK23 or mucosal-dominant PV-IgG both of which are targeting Dsg3, but rather by IgG fractions containing aDsg1 antibodies (17). Here we confirmed these results as we detected increased ERK phosphorylation after incubation with mucocutaneous PV-IgG but not AK23 in NHEK cells. However, the underlying ERK-dependent mechanisms relevant for pemphigus skin blistering are not yet completely understood. Interestingly, upon ST18 overexpression in HaCaT monolayers, ERK was activated under AK23 as well as c-IgG treatment, suggesting that ST18 may generally modulate ERK signaling. Nevertheless, further analysis revealed that baseline adhesion in ST18-transfected cells was unaffected by ERK inhibition (**Figure 4D**) indicating that PV-IgG is required as an additional factor to facilitate ERK-mediated loss of adhesion in response to ST18 overexpression.

Taken together, our study adds new insight on the mechanisms by which ST18 may contribute to pemphigus pathogenesis and indicates that altered signaling mechanisms regulating desmosomal adhesion may render keratinocytes more susceptible to autoantibody-induced loss of cell adhesion.

ETHICS STATEMENT

Human sera were collected and used in accordance with recommendations of the ethics committee of the Philipps-Universität Marburg, Marburg, Germany. Name of the indicated project: Phänotypische und funktionelle Analyse von Immunzellen des peripheren Bluts beim Pemphigus vulgaris.

AUTHOR CONTRIBUTIONS

MR and EW performed the experiments, participated in study design, interpreted results, and wrote the manuscript. RS isolated the primary NHEK cells. JW designed the experiments, interpreted results, revised the manuscript and provided the funding. AY, NS, OS, and ES revised the manuscript and actively participate in the scientific discussions.

ACKNOWLEDGMENTS

The authors thank Martina Hitzenbichler (LMU München) and Mariola Dragan (JMU, Würzburg) for their excellent technical assistance. Additionally, we are very thankful to Prof. Dr. med. Michael Hertl and Prof. Dr. med Rüdiger Eming for providing us with a patients' sera.

REFERENCES

1. Kasperkiewicz M, Ellebrecht CT, Takahashi H, Yamagami J, Zillikens D, Payne AS, et al. Pemphigus. *Nat Rev Dis Primers.* (2017) 3:17026. doi: 10.1038/nrdp.2017.26
2. Spindler V, Heupel WM, Efthymiadis A, Schmidt E, Eming R, Rankl C, et al. Desmocollin 3-mediated binding is crucial for keratinocyte cohesion and is impaired in pemphigus. *J Biol Chem.* (2009) 284:30556–64. doi: 10.1074/jbc.M109.024810
3. Mao X, Nagler AR, Farber SA, Choi EJ, Jackson LH, Leiferman KM, et al. Autoimmunity to desmocollin 3 in pemphigus vulgaris. *Am J Pathol.* (2010) 177:2724–30. doi: 10.2353/ajpath.2010.100483
4. Rafei D, Muller R, Ishii N, Llamazares M, Hashimoto T, Hertl M, et al. IgG autoantibodies against desmocollin 3 in pemphigus sera induce loss of keratinocyte adhesion. *Am J Pathol.* (2011) 178:718–23. doi: 10.1016/j.ajpath.2010.10.016
5. Price AJ, Cost AL, Ungewiss H, Waschke J, Dunn AR, Grashoff C. Mechanical loading of desmosomes depends on the magnitude and orientation of external stress. *Nat Commun.* (2018) 9:5284. doi: 10.1038/s41467-018-07523-0
6. Waschke J. The desmosome and pemphigus. *Histochem Cell Biol.* (2008) 130:21–54. doi: 10.1007/s00418-008-0420-0
7. Johnson JL, Najor NA, Green KJ. Desmosomes: regulators of cellular signaling and adhesion in epidermal health and disease. *Cold Spring Harb Perspect Med.* (2014) 4:a015297. doi: 10.1101/cshperspect.a015297
8. Waschke J. Desmogleins as signaling hubs regulating cell cohesion and tissue/organ function in skin and heart- EFEM lecture 2018. *Ann Anat.* (2018). doi: 10.1016/j.aanat.2018.11.006. [Epub ahead of print].
9. Aoyama Y, Kitajima Y. Pemphigus vulgaris-IgG causes a rapid depletion of desmoglein 3 (Dsg3) from the Triton X-100 soluble pools, leading to the formation of Dsg3-depleted desmosomes in a human squamous carcinoma cell line, DJM-1 cells. *J Invest Dermatol.* (1999) 112:67–71. doi: 10.1046/j.1523-1747.1999.00463.x
10. Spindler V, Endlich A, Hartlieb E, Vielmuth F, Schmidt E, Waschke J. The extent of desmoglein 3 depletion in pemphigus vulgaris is dependent on Ca(2+)-induced differentiation: a role in suprabasal epidermal skin splitting? *Am J Pathol.* (2011) 179:1905–16. doi: 10.1016/j.ajpath.2011.06.043
11. Schlogl E, Radeva MY, Vielmuth F, Schinner C, Waschke J, Spindler V. Keratin retraction and desmoglein3 internalization independently contribute to autoantibody-induced cell dissociation in pemphigus vulgaris. *Front Immunol.* (2018) 9:858. doi: 10.3389/fimmu.2018.00858
12. Vielmuth F, Walter E, Fuchs M, Radeva MY, Buechau F, Magin TM, et al. Keratins Regulate p38MAPK-dependent desmoglein binding properties in Pemphigus. *Front Immunol.* (2018) 9:528. doi: 10.3389/fimmu.2018.00528
13. Berkowitz P, Hu P, Warren S, Liu Z, Diaz LA, Rubenstein DS. p38MAPK inhibition prevents disease in pemphigus vulgaris mice. *Proc Natl Acad Sci USA.* (2006) 103:12855–60. doi: 10.1073/pnas.0602973103
14. Mao X, Sano Y, Park JM, Payne AS. p38 MAPK activation is downstream of the loss of intercellular adhesion in pemphigus vulgaris. *J Biol Chem.* (2011) 286:1283–91. doi: 10.1074/jbc.M110.172874
15. Yoshida K, Ishii K, Shimizu A, Yokouchi M, Amagai M, Shiraishi K, et al. Non-pathogenic pemphigus foliaceus (PF) IgG acts synergistically with a directly pathogenic PF IgG to increase blistering by p38MAPK-dependent desmoglein 1 clustering. *J Dermatol Sci.* (2017) 85:197–207. doi: 10.1016/j.jdermsci.2016.12.010
16. Frusic-Zlotkin M, Raichenberg D, Wang X, David M, Michel B, Milner Y. Apoptotic mechanism in pemphigus autoimmunoglobulins-induced acantholysis–possible involvement of the EGF receptor. *Autoimmunity.* (2006) 39:563–75. doi: 10.1080/08916930600971836
17. Walter E, Vielmuth F, Rotkopf L, Sardy M, Horvath ON, Goebeler M, et al. Different signaling patterns contribute to loss of keratinocyte cohesion dependent on autoantibody profile in pemphigus. *Sci Rep.* (2017) 7:3579. doi: 10.1038/s41598-017-03697-7
18. Jolly PS, Berkowitz P, Bektas M, Lee HE, Chua M, Diaz LA, et al. p38MAPK signaling and desmoglein-3 internalization are linked events in pemphigus acantholysis. *J Biol Chem.* (2010) 285:8936–41. doi: 10.1074/jbc.M109.087999
19. Sayar BS, Ruegg S, Schmidt E, Sibilia M, Siffert M, Suter MM, et al. EGFR inhibitors erlotinib and lapatinib ameliorate epidermal blistering in pemphigus vulgaris in a non-linear, V-shaped relationship. *Exp Dermatol.* (2014) 23:33–8. doi: 10.1111/exd.12290
20. Egu DT, Walter E, Spindler V, Waschke J. Inhibition of p38MAPK signalling prevents epidermal blistering and alterations of desmosome structure induced by pemphigus autoantibodies in human epidermis. *Br J Dermatol.* (2017) 177:1612–8. doi: 10.1111/bjd.15721
21. Tron F, Gilbert D, Mouquet H, Joly P, Drouot L, Makni S, et al. Genetic factors in pemphigus. *J Autoimmun.* (2005) 24:319–28. doi: 10.1016/j.jaut.2005.03.006
22. Sinha AA. The genetics of pemphigus. *Dermatol Clin.* (2011) 29:381–91. doi: 10.1016/j.det.2011.03.020
23. Parameswaran A, Attwood K, Sato R, Seiffert-Sinha K, Sinha AA. Identification of a new disease cluster of pemphigus vulgaris with autoimmune thyroid disease, rheumatoid arthritis and type I diabetes. *Br J Dermatol.* (2015) 172:729–38. doi: 10.1111/bjd.13433
24. Salathiel AM, Brochado MJ, Kim O, Deghaide NH, Donadi EA, Roselino AM. Family study of monozygotic twins affected by pemphigus vulgaris. *Hum Immunol.* (2016) 77:600–4. doi: 10.1016/j.humimm.2016.05.005
25. Vodo D, Sarig O, Sprecher E. The genetics of pemphigus vulgaris. *Front Med.* (2018) 5:226. doi: 10.3389/fmed.2018.00226
26. Yang J, Siqueira MF, Behl Y, Alikhani M, Graves DT. The transcription factor ST18 regulates proapoptotic and proinflammatory gene expression in fibroblasts. *FASEB J.* (2008) 22:3956–67. doi: 10.1096/fj.08-111013
27. Grando SA, Bystryn JC, Chernyavsky AI, Frusic-Zlotkin M, Gniadecki R, Lotti R, et al. Apoptolysis: a novel mechanism of skin blistering in pemphigus vulgaris linking the apoptotic pathways to basal cell shrinkage and suprabasal acantholysis. *Exp Dermatol.* (2009) 18:764–70. doi: 10.1111/j.1600-0625.2009.00934.x
28. Giordano CN, Sinha AA. Cytokine networks in pemphigus vulgaris: an integrated viewpoint. *Autoimmunity.* (2012) 45:427–39. doi: 10.3109/08916934.2012.697593
29. Vodo D, Sarig O, Geller S, Ben-Asher E, Olender T, Bochner R, et al. Identification of a functional risk variant for pemphigus vulgaris in the ST18 gene. *PLoS Genet.* (2016) 12:e1006008. doi: 10.1371/journal.pgen.1006008
30. Sarig O, Bercovici S, Zoller L, Goldberg I, Indelman M, Nahum S, et al. Population-specific association between a polymorphic variant in ST18, encoding a pro-apoptotic molecule, and pemphigus vulgaris. *J Invest Dermatol.* (2012) 132:1798–805. doi: 10.1038/jid.2012.46
31. Etesami I, Seirafi H, Ghandi N, Salmani H, Arabpour M, Nasrollahzadeh A, et al. The association between ST18 gene polymorphism and severe Pemphigus disease among Iranian population. *Exp Dermatol.* (2018) 7:1395–8. doi: 10.1111/exd.13778
32. Heupel WM, Engerer P, Schmidt E, Waschke J. Pemphigus vulgaris IgG cause loss of desmoglein-mediated adhesion and keratinocyte dissociation independent of epidermal growth factor receptor. *Am J Pathol.* (2009) 174:475–85. doi: 10.2353/ajpath.2009.080392
33. Hartlieb E, Kempf B, Partilla M, Vigh B, Spindler V, Waschke J. Desmoglein 2 is less important than desmoglein 3 for keratinocyte cohesion. *PLoS ONE.* (2013) 8:e53739. doi: 10.1371/journal.pone.0053739
34. Waschke J, Bruggeman P, Baumgartner W, Zillikens D, Drenckhahn D. Pemphigus foliaceus IgG causes dissociation of desmoglein 1-containing junctions without blocking desmoglein 1 transinteraction. *J Clin Invest.* (2005) 115:3157–65. doi: 10.1172/JCI23475
35. Tsunoda K, Ota T, Aoki M, Yamada T, Nagai T, Nakagawa T, et al. Induction of pemphigus phenotype by a mouse monoclonal antibody against the amino-terminal adhesive interface of desmoglein 3. *J Immunol.* (2003) 170:2170–8. doi: 10.4049/jimmunol.170.4.2170
36. Petit-Frere C, Capulas E, Lyon DA, Norbury CJ, Lowe JE, Clingen PH, et al. Apoptosis and cytokine release induced by ionizing or ultraviolet B radiation in primary and immortalized human keratinocytes. *Carcinogenesis.* (2000) 21:1087–95. doi: 10.1093/carcin/21.5.087
37. Pasparakis M, Haase I, Nestle FO. Mechanisms regulating skin immunity and inflammation. *Nat Rev Immunol.* (2014) 14:289–301. doi: 10.1038/nri3646
38. Chiurchiu V, Rapino C, Talamonti E, Leuti A, Lanuti M, Gueniche A, et al. Anandamide suppresses proinflammatory T cell responses *in vitro* through type-1 cannabinoid receptor-mediated mTOR inhibition in human keratinocytes. *J Immunol.* (2016) 197:3545–53. doi: 10.4049/jimmunol.1500546

39. Masjedi M, Esmaeil N, Saffaei A, Abtahi-Naeini B, Pourazizi M, Haghjooy Javanmard S, et al. Cytokine indexes in pemphigus vulgaris: perception of its immunpathogenesis and hopes for non-steroidal treatment. *Iran J Pharm Res.* (2017) 16:1223–9.
40. Duncia JV, Santella JB III, Higley CA, Pitts WJ, Wityak J, Frietze WE, et al. MEK inhibitors: the chemistry and biological activity of U0126, its analogs, and cyclization products. *Bioorg Med Chem Lett.* (1998) 8:2839–44.
41. Favata MF, Horiuchi KY, Manos EJ, Daulerio AJ, Stradley DA, Feeser WS, et al. Identification of a novel inhibitor of mitogen-activated protein kinase kinase. *J Biol Chem.* (1998) 273:18623–32.
42. Spindler V, Waschke J. Pemphigus-A disease of desmosome dysfunction caused by multiple mechanisms. *Front Immunol.* (2018) 9:136. doi: 10.3389/fimmu.2018.00136
43. Amber KT, Valdebran M, Grando SA. Non-desmoglein antibodies in patients with pemphigus vulgaris. *Front Immunol.* (2018) 9:1190. doi: 10.3389/fimmu.2018.01190
44. Hertl M. Humoral and cellular autoimmunity in autoimmune bullous skin disorders. *Int Arch Allergy Immunol.* (2000) 122:91–100. doi: 10.1159/000024364
45. Albanesi C, Madonna S, Gisondi P, Girolomoni G. The interplay between keratinocytes and immune cells in the pathogenesis of psoriasis. *Front Immunol.* (2018) 9:1549. doi: 10.3389/fimmu.2018.01549
46. Grone A. Keratinocytes and cytokines. *Vet Immunol Immunopathol.* (2002) 88:1–12. doi: 10.1016/S0165-2427(02)00136-8
47. Matsue H, Bergstresser PR, Takashima A. Reciprocal cytokine-mediated cellular interactions in mouse epidermis: promotion of gamma delta T-cell growth by IL-7 and TNF alpha and inhibition of keratinocyte growth by gamma IFN. *J Invest Dermatol.* (1993) 101:543–8.
48. Konur A, Schulz U, Eissner G, Andreesen R, Holler E. Interferon (IFN)-gamma is a main mediator of keratinocyte (HaCaT) apoptosis and contributes to autocrine IFN-gamma and tumour necrosis factor-alpha production. *Br J Dermatol.* (2005) 152:1134–42. doi: 10.1111/j.1365-2133.2005.06508.x.
49. Baroni A, Perfetto B, Ruocco E, Greco R, Criscuolo D, Ruocco V. Cytokine pattern in blister fluid and sera of patients with pemphigus. *Dermatology.* (2002) 205:116–21. doi: 10.1159/000063895
50. Satyam A, Khandpur S, Sharma VK, Sharma A. Involvement of T(H)1/T(H)2 cytokines in the pathogenesis of autoimmune skin disease-pemphigus vulgaris. *Immunol Invest.* (2009) 38:498–509. doi: 10.1080/08820130902943097
51. Lee SH, Hong WJ, Kim SC. Analysis of serum cytokine profile in pemphigus. *Ann Dermatol.* (2017) 29:438–45. doi: 10.5021/ad.2017.29.4.438
52. Timoteo RP, da Silva MV, Miguel CB, Silva DA, Catarino JD, Rodrigues Junior V, et al. Th1/Th17-Related cytokines and chemokines and their implications in the pathogenesis of pemphigus vulgaris. *Media Inflamm.* (2017) 2017:7151285. doi: 10.1155/2017/7151285
53. Feliciani C, Toto P, Amerio P, Pour SM, Coscione G, Shivji G, et al. *In vitro* and *in vivo* expression of interleukin-1alpha and tumor necrosis factor-alpha mRNA in pemphigus vulgaris: interleukin-1alpha and tumor necrosis factor-alpha are involved in acantholysis. *J Invest Dermatol.* (2000) 114:71–7. doi: 10.1046/j.1523-1747.2000.00835.x
54. Chernyavsky A, Chen Y, Wang PH, Grando SA. Pemphigus vulgaris antibodies target the mitochondrial nicotinic acetylcholine receptors that protect keratinocytes from apoptolysis. *Int Immunopharmacol.* (2015) 29:76–80. doi: 10.1016/j.intimp.2015.04.046
55. Lotti R, Shu E, Petrachi T, Marconi A, Palazzo E, Quadri M, et al. Soluble fas ligand is essential for blister formation in pemphigus. *Front Immunol.* (2018) 9:370. doi: 10.3389/fimmu.2018.00370
56. Jandrig B, Seitz S, Hinzmann B, Arnold W, Micheel B, Koelble K, et al. ST18 is a breast cancer tumor suppressor gene at human chromosome 8q11.2. *Oncogene.* (2004) 23:9295–302. doi: 10.1038/sj.onc.1208131
57. Yue Z, Fu X, Chen M, Wang Z, Wang C, Yang B, et al. Lack of association between the single nucleotide polymorphism of ST18 and pemphigus in Chinese population. *J Dermatol.* (2014) 41:353–4. doi: 10.1111/1346-8138.12363
58. Waschke J, Spindler V. Desmosomes and extradesmosomal adhesive signaling contacts in pemphigus. *Med Res Rev.* (2014) 34:1127–45. doi: 10.1002/med.21310
59. Spindler V, Eming R, Schmidt E, Amagai M, Grando S, Jonkman MF, et al. Mechanisms causing loss of keratinocyte cohesion in pemphigus. *J Invest Dermatol.* (2018) 138:32–7. doi: 10.1016/j.jid.2017.06.022
60. Rotzer V, Breit A, Waschke J, Spindler V. Adducin is required for desmosomal cohesion in keratinocytes. *J Biol Chem.* (2014) 289:14925–40. doi: 10.1074/jbc.M113.527127
61. Shinohara H, Inoue A, Toyama-Sorimachi N, Nagai Y, Yasuda T, Suzuki H, et al. Dok-1 and Dok-2 are negative regulators of lipopolysaccharide-induced signaling. *J Exp Med.* (2005) 201:333–9. doi: 10.1084/jem.20041817
62. Kyriakis JM, Avruch J. Mammalian MAPK signal transduction pathways activated by stress and inflammation: a 10-year update. *Physiol Rev.* (2012) 92:689–737. doi: 10.1152/physrev.00028.2011
63. Sanin DE, Prendergast CT, Mountford AP. IL-10 production in macrophages is regulated by a TLR-driven CREB-mediated mechanism that is linked to genes involved in cell metabolism. *J Immunol.* (2015) 195:1218–32. doi: 10.4049/jimmunol.1500146
64. Chiba S, Hisamatsu T, Suzuki H, Mori K, Kitazume MT, Shimamura K, et al. Glycolysis regulates LPS-induced cytokine production in M2 polarized human macrophages. *Immunol Lett.* (2017) 183:17–23. doi: 10.1016/j.imlet.2017.01.012
65. Wen X, Han XR, Wang YJ, Fan SH, Zhang ZF, Wu DM, et al. Effects of S100A12 gene silencing on serum levels of anti-inflammatory/pro-inflammatory cytokines in septic rats through the ERK signaling pathway. *J Cell Biochem.* (2018) 119:4038–49. doi: 10.1002/jcb.26568.
66. Heupel WM, Zillikens D, Drenckhahn D, Waschke J. Pemphigus vulgaris IgG directly inhibit desmoglein 3-mediated transinteraction. *J Immunol.* (2008) 181:1825–34. doi: 10.4049/jimmunol.181.3.1825

12

Pemphigus: Current and Future Therapeutic Strategies

Dario Didona[1†], Roberto Maglie[1,2,3*†], Rüdiger Eming[1] and Michael Hertl[1‡]*

[1] Department of Dermatology and Allergology, Philipps University, Marburg, Germany, [2] Surgery and Translational Medicine, Section of Dermatology, University of Florence, Florence, Italy, [3] Section of Dermatology, Departement of Health Sciences, University of Florence, Florence, Italy

***Correspondence:**
Dario Didona
dario.didona@uk-gm.de
Roberto Maglie
robertomaglie.med@libero.it*

† These authors share first authorship

‡ Senior authorship

Pemphigus encompasses a heterogeneous group of autoimmune blistering diseases, which affect both mucous membranes and the skin. The disease usually runs a chronic-relapsing course, with a potentially devastating impact on the patients' quality of life. Pemphigus pathogenesis is related to IgG autoantibodies targeting various adhesion molecules in the epidermis, including desmoglein (Dsg) 1 and 3, major components of desmosomes. The pathogenic relevance of such autoantibodies has been largely demonstrated experimentally. IgG autoantibody binding to Dsg results in loss of epidermal keratinocyte adhesion, a phenomenon referred to as acantholysis. This in turn causes intra-epidermal blistering and the clinical appearance of flaccid blisters and erosions at involved sites. Since the advent of glucocorticoids, the overall prognosis of pemphigus has largely improved. However, mortality persists elevated, since long-term use of high dose corticosteroids and adjuvant steroid-sparing immunosuppressants portend a high risk of serious adverse events, especially infections. Recently, rituximab, a chimeric anti CD20 monoclonal antibody which induces B-cell depletion, has been shown to improve patients' survival, as early rituximab use results in higher disease remission rates, long term clinical response and faster prednisone tapering compared to conventional immunosuppressive therapies, leading to its approval as a first line therapy in pemphigus. Other anti B-cell therapies targeting B-cell receptor or downstream molecules are currently tried in clinical studies. More intriguingly, a preliminary study in a preclinical mouse model of pemphigus has shown promise regarding future therapeutic application of Chimeric Autoantibody Receptor T-cells engineered using Dsg domains to selectively target autoreactive B-cells. Conversely, previous studies from our group have demonstrated that B-cell depletion in pemphigus resulted in secondary impairment of T-cell function; this may account for the observed long-term remission following B-cell recovery in rituximab treated patients. Likewise, our data support the critical role of Dsg-specific T-cell clones in orchestrating the inflammatory response and B-cell activation in pemphigus. Monitoring autoreactive T-cells in patients may indeed provide further information on the role of these cells, and would be the starting point for designating therapies aimed at restoring the lost immune tolerance against Dsg. The present review focuses on current advances, unmet challenges and future perspectives of pemphigus management.

Keywords: pemphigus, CAAR T-cell, rituximab, anti-CD 20 antibodies, BTK inhibitors, neonatal Fc receptor (FcRn)

INTRODUCTION

Definition

Pemphigus encompasses a heterogeneous group of autoimmune chronic blistering skin diseases, which affect both mucous membranes and the skin. Pemphigus group diseases are characterized by IgG autoantibodies directed against epidermal adhesion complexes (desmosomes) of keratinocytes, leading to loss of cell–cell adhesion, a phenomenon called acantholysis (1, 2).

Pemphigus can be divided into three major forms: pemphigus vulgaris (PV), pemphigus foliaceus (PF), and paraneoplastic pemphigus (PNP). Autoantibodies directed against Dsg3 and Dsg1 are mainly identified in PV; anti-Dsg1 autoantibodies are the serological hallmark of PF (3). In addition, autoantibodies targeting non-Dsg antigens have been reported in PV patients (4), such as IgG against alpha9 acetylcholine receptor (5), various mitochondrial nicotinic cholinergic receptor subtypes (4) and desmocollins 1-3 (4).

A variety of IgG autoantibodies have been described in PNP patients, including IgG against adhesion proteins of the plakin family, plakophilin 3, desmocollins 1 and 3, Dsg1, and Dsg3 and a 170 kD protein which has been recently identified as the protease inhibitor, alpha-2 macroglobulin-like 1 (A2ML1) (6).

Alike PV, PF and PNP, IgA pemphigus is an extremely rare variant of pemphigus, in which IgA but not IgG autoantibodies against epidermal antigens can be identified (3, 7, 8).

Epidemiology

Epidemiology of Pemphigus Vulgaris

PV is the most common clinical pemphigus variant. The annual incidence rate has been reported between 0.76 and 16.1 per million population, depending on the geographical area and the ethnicity (9, 10), with the highest incidence reported in Ashkenazi Jews (10, 11). This observation has been related to the more frequent occurrence of particular Human Leukocyte Antigen (HLA) class II genes in PV patients of Jewish origin, particularly HLA-DRB1*04:02; while HLA-DQB1*05:03 is more common in non-Jewish PV patients (12) and was also shown to have the strongest association with PV in a Chinese study using next generation sequence analysis (13).

The exact prevalence of pemphigus is unknown. A German analysis reported a point prevalence of 0.009% (14), while a Danish analysis estimated the pemphigus prevalence at 0.006% (15, 16). In addition, in a recent analysis on the US population, an overall standardized point prevalence of 5.2 cases per 100,000 adults has been reported (17). The age at initial PV presentation varies from 36.5 and 72.4 years (12). The mean age of PV onset is 50–60 years, although several cases of PV in children have been described (12). A female predominance has been globally reported, with an estimated female to male ratio of 5.0 in the American PV population (11).

Epidemiology of Pemphigus Foliacues

The annual incidence of sporadic PF in the Caucasian population is ~0.04 per 100.000 inhabitants (10, 12). Sporadic PF corresponding to ~20% of pemphigus cases (10, 12). People in the fifth decade are mainly affected, without sex preference (10, 12). HLA-DRB1*04:01, HLA-DRB1*04:06, HLA-DRB1*14, DRB1*01:01, have been associated with a higher risk of PF (13, 18). No ethnic predisposition has been reported (10, 12).

Endemic PF (*fogo selvagem*) has been reported in some areas of Brazil, Colombia, and Tunisia (19). Most of the patients are young rural workers, who live in forest areas adjacent to rivers and streams (19). In these areas, some insects including black fly (simulium species), are though to trigger the disease, leading to an immune reaction against Dsg1 via molecular mimicry (20, 21). This hypothesis is supported by high positivity rates of anti-Dsg1 IgG autoantibodies in the sera of healthy individuals living in endemic regions of *fogo selvagem* (21). In Brazilian population HLA-DRB1 alleles *04:04, *14:02, *14:06, and *01:02 have been reported as risk factors for *fogo selvagem* (22).

Epidemiology of Paraneoplastic Pemphigus

PNP is considered a rare disease, with about 500 cases reported in the literature (6, 23). Patients between 45 and 70 years of age are usually affected (6, 23). PNP accounts for 3–5% of all pemphigus cases (6, 23). Furthermore, PNP can affect also children and adolescents, particularly in association with Castleman's disease (6, 23). In this sub-group of patients, a predisposition in patients with Hispanic roots was described (24). An association with HLA class II DRB1*03 and HLA Cw*14, respectively, was reported in Caucasian and in Han Chinese patients (25, 26).

Major Clinical Variants

Pemphigus Vulgaris

More than half of the patients develop flaccid cutaneous blisters (3, 8, 27) (**Figure 1A**), which evolve into oozing erosions on erythematous skin. The entire skin may be affected, although lesions mostly occurs in areas exposed to increased mechanical stress (e.g., intertriginous areas) (3, 8, 27) and seborrheic areas (3, 8, 27). Bacterial or viral superinfections of cutaneous and mucosal lesions are fairly common. Cutaneous blisters and erosions usually transform into crusts followed by re-epithelisation without scars. Post-inflammatory hypo and/or hyperpigmentation are common.

In most instances, PV initially manifests with extremely painful erosions of the oral mucosa, particularly the buccal mucosa, the gingiva, the tongue, and the hard and soft palate (3, 8, 27) (**Figure 1B**). These lesions lead impaired food uptake which results in progressive weight loss. Hoarseness of the voice may be indicative of laryngeal involvement. In the early stages, oral lesions may be misinterpreted as recurrent aphthae, herpetic gingivostomatitis, or erosive lichen planus (3, 8, 27). Other mucous membranes might be less frequently involved, such as laryngeal, esophageal, conjunctival, nasal, anal, and genital mucosa (28).

PV may also involve the nail apparatus. In one study, nail involvement occurred in circa 13% of PV patients. Nail alterations included paronychia, nail discoloration, onychorrhexis, periungual hemorrhages, and onycholysis (29).

Erosions of the intertriginous areas, the scalp and face might evolve into papillomatous or vegetative lesions characterized by abnormal growth of keratinocytes (30) (**Figure 2**). This

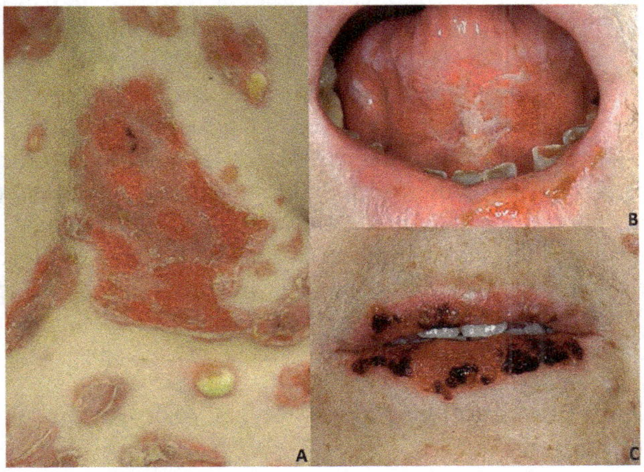

FIGURE 1 | Pemphigus vulgaris: **(A)** Flaccid cutaneous blisters associated with erosions; **(B)** Multiple erosions of the tongue and of the lips; Paraneoplastic pemphigus: **(C)** haemorrhagic crusts and erosion of the lips. All the patients gave written informed consent for the publication of the pictures.

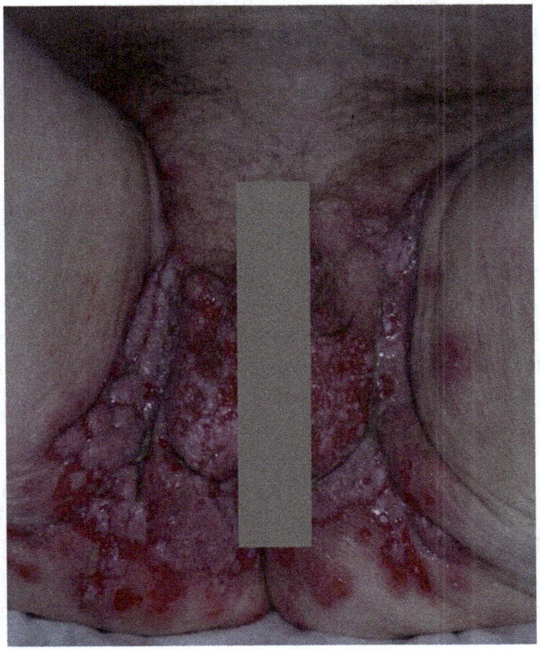

FIGURE 2 | Pemphigus vegetans: vegetative lesions and erosions of the groin and genitals.

phenomenon represents the clinical hallmark of pemphigus vegetans (PVe) (30), which accounts for <5% of pemphigus cases (30).

A substantial number of PV patients shows a transition from a mucosal dominant to a mucocutaneous phenotype with skin lesions characteristic of PF as a result of epitope spreading, a process of diversification of B and/or T-cell responses from the initial dominant epitope (i.e., Dsg3) to a secondary one (i.e., Dsg1) (31). Based on the involved area, PV can be clinically divided in mucosal dominant, mucocutaneous, and, less frequently, cutaneous dominant (3, 8, 27).

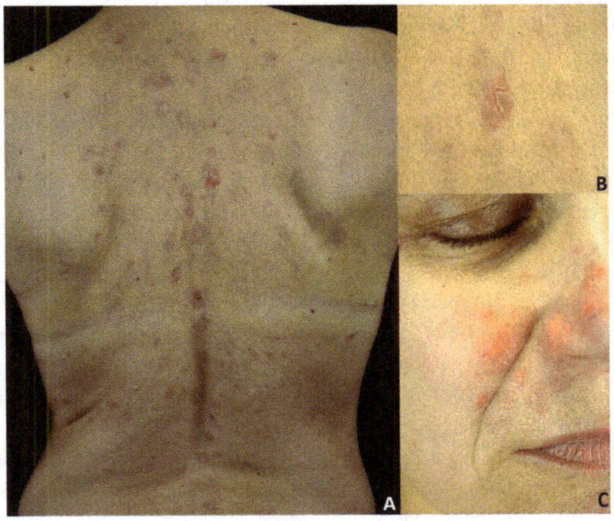

FIGURE 3 | Pemphigus foliaceus: **(A)** Scaly and crusted erythematous plaques on the seborrheic areas; **(B)** Leafy and crusted circumscribed erosion on the back; **(C)** Scaly erythematous plaques on the seborrheic areas. All the patients gave written informed consent for the publication of the pictures.

Pemphigus Foliaceus

Sporadic PF is characterized by the absence of mucosal involvement (3, 8, 27). It presents with leafy, scaly and crusted circumscribed erosions on erythematous skin (3, 8, 27) (**Figure 3**). Seborrheic areas, including the upper trunk and the face, are mainly involved. Flaccid, fragile blisters are rarely seen because of their fragility. Skin lesions can dramatically progress leading to exfoliative erythroderma. PF onset is often subtle, with a few scattered crusted lesions that resembling impetigo. Furthermore, the scaly erythema on the scalp may be misdiagnosed for seborrheic dermatitis. The endemic variant of PF *(fogo selvagem)* is clinically and pathologically indistinguishable from the sporadic one (3, 8, 27). Pemphigus erythematosus (Senear-Usher syndrome) is a rare clinical variant of PF (3, 8, 27), characterized by malar erythemato-squamous plaques and vesicles involving the face in a butterfly-like distribution pattern, the trunk and sun-exposed areas resembling lupus erythematosus (32). In addition, a diagnosis of psoriasis should be also ruled out. Pemphigus seborrhoicus is a very superficial variant of PF with extensive superficial, crusty erosions and erythematous plaques affecting seborrheic areas, particularly the face (3, 27).

Paraneoplastic Pemphigus

PNP is a rare pemphigus variant which is always associated with underlying neoplasms, both malignant and benign. Up to 84% of all PNP cases are secondary to hematologic malignancies (33), including non-Hodgkin lymphomas (38.6%), chronic lymphocytic leukemia (18.4%), Castleman's disease (18.4%), thymoma (5.5%), Waldenstrom's macroglobulinemia (1.2%),

Hodgkin lymphoma (0.6%), and monoclonal gammopathy (0.6%) (6, 33). Less frequently, epithelial carcinomas (8.6%), sarcomas (6.2%) and gastric cancers have been described in association with PNP (6, 33–35). Some cases of PNP have been reported to be triggered by anti-neoplastic drugs, including fludarabin and bendamustine (36) or radiotherapy (37). PNP has a polymorphic clinical appearance, probably related to the variable presence of different IgG autoantibodies in addition to anti Dsg3/Dsg1 IgG (38). PNP typically presents with a painful stomatitis, and with extensive erosions of the oral cavity and oropharynx (**Figure 1C**). Usually, the vermillion border of the lips is involved (6). Differential diagnosis includes erythema multiforme (EM), toxic epidermal necrolysis (TEN) and Stevens-Johnson's syndrome; in pediatric cases, oral involvement may be mistaken for a herpetic stomatitis (6).

The nasopharynx, anogenital region, and esophagus may be also affected. Ocular involvement occurs in about 70% of cases (39). Usually, skin lesions, including diffuse erythema, vesicles, blisters, papules, scaly plaques, exfoliative erythroderma, erosions or ulcerations, appear after the onset of the mucosal lesions (38). Moreover, erythema may appear as macular, urticarial, targetoid or polymorphous lesions and a single patient may present different types of lesions, that could evolve from one type to another (40). Lichenoid lesions are also common and occur more frequently in children (24).

The peculiar clinical features of PNP can be explained by both, antibody-driven and cell-mediated pathogenetic mechanisms (41). The first usually determine a PV-like clinical phenotype, while the second features lead to a lichenoid phenotype. More than 90% of PNP cases show an involvement of the respiratory epithelium with dyspnea, obstructive lung disease, and bronchiolitis obliterans, which is one of the main causes of death in PNP (6, 42, 43). Recently, a correlation between bronchiolitis obliterans and anti-epiplakin Ig Abs was found in Japanese PNP patients (42).

IgA Pemphigus

IgA pemphigus is characterized by intraepidermal pustules or vesicles with neutrophilic infiltration (3, 7, 8). Acantholysis is usually absent. Depending on the level of pustule formation, IgA pemphigus is divided into two major subtypes, namely subcorneal pustular dermatosis type (IgA-SPD), characterized by subcorneal pustules in the upper epidermis, and intraepidermal neutrophilic type (IgA-IEN), characterized by suprabasilar pustules located at the lower or entire epidermis (3, 7, 8).

Pathogenesis

Dsg1/Dsg3 Compensation Theory

Because of the different expression of the pemphigus autoantigens (Dsg1 and Dsg3) in the cornified and non-cornified epithelium, skin and mucosae are differentially affected by anti-Dsg IgG autoantibodies. PF patients show only anti-Dsg1 IgG autoantibodies; whilst, patients affected by mucosal-dominant PV have only anti-Dsg3 IgG autoantibodies. Furthermore, in patients with mucocutaneous PV both anti-Dsg3 and anti-Dsg1 IgG autoantibodies are detected (44). In the skin and mucosae, the expression of Dsg1 and Dsg3 is different: cutaneous Dsg1 is expressed in the entire epidermis, but more strongly in the superficial layers; cutaneous Dsg3 is expressed in the lower epidermis, mainly in the basal and parabasal layers. On the contrary, mucosal Dsg1 and Dsg3 are expressed in the entire squamous layer, but the expression of Dsg3 is much higher.

Therefore, sera with only anti-Dsg1 IgG lead to superficial blisters and only in the skin, as in PF, because Dsg3 compensates for the loss of Dsg1. In contrast, anti-Dsg3 IgG lead to impairment of mucosal epidermal adhesion because of the low expression of Dsg1, that is not adequate to compensate the loss of Dsg3 adhesion. When anti-Dsg1 and anti-Dsg3 IgG is present, skin and mucous membranes are affected (45).

Blister Formation and Acantholysis: Auto-Antibody Dependent Factors

Ig autoantibodies directed against Dsg antigens lead to epithelial acantholysis presumably through several synergistic mechanisms. A model in which acantholysis is produced by interference through antibodies in desmosome adhesion and/or assembly has been proposed. Furthermore, an altered outside-in-signaling caused by antibodies has been thought to cooperate in damaging the desmosomal integrity (46).

The pivotal role of antibodies in pemphigus has been extensively reported (47). Furthermore, it has been highlighted that the sole monovalent antibody fragments can lead to skin lesions (48). In addition, IgG4 antibodies have been mainly reported in pemphigus, which do not involve the complement cascade (49).

The most important targets for Ig antibodies in pemphigus are extracellular domains of Dsg. Dsg show five extracellular cadherin repeats domains (EC1-EC5); the amino-terminal EC1 and EC2 domains, which play a pivotal role in adhesive interactions, are usually targeted by pemphigus antibodies. Indeed, anti-Dsg3 autoantibodies form PV patients and model mice bind directly to residues involved in trans-adhesion (50) and cis-adhesion (51). Thus, antibodies to the NH2-terminal cadherin domains likely compete with or block cellular cohesion. Di Zenzo et al. (51) propose that human anti-Dsg3 autoantibodies bind to the cis-adhesive Dsg3 interface inducing acantholysis. Furthermore, in contrast to IgG autoantibodies directed against other epitopes of Dsg1 and Dsg3, the serum concentrations of these IgG Abs correlate with disease activity (52, 53).

Depletion of Dsg results from several steps: desmosomes lose adhesive properties, probably through a direct interference of trans-interaction of Dsg; further, different signaling pathways cause Dsg endocytosis and depletion, leading to loss of demosomal integrity and adhesion (45). Moreover, the depletion of extradesmosomal Dsg located in association with lipid raft components may affect the *ex novo* expression of desmosomes (54). Furthermore, it has been reported that polyclonal IgG antibodies from PV patients can directly inhibit homophilic Dsg3 trans-interactions. These evidences provide support for the steric hindrance model of pemphigus pathogenesis (52, 53).

Further mechanisms have been thought to be involved in pemphigus acantholysis. Dsg endocytosis and desmosome disassembly have been reported as triggered by both

IgG autoantibodies from PV patients and recombinant monovalent human anti-Dsg3 autoantibodies (55, 56). In addition, intercellular widening at non-acantholytic cell layers induced by pathogenic pemphigus antibodies have been detected by both immunofluorescence and electron microscopy findings (57, 58).

Autoantibody-triggered cellular signaling pathways have been also reported as pathogenetic co-mechanisms in pemphigus. Specifically, it has been shown that polyclonal IgG antibodies from serum of PF patients can lead to dissociation of Dsg1 junctions without blocking homophilic Dsg1 trans-interactions (59). In addition, several molecules and signaling pathways have been reported as playing a role in pemphigus acantholysis, including p38 mitogen-activated protein kinase (MAPK) and MAPK-activated protein kinase 2 (MK2) (60, 61). p38MAPK directly modulates intermediate filament formation and the maintenance of the desmosomal structure. It was recently reported that p38 MAPK signaling and Dsg3 internalization play a pivotal role in pemphigus acantholysis (62); however, it has been also highlighted that blisters induced by monoclonal autoantibodies from PV patients are not affected by p38 or MK2 inhibition, indicating that this mechanism of blisters formation might be mainly related to steric hindrance (60, 61, 63).

Furthermore, Saito et al. (63) demonstrated that monoclonal and polyclonal autoantibodies are both complementary involved in acantholysis; indeed, an inducible Dsg clustering has been reported with polyclonal serum IgG, but not with monoclonal antibodies. Furthermore, several other signaling molecules and pathways have been reported as altered by anti-Dsg autoantibodies in pemphigus acantholysis, such as EGFR, caspases (64), and MYC (65). However, none of these events can solely induce acantholysis.

TABLE 1 | Diagnostic algorithm in pemphigus [adapted from Witte et al. (76)].

HISTOPATHOLOGY
Suprabasal acantholysis (IgA-IEN, PNP, PV)
Subcorneal acantholysis (IgA-SPD, PF)
Interface dermatitis with vacuolization of the basal cells and lichenoid infiltrate at the DEJ (PNP)
DIF
Reticular binding of IgG and/or C3 to the surface of epidermal keratinocytes (PF, PV)
Reticular binding of IgA and/or C3 to the surface of epidermal keratinocytes (IgA-IEN, IgA-SPD)
Linear deposits of IgG and/or C3 at the BMZ (PNP)
Net-like IgG and/or C3 deposits on the surface of epidermal keratinocytes and along the DEJ (PNP)
IIF
Reticular pattern of cell surface reactivity of IgG antibodies on the epithelium of monkey esophagus (PF, PNP, PV)
Reticular pattern of cell surface reactivity of IgA antibodies on the epithelium of monkey esophagus (IgA-IEN, IgA-SPD)
Net-like pattern of cell surface reactivity of IgG antibodies on monkey esophagus epithelia, normal human skin, and plakin-rich urinary bladder (PNP)
ELISA
Alpha-2-macroglobulin-like-1 (PNP)
BP230 (PNP)
Desmocollin 1 (IgA-SPD)
Desmocollin 3 (IgA-SPD, PNP)
Desmoglein 1 (IgA-IEN, PF, PNP, PV)
Desmoglein 3 (IgA-IEN, PV, PNP)
Periplakin/Envoplakin (PNP)

BMZ, Basal membrane zone; DEJ, dermo-epidermal junction; DIF, direct immunofluorescence; ELISA, enzyme-linked immunosorbent assay; IgA-IEN, intraepidermal neutrophilic type of IgA pemphigus; IgA-SPD, subcorneal pustular dermatosis type of IgA pemphigus; IIF, indirect immunofluorescence; PF, pemphigus foliaceus; PNP, paraneoplastic pemphigus; PV, pemphigus vulgaris.

Blister Formation and Acantholysis: IgG-Independent Factors

Beside of the Abs role in acantholysis, several autoantibody-independent factors have been thought to be involved in acantholysis. However, the distinct role of these factors is not completely understood.

An increment of Th2 cytokines, such as interleukin (IL)-4, IL-6, and IL-10, has been extensively reported in sera of PV patients, while a reduction of Th1 cytokines, such as IL-2 and Interferon-gamma (IFN-γ) has been also reported (66). In addition, an increase of IL-17a, produced by Th17-cells, and IL-21 and IL-27, synthesized by T follicular helper cell, has been detected (67). Of note, IL-17a was also shown in PV blisters (67). Furthermore, complement activation, cytotoxic proteases and high levels of IL-4 and IL-10 were observed (66, 68). In addition, Tumor Necrosis Factor-alpha (TNF-α) RNA is widely expressed in PV skin lesions and TNF-α serum concentrations correlate with disease activity and IgG autoantibody titers (69, 70).

The importance of apoptosis of epidermal keratinocytes in acantholysis is still under debate. Indeed, some groups considered this process a downstream event after loss of cell–cell adhesion (71), while others suggested it as an upstream event (72). Caspase 8 activation induced by Fas ligand (FasL) detected in PV sera was described to induce apoptosis in keratinocytes. It has been reported *in vitro* and *in vivo* that hindrance of FasL protein causes an inhibition of PV IgG-induced apoptosis of epidermal keratinocytes, suggesting a pivotal role of that FasL in PV pathogenesis (73, 74). Moreover, Lotti et al. (73) highlighted that apoptosis precedes acantholysis, as Fas overexpression, caspase activation before cell detachment *in vivo*.

Furthermore, it was reported that the secretion of cytokines from keratinocytes could be stimulated by PV-IgG (75). Indeed, the expression of the transcription factor ST18 in keratinocytes was reported in response to PV-IgG, leading to both secretion of cytokines and loss of keratinocyte cohesion; therefore, it has been concluded that that cytokines contribute to blistering downstream of autoantibodies (75).

Diagnostics

The proper diagnosis of pemphigus is based on four criteria, namely clinics, histopathology of the lesional skin, direct immunofluorescence microscopy (DIF) of perilesional skin, and detection of serum autoantibodies by indirect immunofluorescence microscopy (IIF), enzyme-linked immunosorbent assay (ELISA) and/or additional techniques such as Biochip, immunoblot analysis or immunoprecipitation (7, 76) (**Table 1**).

Histopathologically, PV is characterized by intraepidermal acantholysis (7) (**Figure 4A**), with basal keratinocytes still attached to the basement membrane zone assuming a characteristic tombstone-like morphology. In contrast to PV, PF lesions show a more superficial, subcorneal acantholysis (**Figure 4B**). In PNP, the histopathological features are polymorphic. Bullous lesions show suprabasal acantholysis with dyskeratosis and a scattered inflammatory infiltrate (6). In maculopapular lesions, a lichenoid interface dermatitis is more frequently observed (6). Clinically mixed maculopapular and bullous lesions show both acantholysis and lichenoid interface dermatitis (23). IgA pemphigus is characterized by intraepidermal pustules or vesicles with neutrophilic infiltration whereas acantholysis is usually absent (7).

In all pemphigus variants, DIF of perilesional skin shows reticular binding of IgG and/or C3 to the surface of epidermal keratinocytes (7, 77) (**Figure 4C**). In IgA pemphigus, DIF detects IgA instead of IgG (7, 77). In PNP, net-like IgG and/or C3 deposits on the surface of epidermal keratinocytes and along the dermo-epidermal junction can be detected in <50% of cases (6). In contrast to PV and PF, PNP lesions show linear deposits of IgG and/or C3 at the basal membrane zone by DIF (6).

In IIF routine diagnostics, monkey esophagus is used as the major tissue substrate. A reticular pattern of cell surface reactivity of IgG antibodies with epithelial cells is characteristic (7, 77). In IgA pemphigus, intercellular deposits of IgA directed against Dsg 1 and Dsg 3 (IgA-IEN), as well as against Dsc 1 and Dsc 3 (IgA-SPD) are detected by IIF (7, 77). IgA autoantibodies in IgA-SPD may be detected by IIF on Dsc1-transfected COS-7 cells (78).

In PNP, IgG antibodies directed against plakins can be detected; among those, IgG against envoplakin and periplakin are the most common (23). In PNP, IIF also shows a net-like staining pattern with normal human skin and plakin-rich urinary bladder, the latter being the substrate of choice since it shows for the detection of plakin-reactive IgG autoantibodies (83%) (6, 23, 76).

In PV, IgG autoantibodies against Dsg 1 and Dsg 3 can be detected by ELISA. Patients affected by dominant cutaneous PV show only or preferentially anti-Dsg 1 autoantibodies, while patients with mucosal dominant PV show only or preferably anti-Dsg 3 IgG autoantibodies. In muco-cutaneous PV, both anti-Dsg 1 and anti-Dsg 3 autoantibodies can be detected. In contrast to PV, patients with PF show only IgG against Dsg 1 in the vast majority of cases (7, 77). In general, anti-Dsg 1 and anti-Dsg 3 serum antibody concentrations correlate with disease activity (7, 77). However, in case of atypical pemphigus, autoantibodies against Dscs are detected, while reactivity against Dsg 3 and/or Dsg 1 lacks. In atypical pemphigus, both IgA and IgG against different Dscs are detected (79). However, routine evaluation of serum IgG and IgA against Dscs does not play a significant role in making the diagnosis of PV and PF (79).

Depending on the subtype, different IgA autoantibodies are detected in IgA pemphigus by ELISA, including IgA against Dsc 1, Dsg 1, and Dsg 3.

The spectrum of IgG autoantibodies is more diverse in PNP, including IgG autoantibodies against Dsg 1, Dsg 3, desmoplakin 1, desmoplakin 2, Dsc 1, Dsc 3, envoplakin, periplakin, plectin, BP180, BP230, and the protease inhibitor, alpha-2-macroglobulin-like-1 (6, 80). However, ELISA lacks sensitivity in PNP patients due to the wide range of autoantigens targeted by Ig autoantibodies (81).

Immunoblotting and immunoprecipitation are considered useful techniques for diagnosing PNP and can show IgG antibodies against several antigens, including plakins, periplakin, desmoplakin, BP180, BP230, and alpha-2-macroglobulin-like-1 (6, 80). Indeed, IgG autoantibodies against envoplakin and periplakin and/or alpha-2 macroglobulin-like-1 confirm the diagnosis of PNP. Therefore, in PNP patients two of three serological techniques (IIF on rat bladder, immunoblot and immunoprecipitation) should be performed to establish the correct diagnosis (76).

Immunoblot analysis is performed with recombinant proteins or extracts of dermis, epidermis, bovine gingiva, amnion membrane or cultured keratinocytes (76). They can be used for the detection of several autoantibodies, such as anti-envoplakin, anti-periplakin, anti-desmoplakin, anti-BP180, and anti-BP230 Ig (76).

Recently, a novel lateral flow immunoassay (LFIA) was developed (82). It detects anti-Dsg 3 IgG in human sera. In contrast to other diagnostic procedures, the assay is simpler and faster. LFIA was validated on a collection of 200 sera and showed a sensitivity and specificity of 78.1 and 97.1%, respectively (82).

TREATMENT

Since the advent of targeted therapies, the management of pemphigus has gradually changed. Until now, systemic corticosteroids (CS) and immunosuppressants have been the mainstay of pemphigus therapy. Among conventional adjuvant immunosuppressants, both EADV and BAD guidelines suggest azathioprine (AZA) and mycophenolate mofetil (MMF) as a first line steroid-sparing agent (83, 84). However, different variables, including patients' comorbidities, single institutional experience and costs have to be taken into account, and other drugs, such as methotrexate and cyclophosphamide, also demonstrate efficacy. Notably, these drugs have mainly a CS-sparing rather than a morbostatic effect (85–87). Accordingly, they do not lead to an improvement in achieving remission, but reduce the risk of relapse by 29% in comparison to CS alone (85). A recent prospective multicentre study by Joly et al. (88), now supports using RTX as a first line adjuvant therapy for pemphigus, showing superior efficacy compared to CS alone and reduced incidence of CS-related serious adverse events and overall mortality. The administration of intravenous immunoglobulin (IVIg) or immunoadsorption (IA) is a therapeutic option in patients with severe/refractory PV. Proposed algorithms for the induction and maintenance therapy as well as therapy of relapse are summarized in **Figures 5–7**.

Corticosteroids and Immunosuppressants

Corticosteroids

In pemphigus, prednisolone is recommended as a first-line therapy in combination with an immunosuppressive agent, such as azathioprine (AZA) and mycophenolate mofetil (MMF), or RTX (83, 84). In addition, prednisolone alone at a dose of

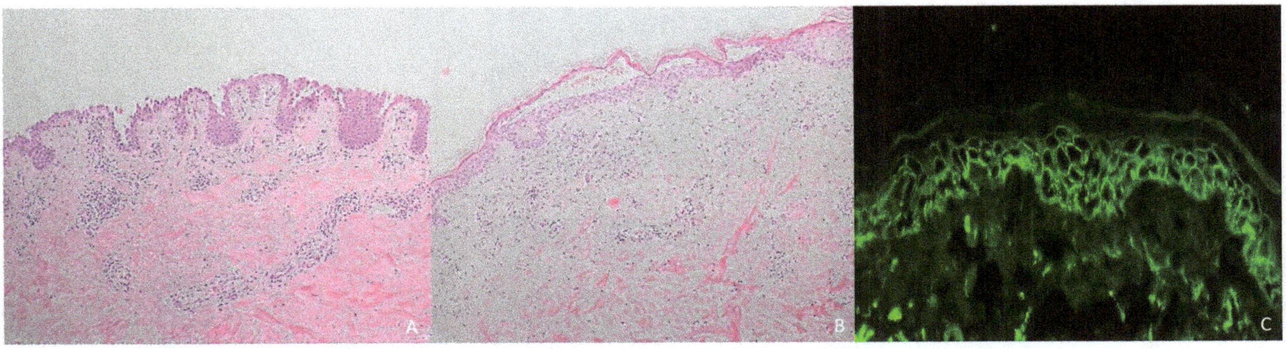

FIGURE 4 | Diagnostic of pemphigus: **(A)** Intraepidermal acantholysis in pemphigus vulgaris; **(B)** Subcorneal loss of adhesion in pemphigus foliaceus; **(C)** Reticular binding of IgG in pemphigus vulgaris.

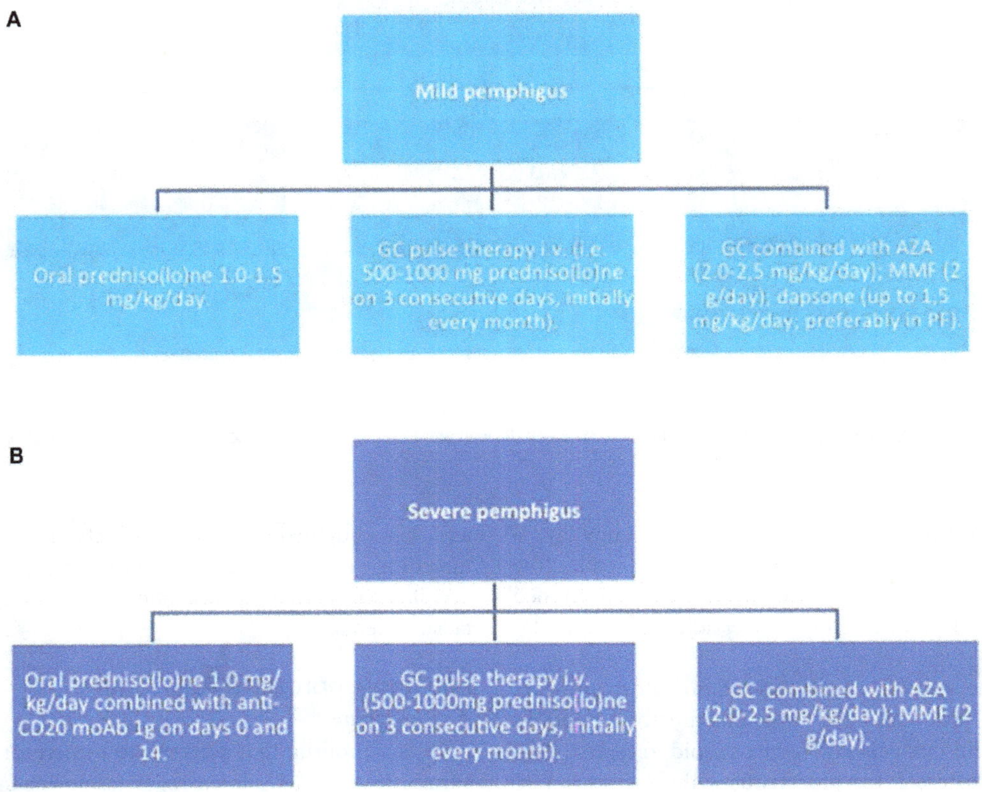

FIGURE 5 | Induction therapy in pemphigus. **(A)** mild pemphigus; **(B)** severe pemphigus. AZA, azathioprine; GC, glucocorticoids; MMF, mycophenolate mofetil; moAb, monoclonal antibody.

1–1.5 mg/kg/day is still recommended as first line therapy in patients who are not eligible for treatment with RTX or other immunosuppressive adjuvants.

Higher CS doses (up to 1.5 mg/kg) may be administered, if disease control is not achieved within 3 weeks. As soon as disease control is reached, the doses should be tapered by a 25% reduction every other week. If lesions reappear, CS should be increased until two steps back at the previous dose to lead to disease control (84). However, the optimal dose has not been validated by randomized clinical trials RCT.

No significant differences regarding the duration of remissions and relapse rates have been reported in PV patients receiving low-dose oral prednisolone (45–60 mg/day) or high-dose oral prednisolone (120–180 mg/day) (89). In the maintenance period of PV, no advantages in terms of remission, death, relapse or withdrawal rates have been reported in patients on a pulsed CS therapy in comparison to conventional oral CS therapy. Indeed, the two RCTs about this topic reported opposite results (90, 91).

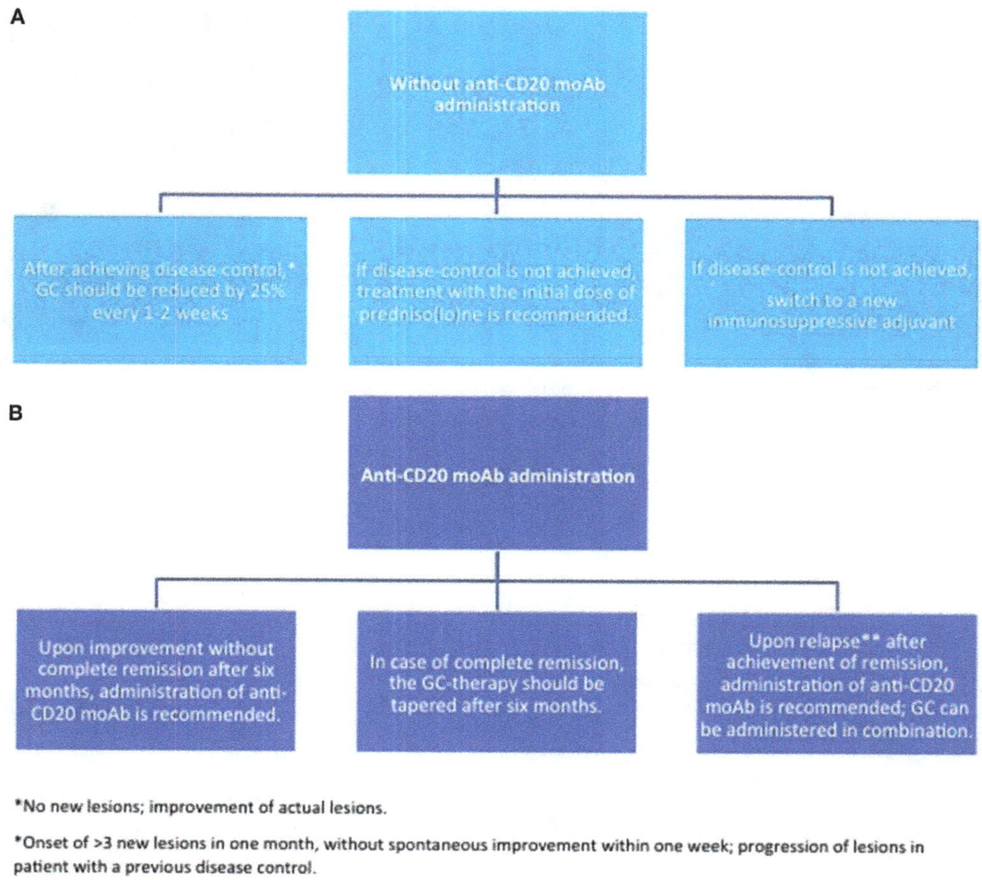

FIGURE 6 | Maintenance therapy in pemphigus. **(A)** without anti-CD20 moAb; **(B)** with anti-CD20 moAb. GC, glucocorticoids; moAb, monoclonal antibody.

If the required CS dose is higher than 100 mg/day, a pulse therapy should be considered, in order to reduce the risk of adverse effects (92). Still, the advantage of combined oral CS pulses and immunosuppressive adjuvants is under debate (90, 93).

CS increase the expression of anti-inflammatory proteins and inhibit the production of pro-inflammatory proteins interacting with the cytoplasmic corticosteroid receptor (94). Indeed, the corticosteroid receptor reduces the expression of transcription factors as well as their co-activator molecules, such as NF-κB and activator protein 1 (94). In addition, CS induce the downregulation of IL-2, leading to a reduction in both B-cell clone expansion and autoantibodies synthesis (94). Furthermore, the reduction IL-2 expression inhibits the cell-mediated immunity and reduces T-cell proliferation (95). Therefore, CS lead to multiple signal transduction pathways producing anti-inflammatory, immunosuppressive, antiproliferative, and vasoconstrictive effects.

Several adverse effects have been described in patients undergoing long-time CS therapy, including increased overall susceptibility to infections and infestations, secondary adrenal insufficiency, osteoporosis, transient hyperglycaemia, hypertension, and posterior subcapsular cataract (96). In addition, cutaneous adverse effects have been described, including purpura, telangiectasias, atrophy, striae rubrae, acneiform or rosacea-like eruptions, infections, stern obesity and facial oedema.

Immunosuppressive Adjuvants

Azathioprine

AZA is a prodrug that converts to 6-mercaptopurine after oral administration. AZA down-regulates purine metabolism leading to a block of DNA, RNA and proteins synthesis. Furthermore, AZA inhibits mitosis and leads to immunosuppression in several ways (97). AZA reduces the number of monocytes and Langerhans cells, decreases γ-globulin production, and lower T-cell as well as suppressor B cell activity. Furthermore, it blocks T-helper-cell dependent responses of B cells (97, 98). 6-mercaptopurine can be inactivated to 6-methyl-mercaptopurine by thiopurine methyltransferase (TPMT) enzyme (96).

AZA is a safe CS-sparing agent, recommended as a first-line adjuvant immunosuppressant (83). The dosage of AZA is adapted to the TPMT activity and measurement of TPMT activity should be performed before AZA administration (99). Usually, 2.0 mg AZA kg/day are recommended by normal TPMT activity, while 1 mg AZA kg/day is recommended for patients

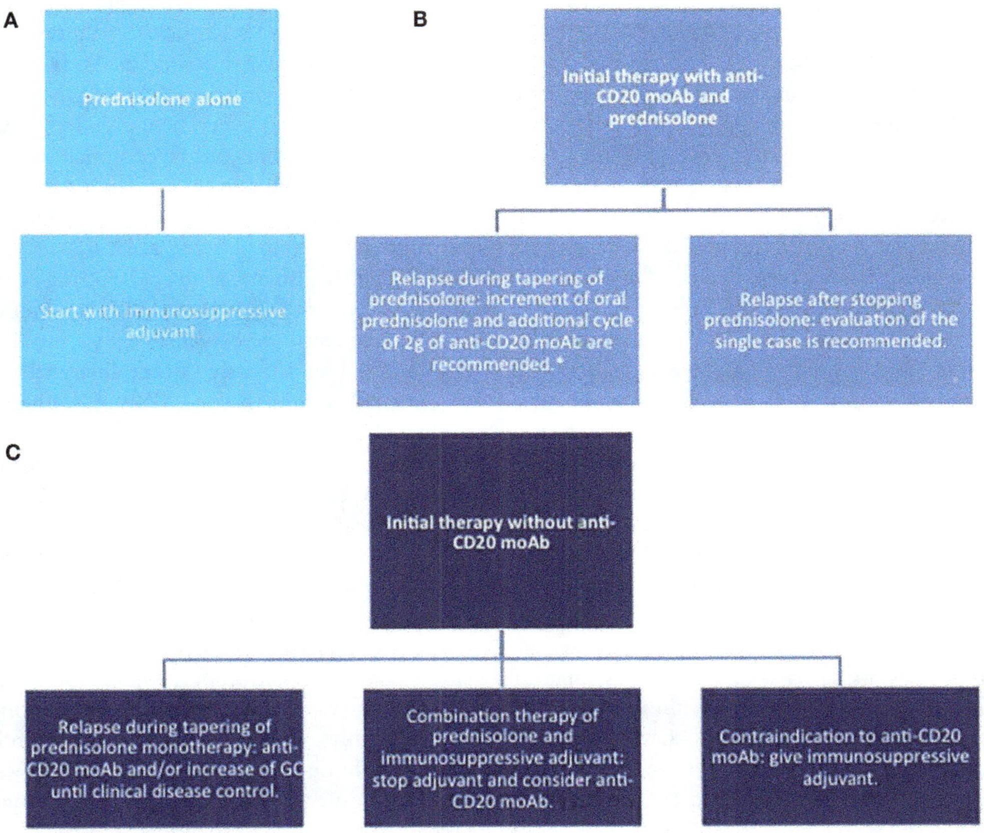

FIGURE 7 | Therapy of relapse. **(A)** with corticosteroids only; **(B)** systemic corticosteroids combined with anti CD20 moAb; **(C)** systemic corticosteroids combined with other immunosuppressive agents. moAb, monoclonal antibody.

with TPMT enzyme mutations (84). A dose of 50 mg AZA per day is recommended as initial therapy; the dose can be increased to the optimal dose based on TPMT activity (84). Adverse effects have been reported in 15–30% of patients. Severe adverse effects include myelosuppression and pancytopenia, and hepatotoxicity (99). However, myelosuppression may occur despite normal TPMT. Therefore, despite normal TPMT activity, a routine complete blood count including liver enzymes throughout the treatment period should be performed (99). In addition, long-term immunosuppression raises the risk of infections and cancer (100). Indeed, AZA shows a mutagenic potential that might provoke hematologic malignancies (100). Therefore, AZA is not recommended in pregnancy and breastfeeding (101). Other adverse effects include nausea, pancreatitis, diarrhea, aphthous stomatitis, maculopapular rashes, and anaphylaxis (99).

In a RCT involving 120 PV patients, a combined therapy of CS and adjuvant AZA (2.5 mg/kg daily) showed a higher CS-sparing effect than CS alone and a combination therapy with MMF (102). Furthermore, in a previous RCT study, adjuvant AZA (2.5 mg/kg daily) was compared to CS alone (103). During 1-year follow-up, a significant CS-sparing effect has been shown only in the last 3 months. Furthermore, disease activity was also significantly lower in the AZA group only in the last 3 months in comparison to the CS only. In addition, in a non-randomized study on PV patients, high-dose oral prednisone daily (1.5 mg/kg/day) vs. low-dose oral prednisone (40 mg every other day) plus AZA (100 mg/day) have been compared. It was shown a shorter main time to remission in high-dose oral prednisone monotherapy group, although the rate of adverse effects was higher (104). In summary, there is good evidence for a higher CS-sparing effect of AZA than CS monotherapy and MMF (83).

Mycophenolate mofetil

MMF is a prodrug that converts to mycophenolic acid (MPA) upon oral administration. MPA downregulates the immune system by selective impairment of inosine monophosphate dehydrogenase, leading to a blockade of the *de novo* pathway of purine synthesis in T and B cells, affecting both cellular and humoral immunity. Because lymphocytes are mainly dependent on the *de novo* pathway for purine biosynthesis, lymphocytes are the primary target of MPA. Because this target profile, MMF shows a safer profile in comparison to other less selective immunosuppressants, such as AZA (105).

As AZA, MMF is also recommended as a first-line adjuvant immunosuppressant (83, 84). The recommended dose of 2 g/day divided in two doses. In patients with a reduced renal function a reduced dosage should be administered (106). Initially, a dose of 500 mg MMF/day should be administered and an increase by

500 mg may be possible. A final dose of 2 g/day has been proposed in order to reach a better gastrointestinal tolerance (97).

Severe adverse effects have been rarely reported. Mild gastrointestinal symptoms, such as nausea, vomiting, and diarrhea are commonly seen. Rare are opportunistic infections, hematologic abnormalities, esophagitis, and gastritis (107). Studies on transplant recipients in therapy with MMF have demonstrated an increased risk of developing lymphomas and skin cancer (86). MMF is not recommended in pregnancy and breastfeeding, because of an increased risk of spontaneous abortion and congenital malformations (101).

Beissert et al. (108) compared CS plus MMF with CS plus placebo in PV patients. It has been highlighted that the MMF group showed a faster response to therapy, a longer disease-free interval, and a statistically significant CS-sparing. However, adjuvant MMF was not superior to CS in inducing disease control (108). Furthermore, no significant differences in cumulative CS dose, efficacy, or adverse effects were reported between AZA plus oral methylprednisolone and MMF plus oral methylprednisolone (109). In addition, Chams-Davatchi et al. (102) showed no significant difference in efficacy or safety between a combination therapy of prednisolone plus MMF (2 g/day) and prednisolone plus AZA. Regarding the CS-sparing effect, MMF was superior to prednisolone alone, but inferior to AZA, while compared to Cyclophosphamide (CYP), non-conclusive data were reported (102). The optimal MMF dose in PV has not yet been found. In a multicentric randomized controlled trial (RCT), no clear conclusions regarding the use of standard MMF dose (2 g daily) vs. a high one (3 g daily) were reported (108).

Cyclophosphamide

CYP is an alkylating prodrug with antineoplastic and immunosuppressive properties. CYP is converted in the liver into two active metabolites, phosphoramide mustard and aldophosphamide, which downregulate DNA replication and induce cell death. CYP shows also a blocking activity on proliferation, cytokine production, and lymphocyte-induced inflammation (85, 92).

The recommended oral dose is 2 mg/kg/day (97). Because of its rather unfavorable safety profile, CYP is not recommended as a first-line CS-sparing agent but rather as a rescue drug.

Several frequent adverse effects have been reported, including nausea, vomiting, diarrhea, hyperpigmentation of the skin/nails, and alopecia. Leukopenia, anemia, and thrombocytopenia may also occur. A severe complication is haemorrhagic cystitis, which may be prevented by adequate fluid intake and sodium 2-mercaptoethane sulfonate.

CYP shows a carcinogenic and teratogenic activity (86). As a result CYP administration is not allowed in pregnancy and breastfeeding (101). Moreover, temporary or permanent gonadal dysfunction has been described.

Three RCTs evaluated the CS-sparing effect of CYP. Chrysomallis et al. (110) compared oral CS monotherapy with a combined therapy of oral CYP and CS as well as a combined therapy of cyclosporine and CS. No difference in efficacy between these treatments were observed, but adverse events were higher in patients on combination treatment. An RCT comparing intravenous CYP pulse therapy (15 mg/kg monthly) plus CS vs. CS alone showed no conclusive difference in remission and relapse rates, cumulative steroid doses, and adverse events (111). Moreover, RCT regarding CYP pulse therapy (1 g monthly for 6 months, then 1 g every 2 months) plus CS in comparison to prednisolone alone and in combination with adjuvant AZA or MMF showed inconclusive results regarding efficacy and CS-sparing effect (102). Finally, oral methylprednisolone (2 mg/kg/day) combined with AZA (2–2.5 mg/kg/day) and a pulse CYP treatment protocol (500 mg intravenous CYP in combination with 100 mg intravenous dexamethasone for 3 consecutive days) were evaluated in a multicentric prospective RCT and did not show significant differences (112).

Different dexamethasone–CYP pulse therapy regimens were evaluated in two RCTs. In the first study, a combination of dexamethasone i.v. (100 mg on three consecutive days per months), CYP i.v. (500 mg once a month), and oral CYP (50 mg/day) was compared with CYP pulse therapy (15 mg/kg monthly) and prednisolone. In the first group a cutaneous, but not mucosal, response was faster achieved, while in the second group, the remission was seen earlier, but more severe CS-related adverse effects were reported (113). In the second study, patients under oral CYP alone (50 mg daily) and under a combination of dexamethasone i.v. (100 mg on three consecutive days monthly) with CYP i.v. (500 mg monthly) or oral CYP (50 mg daily on days between the pulses) were evaluated. No significant differences were reported regarding relapse rate, anti-Dsg1 and anti-Dsg3 autoantibodies titres, and the presence of tissue-binding autoantibodies by DIF (114).

Dapsone

Dapsone is used alone or in combination with topical clobetasol as first-line therapy in mild PF. Evaluation of serum glucose-6-phosphate dehydrogenase (G6PD) activity is mandatory before administration. The role of DA in the maintenance phase of PV has been evaluated only in one RCT, showing no statistical significance (115).

Methotrexate

Methotrexate (MTX) (10–20 mg/week) is considered a third-line CS-sparing drug in PV (83). In a retrospective single-center study, it has been reported that >80% of PV patients were able to reduce CS after 6 months on adjuvant MTX (15 mg/week) (116). Furthermore, Tran et al. (117) reported in a retrospective single-center study that 70% of PV patients stopped completely CS, mainly after 18 months. These findings support the concept that MTX has a CS-sparing effect in PV.

Cyclosporine

There are only limited data regarding the adjuvant use of cyclosporine in PV. Chrysomallis et al. (110) reported an inconclusive effect of adjuvant cyclosporine and a higher incidence of toxicities in combination treatment with prednisolone. Ioannides et al. (118) showed no advantage of this adjuvant drug over treatment with CS alone. Based on this data, CS is not recommended as adjuvant therapy in PV by the EADV or BAD guidelines (83, 84).

Rituximab

Rituximab—Mode of Action

The putative mode of action of RTX in pemphigus is shown in **Figure 8**. RTX is a chimeric type I monoclonal anti CD20 antibody, consisting of a human Fc portion and a murine variable region which serve as CD20 binding site (119). RTX was first licensed for use in B-cell malignancies (120), however, it is currently used in several autoimmune disorders, and has been recently licensed as first-line treatment in pemphigus (121–124). RTX target, CD20, is a transmembrane receptor, that is expressed across various developmental stages of the B-cell, from the pre-B cell to the mature; while, early precursor pro-B cells and antibody-producing plasma cells do not express it (125). Probably, it functions as a Ca^{2+} channel, that regulates intracellular Ca^{2+} influx through interaction between the intracytoplasmic domain and the activated B-cell receptor (119, 126). Noteworthy, $CD20^{-/-}$ mice display normal B-cell development and function, and no enhanced susceptibility to infections (127). RTX binds near the large extracellular loop of CD20 (128). RTX binding to CD20 induces B-cell depletion by, at least, four different mechanisms: (i) direct induction of programmed cell death, which is dependent on activation of caspases and involves intracellular molecules, including Src kinases, p38 MAPK and NFkB (129–131); (ii) complement-dependent cytotoxicity, that happens when C1s binds to RTX opsonized cells and triggers complement activation and formation of the membrane attack complex (MAC), which eventually induces cell lysis (132); (iii) antibody-dependent cytotoxicity, which consists of activation of NK cells through binding the human Fc portion of RTX to the FcRIII receptor: this activates NK cells to release cytotoxic mediators, including perforins and granzyme B, which induces caspases-dependent cell death in the target lymphocyte (133); (iv) antibody-dependent phagocytosis, in which neutrophils, monocytes and macrophages bind RTX opsonized B-cells through the Fcγ Receptor (132). Recently, a new mechanism, referred to as trogocytosis, or shaving, has been characterized. In trogocytosis, macrophages remove RTX-CD20 complexes by transferring plasma membrane; this triggers cell death through a yet-to-be identified mechanism (134).

RTX is a highly effective therapy in pemphigus (1). By depleting B-cells, RTX leads to marked decrease of circulating anti-Dsg autoantibodies, and, since the pathogenic role of such autoantibodies, significant amelioration of the lesions (135). Multiple lines of evidence, however, suggest that RTX exerts a deep modulation of both humoral and acquired immune function in pemphigus, explaining the fact that, in many cases, disease amelioration lasts longer than B-cell re-appearance in the peripheral blood of the patients (136). First, it should be noted that RTX, in parallel with a drastic decrease of pathogenic autoantibodies, induces drop of total serum IgM, but does not modify total serum IgG, thus suggesting that long-lived plasmablasts accounting for antibody production against microbes are not affected (137). Previously, we showed that in PV patients, RTX induced elevation of B-cell activating factor (BAFF) in parallel with decreasing pathogenic antibody levels and increased IgG titer against Varicella Zoster virus and Epstein Barr virus: thus elevation of BAFF may at least partly exerts a stimulatory role on long-lived plasma blasts (124). Likewise, one study recently showed that while autoimmune blistering disease patients receiving RTX showed reduced circulating memory B-cells against the influenza virus compared to healthy people, they showed comparable recall response to vaccination, suggesting the existence of a memory B-cell compartment, probably resident in lymphoid tissues, which is not depleted by RTX (138). Interestingly, when B-cells re-appear following RTX treatment, there is a substantial increase in the proportion of naive and transitional B-cells and an increased naive/memory B-cell ratio (137). Patients in complete clinical response also display increased number of IL-10-producing regulatory B-cells and absence of Dsg3-IgG^+ B-cells (136). Altogether, these findings suggest that RTX induces a complete reset of the B-cell repertoire in pemphigus, favoring early appearance of immature B-cells and anti-inflammatory regulatory B (Breg) cells, and delayed reappearance of Dsg-specific memory B-cells, which eventually account for disease relapse (136, 139).

Our group demonstrated that, besides pleiotropic effects on B-cells, RTX inhibits auto-reactive Th1 and Th2 cells, by interfering with the T-B cell cross-talk, in which Dsg-specific B-cells probably serve as antigen presenting cells. Decreasing Th1 and Th2 functions occurred early following RTX and lasted around 6 and 12 months, respectively. Conversely, we did not observe inhibition of Dsg-specific regulatory T (Treg)-cells, which account for maintaining peripheral tolerance against Dsg antigens. Finally, we demonstrated that T-cells specific for the tetanus toxoid as well as the total count of $CD3^+CD4^+$ T cells were not decreased by RTX (140). Similar results were found in a subsequent study by Leshem et al. (141), confirming that RTX impairs autoreactive, rather than global T-cell function in pemphigus.

RTX side effects mostly include infections and infusion-related adverse events. In fact, while single RTX infusions may not impair significantly memory responses against previously encountered pathogens (138), patients mounts a defective immune reactions against newly encountered pathogens and serious and life-threatening infections, including sepsis, following RTX treatment have been variously reported (120, 142–147). Opportunistic infections can also occur, including cytomegalovirus and *Pneumocytic jiroveci* infections (148–153). In this regard, it is not known yet whether pemphigus patients receiving RTX may benefit from prophylaxis against *Pneumocystis jiroveci* infection (154). A theoretical risk of reactivation of hepatitis B and C viruses as well as tuberculosis should be also taken into account (138, 155–157). Infusion-related adverse events mostly occur during the time of infusion and include type I hypersensitivity reaction and anaphylaxis, and cytokine release syndrome (158–162), although the latter has never been reported in pemphigus patients (142, 163). Delayed reactions include serum sickness, vasculitis and Steven Johnson syndrome (164–167). Interestingly, there have been some cases of paradoxical pemphigus flares following RTX treatment. In one case, paradoxical pemphigus flare

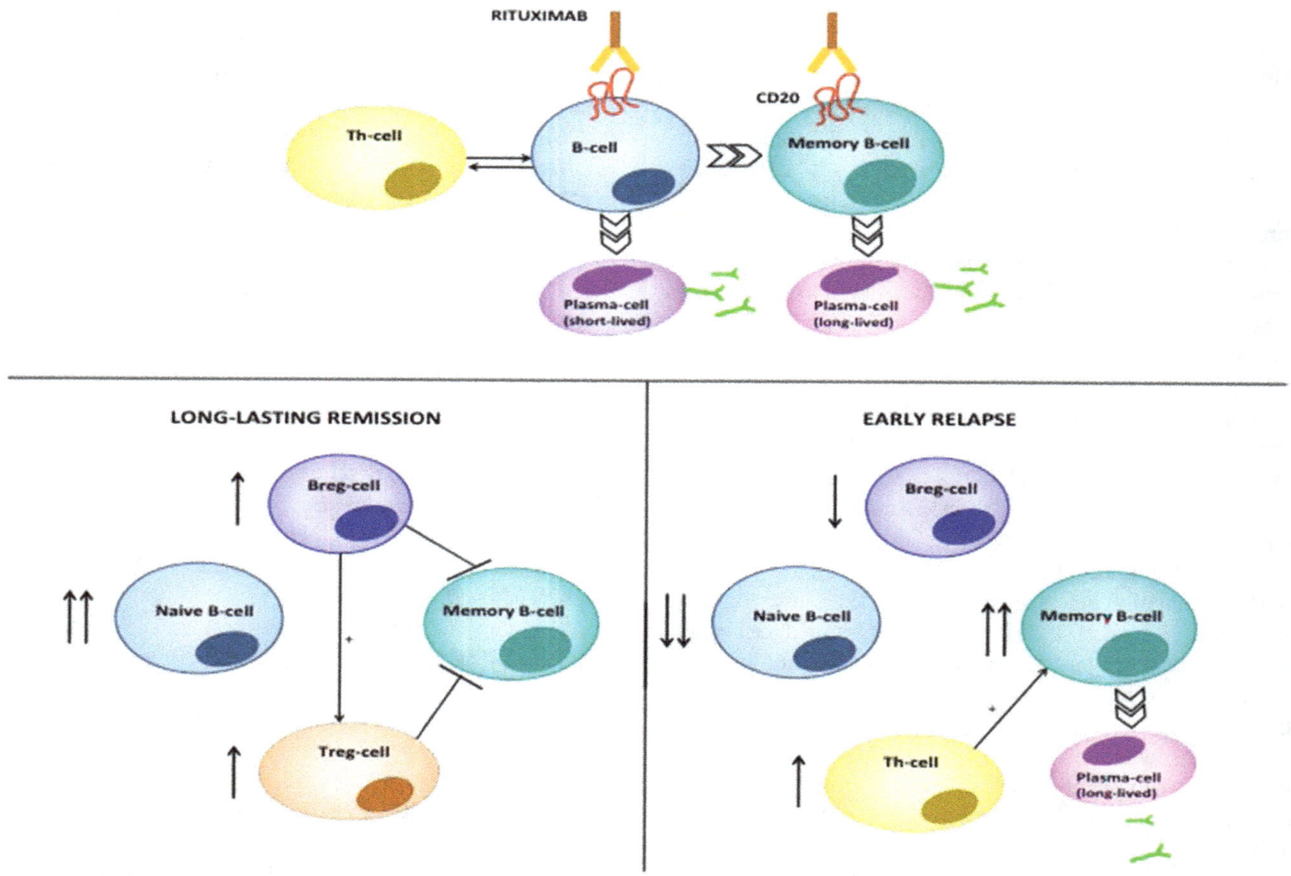

FIGURE 8 | Mode of action of RTX in pemphigus. RTX induces depletion of B-cells and lymphoid resident memory B-cells by different mechanisms, including direct cell apoptosis, complement-dependent cytotoxicity and antibody-dependent cytotoxicity. The latter consists of the phagocytosis of opsonized B-cells by neutrophils, monocytes and macrophages, which express the Fcγ Receptor. Moreover, RTX significantly decreases T-cell function, by depleting antigen presenting B cells. Patients achieving durable responses have an increased naïve/memory B-cell ratio. Regulatory B-cells (B-regs) and regulatory T-cells (T-regs) are also increased, and are inhibitory on Dsg3-specific memory B-cells. On the contrary, patients with early relapses following B-cell repopulation have a decreased naïve/memory B-cell ratio. Reappearance of auto-reactive, Dsg3-specific T-cells contributes to activation of autoreactive B-cells and subsequent anti-Dsg IgG production.

was accompanied by increased serum concentrations of anti-Dsg3 IgG autoantibodies (168). In any case, disease flare predicted treatment failure. Suggested underlying mechanisms include increased cytokine release from apoptotic B-cells, immediate depletion of regulatory B-cells or a transient lymphocyte activation following RTX-CD20 interaction (141, 163, 168–171).

There is much controversy about the optimal RTX dose in pemphigus. Two main protocols are used: the rheumatoid arthritis protocol, which consists of two 1,000 mg infusions 2 weeks apart, and the lymphoma protocol, which consists of four 500 mg infusions once a week (135). There are not yet randomized trials assessing which protocol is better in terms of efficacy and safety. On the other hand, high dose regimens should be preferred instead of low-dose regimens, due to longer disease response (163). Nowadays, one study recently reported on a pemphigus patient achieving successful disease remission with an ultra-low dose of RTX (200 mg in a single infusion), with persistent B-cell depletion after 6-month follow-up (172, 173). This highlights the need of further investigating individual factors that may influence RTX efficacy in an effort to personalize treatment schedules and optimize the safety.

Rituximab in Pemphigus Vulgaris and Pemphigus Foliaceus

RTX was initially shown to be effective for pemphigus patients resistant to standard immunosuppressive therapies. In one study in 2006, Ahmed et al. (174) reported complete clinical remission, allowing successful tapering of immunosuppressive therapies, in 9 out of 11 patients with refractory pemphigus following a protocol combining IVIg and 10 RTX infusions over a 6 months period (**Table 1**). After 10-year follow-up most patients were shown to maintain clinical remission (175). In 2007, in a larger clinical series, Joly et al. (176) reported durable clinical response with significant corticosteroid sparing effects in 86% of 21 patients with refractory pemphigus following a single cycle of RTX. Similar results were reported in a series of 42 patients by Cianchini et al. (177), they also observed that a recall infusion of 500 mg was effective for patients who relapsed following initial disease control. One study including 136 patients with refractory pemphigus from four different European countries reported a 95% overall response rate, with two third of patients achieving complete remission (178). Likewise, review articles and meta-analysis estimated complete clinical remission occurring in 76–90% of patients within a median time of ~6 months (146, 163). Mean remission duration ranged from 15 to 17 months, although only a small percentage of patients maintained remission off therapy (146, 163). In two studies, RTX use early in the disease course resulted in significantly higher and longer clinical response (136, 179). The same finding emerged also in a study by Amber and Hertl, reviewing clinical outcomes of 155 pemphigus patients treated with a single cycle of RTX (179, 180). These preliminary observations have lead different research groups to investigate the potential benefit of RTX applied as a first line therapy in pemphigus. Indeed, first-line therapy with RTX, combined either with high potency topical corticosteroids or IVIg, was shown to be effective in pemphigus patients with contraindication to systemic steroids (181, 182). One retrospective study found significantly higher rate of complete remission off immunosuppressive therapy in patients who were administered RTX as a first-line steroid sparing agent compared to patients who received RTX after failing other immunosuppressants (183). In 2017 a large prospective randomized trial, comparing RTX combined with a short course of prednisone vs. prednisone alone in patients with newly diagnosed pemphigus, demonstrated significantly higher complete remission rate off therapy in patients receiving RTX, resulting in a dramatic decrease of the cumulative steroid dose and significantly fewer adverse events. Furthermore, re-treatment with a single RTX dose of 500 mg after 12 and 18 months was highly effective and well-tolerated in achieving long-term clinical remissions (88). Interestingly, also patients with PF, in whom the rate of remission with RTX was estimated around 50% in the refractory setting, were shown to respond well to RTX when applied as a first line therapy (88, 184–186). In summary, while RTX was initially recommended as a third line therapy in patients without adequate disease control with standard immunosuppressants, several studies have definitively demonstrated that patients may benefit from early RTX treatment, in terms of both clinical efficacy and safety, leading current guidelines to recommend it as the gold standard for new onset pemphigus (187, 188).

Rituximab in Paraneoplastic Pemphigus

PNP usually occurs secondary to B-cell neoplasms, hence RTX appears to be a reasonable treatment, targeting both autoreactive and malignant B-cells (189–191). Several cases in the literature have shown remarkable responses in B-cell malignancies-associated PNP using RTX either alone or in combination with immunosuppressants or chemotherapy (192–195). However, the overall efficacy of RTX in PNP is much less consistent than PV and PF (196); mucosal lesions were shown to be particularly resistant to RTX treatment (197). Moreover, some authors pointed out that RTX treatment of the underlying malignancy may paradoxically trigger PNP (198).

PNP combines clinical and histologic features of PV and lichenoid/interface dermatitis, reflecting a mixed B- and T-cell response against epidermal autoantigens. Indeed, while declining B-cells autoreactivity, RTX may be ineffective against clinical manifestations secondary to auto-reactive T-cells activation (199). Indeed, RTX use to treat the underlying malignancy may lead to overlook the diagnosis of PNP in patients presenting with lichenoid dermatitis or toxic epidermal necrolysis-like lesions without detectable circulating autoantibodies and negative DIF. This was recently hypothesized in an interesting study by Kwatra et al. where the authors observed a significant reduction in the cases of B-cell lymphoma-associated PNP from 2011 to 2017 compared to the period from 2003 to 2010. All the patients diagnosed with PNP during or after 2011 had already received RTX; whereas, most of the cases before 2011 did not (199).

Is There Evidence for a Maintenance Therapy With Rituximab in Pemphigus?

Relapse following RTX occurs in about 40–80% of the patients (163), within a mean time ranging from 6 to 24 months (153, 200). Additional cycles of RTX were shown to be effective in relapsed patients, suggesting that patients may benefit from maintenance with RTX (88, 176, 177). However, the exact timing of RTX re-treatment to prevent relapse is uncertain (187). Re-treatment at 6 months has been adopted empirically, but it is not currently validated in the setting of randomized trials (201). Noteworthy, there is a subset of patients who achieves long-lasting remission even with a single cycle of RTX (136, 176, 202). In these patients, additional prophylactic cycles of RTX not only result in unneeded costs, but also substantially increase the risk of adverse events. Developing biomarkers that could identify patients at higher risk of relapse following RTX is therefore an urgent need.

Relapse following RTX can be attributed to persistence of autoreactive B-cells, because of incomplete B-cell depletion, or re-appearance of Dsg-specific B-cell clones during B-cell repopulation. Thus, monitoring the B-cell repertoire appears to be a suitable tool to predict the risk of relapse following RTX. In one study, shorter time to relapse was found in patients receiving adjuvant immunosuppressants during and following RTX treatment, suggesting a possible effect of prolonged immunosuppression on immunosurveillance, favoring an early re-appearance of autoreactive B-cells (203). In 2008, a consensus of German experts recommended checking the number of $CD19^+$ B-cells in the blood at baseline and after RTX treatment (204). In one retrospective study by Albers et al. (200) including 62 pemphigus patients treated with a total of 99 RTX cycles, the number of $CD19^+$ B-cells were shown to be a useful predictor of relapse. A time to B-cell repopulation lower than 12 months also correlated with the risk of relapse. However, relapse has reportedly occurred even before B-cell re-population (205). In these cases, it is conceivable that lymphoid tissues served as a reservoir for autoreactive B-cells and protected them from RTX.

Longitudinal analysis of the naïve/memory B-cells ratio and the number of B-regs may also provide useful information (206). Interestingly, Albers et al. (200) found an inverted correlation between $CD4^+$ T-cell counts following RTX and the risk of relapse. Autoreactive T-cells are essential in pemphigus to orchestrate the B-cell responses and autoantibody production against Dsgs. RTX also is effective in decreasing peripheral T-cell response against Dsgs (140). Thus, high $CD4^+$ T-cells count would be expected to predict relapse. However, Albers et al. (200) speculated that the protective role of $CD4^+$ T-cells could be attributed to Treg cells, which prevented further expansion of autoreactive B-cell clones. Levels of circulating anti-Dsg autoantibodies were also shown to be involved in the relapse of patients with pemphigus (207). In Albers et al. (200), levels of anti-Dsg3 IgG were predictive of relapse in patients with mucocutaneous and mucosal disease, whereas anti-Dsg1 IgG were predictive for the subset of mucosal PV patients with cutaneous involvement. However, in other studies, elevation of anti-Dsg3 IgG was also noted in patients maintaining a clinical remission, suggesting that in some cases anti-Dsg3 IgG may target non-pathogenic epitopes of the Dsg3 ectodomain (208). Mouquet et al. (137) found that elevation of Dsg1 autoantibodies was associated with early relapse following RTX.

In a prospective study, a high baseline index of anti-Dsg1 IgG was found in early relapsing patients compared to late relapsing patients following RTX. Baseline anti-Dsg1 IgG, but not Dsg3-IgG, indeed showed a significant positive correlation with a risk of relapse within 12 months after RTX treatment, thus suggesting that patients with high anti-Dsg1 IgG before treatment deserve a close monitoring during the 12 months following treatment, or at least may benefit from a prophylactic RTX dose during the first 12 months. Also in this study, later B-cell repopulation was found in patients experiencing a late relapse compared to patients experiencing an early relapse (209). By contrast, in a retrospective study including 40 pemphigus patients treated with RTX, mucosal involvement was found to be associated with a poor clinical outcome and relapse (210).

Intravenous Immunoglobulin

IVIg consist of human plasma-derived IgG, sugars, salts and solvents. IVIg derived from large plasma pools. Albeit not immunosuppressive, they exerts various anti-inflammatory effects, including Fc receptor blockade, stimulation of antibodies production against different subclasses of T lymphocytes, inhibition of different T-cell functions, complement hindrance via inactivating C3 precursors, dendritic cell downregulation, B-lymphocyte apoptosis, inhibition of phagocytosis, and increment of response to steroids (211). However, the main mode of action is an increased catabolism of immunoglobulins via binding to the neonatal Fc receptor (FcRn) (211).

A dose of 2 g per kg body weight per treatment cycle is recommended. High-dose IVIg was shown to independently increase disease control in pemphigus (85). IVIg is mostly used as an adjuvant therapy to CS and immunosuppressive drugs in recalcitrant PV. Indeed, Amagai et al. (212) reported that high dose IVIg (0.4 g/kg per day) over 5 days resulted in significantly reduced disease activity and autoantibody titres in 51 patients with CS-resistant PV. Furthermore, Svecova et al. (213) reported a significant improvement in Pemphigus Disease Area Index (PDAI) and a reduction of 90% of the CS dose in a cohort of 10 CS-resistant PV. Combination of IVIg and RTX also demonstrated efficacy (**Table 2**).

Adverse effects have been reported in < 5% of patients and occur more often in patients who are IVIg-naive or at risk of bacterial infections (217, 218). Immediate adverse effects (occurring within the first hour of infusion) include headache, nausea, fever, tachycardia, malaise, arthralgia, and dyspnoea. Delayed reactions include headache, acute renal failure, thromboembolic events, and pseudohyponatremia (218). Myocardial infarction, thrombosis, pulmonary embolus and Stevens–Johnson syndrome, have been also described. Thrombosis can be provoked by hypercoagulability due to increased blood viscosity, augmented fibrinogen production, and raised platelet activity (219). Therefore, high-risk patients, such as elderly or people affected by hypertension or coronary heart disease, should be screened appropriately and prophylactic anticoagulation need to be considered. In a series of 54 patients on IVIg treatment, an incidence of aseptic meningitis of 11% has been reported. Risk factors were a previous history of migraine and high-dose IVIg regimen (220). Finally transient acute kidney injury has been also described (221).

Immunoadsorption

IA consists of the passive removal of IgG from the patient's systemic circulation. In IA, the blood is passed through adsorber columns, in which molecules with high affinity for IgG, i.g. protein A (Immunosorba®) or the synthetic peptide PGAM146 (Globaffin®), function as a ligand (135, 222). Basic principles of IA are, indeed, similar to plasmapheresis, but, compared to the latter, IA does not remove plasma proteins, such as albumin and clotting factors. The use of plasmapheresis in pemphigus has been largely abandoned due to significant incidence of serious adverse events, such as sepsis (223). The fact that IA does not require replacement of fresh frozen plasma and albumins allows processing higher plasma volume per treatment session, resulting in a lower, albeit not abolished, risk of adverse events. Nevertheless, infections are still the most frequently encountered complication and can occur either secondary to the IA procedure, i.g. cathether-associated infections, or secondary to decreased serum concentrations of protective antibodies (224–226).

IA is an ideal treatment for pemphigus patients with severe and extensive disease at baseline. Combining IA with immunosuppressive therapies provides faster clinical responses compared to the immunosuppressive therapy alone, since IA allows immediate removal of pathogenic antibodies, whose serum concentration reflects both disease activity and severity. Once circulating antibodies are removed, a positive gradient between the skin and blood leads skin-bound autoantibodies to move into the systemic circulation. To avoid a rebound increase of the autoantibody titer, IA is therefore performed on 3 or 4 consecutive days, and then repeated on a monthly base based on the disease response, autoantibody serum concentrations and treatment tolerability (227).

Current guidelines indicate IA as a reliable first-line treatment in pemphigus patients, in whom lesions cover (1) > 30% of the body surface or (2) > 25% of oral or genital mucous membranes or involve (3) the conjunctiva or (4) the esophagus; it can

TABLE 2 | Combination therapy of rituximab with intravenous immunoglobulins (IVIg) or immunoadsorption (IA).

Study	Study design	Synopsis	Adverse events
RTX PLUS IVIg			
Ahmed et al. (174)	Prospective, including 11 refractory PV patients, treated with 2 cycles of RTX 375 mg/Kg/m^2 once a week for 3 weeks followed by a cycle of IVIg 2 g/Kg in the fourth week. Maintenance with RTX and IVIg infusions once a month for 4 months	9 out of 11 patients achieved a complete remission in parallel with a rapid decreasing of the serum concentrations of anti-Dsg autoantibodies, which allowed successful discontinuation of steroids and adjuvant immunosuppressants. Clinical responses lasted 22–37 months (follow-up after discontinuation of RTX: 15–37 months). In 2 patients experiencing a relapse, retreatment with RTX was effective	No relevant side effects reported, including infections or infusion-related reactions
Ahmed et al. (175)	10-year follow-up study of Ahmed et al. (174)	All the 10 patients previously treated with RTX and IVIg retained clinical remission after 10 years from the last RTX infusion	Not observed
Feldman et al. (205)	Retrospective, including 19 patients with refractory pemphigus. RTX was given at week 1, 2, 3, 4, 5, 6, 7, 8, 12, 16, 20, 24. IVIg were given at week 0, 4, 8, 12, 16, 20, 24	11 patients achieved long-term remission, allowing discontinuation of corticosteroids and other immunosuppressants. 8 suffered at total of 15 relapses. Re-treatment with RTX and IVIg was effective in achieving a long-term remission. Relapse was associated with incomplete B-cell depletion, B-cell repopulation and raise of serum anti-Dsg autoantibodies	Not reported
RTX PLUS IA			
Behzad et al. (208)	Retrospective, including 10 patients with refractory PV. IA was administered at 4-week intervals, followed by RTX according to either the lymphoma protocol or the RA protocol	8 out of 10 patients obtained a complete remission on therapy at 6 months following the first IA treatment. In 6 of them complete remission on therapy persisted at 12 months. Treatment with IA and RTX leads to a successful tapering of oral prednisone	No serious adverse events reported
Kasperkiewicz et al. (214)	Clinical series including 23 consecutive patients. IA was given on 3 consecutive days and repeated at initially 3 and then 4 weeks until lesions clearance of 90%. RTX 1,000 mg was infused at weeks 1 and 3. Patients also received intravenous dexamethasone pulses and oral azathioprine or mycophenolic acid	19 patients achieved long-term complete remission. Over a period of a mean of 29-month follow-up, 6 patients suffered a relapse	A *Staphylococcus aureus sepsis* associated with an infected central intravenous line and an episode of extensive herpes simplex infection
Kolesnik et al. (215)	Retrospective, including 4 patients with PV and 2 with PF. The treatment protocol included a combination of protein A IA and RTX (375 mg/m^2 once a week the day after each IA session) (Magdeburg treatment protocol). Patients with sub-epidermal blistering dermatoses were also included	Complete or partial remission was observed in 88 and 12% of patients, respectively, within an average follow-up of 22 months. Relapse occurred in one patient with PF. Treatment was associated with a substantial decrease of serum autoantibody concentrations	Erysipelas at the lower leg of one patient due to trauma
RTX PLUS IVIg PLUS IA			
Shimanovich et al. (216)	Clinical series, including 5 patients with PV and 2 with PF. Treatment included a combination of protein A IA and RTX (375 mg/m^2 once a week per 4 consecutive weeks). All patients received adjuvant immunosuppressive therapies. IVIg were given in non-responder patients	Long-term remission was achieved by 3 patients. Partial remission was induced in 1. Three refractory patients achieved long-term disease control following IVIg therapy	*Staphylococcus aureus* bacteremia, deep venous thrombosis and *P. carinii* pneumonia

RTX, rituximab; IA, immunoadsorption; IVIG, intravenous immunoglobulins; PV, pemphigus vulgaris; PF, pemphigus foliaceus; RA, rheumatoid arthritis.

be also recommended in refractory patients with more than 3 months of active disease despite at least two immunosuppressive therapies (84, 187, 188).

Possibly, IA may also exert immunomodulating properties, which account for its synergistic effect in combination with RTX (**Table 2**). Accordingly, in a study by Amber and Hertl, IA was the only adjuvant treatment resulting in a lower risk of relapse following RTX (180). Indeed two studies, including one by our group, demonstrated rapid and durable clinical response combining RTX and IA with or without oral immunosuppressants (208, 214). Moreover, a yet unpublished German multicentric prospective randomized trial comparing IA plus the best medical therapy vs. the best medical therapy alone found that the adjunct of IA resulted in faster withdrawing prednisone and reduced cumulative steroid dose to achieve pemphigus remission (DRKS 00000566).

Langenhan et al. (228) developed specific adsorbers using Dsg1 and Dsg3 ectodomains as a ligand which were shown to efficiently remove pathogenic autoantibodies by 25 and 21%, respectively, without significant variation of anti-EBNA 1 IgG. The same group demonstrated that Dsg3/Dsg1 specific IA eliminated the capacity of PV sera to induce Dsg3 internalization *in vitro* and blistering in neonatal mice (229). Hopefully, future clinical application of these absorbers would lead to increase the safety of IA, reducing the incidence of infections secondary to hypogammaglobulinemia.

Double filtration plasmapheresis (DFPP) is a relatively new procedure that, similar to IA, removes selectively immunoglobulins, while minimizing the loss of albumin. In small case series and one retrospective study DFPP also demonstrated efficacy in drug resistant pemphigus (230–232).

EMERGING THERAPIES

B-Cell Therapies Other Than Rituximab

Although RTX has dramatically improved the overall prognosis of pemphigus, treatment failure or early relapse may be observed. RTX is a chimeric monoclonal antibody, whose murine component is thought to be responsible for the observed allergic reactions during the infusion. However, it also accounts for the appearance of human anti-chimeric antibodies (HACAT), which may potentially limit the efficacy of the drug (233). Over the recent years, different monoclonal antibodies targeting CD20 have been developed. Second generation anti-CD20 mAb differ from RTX in that they are humanized or fully human, taking advantage of being less immunogenic (234) (**Figure 9**). Amongst second-generation anti-CD20 monoclonal antibodies, ofatumumab has been the first to be approved. It is a type I anti-CD20 monoclonal antibodies that targets the extracellular portion of CD20 close to the B-cell membrane, resulting in a more potent complement-dependent cytotoxicity compared to RTX (235). Ofatumumab demonstrated efficacy in a patient with pemphigus, in whom RTX loses efficacy presumably because of the appearance of HACAT (236). Unfortunately, a randomized controlled trial of ofatumumab in pemphigus has been prematurely terminated due to financial restrictions (186). Similarly, Ellebrecht et al. (237) described successful treatment with subcutaneous veltuzmab in a pemphigus patient who only achieved a partial remission with RTX. Veltuzumab is a type I humanized anti CD20 monoclonal antibody that has similar complementary-determining regions of RTX, but a 2.7-fold greater binding avidity and effect on complement-dependent cytotoxicity than RTX. It can be also administered subcutaneously, resulting in lower side effects than intravenous RTX (234).

Obinutuzumab is a third generation glycoenginereed type II humanized anti-CD20 monoclonal antibody. Differently from type I monoclonal antibodies, obinutuzumab shows enhanced capacity to induce direct apoptosis (via a caspase-independent factor) and antibody-dependent cytotoxicity, whereas it does not induce complement-dependent cytotoxicity (238–240). Obinutuzumab has shown to induce superior B-cell depletion compared to RTX in blood samples from patients with rheumatoid arthritis and systemic lupus erythematosus. More intriguingly, it has been shown to induce significant cytotoxicicty also in naive and class-switched memory B-cells, a high number of which may be implicated in early relapse following RTX treatment in pemphigus (241). Other therapies of interest include belimumab and atacicept, a monoclonal human IgG1 antibody and a fully human recombinant fusion protein, which respectively, target BAFF and a proliferating-induced ligand (APRIL), which are involved in B-cell differentiation in antibody producing plasma cells (242, 243). It is worth mentioning that a monoclonal anti-BAFF-receptor antibody (VAY736) is being investigated in a randomized, partial-blind, placebo- controlled multicentre trial (NCT01930175) (125).

Bruton kinase (BTK) inhibitors are also a promising B-cell targeting therapy in pemphigus. BTK is a member of the Tec family of kinases, which is mainly expressed on B-cells, excluding antibody-producing plasma cells. Activation of BTK following antigen-recognition by the BCR activates different downstream molecules including p38MAPK, MEK/ERK, and NFkB, whose related signals are key regulator of B-cells survival, proliferation, maturation and antigen-presentation (244, 245). BTK inhibitors such as ibrutinib have shown impressive clinical responses in patients with B-cell malignancies, but also hold promise for the treatment of autoimmune disorders. In particular, over-activation of BTK have been shown to drive autoimmunity by enhancing autoantibody production and class switching, promoting B-T cell cross talk and peripheral B-cell loss of tolerance (244). Furthermore, enhanced expression of BTK in B-cells induces differentiation of T follicular helper cells, which have been shown to be involved in the pathogenesis of pemphigus (67, 246). Interestingly, ibrutinib has been successfully used in two cases of PNP associated with B-cell malignancies (247, 248). The efficacy of PRN1008, an oral inhibitor of BTK is currently being evaluated in a clinical trial (NCT02704429) (125, 249).

Monoclonal antibodies targeting $CD19^+$ (a B-cell surface molecule which is also expressed on antibody producing plasma cells) such as inebilizumab, would be an effective strategy in pemphigus, since persistence of long-lived plasmablasts producing anti-Dsg IgG autoantibodies is presumably amongst the mechanisms of disease resistance to RTX treatment (125). **Figure 9** summarizes how emerging anti-B-cell therapies works in pemphigus.

Chimeric Autoantibody Receptor (CAAR)-T Cell: A Most Promising Treatment Approach in Pemphigus

Chimeric antigen receptor (CAR)-T-cell therapy has shown remarkable efficacy in otherwise untreatable hematologic malignancies (250). Currently, two CD19-directed CAR-T-cell therapy, tisagenlecleucel and axicabtagene ciloleucel have been approved for treatment of heavily refractory/relapsed acute lymphoblastic leukemia and B-cell aggressive lymphomas (251–254). The noteworthy antitumor activity of CAR-T cells in hematologic malignancies has recently led to

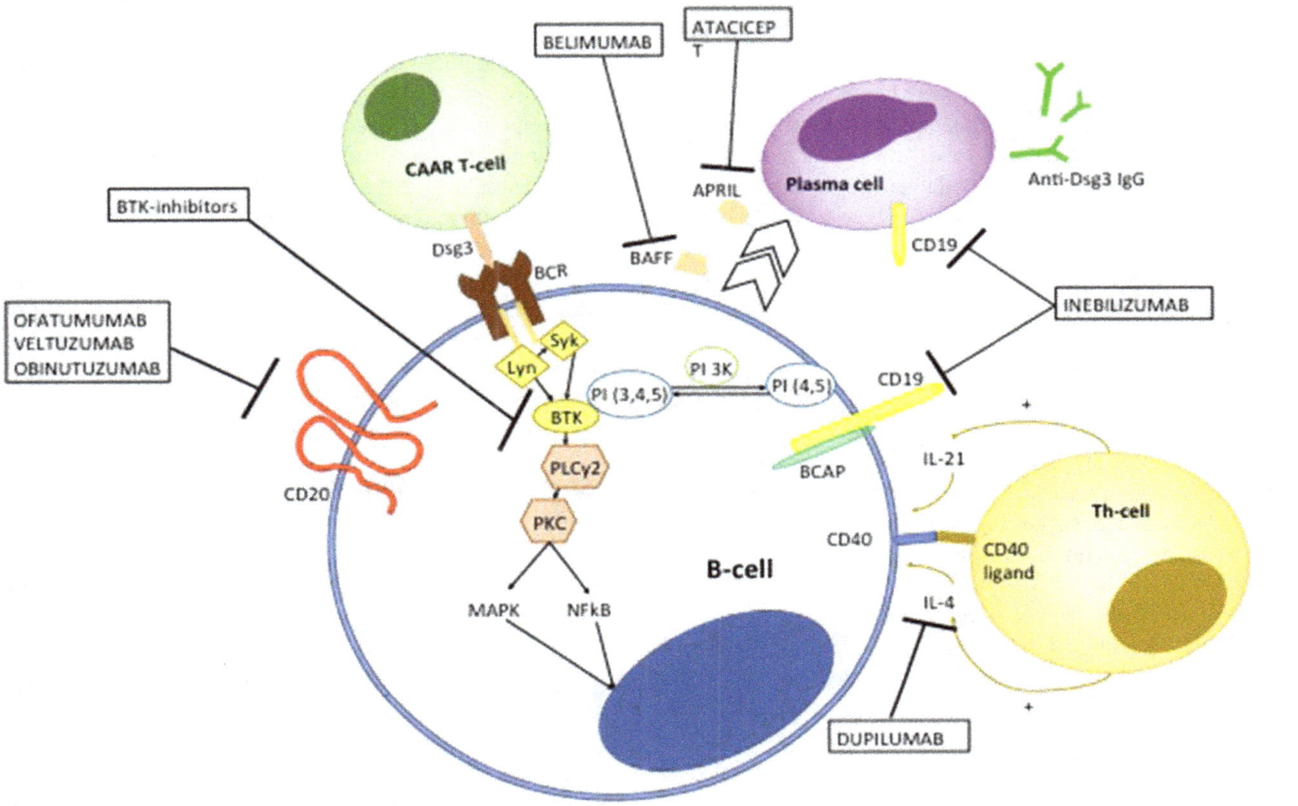

FIGURE 9 | Emerging therapies targeting auto-reactive B and T-cells in pemphigus. Ofatumumab, veltuzumab, and obinutuzumab are fully human or humanized monoclonal antibodies targeting CD20. Ofatumumab and veltuzumab are class I anti-CD20 monoclonal antibody, with a higher capacity of binding CD20 and inducing complement-dependent cytotoxicity compared to RTX. Obinutuzumab is a class II anti-CD20 monoclonal antibody, that has an increased affinity to the FcγIII receptor, resulting in a more potent antibody-dependent cytotoxicity. Bruton kinase (BTK) inhibitors interfere with B cell activation. BCR signaling induces migration of BTK from the cytosol to the cell membrane, though the interaction with phosphatidylinositol 3,4,5-triphosfate generated by phosphoinositide 3-kinase (PI3K). BTK is activated by Lyn and Syk and then actives downstream molecules including phospholipase C gamma 2 (PLCγ2) and Protein kinase C. The latter in turns activate different pro-inflammatory pathways including mitogen associated protein kinases (MAPK) and Nuclear Factor k B (NFkB). Chimeric autoantibody receptor (CAAR)-T-cells are engineered T-lymphocytes which express Dsg3 ectodomain, which allows recognition and subsequent killing of B-cells targeting Dsg3. Belimumab and atacicept target B-cell derived B-cell activating factor (BAFF) and a proliferation-inducing ligand (APRIL), respectively, which promote differentiation toward autoantibody-producing plasma cells. Inebilizumab is a monoclonal antibody targeting CD19 which is not only expressed on B cells but also plasma cells. Dupilumamb is a monoclonal antibody targeting interleukin (IL-4), which is one the main cytokine produced by T helper 2 cells and T follicular helper cell which induces autoantibody production by autoreactive B-cells.

investigate potential clinical application of such a therapy in solid tumors (255–257); an intriguing scenario has been also opened with regard to autoimmune diseases (258). CAR-T cell therapy represents an example of adoptive cell transfer therapy: patient's derived T-cells are modified *ex-vivo* to express a CAR, which allows selective recognition of the antigen of interest and consequent killing, via an MHC-unrestricted manner, of the antigen-bearing cells (259–261).

CARs are fusion proteins whose structure comprises three domains: (i) the extracellular domain, which consists of a single chain variable fragment and serves as antigen recognition domain; (ii) the transmembrane domain; and (iii) the intracellular domain, which consists of the zeta (ζ) chain of the CD3, a component of the endogenous T-cell receptor (262). In second and third-generation CARs, the intracellular domain is linked to co-stimulatory molecules, specifically 4-IBB and CD28, which promote survival and proliferation of CAR-T cells following antigen recognition, resulting in higher clinical efficacy (263). Production of CAR-T-cells requires different steps. Briefly, the CAR protein is cloned into lentiviral or retroviral plasmids. Viral vectors are then transfected to packaging cell lines, such as HEK293 cells, in order to obtain large amounts of the CAR-bearing plasmids. Patient's T-cells, which are obtained by leukapheresis, are incubated with the viral vector, which enters into the cells and introduces the CAR encoding-RNA. The latter is reverse-transcribed in DNA and stably integrates into the T-cell genome. The CAR protein can be then transcribed and translated and eventually expressed on the T-cell surface. CAR T-cells are finally expanded, concentrated and cryopreserved to be then re-infused into the patient (263, 264).

Recently, Ellebrecht et al. (265) created a "chimeric autoantibody receptor" (CAAR), whose extracellular domain consisted of Dsg3 fragments. T-cells engineered to express Dsg3 CAAR were shown to selectively target human anti-Dsg3 B-cells *in vitro*. Anti-Dsg3 antibodies derived from patients' sera did not abolish CAAR-T cells activity. In a PV murine model, CAAR-T cells reduced pathogenic IgG antibodies and ameliorated disease severity. Interestingly CAAR-T-cells were shown to target B-cells bearing antibodies against different Dsg3 epitopes, providing support for their efficacy in a disease typically characterized by oligo-clonality (265, 266). Apart from the possibility that Dsg3-CAAR T-cells could potentially target keratinocytes expressing desmocollins and desmogleins, which physiologically binds to Dsg3, the authors did not observe any significant toxicity (the so-called off-target toxicity) against keratinocytes. Finally, the authors reported similar activity against anti-Dsg3 B-cells between CAAR-T-cells and $CD19^{+}$ CAR T-cells, hence suggesting that selective target of self-reactive B-lymphocytes does not result in reduced treatment efficacy (265).

A major advantage of CAAR-T cell therapy in PV involves the possibility to target memory B cells, which still accounts for the observed relapse following anti CD20 therapies (136, 267). Moreover, since part of CAAR-T-cells differentiates toward memory cells (267), this may prevent future formation and expansion of Dsg 3-reactive B-cells, conferring such a kind of "immunity against autoimmunity." A second advantage of CAAR-T-cell therapy is reduced immunosuppression, since normal B-cells are not expected to be killed (265).

Since auto-reactive B-cells in pemphigus account for only a minor subset of total B-cells, it is unlikely that CAAR-T-cell therapy may lead to serious adverse events as has been observed in the onco-hematologic setting (265, 268).

One potential limitation of Dsg3 CAAR-T-cell therapy in pemphigus IgG-driven autoimmunity not only against Dsg3 but also against Dsg1. Moreover, patients with Dsg3 mucosal dominant-PV were shown to possibly relapse as PF (or vice versa), probably via intermolecular epitope spreading (269, 270). These findings highlight the importance of targeting simultaneously both Dsg1 and Dsg3 reactive B-cells. A major challenge of CAR-T cell therapy in cancer is the ability of neoplastic cells to escape by down-regulating the expression of the target antigen. A novel strategy to overcome tumor antigen loss is modifying individual T cells with two distinct CAR molecules (dual-signaling CAR) or with one CAR molecule containing two different binding domains, referred to as Tandem CAR (271, 272). A similar strategy could be adopted to develop CAAR-T-cells targeting at the same time Dsg1 and Dsg3 reactive B-cells.

Also, another intriguing therapeutic perspective would be developing CAR-Treg cells to down-regulate ongoing immune reaction against Dsg (273, 274). In this regard, of interest is a study by Fransson et al. involving a murine model of autoimmune encephalitis, in which mouse $CD4^{+}$ T cells were modified to express a CAR targeting myelin oligodendrocyte glycoprotein (MOG) in trans with the murine FoxP3 gene promoting Treg differentiation. Myelin targeting Treg cells successfully suppressed inflammation and improved symptoms in the treated mice (275).

Another potential limitation of CAAR-T-cell therapy in pemphigus includes prohibitive costs. For example, one single infusion of the CD19 CAR T-cell products costs around $ 373,000–475,000 (276). However, taking into account the economic impact of a virtually life-long immunosuppressive therapy, if the aim of pemphigus cure with front-line CAAR T-cell therapy were to be realized, reductions in cumulative spending may conceivably occur. **Figure 9** represents how CAAR-T cells works in pemphigus.

Targeting the Neonatal Fc Receptor in Pemphigus

FcRn is a heterodimer including the MHC class I-like H chain and the β_2-microglobulin L chain (277). This receptor is involved in the transport of IgG from mother to fetus; different studies however have shown that FcRn also plays a critical role in regulating IgG homeostasis; accordingly, when IgG enter into FcRn-expressing cells, the IgG-FcRn binding in acidified endosomes avoids degradation of IgG and allows subsequent recycle and release of IgG in the extracellular space at a near-neutral pH. IgM and IgA do not bind to FcRn and consequently have a reduced half-life compared to IgG (278, 279). Blocking the interaction between FcRn and pathogenic autoantibodies in autoimmune diseases may thereby accelerate pathogenic autoantibody catabolism (280). Interestingly, keratinocytes have been shown to express FcRn (281). Indeed, different studies have demonstrated a critical role of FcRn in pemphigus. Knock-out mouse lacking FcRn do not develop acantholysis by passive transfer of anti-Dsg antibodies (282). Therapeutic efficacy of IVIg can be at least in part attributed to saturation of FcRn, allowing faster degradation of anti-Dsg autoantibodies (282). *In vitro*, an excess of normal IgG accordingly protects cultured keratinocytes from anti-Dsg autoantibodies-induced apoptolysis (283). One recent study demonstrated that FcRn induces enter of anti-mitochondrial antibodies, which are also found in pemphigus sera and contribute to keratinocyte shrinkage due to mithocondial damage. In this study, blocking of FcRn abolished the capacity of PV sera to cause detachment of keratinocytes *in vitro* (284). In another study, Recke et al. (285) found that an allelic variant harboring an amino acid replacement of His435 to Arg favoring high affinity of IgG3 to FcRn was associated with an increase risk of PV. Altogether these studies raise evidence for a potential benefit of targeting FcRn in pemphigus. In 2018, the results of a randomized double-blind placebo-controlled first in-human study on efgartigimod, an antagonist of FcRN, including 62 healthy volunteers showed that the drug was effective in reducing IgG levels by about 75% on after multiple dosing (286). The treatment was well-tolerated and no serious adverse events were recorded (286). A phase II study evaluating the safety and efficacy of ARGX-113, a human IgG1-derived Fc fragments binding to FcRn in patients with PV and PF is currently ongoing (NCT03334058) (287).

Targeting T-Cells and the T-B Cell Cross Talk in Pemphigus

Autoreactive T-cells are critically involved in the pathogenesis of pemphigus (288). Both Th1 and Th2 cells reacting against Dsg were detected in patients with pemphigus at different stages of the disease. However, while Dsg3-reactive Th1 cells can be found in healthy individuals carrying PV predisposing HLA class II alleles, Dsg3-reactive Th2 cells are restricted to pemphigus patients (289, 290). In a recent study by our group, we demonstrated that patients with PV developed a predominant Th2-type response against Dsg3, in contrast to patients with lichen planus, who developed a Th1-type response against the identical autoantigen (291). Indeed, high amount of serum IL-4 sustaining autoantibody production by autoreactive B-cells have been found in pemphigus patients (292). Our group demonstrated the presence of IgE targeting Dsg3 in patients with pemphigus, which further supports the critical role of Th2 cells in orchestrating the inflammatory response and autoantibody production in pemphigus (293). Interestingly, dupilumab, a monoclonal antibody targeting IL-4 has been recently shown to be effective in bullous pemphigoid, a disease in which Th2 cells targeting BP180 and both IgG and IgE against BP180 have also a prominent pathogenic role (294, 295). As far as we are aware, no studies have yet investigated the efficacy of dupilumab in pemphigus. However, pathogenic evidence suggests that the drug may be of potential benefit (**Figure 6**). In parallel to activation of Th2 cells, in pemphigus there is a marked down-regulation of Dsg-specific Foxp3-expressing Treg cells (289). In mouse experiments, Treg cells created in Dsg3$^{-/-}$ mice and transferred into mice with PV were able to reduce autoantibody production (296). Thus, enhancing Treg functions in pemphigus appears to be a promising strategy to restore the lost immune tolerance against Dsg. Infusion of autologous polyclonal regulatory T cells is currently being studied in a phase 1 open-label multicenter trial in patients with active pemphigus vulgaris and pemphigus foliaceus (NCT03239470) (135, 296).

Current work of our group aims at restoring immune tolerance to Dsg3 via targeting of autoreactive T cells. Specifically, we observed in a preclinical mouse model of pemphigus that injections of immunodominant HLA-DRß1*04:02-binding T cell epitopes of Dsg3 conjugated either to antigen-presenting cells lacking a second co-stimulatory signal or to nanoparticles prevented the production of pathogenic anti-Dsg3 IgG.

As previously mentioned, RTX has an inhibitory effect on the co-stimulation of autoreactive B and T-cells in pemphigus by depletion B cells which act as antigen presenting cells (140). In this process, the interaction between CD40 expressed on the surface of B-cells and CD40 L expressed on the surface of T-cells is thought to play an essential role (297). Interestingly, targeting CD40 L demonstrated efficacy in an active mouse PV model. Specifically, Rag2-deficient mice expressing Dsg3 and treated with a monoclonal antibody targeting CD40L did not develop PV after having received splenocytes from Dsg3 deficient mice. However, this preventive effect did not occur when the monoclonal antibody was given after the adoptive cell transfer suggesting that targeting T-B-cell cross-talk may be an effective tool to prevent disease recurrences in patients who have already achieved disease remission (**Figure 9**) (297–299).

Is There a Possibility for a Local Targeted Therapy in Pemphigus?

Vinaj et al. (300) reported on 3 patients with oral PV lesions refractory to immunosuppressants, including intravenous RTX, in whom intralesional RTX injections led to meaningful clinical improvement, suggesting a local immunomodulating effect of the drug. A landmark paper by Yuan et al. (301) demonstrated an accumulation of Dsg-3 and Dsg-1 specific B-cells in the skin of pemphigus lesions. Additionally they showed that the skin in pemphigus serves as a tertiary lymphoid organ in which a close interaction between IL-21- and IL17A-producing CD4$^+$ T cells leads to in loco production of anti-Dsg autoantibodies by auto-reactive B-cells. It is possible that the formation of this tertiary lymphoid organ in the skin may contribute to the resistance of pemphigus lesions to immunosuppressive treatments, including RTX. The discovery by Yuan et al. (301) may also provide a plausible explanation for the successful use of intralesional RTX in oral pemphigus lesions observed by Vinaj et al. (300). It is interesting to note that secretion of IL-21 is associated with activation of JAK1 and JAK3. Tofacinib, an inhibitor of both JAK1 and JAK3, was suggested as a possible therapeutic in pemphigus (302). Interestingly, tofacinib has been successfully applied in different autoimmune disorders (303, 304). Moreover, a topical preparation of tofacinib was shown to be effective in alopecia areata (305). Based on these findings, it would be intriguing to evaluate the potential benefit of topical JAK inhibitors as a local adjuvant therapy in pemphigus.

We have previously shown that mechanisms of acantholysis in pemphigus require activation of different intracellular signaling, including p38MAPK. *In vitro* studies showed that inhibition of p38MAPK eliminated PV IgG-induced blister formation in human skin biopsies (306). Oral p38MAPK inhibitors have been tried in clinical trials in rheumatoid arthritis, Crohn's disease and psoriasis, as well as in pemphigus, but had resulted in severe adverse events (1). Nevertheless, topical p38MAPK inhibitors have been shown to exert potent anti-inflammatory effects in the skin of mice following burn injury (307). Indeed, topical p38MAPK inhibitors may represent a therapeutic strategy in pemphigus to overcome the significant toxicity observed with the systemic counterpart. Finally in a study by Mao et al. (308), inhibition of STAT3 by hydrocortisone, rapamicin, an inhibitor of mTOR, or Stat3 inhibitor XVIII prevented blister formation in a passive transfer PV mouse model by up-regulating the expression of Dsg3. Interestingly, sirolimus, a systemic inhibitor of mTOR, was shown to be effective in PV, whereas topical rapamicin did not (309, 310). Notably, intratumoral injection of Stat3 oligonucletide decoy demonstrated mild efficacy in a trial including patients with head and neck tumors (311). Due to its pivotal implication in the mechanisms of acantholysis in pemphigus, Pharmacologic inhibition of Stat3 through topical drugs may also hold promise in the field of targeted therapy in pemphigus.

DEDICATION

This article is dedicated to Stephen I. Katz, MD, PhD, who enormously contributed to a better understanding of autoimmune bullous skin diseases and immunological skin disorders in general. It was his institute which identified desmoglein 3 as the autoantigen of pemphigus vulgaris and firstly described the central role of autoreactive T cells in this disorder. Steve Katz trained world leaders in immunodermatology from all over the world and will be unforgotten as a superb mentor and wonderful person.

AUTHOR CONTRIBUTIONS

RM and MH designed the manuscript. DD, RM, RE, and MH drafted the manuscript and approved the final version of the manuscript. MH revised critically the final version of the manuscript.

ACKNOWLEDGMENTS

We are grateful to Hazem A. Juratli for help with the histopathological images.

REFERENCES

1. Pollmann R, Schmidt T, Eming R, Hertl M. Pemphigus: a comprehensive review on pathogenesis, clinical presentation and novel therapeutic approaches. *Clin Rev Allergy Immunol.* (2018) 54:1–25. doi: 10.1007/s12016-017-8662-z
2. Ludwig RJ, Vanhoorelbeke K, Leypoldt F, Kaya Z, Bieber K, McLachlan SM, et al. Mechanisms of autoantibody-induced pathology. *Front Immunol.* (2017) 8:603. doi: 10.3389/fimmu.2017.00603
3. Kasperkiewicz M, Ellebrecht CT, Takahashi H, Yamagami J, Zillikens D, Payne AS, et al. Pemphigus. *Nat Rev Dis Primers.* (2017) 3:17026. doi: 10.1038/nrdp.2017.26
4. Sinha AA, Sajda T. The evolving story of autoantibodies in pemphigus vulgaris: development of the "super compensation hypothesis". *Front Med.* (2018) 5:218. doi: 10.3389/fmed.2018.00218
5. Vu TN, Lee TX, Ndoye A, Shultz LD, Pittelkow MR, Dahl MV, et al. The pathophysiological significance of nondesmoglein targets of pemphigus autoimmunity. Development of antibodies against keratinocyte cholinergic receptors in patients with pemphigus vulgaris and pemphigus foliaceus. *Arch Dermatol.* (1998) 134:971–80. doi: 10.1001/archderm.134.8.971
6. Paolino G, Didona D, Magliulo G, Iannella G, Didona B, Mercuri SR, et al. Paraneoplastic pemphigus: insight into the autoimmune pathogenesis, clinical features and therapy. *Int J Mol Sci.* (2017) 18:2532. doi: 10.3390/ijms18122532
7. Kneisel A, Hertl M. Autoimmune bullous skin diseases. Part 2: diagnosis and therapy. *J Dtsch Dermatol Ges.* (2011) 9:927–47. doi: 10.1111/j.1610-0387.2011.07809.x
8. Kneisel A, Hertl M. Autoimmune bullous skin diseases. Part 1: clinical manifestations. *J Dtsch Dermatol Ges.* (2011) 9:844–56; quiz 57. doi: 10.1111/j.1610-0387.2011.07793.x
9. Pisanti S, Sharav Y, Kaufman E, Posner LN. Pemphigus vulgaris: incidence in Jews of different ethnic groups, according to age, sex, and initial lesion. *Oral Surg Oral Med Oral Pathol.* (1974) 38:382–7. doi: 10.1016/0030-4220(74)90365-X
10. Kridin K, Zelber-Sagi S, Bergman R. Pemphigus vulgaris and pemphigus foliaceus: differences in epidemiology and mortality. *Acta Derm Venereol.* (2017) 97:1095–9. doi: 10.2340/00015555-2706
11. Simon DG, Krutchkoff D, Kaslow RA, Zarbo R. Pemphigus in Hartford County, Connecticut, from 1972 to 1977. *Arch Dermatol.* (1980) 116:1035–7. doi: 10.1001/archderm.1980.01640330073017
12. Kridin K. Pemphigus group: overview, epidemiology, mortality, and comorbidities. *Immunol Res.* (2018) 66:255–70. doi: 10.1007/s12026-018-8986-7
13. Sun Y, Liu H, Yang B, Wang C, Foo JN, Bao F, et al. Investigation of the predisposing factor of pemphigus and its clinical subtype through a genome-wide association and next generation sequence analysis. *J Eur Acad Dermatol Venereol.* (2019) 33:410–5. doi: 10.1111/jdv.15227
14. Hubner F, Recke A, Zillikens D, Linder R, Schmidt E. Prevalence and age distribution of pemphigus and pemphigoid diseases in Germany. *J Invest Dermatol.* (2016) 136:2495–8. doi: 10.1016/j.jid.2016.07.013
15. Eaton WW, Pedersen MG, Atladottir HO, Gregory PE, Rose NR, Mortensen PB. The prevalence of 30 ICD-10 autoimmune diseases in Denmark. *Immunol Res.* (2010) 47:228–31. doi: 10.1007/s12026-009-8153-2
16. Eaton WW, Rose NR, Kalaydjian A, Pedersen MG, Mortensen PB. Epidemiology of autoimmune diseases in Denmark. *J Autoimmun.* (2007) 29:1–9. doi: 10.1016/j.jaut.2007.05.002
17. Wertenteil S, Garg A, Strunk A, Alloo A. Prevalence estimates for pemphigus in the United States: a sex- and age-adjusted population analysis. *JAMA Dermatol.* (2019) 155:627–9. doi: 10.1001/jamadermatol.2018.5954
18. del Mar Saez-de-Ocariz M, Vega-Memije ME, Zuniga J, Salgado N, Ruiz J, Balbuena A, et al. HLA-DRB1*0101 is associated with foliaceous pemphigus in Mexicans. *Int J Dermatol.* (2005) 44:350. doi: 10.1111/j.1365-4632.2005.02038.x
19. Diaz LA, Sampaio SA, Rivitti EA, Martins CR, Cunha PR, Lombardi C, et al. Endemic pemphigus foliaceus (*fogo selvagem*). I. Clinical features and immunopathology. *J Am Acad Dermatol.* (1989) 20:657–69.
20. Culton DA, Qian Y, Li N, Rubenstein D, Aoki V, Filhio GH, et al. Advances in pemphigus and its endemic pemphigus foliaceus (*fogo selvagem*) phenotype: a paradigm of human autoimmunity. *J Autoimmun.* (2008) 31:311–24. doi: 10.1016/j.jaut.2008.08.003
21. Diaz LA, Arteaga LA, Hilario-Vargas J, Valenzuela JG, Li N, Warren S, et al. Anti-desmoglein-1 antibodies in onchocerciasis, leishmaniasis and Chagas disease suggest a possible etiological link to *fogo selvagem*. *J Invest Dermatol.* (2004) 123:1045–51. doi: 10.1111/j.0022-202X.2004.23438.x
22. Aoki V, Millikan RC, Rivitti EA, Hans-Filho G, Eaton DP, Warren SJ, et al. Environmental risk factors in endemic pemphigus foliaceus (*fogo selvagem*). *J Investig Dermatol Symp Proc.* (2004) 9:34–40. doi: 10.1111/j.1087-0024.2004.00833.x
23. Zimmermann J, Bahmer F, Rose C, Zillikens D, Schmidt E. Clinical and immunopathological spectrum of paraneoplastic pemphigus. *J Dtsch Dermatol Ges.* (2010) 8:598–606. doi: 10.1111/j.1610-0387.2010.07380.x
24. Mimouni D, Anhalt GJ, Lazarova Z, Aho S, Kazerounian S, Kouba DJ, et al. Paraneoplastic pemphigus in children and adolescents. *Br J Dermatol.* (2002) 147:725–32. doi: 10.1046/j.1365-2133.2002.04992.x
25. Martel P, Loiseau P, Joly P, Busson M, Lepage V, Mouquet H, et al. Paraneoplastic pemphigus is associated with the DRB1*03

allele. *J Autoimmun.* (2003) 20:91–5. doi: 10.1016/S0896-8411(02)00092-6
26. Liu Q, Bu DF, Li D, Zhu XJ. Genotyping of HLA-I and HLA-II alleles in Chinese patients with paraneoplastic pemphigus. *Br J Dermatol.* (2008) 158:587–91. doi: 10.1111/j.1365-2133.2007.08361.x
27. Hofmann SC, Juratli HA, Eming R. Bullous autoimmune dermatoses. *J Dtsch Dermatol Ges.* (2018) 16:1339–58. doi: 10.1111/ddg.13688
28. Grando SA, Grando AA, Glukhenky BT, Doguzov V, Nguyen VT, Holubar K. History and clinical significance of mechanical symptoms in blistering dermatoses: a reappraisal. *J Am Acad Dermatol.* (2003) 48:86–92. doi: 10.1067/mjd.2003.39
29. Pietkiewicz P, Bowszyc-Dmochowska M, Gornowicz-Porowska J, Dmochowski M. Involvement of nail apparatus in pemphigus vulgaris in ethnic poles is infrequent. *Front Med.* (2018) 5:227. doi: 10.3389/fmed.2018.00227
30. Zaraa I, Sellami A, Bouguerra C, Sellami MK, Chelly I, Zitouna M, et al. Pemphigus vegetans: a clinical, histological, immunopathological and prognostic study. *J Eur Acad Dermatol Venereol.* (2011) 25:1160–7. doi: 10.1111/j.1468-3083.2010.03939.x
31. Didona D, Di Zenzo G. Humoral epitope spreading in autoimmune bullous diseases. *Front Immunol.* (2018) 9:779. doi: 10.3389/fimmu.2018.00779
32. Gomi H, Kawada A, Amagai M, Matsuo I. Pemphigus erythematosus: detection of anti-desmoglein-1 antibodies by ELISA. *Dermatology.* (1999) 199:188–9. doi: 10.1159/000018239
33. Czernik A, Camilleri M, Pittelkow MR, Grando SA. Paraneoplastic autoimmune multiorgan syndrome: 20 years after. *Int J Dermatol.* (2011) 50:905–14. doi: 10.1111/j.1365-4632.2011.04868.x
34. Ahmed AR, Avram MM, Duncan LM. Case records of the Massachusetts General Hospital. Weekly clinicopathological exercises. Case 23-2003. A 79-year-old woman with gastric lymphoma and erosive mucosal and cutaneous lesions. *N Engl J Med.* (2003) 349:382–91. doi: 10.1056/NEJMcpc030016
35. Basir N, Telisinghe PU, Chong VH. Gastric cancer and paraneoplastic pemphigus. *Indian J Surg.* (2015) 77:545–6. doi: 10.1007/s12262-015-1311-y
36. Anhalt GJ. Paraneoplastic pemphigus: the role of tumours and drugs. *Br J Dermatol.* (2001) 144:1102–4. doi: 10.1046/j.1365-2133.2001.04272.x
37. Lee MS, Kossard S, Ho KK, Barnetson RS, Ravich RB. Paraneoplastic pemphigus triggered by radiotherapy. *Australas J Dermatol.* (1995) 36:206–10. doi: 10.1111/j.1440-0960.1995.tb00976.x
38. Sehgal VN, Srivastava G. Paraneoplastic pemphigus/paraneoplastic autoimmune multiorgan syndrome. *Int J Dermatol.* (2009) 48:162–9. doi: 10.1111/j.1365-4632.2009.03995.x
39. Broussard KC, Leung TG, Moradi A, Thorne JE, Fine JD. Autoimmune bullous diseases with skin and eye involvement: cicatricial pemphigoid, pemphigus vulgaris, and pemphigus paraneoplastica. *Clin Dermatol.* (2016) 34:205–13. doi: 10.1016/j.clindermatol.2015.11.006
40. Vassileva S, Drenovska K, Manuelyan K. Autoimmune blistering dermatoses as systemic diseases. *Clin Dermatol.* (2014) 32:364–75. doi: 10.1016/j.clindermatol.2013.11.003
41. Wade MS, Black MM. Paraneoplastic pemphigus: a brief update. *Australas J Dermatol.* (2005) 46:1–8; quiz 9–10. doi: 10.1111/j.1440-0960.2005.126_1.x
42. Tsuchisaka A, Numata S, Teye K, Natsuaki Y, Kawakami T, Takeda Y, et al. Epiplakin is a paraneoplastic pemphigus autoantigen and related to bronchiolitis obliterans in Japanese patients. *J Invest Dermatol.* (2016) 136:399–408. doi: 10.1038/JID.2015.408
43. Maldonado F, Pittelkow MR, Ryu JH. Constrictive bronchiolitis associated with paraneoplastic autoimmune multi-organ syndrome. *Respirology.* (2009) 14:129–33. doi: 10.1111/j.1440-1843.2008.01397.x
44. Amagai M, Stanley JR. Desmoglein as a target in skin disease and beyond. *J Invest Dermatol.* (2012) 132 (3 Pt 2):776–84. doi: 10.1038/jid.2011.390
45. Kitajima Y. 150(th) anniversary series: desmosomes and autoimmune disease, perspective of dynamic desmosome remodeling and its impairments in pemphigus. *Cell Commun Adhes.* (2014) 21:269–80. doi: 10.3109/15419061.2014.943397
46. Waschke J, Spindler V. Desmosomes and extradesmosomal adhesive signaling contacts in pemphigus. *Med Res Rev.* (2014) 34:1127–45. doi: 10.1002/med.21310
47. Anhalt GJ, Till GO, Diaz LA, Labib RS, Patel HP, Eaglstein NF. Defining the role of complement in experimental pemphigus vulgaris in mice. *J Immunol.* (1986) 137:2835–40.
48. Mascaro JM Jr, Espana A, Liu Z, Ding X, Swartz SJ, Fairley JA, et al. Mechanisms of acantholysis in pemphigus vulgaris: role of IgG valence. *Clin Immunol Immunopathol.* (1997) 85:90–6. doi: 10.1006/clin.1997.4408
49. Futei Y, Amagai M, Ishii K, Kuroda-Kinoshita K, Ohya K, Nishikawa T. Predominant IgG4 subclass in autoantibodies of pemphigus vulgaris and foliaceus. *J Dermatol Sci.* (2001) 26:55–61. doi: 10.1016/S0923-1811(00)00158-4
50. Tsunoda K, Ota T, Aoki M, Yamada T, Nagai T, Nakagawa T, et al. Induction of pemphigus phenotype by a mouse monoclonal antibody against the amino-terminal adhesive interface of desmoglein 3. *J Immunol.* (2003) 170:2170–8. doi: 10.4049/jimmunol.170.4.2170
51. Di Zenzo G, Di Lullo G, Corti D, Calabresi V, Sinistro A, Vanzetta F, et al. Pemphigus autoantibodies generated through somatic mutations target the desmoglein-3 cis-interface. *J Clin Invest.* (2012) 122:3781–90. doi: 10.1172/JCI64413
52. Heupel WM, Zillikens D, Drenckhahn D, Waschke J. Pemphigus vulgaris IgG directly inhibit desmoglein 3-mediated transinteraction. *J Immunol.* (2008) 181:1825–34. doi: 10.4049/jimmunol.181.3.1825
53. Muller R, Svoboda V, Wenzel E, Gebert S, Hunzelmann N, Muller HH, et al. IgG reactivity against non-conformational NH-terminal epitopes of the desmoglein 3 ectodomain relates to clinical activity and phenotype of pemphigus vulgaris. *Exp Dermatol.* (2006) 15:606–14. doi: 10.1111/j.1600-0625.2006.00451.x
54. Vollner F, Ali J, Kurrle N, Exner Y, Eming R, Hertl M, et al. Loss of flotillin expression results in weakened desmosomal adhesion and Pemphigus vulgaris-like localisation of desmoglein-3 in human keratinocytes. *Sci Rep.* (2016) 6:28820. doi: 10.1038/srep28820
55. Calkins CC, Setzer SV, Jennings JM, Summers S, Tsunoda K, Amagai M, et al. Desmoglein endocytosis and desmosome disassembly are coordinated responses to pemphigus autoantibodies. *J Biol Chem.* (2006) 281:7623–34. doi: 10.1074/jbc.M512447200
56. Mao X, Choi EJ, Payne AS. Disruption of desmosome assembly by monovalent human pemphigus vulgaris monoclonal antibodies. *J Invest Dermatol.* (2009) 129:908–18. doi: 10.1038/jid.2008.339
57. Oktarina DA, van der Wier G, Diercks GF, Jonkman MF, Pas HH. IgG-induced clustering of desmogleins 1 and 3 in skin of patients with pemphigus fits with the desmoglein nonassembly depletion hypothesis. *Br J Dermatol.* (2011) 165:552–62. doi: 10.1111/j.1365-2133.2011.10463.x
58. Sokol E, Kramer D, Diercks GFH, Kuipers J, Jonkman MF, Pas HH, et al. Large-scale electron microscopy maps of patient skin and mucosa provide insight into pathogenesis of blistering diseases. *J Invest Dermatol.* (2015) 135:1763–70. doi: 10.1038/jid.2015.109
59. Waschke J, Bruggeman P, Baumgartner W, Zillikens D, Drenckhahn D. Pemphigus foliaceus IgG causes dissociation of desmoglein 1-containing junctions without blocking desmoglein 1 transinteraction. *J Clin Invest.* (2005) 115:3157–65. doi: 10.1172/JCI23475
60. Mao X, Li H, Sano Y, Gaestel M, Mo Park J, Payne AS. MAPKAP kinase 2 (MK2)-dependent and -independent models of blister formation in pemphigus vulgaris. *J Invest Dermatol.* (2014) 134:68–76. doi: 10.1038/jid.2013.224
61. Mao X, Sano Y, Park JM, Payne AS. p38 MAPK activation is downstream of the loss of intercellular adhesion in pemphigus vulgaris. *J Biol Chem.* (2011) 286:1283–91. doi: 10.1074/jbc.M110.172874
62. Jolly PS, Berkowitz P, Bektas M, Lee HE, Chua M, Diaz LA, et al. p38MAPK signaling and desmoglein-3 internalization are linked events in pemphigus acantholysis. *J Biol Chem.* (2010) 285:8936–41. doi: 10.1074/jbc.M109.087999
63. Saito M, Stahley SN, Caughman CY, Mao X, Tucker DK, Payne AS, et al. Signaling dependent and independent mechanisms in pemphigus vulgaris blister formation. *PLoS ONE.* (2012) 7:e50696. doi: 10.1371/journal.pone.0050696
64. Li N, Zhao M, Wang J, Liu Z, Diaz LA. Involvement of the apoptotic mechanism in pemphigus foliaceus autoimmune injury of the skin. *J Immunol.* (2009) 182:711–7. doi: 10.4049/jimmunol.182.1.711

65. Williamson L, Raess NA, Caldelari R, Zakher A, de Bruin A, Posthaus H, et al. Pemphigus vulgaris identifies plakoglobin as key suppressor of c-Myc in the skin. *EMBO J.* (2006) 25:3298–309. doi: 10.1038/sj.emboj.7601224
66. Satyam A, Khandpur S, Sharma VK, Sharma A. Involvement of T(H)1/T(H)2 cytokines in the pathogenesis of autoimmune skin disease-Pemphigus vulgaris. *Immunol Invest.* (2009) 38:498–509. doi: 10.1080/08820130902943097
67. Hennerici T, Pollmann R, Schmidt T, Seipelt M, Tackenberg B, Mobs C, et al. Increased frequency of T follicular helper cells and elevated interleukin-27 plasma levels in patients with pemphigus. *PLoS ONE.* (2016) 11:e0148919. doi: 10.1371/journal.pone.0148919
68. Bhol KC, Rojas AI, Khan IU, Ahmed AR. Presence of interleukin 10 in the serum and blister fluid of patients with pemphigus vulgaris and pemphigoid. *Cytokine.* (2000) 12:1076–83. doi: 10.1006/cyto.1999.0642
69. Feliciani C, Toto P, Amerio P, Pour SM, Coscione G, Shivji G, et al. *In vitro* and *in vivo* expression of interleukin-1alpha and tumor necrosis factor-alpha mRNA in pemphigus vulgaris: interleukin-1alpha and tumor necrosis factor-alpha are involved in acantholysis. *J Invest Dermatol.* (2000) 114:71–7. doi: 10.1046/j.1523-1747.2000.00835.x
70. Lopez-Robles E, Avalos-Diaz E, Vega-Memije E, Hojyo-Tomoka T, Villalobos R, Fraire S, et al. TNFalpha and IL-6 are mediators in the blistering process of pemphigus. *Int J Dermatol.* (2001) 40:185–8. doi: 10.1046/j.1365-4362.2001.01083.x
71. Janse IC, van der Wier G, Jonkman MF, Pas HH, Diercks GFH. No evidence of apoptotic cells in pemphigus acantholysis. *J Invest Dermatol.* (2014) 134:2039–41. doi: 10.1038/jid.2014.60
72. Schmidt E, Waschke J. Apoptosis in pemphigus. *Autoimmun Rev.* (2009) 8:533–7. doi: 10.1016/j.autrev.2009.01.011
73. Lotti R, Shu E, Petrachi T, Marconi A, Palazzo E, Quadri M, et al. Soluble fas ligand is essential for blister formation in pemphigus. *Front Immunol.* (2018) 9:370. doi: 10.3389/fimmu.2018.00370
74. Puviani M, Marconi A, Cozzani E, Pincelli C. Fas ligand in pemphigus sera induces keratinocyte apoptosis through the activation of caspase-8. *J Invest Dermatol.* (2003) 120:164–7. doi: 10.1046/j.1523-1747.2003.12014.x
75. Vodo D, Sarig O, Geller S, Ben-Asher E, Olender T, Bochner R, et al. Identification of a functional risk variant for pemphigus vulgaris in the ST18 gene. *PLoS Genet.* (2016) 12:e1006008. doi: 10.1371/journal.pgen.1006008
76. Witte M, Zillikens D, Schmidt E. Diagnosis of autoimmune blistering diseases. *Front Med.* (2018) 5:296. doi: 10.3389/fmed.2018.00296
77. Hoffmann K, Hertl M, Sitaru C. [Molecular diagnosis of autoimmune dermatoses]. *Hautarzt.* (2016) 67:33–9. doi: 10.1007/s00105-015-3723-9
78. Otten JV, Hashimoto T, Hertl M, Payne AS, Sitaru C. Molecular diagnosis in autoimmune skin blistering conditions. *Curr Mol Med.* (2014) 14:69–95. doi: 10.2174/15665240113136660079
79. Mindorf S, Dettmann IM, Kruger S, Fuhrmann T, Rentzsch K, Karl I, et al. Routine detection of serum antidesmocollin autoantibodies is only useful in patients with atypical pemphigus. *Exp Dermatol.* (2017) 26:1267–70. doi: 10.1111/exd.13409
80. Maier L, Udvardi A, Hertl M, Eming R, Schmidt E, Zillikens D, et al. Paraneoplastic pemphigus with anti-BP180 autoantibodies and Castleman disease. *Br J Dermatol.* (2017) 176:824–6. doi: 10.1111/bjd.14877
81. Kelly S, Culican S, Silvestrini RA, Vu J, Schifter M, Fulcher DA, et al. Comparative study of five serological assays for the diagnosis of paraneoplastic pemphigus. *Pathology.* (2015) 47:58–61. doi: 10.1097/PAT.0000000000000196
82. Schmidt T, Mauracher S, Bender L, Greene B, Kurzhals J, Eming R, et al. A novel lateral flow immunoassay for the rapid detection of anti-Dsg3 IgG serum autoantibodies in pemphigus vulgaris. *Exp Dermatol.* (2018) 27:233–7. doi: 10.1111/exd.13488
83. Harman KE, Brown D, Exton LS, Groves RW, Hampton PJ, Mohd Mustapa MF, et al. British Association of Dermatologists' guidelines for the management of pemphigus vulgaris 2017. *Br J Dermatol.* (2017) 177:1170–201. doi: 10.1111/bjd.15930
84. Hertl M, Jedlickova H, Karpati S, Marinovic B, Uzun S, Yayli S, et al. Pemphigus. S2 Guideline for diagnosis and treatment–guided by the European Dermatology Forum (EDF) in cooperation with the European Academy of Dermatology and Venereology (EADV). *J Eur Acad Dermatol Venereol.* (2015) 29:405–14. doi: 10.1111/jdv.12772
85. Atzmony L, Hodak E, Leshem YA, Rosenbaum O, Gdalevich M, Anhalt GJ, et al. The role of adjuvant therapy in pemphigus: a systematic review and meta-analysis. *J Am Acad Dermatol.* (2015) 73:264–71. doi: 10.1016/j.jaad.2015.04.038
86. Meurer M. Immunosuppressive therapy for autoimmune bullous diseases. *Clin Dermatol.* (2012) 30:78–83. doi: 10.1016/j.clindermatol.2011.03.013
87. Martin LK, Werth VP, Villaneuva EV, Murrell DF. A systematic review of randomized controlled trials for pemphigus vulgaris and pemphigus foliaceus. *J Am Acad Dermatol.* (2011) 64:903–8. doi: 10.1016/j.jaad.2010.04.039
88. Joly P, Maho-Vaillant M, Prost-Squarcioni C, Hebert V, Houivet E, Calbo S, et al. First-line rituximab combined with short-term prednisone versus prednisone alone for the treatment of pemphigus (Ritux 3): a prospective, multicentre, parallel-group, open-label randomised trial. *Lancet.* (2017) 389:2031–40. doi: 10.1016/S0140-6736(17)30070-3
89. Ratnam KV, Phay KL, Tan CK. Pemphigus therapy with oral prednisolone regimens. A 5-year study. *Int J Dermatol.* (1990) 29:363–7. doi: 10.1111/j.1365-4362.1990.tb04765.x
90. Mentink LF, Mackenzie MW, Toth GG, Laseur M, Lambert FP, Veeger NJ, et al. Randomized controlled trial of adjuvant oral dexamethasone pulse therapy in pemphigus vulgaris: PEMPULS trial. *Arch Dermatol.* (2006) 142:570–6. doi: 10.1001/archderm.142.5.570
91. Femiano F, Gombos F, Scully C. Pemphigus vulgaris with oral involvement: evaluation of two different systemic corticosteroid therapeutic protocols. *J Eur Acad Dermatol Venereol.* (2002) 16:353–6. doi: 10.1046/j.1468-3083.2002.00461.x
92. Dick SE, Werth VP. Pemphigus: a treatment update. *Autoimmunity.* (2006) 39:591–9. doi: 10.1080/08916930600972008
93. Toth GG, Westerlaken BO, Eilders M, Laseur M, Jonkman MF, Uges DR. Dexamethasone pharmacokinetics after high-dose oral therapy for pemphigus. *Ann Pharmacother.* (2002) 36:1108–9. doi: 10.1345/aph.1A047
94. Barnes PJ. Corticosteroids: the drugs to beat. *Eur J Pharmacol.* (2006) 533:2–14. doi: 10.1016/j.ejphar.2005.12.052
95. Ito K, Chung KF, Adcock IM. Update on glucocorticoid action and resistance. *J Allergy Clin Immunol.* (2006) 117:522–43. doi: 10.1016/j.jaci.2006.01.032
96. Kridin K. Emerging treatment options for the management of pemphigus vulgaris. *Ther Clin Risk Manag.* (2018) 14:757–78. doi: 10.2147/TCRM.S142471
97. Tavakolpour S. Current and future treatment options for pemphigus: is it time to move towards more effective treatments? *Int Immunopharmacol.* (2017) 53:133–42. doi: 10.1016/j.intimp.2017.10.027
98. Maltzman JS, Koretzky GA. Azathioprine: old drug, new actions. *J Clin Invest.* (2003) 111:1122–4. doi: 10.1172/JCI18384
99. Meggitt SJ, Anstey AV, Mohd Mustapa MF, Reynolds NJ, Wakelin S. British Association of Dermatologists' guidelines for the safe and effective prescribing of azathioprine 2011. *Br J Dermatol.* (2011) 165:711–34. doi: 10.1111/j.1365-2133.2011.10575.x
100. Mabrouk D, Gurcan HM, Keskin DB, Christen WG, Ahmed AR. Association between cancer and immunosuppressive therapy–analysis of selected studies in pemphigus and pemphigoid. *Ann Pharmacother.* (2010) 44:1770–6. doi: 10.1345/aph.1P309
101. Tavakolpour S, Mirsafaei HS, Delshad S. Management of pemphigus disease in pregnancy. *Am J Reprod Immunol.* (2017) 77:12601. doi: 10.1111/aji.12601
102. Chams-Davatchi C, Esmaili N, Daneshpazhooh M, Valikhani M, Balighi K, Hallaji Z, et al. Randomized controlled open-label trial of four treatment regimens for pemphigus vulgaris. *J Am Acad Dermatol.* (2007) 57:622–8. doi: 10.1016/j.jaad.2007.05.024
103. Chams-Davatchi C, Mortazavizadeh A, Daneshpazhooh M, Davatchi F, Balighi K, Esmaili N, et al. Randomized double blind trial of prednisolone and azathioprine, vs. prednisolone and placebo, in the treatment of pemphigus vulgaris. *J Eur Acad Dermatol Venereol.* (2013) 27:1285–92. doi: 10.1111/j.1468-3083.2012.04717.x
104. Chaidemenos G, Apalla Z, Koussidou T, Papagarifallou I, Ioannides D. High dose oral prednisone vs. prednisone plus azathioprine for the treatment of oral pemphigus: a retrospective, bi-centre, comparative study. *J Eur Acad Dermatol Venereol.* (2011) 25:206–10. doi: 10.1111/j.1468-3083.2010.03753.x

105. Allison AC. Mechanisms of action of mycophenolate mofetil. *Lupus.* (2005) 14 (Suppl. 1):S2–8. doi: 10.1177/096120330501400102
106. Orvis AK, Wesson SK, Breza TS Jr, Church AA, Mitchell CL, Watkins SW. Mycophenolate mofetil in dermatology. *J Am Acad Dermatol.* (2009) 60:183–99; quiz 200–2. doi: 10.1016/j.jaad.2008.08.049
107. Nousari HC, Sragovich A, Kimyai-Asadi A, Orlinsky D, Anhalt GJ. Mycophenolate mofetil in autoimmune and inflammatory skin disorders. *J Am Acad Dermatol.* (1999) 40 (2 Pt 1):265–8. doi: 10.1016/S0190-9622(99)70203-3
108. Beissert S, Mimouni D, Kanwar AJ, Solomons N, Kalia V, Anhalt GJ. Treating pemphigus vulgaris with prednisone and mycophenolate mofetil: a multicenter, randomized, placebo-controlled trial. *J Invest Dermatol.* (2010) 130:2041–8. doi: 10.1038/jid.2010.91
109. Beissert S, Werfel T, Frieling U, Bohm M, Sticherling M, Stadler R, et al. A comparison of oral methylprednisolone plus azathioprine or mycophenolate mofetil for the treatment of pemphigus. *Arch Dermatol.* (2006) 142:1447–54. doi: 10.1001/archderm.142.11.1447
110. Chrysomallis F, Ioannides D, Teknetzis A, Panagiotidou D, Minas A. Treatment of oral pemphigus vulgaris. *Int J Dermatol.* (1994) 33:803–7. doi: 10.1111/j.1365-4362.1994.tb01003.x
111. Sharma VK, Khandpur S. Evaluation of cyclophosphamide pulse therapy as an adjuvant to oral corticosteroid in the management of pemphigus vulgaris. *Clin Exp Dermatol.* (2013) 38:659–64. doi: 10.1111/ced.12073
112. Rose E, Wever S, Zilliken D, Linse R, Haustein UF, Brocker EB. Intravenous dexamethasone-cyclophosphamide pulse therapy in comparison with oral methylprednisolone-azathioprine therapy in patients with pemphigus: results of a multicenter prospectively randomized study. *J Dtsch Dermatol Ges.* (2005) 3:200–6. doi: 10.1111/j.1610-0378.2005.04747.x
113. Sethy PK, Khandpur S, Sharma VK. Randomized open comparative trial of dexamethasone-cyclophosphamide pulse and daily oral cyclophosphamide versus cyclophosphamide pulse and daily oral prednisolone in pemphigus vulgaris. *Indian J Dermatol Venereol Leprol.* (2009) 75:476–82. doi: 10.4103/0378-6323.55390
114. Parmar NV, Kanwar AJ, Minz RW, Parsad D, Vinay K, Tsuruta D, et al. Assessment of the therapeutic benefit of dexamethasone cyclophosphamide pulse versus only oral cyclophosphamide in phase II of the dexamethasone cyclophosphamide pulse therapy: a preliminary prospective randomized controlled study. *Indian J Dermatol Venereol Leprol.* (2013) 79:70–6. doi: 10.4103/0378-6323.104672
115. Werth VP, Fivenson D, Pandya AG, Chen D, Rico MJ, Albrecht J, et al. Multicenter randomized, double-blind, placebo-controlled, clinical trial of dapsone as a glucocorticoid-sparing agent in maintenance-phase pemphigus vulgaris. *Arch Dermatol.* (2008) 144:25–32. doi: 10.1001/archderm.144.1.25
116. Baum S, Greenberger S, Samuelov L, Solomon M, Lyakhovitsky A, Trau H, et al. Methotrexate is an effective and safe adjuvant therapy for pemphigus vulgaris. *Eur J Dermatol.* (2012) 22:83–7. doi: 10.1684/ejd.2011.1611
117. Tran KD, Wolverton JE, Soter NA. Methotrexate in the treatment of pemphigus vulgaris: experience in 23 patients. *Br J Dermatol.* (2013) 169:916–21. doi: 10.1111/bjd.12474
118. Ioannides D, Chrysomallis F, Bystryn JC. Ineffectiveness of cyclosporine as an adjuvant to corticosteroids in the treatment of pemphigus. *Arch Dermatol.* (2000) 136:868–72. doi: 10.1001/archderm.136.7.868
119. Pierpont TM, Limper CB, Richards KL. Past, present, and future of rituximab-the world's first oncology monoclonal antibody therapy. *Front Oncol.* (2018) 8:163. doi: 10.3389/fonc.2018.00163
120. Kasperkiewicz M, Eming R, Behzad M, Hunzelmann N, Meurer M, Schulze-Koops H, et al. Efficacy and safety of rituximab in pemphigus: experience of the German Registry of Autoimmune Diseases. *J Dtsch Dermatol Ges.* (2012) 10:727–32. doi: 10.1111/j.1610-0387.2012.07931.x
121. Wang KC, Liao HT, Chen WS, Lai CC, Chou CT, Chen MH, et al. Real-world effectiveness and safety of rituximab in the treatment of rheumatoid arthritis: a single-center experience in Taiwan. *Int J Rheum Dis.* (2019) 22:860–8. doi: 10.1111/1756-185X.13511
122. MacIsaac J, Siddiqui R, Jamula E, Li N, Baker S, Webert KE, et al. Systematic review of rituximab for autoimmune diseases: a potential alternative to intravenous immune globulin. *Transfusion.* (2018) 58:2729–35. doi: 10.1111/trf.14841
123. So H, Wong VTL, Lao VWN, Pang HT, Yip RML. Rituximab for refractory rapidly progressive interstitial lung disease related to anti-MDA5 antibody-positive amyopathic dermatomyositis. *Clin Rheumatol.* (2018) 37:1983–9. doi: 10.1007/s10067-018-4122-2
124. Nagel A, Podstawa E, Eickmann M, Muller HH, Hertl M, Eming R. Rituximab mediates a strong elevation of B-cell-activating factor associated with increased pathogen-specific IgG but not autoantibodies in pemphigus vulgaris. *J Invest Dermatol.* (2009) 129:2202–10. doi: 10.1038/jid.2009.27
125. Musette P, Bouaziz JD. B cell modulation strategies in autoimmune diseases: new concepts. *Front Immunol.* (2018) 9:622. doi: 10.3389/fimmu.2018.00622
126. Li H, Ayer LM, Lytton J, Deans JP. Store-operated cation entry mediated by CD20 in membrane rafts. *J Biol Chem.* (2003) 278:42427–34. doi: 10.1074/jbc.M308802200
127. Uchida J, Lee Y, Hasegawa M, Liang Y, Bradney A, Oliver JA, et al. Mouse CD20 expression and function. *Int Immunol.* (2004) 16:119–29. doi: 10.1093/intimm/dxh009
128. Butler LA, Tam CS, Seymour JF. Dancing partners at the ball: rational selection of next generation anti-CD20 antibodies for combination therapy of chronic lymphocytic leukemia in the novel agents era. *Blood Rev.* (2017) 31:318–27. doi: 10.1016/j.blre.2017.05.002
129. Bezombes C, Fournie JJ, Laurent G. Direct effect of rituximab in B-cell-derived lymphoid neoplasias: mechanism, regulation, and perspectives. *Mol Cancer Res.* (2011) 9:1435–42. doi: 10.1158/1541-7786.MCR-11-0154
130. Unruh TL, Li H, Mutch CM, Shariat N, Grigoriou L, Sanyal R, et al. Cholesterol depletion inhibits src family kinase-dependent calcium mobilization and apoptosis induced by rituximab crosslinking. *Immunology.* (2005) 116:223–32. doi: 10.1111/j.1365-2567.2005.02213.x
131. Seyfizadeh N, Seyfizadeh N, Hasenkamp J, Huerta-Yepez S. A molecular perspective on rituximab: a monoclonal antibody for B cell non Hodgkin lymphoma and other affections. *Crit Rev Oncol Hematol.* (2016) 97:275–90. doi: 10.1016/j.critrevonc.2015.09.001
132. Golay J, Introna M. Mechanism of action of therapeutic monoclonal antibodies: promises and pitfalls of *in vitro* and *in vivo* assays. *Arch Biochem Biophys.* (2012) 526:146–53. doi: 10.1016/j.abb.2012.02.011
133. Clynes RA, Towers TL, Presta LG, Ravetch JV. Inhibitory Fc receptors modulate *in vivo* cytotoxicity against tumor targets. *Nat Med.* (2000) 6:443–6. doi: 10.1038/74704
134. Velmurugan R, Challa DK, Ram S, Ober RJ, Ward ES. Macrophage-mediated trogocytosis leads to death of antibody-opsonized tumor cells. *Mol Cancer Ther.* (2016) 15:1879–89. doi: 10.1158/1535-7163.MCT-15-0335
135. Amber KT, Maglie R, Solimani F, Eming R, Hertl M. Targeted therapies for autoimmune bullous diseases: current status. *Drugs.* (2018) 78:1527–48. doi: 10.1007/s40265-018-0976-5
136. Colliou N, Picard D, Caillot F, Calbo S, Le Corre S, Lim A, et al. Long-term remissions of severe pemphigus after rituximab therapy are associated with prolonged failure of desmoglein B cell response. *Sci Transl Med.* (2013) 5:175ra30. doi: 10.1126/scitranslmed.3005166
137. Mouquet H, Musette P, Gougeon ML, Jacquot S, Lemercier B, Lim A, et al. B-cell depletion immunotherapy in pemphigus: effects on cellular and humoral immune responses. *J Invest Dermatol.* (2008) 128:2859–69. doi: 10.1038/jid.2008.178
138. Cho A, Bradley B, Kauffman R, Priyamvada L, Kovalenkov Y, Feldman R, et al. Robust memory responses against influenza vaccination in pemphigus patients previously treated with rituximab. *JCI Insight.* (2017) 2:93222. doi: 10.1172/jci.insight.93222
139. Maglie R, Antiga E, Vannucchi M, Del Bianco E, Bianchi B, Massi D, et al. Bullous eruption in a patient with B-cell chronic lymphocytic leukemia: a diagnostic challenge. *Int J Dermatol.* (2017) 56:1445–7. doi: 10.1111/ijd.13807
140. Eming R, Nagel A, Wolff-Franke S, Podstawa E, Debus D, Hertl M. Rituximab exerts a dual effect in pemphigus vulgaris. *J Invest Dermatol.* (2008) 128:2850–8. doi: 10.1038/jid.2008.172
141. Leshem YA, David M, Hodak E, Waitman DA, Vardy D, Israeli M, et al. A prospective study on clinical response and cell-mediated immunity of pemphigus patients treated with rituximab. *Arch Dermatol Res.* (2014) 306:67–74. doi: 10.1007/s00403-013-1355-4

142. Williams M, Khalid T, Hughes S, Bonney D, Wynn R. Rituximab-induced cytokine storm in the absence of overt lymphoproliferative disease. *J Pediatr Hematol Oncol.* (2016) 38:e29–31. doi: 10.1097/MPH.0000000000000485
143. Kanwar AJ, Tsuruta D, Vinay K, Koga H, Ishii N, Dainichi T, et al. Efficacy and safety of rituximab treatment in Indian pemphigus patients. *J Eur Acad Dermatol Venereol.* (2013) 27:e17–23. doi: 10.1111/j.1468-3083.2011.04391.x
144. Ferranti M, Tadiotto Cicogna G, Sattin A, Alaibac M. Citrobacter freundii sepsis in an immunosuppressed patient with pemphigus vulgaris. *BMJ Case Rep.* (2018) 11:e227091. doi: 10.1136/bcr-2018-227091
145. Corbaux C, Joly P. Bullous diseases. *Curr Probl Dermatol.* (2018) 53:64–9. doi: 10.1159/000478078
146. Ahmed AR, Shetty S. A comprehensive analysis of treatment outcomes in patients with pemphigus vulgaris treated with rituximab. *Autoimmun Rev.* (2015) 14:323–31. doi: 10.1016/j.autrev.2014.12.002
147. Chotaliya KK, Gupta R, Marfatia YS. Rituximab therapy in a case of pemphigus vulgaris triggering herpes simplex infection at varied sites. *Indian Dermatol Online J.* (2015) 6:444–6. doi: 10.4103/2229-5178.169722
148. Chiu HY, Chang CY, Hsiao CH, Wang LF. Concurrent cytomegalovirus and herpes simplex virus infection in pemphigus vulgaris treated with rituximab and prednisolone. *Acta Derm Venereol.* (2013) 93:200–1. doi: 10.2340/00015555-1429
149. Wei KC, Chen W, Tang PL, Huang YT. *Pneumocystis jirovecii* pneumonia infection in pemphigus patients treated with rituximab: an observational nationwide epidemiological study in Taiwan. *Eur J Dermatol.* (2018) 28:713–5. doi: 10.1684/ejd.2018.3373
150. Wei KC, Sy C, Wu SY, Chuang TJ, Huang WC, Lai PC. *Pneumocystis jirovecii* pneumonia in HIV-uninfected, rituximab treated non-Hodgkin lymphoma patients. *Sci Rep.* (2018) 8:8321. doi: 10.1038/s41598-018-26743-4
151. Lu YM, Lee YT, Chang HC, Yang HS, Chang CY, Huang CM, et al. Combination of echinocandins and trimethoprim/sulfamethoxazole for the treatment of *pneumocystis jiroveci* pneumonia after heart transplantation. *Transplant Proc.* (2017) 49:1893–8. doi: 10.1016/j.transproceed.2017.04.020
152. Wei KC, Wang YH, Wang WH, Chen W. Fatal infection of *Pneumocystis jiroveci* pneumonia in a pemphigus patient treated with rituximab. *J Eur Acad Dermatol Venereol.* (2017) 31:e350-e1. doi: 10.1111/jdv.14144
153. Tavakolpour S, Mahmoudi H, Balighi K, Abedini R, Daneshpazhooh M. Sixteen-year history of rituximab therapy for 1085 pemphigus vulgaris patients: a systematic review. *Int Immunopharmacol.* (2018) 54:131–8. doi: 10.1016/j.intimp.2017.11.005
154. Maglie R, Hertl M. Assessment of serious infections in pemphigus and pemphigoid by a national registry. *J Eur Acad Dermatol Venereol.* (2018) 32:1623–4. doi: 10.1111/jdv.15237
155. van der Kolk LE, Baars JW, Prins MH, van Oers MH. Rituximab treatment results in impaired secondary humoral immune responsiveness. *Blood.* (2002) 100:2257–9.
156. Keith PJ, Wetter DA, Wilson JW, Lehman JS. Evidence-based guidelines for laboratory screening for infectious diseases before initiation of systemic immunosuppressive agents in patients with autoimmune bullous dermatoses. *Br J Dermatol.* (2014) 171:1307–17. doi: 10.1111/bjd.13355
157. Amber KT, Kodiyan J, Bloom R, Hertl M. The controversy of hepatitis C and rituximab: a multidisciplinary dilemma with implications for patients with pemphigus. *Indian J Dermatol Venereol Leprol.* (2016) 82:182–3. doi: 10.4103/0378-6323.168912
158. Khan DA. Hypersensitivity and immunologic reactions to biologics: opportunities for the allergist. *Ann Allergy Asthma Immunol.* (2016) 117:115–20. doi: 10.1016/j.anai.2016.05.013
159. Levin AS, Otani IM, Lax T, Hochberg E, Banerji A. Reactions to rituximab in an outpatient infusion center: a 5-year review. *J Allergy Clin Immunol Pract.* (2017) 5:107–13.e1. doi: 10.1016/j.jaip.2016.06.022
160. Salmon JH, Perotin JM, Morel J, Drame M, Cantagrel A, Ziegler LE, et al. Serious infusion-related reaction after rituximab, abatacept and tocilizumab in rheumatoid arthritis: prospective registry data. *Rheumatology.* (2018) 57:134–9. doi: 10.1093/rheumatology/kex403
161. Crowley MP, McDonald V, Scully M. Ofatumumab for TTP in a patient with anaphylaxis associated with rituximab. *N Engl J Med.* (2018) 378:92–3. doi: 10.1056/NEJMc1714146
162. Hong DI, Bankova L, Cahill KN, Kyin T, Castells MC. Allergy to monoclonal antibodies: cutting-edge desensitization methods for cutting-edge therapies. *Expert Rev Clin Immunol.* (2012) 8:43–52; quiz 3–4. doi: 10.1586/eci.11.75
163. Wang HH, Liu CW, Li YC, Huang YC. Efficacy of rituximab for pemphigus: a systematic review and meta-analysis of different regimens. *Acta Derm Venereol.* (2015) 95:928–32. doi: 10.2340/00015555-2116
164. Karmacharya P, Poudel DR, Pathak R, Donato AA, Ghimire S, Giri S, et al. Rituximab-induced serum sickness: a systematic review. *Semin Arthritis Rheum.* (2015) 45:334–40. doi: 10.1016/j.semarthrit.2015.06.014
165. Vendramin C, Thomas M, Westwood JP, McGuckin S, Scully M. Rituximab-induced acute and delayed serum sickness in thrombotic thrombocytopenic purpura: the role of anti-rituximab antibodies. *Br J Haematol.* (2018) 184:858–61. doi: 10.1111/bjh.15177
166. Succaria F, Sahni D, Wolpowitz D. Rituximab-induced serum sickness-like reaction: a histopathologic viewpoint. *Am J Dermatopathol.* (2016) 38:321–2. doi: 10.1097/DAD.0000000000000356
167. Didona D, Paolino G, Garcovich S, Caposiena Caro RD, Didona B. Successful use of etanercept in a case of toxic epidermal necrolysis induced by rituximab. *J Eur Acad Dermatol Venereol.* (2016) 30:e83-e4. doi: 10.1111/jdv.13330
168. Feldman RJ. Paradoxical worsening of pemphigus vulgaris following rituximab therapy. *Br J Dermatol.* (2015) 173:858–9. doi: 10.1111/bjd.13823
169. Belgi AS, Azeez M, Hoyle C, Williams RE. Response of pemphigus vulgaris to anti-CD20 antibody therapy (rituximab) may be delayed. *Clin Exp Dermatol.* (2006) 31:143. doi: 10.1111/j.1365-2230.2005.01941.x
170. Leshem YA, Hodak E, David M, Anhalt GJ, Mimouni D. Successful treatment of pemphigus with biweekly 1-g infusions of rituximab: a retrospective study of 47 patients. *J Am Acad Dermatol.* (2013) 68:404–11. doi: 10.1016/j.jaad.2012.08.010
171. Sharma VK, Bhari N, Gupta S, Sahni K, Khanna N, Ramam M, et al. Clinical efficacy of rituximab in the treatment of pemphigus: a retrospective study. *Indian J Dermatol Venereol Leprol.* (2016) 82:389–94. doi: 10.4103/0378-6323.174379
172. Alaibac M. Ultra-low dosage regimen of rituximab in autoimmune blistering skin conditions. *Front Immunol.* (2018) 9:810. doi: 10.3389/fimmu.2018.00810
173. Lazzarotto A, Ferranti M, Meneguzzo A, Sacco G, Alaibac M. Persistent B lymphocyte depletion after an ultralow dose of rituximab for pemphigus vulgaris. *J Investig Allergol Clin Immunol.* (2018) 28:347–8. doi: 10.18176/jiaci.0283
174. Ahmed AR, Spigelman Z, Cavacini LA, Posner MR. Treatment of pemphigus vulgaris with rituximab and intravenous immune globulin. *N Engl J Med.* (2006) 355:1772–9. doi: 10.1056/NEJMoa062930
175. Ahmed AR, Kaveri S, Spigelman Z. Long-term remissions in recalcitrant pemphigus vulgaris. *N Engl J Med.* (2015) 373:2693–4. doi: 10.1056/NEJMc1508234
176. Joly P, Mouquet H, Roujeau JC, D'Incan M, Gilbert D, Jacquot S, et al. A single cycle of rituximab for the treatment of severe pemphigus. *N Engl J Med.* (2007) 357:545–52. doi: 10.1056/NEJMoa067752
177. Cianchini G, Lupi F, Masini C, Corona R, Puddu P, De Pita O. Therapy with rituximab for autoimmune pemphigus: results from a single-center observational study on 42 cases with long-term follow-up. *J Am Acad Dermatol.* (2012) 67:617–22. doi: 10.1016/j.jaad.2011.11.007
178. Schmidt E, Goebeler M, Zillikens D. Rituximab in severe pemphigus. *Ann N Y Acad Sci.* (2009) 1173:683–91. doi: 10.1111/j.1749-6632.2009.04744.x
179. Lunardon L, Tsai KJ, Propert KJ, Fett N, Stanley JR, Werth VP, et al. Adjuvant rituximab therapy of pemphigus: a single-center experience with 31 patients. *Arch Dermatol.* (2012) 148:1031–6. doi: 10.1001/archdermatol.2012.1522
180. Amber KT, Hertl M. An assessment of treatment history and its association with clinical outcomes and relapse in 155 pemphigus patients with response to a single cycle of rituximab. *J Eur Acad Dermatol Venereol.* (2015) 29:777–82. doi: 10.1111/jdv.12678
181. Ingen-Housz-Oro S, Valeyrie-Allanore L, Cosnes A, Ortonne N, Hue S, Paul M, et al. First-line treatment of pemphigus vulgaris with a combination of rituximab and high-potency topical corticosteroids. *JAMA Dermatol.* (2015) 151:200–3. doi: 10.1001/jamadermatol.2014.2421
182. Ahmed AR, Nguyen T, Kaveri S, Spigelman ZS. First line treatment of pemphigus vulgaris with a novel protocol in patients with contraindications to systemic corticosteroids and immunosuppressive agents: preliminary

retrospective study with a seven year follow-up. *Int Immunopharmacol.* (2016) 34:25–31. doi: 10.1016/j.intimp.2016.02.013
183. Vinay K, Cazzaniga S, Amber KT, Feldmeyer L, Naldi L, Borradori L. Rituximab as first-line adjuvant therapy for pemphigus: retrospective analysis of long-term outcomes at a single center. *J Am Acad Dermatol.* (2018) 78:806–8. doi: 10.1016/j.jaad.2017.11.024
184. Palacios-Alvarez I, Riquelme-Mc Loughlin C, Curto-Barredo L, Iranzo P, Garcia-Diez I, Espana A. Rituximab treatment of pemphigus foliaceus—a retrospective study of 12 patients. *J Am Acad Dermatol.* (2018) 5:1252. doi: 10.1016/j.jaad.2018.05.1252
185. de Sena Nogueira Maehara L, Huizinga J, Jonkman MF. Rituximab therapy in pemphigus foliaceus: report of 12 cases and review of recent literature. *Br J Dermatol.* (2015) 172:1420–3. doi: 10.1111/bjd.13586
186. Murrell DF, Sprecher E. Rituximab and short-course prednisone as the new gold standard for new-onset pemphigus vulgaris and pemphigus foliaceus. *Br J Dermatol.* (2017) 177:1143–4. doi: 10.1111/bjd.15947
187. Murrell DF, Pena S, Joly P, Marinovic B, Hashimoto T, Diaz LA, et al. Diagnosis and management of pemphigus: recommendations by an international panel of experts. *J Am Acad Dermatol.* (2018) 2:21. doi: 10.1016/j.jaad.2018.02.021
188. Eming R, Sticherling M, Hofmann SC, Hunzelmann N, Kern JS, Kramer H, et al. S2k guidelines for the treatment of pemphigus vulgaris/foliaceus and bullous pemphigoid. *J Dtsch Dermatol Ges.* (2015) 13:833–44. doi: 10.1111/ddg.12606
189. Vezzoli P, Berti E, Marzano AV. Rationale and efficacy for the use of rituximab in paraneoplastic pemphigus. *Expert Rev Clin Immunol.* (2008) 4:351–63. doi: 10.1586/1744666X.4.3.351
190. Borradori L, Lombardi T, Samson J, Girardet C, Saurat JH, Hugli A. Anti-CD20 monoclonal antibody (rituximab) for refractory erosive stomatitis secondary to $CD20^{+}$ follicular lymphoma-associated paraneoplastic pemphigus. *Arch Dermatol.* (2001) 137:269–72.
191. Heizmann M, Itin P, Wernli M, Borradori L, Bargetzi MJ. Successful treatment of paraneoplastic pemphigus in follicular NHL with rituximab: report of a case and review of treatment for paraneoplastic pemphigus in NHL and CLL. *Am J Hematol.* (2001) 66:142–4. doi: 10.1002/1096-8652(200102)66:2<142::aid-ajh1032>3.0.co;2-0
192. Barnadas M, Roe E, Brunet S, Garcia P, Bergua P, Pimentel L, et al. Therapy of paraneoplastic pemphigus with Rituximab: a case report and review of literature. *J Eur Acad Dermatol Venereol.* (2006) 20:69–74. doi: 10.1111/j.1468-3083.2005.01345.x
193. Lee S, Yamauchi T, Ishii N, Hashimoto T, Kinoshita K, Imamura S, et al. Achievement of the longest survival of paraneoplastic pemphigus with bronchiolitis obliterans associated with follicular lymphoma using R-CHOP chemotherapy. *Int J Hematol.* (2017) 106:852–9. doi: 10.1007/s12185-017-2305-2
194. Kikuchi T, Mori T, Shimizu T, Koda Y, Abe R, Kurihara Y, et al. Successful treatment with bendamustine and rituximab for paraneoplastic pemphigus. *Ann Hematol.* (2017) 96:1221–2. doi: 10.1007/s00277-017-3008-8
195. Hirano T, Higuchi Y, Yuki H, Hirata S, Nosaka K, Ishii N, et al. Rituximab monotherapy and rituximab-containing chemotherapy were effective for paraneoplastic pemphigus accompanying follicular lymphoma, but not for subsequent bronchiolitis obliterans. *J Clin Exp Hematop.* (2015) 55:83–8. doi: 10.3960/jslrt.55.83
196. Amber KT, Valdebran M, Grando SA. Paraneoplastic autoimmune multiorgan syndrome (PAMS): beyond the single phenotype of paraneoplastic pemphigus. *Autoimmun Rev.* (2018) 17:1002–10. doi: 10.1016/j.autrev.2018.04.008
197. Schierl M, Foedinger D, Geissler K, Rappersberger K, Feldmann R. Paraneoplastic pemphigus despite treatment with rituximab, fludarabine and cyclophosphamide in chronic lymphocytic leukemia. *Eur J Dermatol.* (2008) 18:717–8. doi: 10.1684/ejd.2008.0528
198. Baykal C, Kilic S, Kucukoglu R. Paraneoplastic pemphigus seen in four patients with haematological malignancies formerly treated with rituximab. *J Eur Acad Dermatol Venereol.* (2018) 32:e50-e2. doi: 10.1111/jdv.14500
199. Kwatra SG, Boozalis E, Pasieka H, Anhalt GJ. Decreased recognition of paraneoplastic pemphigus in patients previously treated with anti-CD 20 monoclonal antibodies. *Br J Dermatol.* (2019) 180:1238–9. doi: 10.1111/bjd.17577
200. Albers LN, Liu Y, Bo N, Swerlick RA, Feldman RJ. Developing biomarkers for predicting clinical relapse in pemphigus patients treated with rituximab. *J Am Acad Dermatol.* (2017) 77:1074–82. doi: 10.1016/j.jaad.2017.07.012
201. Gregoriou S, Giatrakou S, Theodoropoulos K, Katoulis A, Loumou P, Toumbis-Ioannou E, et al. Pilot study of 19 patients with severe pemphigus: prophylactic treatment with rituximab does not appear to be beneficial. *Dermatology.* (2014) 228:158–65. doi: 10.1159/000357031
202. Hebert V, Joly P. Rituximab in pemphigus. *Immunotherapy.* (2018) 10:27–37. doi: 10.2217/imt-2017-0104
203. Heelan K, Al-Mohammedi F, Smith MJ, Knowles S, Lansang P, Walsh S, et al. Durable remission of pemphigus with a fixed-dose rituximab protocol. *JAMA Dermatol.* (2014) 150:703–8. doi: 10.1001/jamadermatol.2013.6739
204. Hertl M, Zillikens D, Borradori L, Bruckner-Tuderman L, Burckhard H, Eming R, et al. Recommendations for the use of rituximab (anti-CD20 antibody) in the treatment of autoimmune bullous skin diseases. *J Dtsch Dermatol Ges.* (2008) 6:366–73. doi: 10.1111/j.1610-0387.2007.06602.x
205. Feldman RJ, Christen WG, Ahmed AR. Comparison of immunological parameters in patients with pemphigus vulgaris following rituximab and IVIG therapy. *Br J Dermatol.* (2012) 166:511–7. doi: 10.1111/j.1365-2133.2011.10658.x
206. Nagel A, Hertl M, Eming R. B-cell-directed therapy for inflammatory skin diseases. *J Invest Dermatol.* (2009) 129:289–301. doi: 10.1038/jid.2008.192
207. Ujiie I, Ujiie H, Iwata H, Shimizu H. Clinical and immunological features of pemphigus relapse. *Br J Dermatol.* (2018) 180:1498–505. doi: 10.1111/bjd.17591
208. Behzad M, Mobs C, Kneisel A, Moller M, Hoyer J, Hertl M, et al. Combined treatment with immunoadsorption and rituximab leads to fast and prolonged clinical remission in difficult-to-treat pemphigus vulgaris. *Br J Dermatol.* (2012) 166:844–52. doi: 10.1111/j.1365-2133.2011.10732.x
209. Saleh MA. A prospective study comparing patients with early and late relapsing pemphigus treated with rituximab. *J Am Acad Dermatol.* (2018) 79:97–103. doi: 10.1016/j.jaad.2018.01.029
210. Cho SI, Kim JW, Lim JS, Chung JH. Mucosal involvement is a risk factor for poor clinical outcomes and relapse in patients with pemphigus treated with rituximab. *Dermatol Ther.* (2019) 32:e12814. doi: 10.1111/dth.12814
211. Dourmishev LA, Guleva DV, Miteva LG. Intravenous immunoglobulins: mode of action and indications in autoimmune and inflammatory dermatoses. *Int J Inflamm.* (2016) 2016:3523057. doi: 10.1155/2016/3523057
212. Amagai M, Ikeda S, Shimizu H, Iizuka H, Hanada K, Aiba S, et al. A randomized double-blind trial of intravenous immunoglobulin for pemphigus. *J Am Acad Dermatol.* (2009) 60:595–603. doi: 10.1016/j.jaad.2008.09.052
213. Svecova D. IVIG therapy in pemphigus vulgaris has corticosteroid-sparing and immunomodulatory effects. *Australas J Dermatol.* (2016) 57:141–4. doi: 10.1111/ajd.12422
214. Kasperkiewicz M, Shimanovich I, Meier M, Schumacher N, Westermann L, Kramer J, et al. Treatment of severe pemphigus with a combination of immunoadsorption, rituximab, pulsed dexamethasone and azathioprine/mycophenolate mofetil: a pilot study of 23 patients. *Br J Dermatol.* (2012) 166:154–60. doi: 10.1111/j.1365-2133.2011.10585.x
215. Kolesnik M, Becker E, Reinhold D, Ambach A, Heim MU, Gollnick H, et al. Treatment of severe autoimmune blistering skin diseases with combination of protein A immunoadsorption and rituximab: a protocol without initial high dose or pulse steroid medication. *J Eur Acad Dermatol Venereol.* (2014) 28:771–80. doi: 10.1111/jdv.12175
216. Shimanovich I, Nitschke M, Rose C, Grabbe J, Zillikens D. Treatment of severe pemphigus with protein A immunoadsorption, rituximab and intravenous immunoglobulins. *Br J Dermatol.* (2008) 158:382–8. doi: 10.1111/j.1365-2133.2007.08358.x
217. Gelfand EW. Intravenous immune globulin in autoimmune and inflammatory diseases. *N Engl J Med.* (2013) 368:777. doi: 10.1056/NEJMc1215489
218. Prins C, Gelfand EW, French LE. Intravenous immunoglobulin: properties, mode of action and practical use in dermatology. *Acta Derm Venereol.* (2007) 87:206–18. doi: 10.2340/00015555-0249
219. Paran D, Herishanu Y, Elkayam O, Shopin L, Ben-Ami R. Venous and arterial thrombosis following administration of intravenous

immunoglobulins. *Blood Coagul Fibrinolysis.* (2005) 16:313–8. doi: 10.1097/01.mbc.0000172694.85233.a8

220. Sekul EA, Cupler EJ, Dalakas MC. Aseptic meningitis associated with high-dose intravenous immunoglobulin therapy: frequency and risk factors. *Ann Intern Med.* (1994) 121:259–62. doi: 10.7326/0003-4819-121-4-199408150-00004
221. Cantu TG, Hoehn-Saric EW, Burgess KM, Racusen L, Scheel PJ. Acute renal failure associated with immunoglobulin therapy. *Am J Kidney Dis.* (1995) 25:228–34. doi: 10.1016/0272-6386(95)90003-9
222. Schmidt E, Klinker E, Opitz A, Herzog S, Sitaru C, Goebeler M, et al. Protein A immunoadsorption: a novel and effective adjuvant treatment of severe pemphigus. *Br J Dermatol.* (2003) 148:1222–9. doi: 10.1046/j.1365-2133.2003.05302.x
223. Sinha AA, Hoffman MB, Janicke EC. Pemphigus vulgaris: approach to treatment. *Eur J Dermatol.* (2015) 25:103–13. doi: 10.1684/ejd.2014.2483
224. Eming R, Hertl M. Immunoadsorption in pemphigus. *Autoimmunity.* (2006) 39:609–16. doi: 10.1080/08916930600972040
225. Schmidt E, Zillikens D. Immunoadsorption in dermatology. *Arch Dermatol Res.* (2010) 302:241–53. doi: 10.1007/s00403-009-1024-9
226. Meyersburg D, Schmidt E, Kasperkiewicz M, Zillikens D. Immunoadsorption in dermatology. *Ther Apher Dial.* (2012) 16:311–20. doi: 10.1111/j.1744-9987.2012.01075.x
227. Zillikens D, Derfler K, Eming R, Fierlbeck G, Goebeler M, Hertl M, et al. Recommendations for the use of immunoapheresis in the treatment of autoimmune bullous diseases. *J Dtsch Dermatol Ges.* (2007) 5:881–7. doi: 10.1111/j.1610-0387.2007.06342.x
228. Langenhan J, Dworschak J, Saschenbrecker S, Komorowski L, Schlumberger W, Stocker W, et al. Specific immunoadsorption of pathogenic autoantibodies in pemphigus requires the entire ectodomains of desmogleins. *Exp Dermatol.* (2014) 23:253–9. doi: 10.1111/exd.12355
229. Hofrichter M, Dworschak J, Emtenani S, Langenhan J, Weiss F, Komorowski L, et al. Immunoadsorption of desmoglein-3-specific IgG abolishes the blister-inducing capacity of pemphigus vulgaris IgG in neonatal mice. *Front Immunol.* (2018) 9:1935. doi: 10.3389/fimmu.2018.01935
230. Yeh JH, Chen WH, Chiu HC, Bai CH. Clearance studies during subsequent sessions of double filtration plasmapheresis. *Artif Organs.* (2006) 30:111–4. doi: 10.1111/j.1525-1594.2006.00189.x
231. Kasuya A, Moriki M, Tatsuno K, Hirakawa S, Tokura Y. Clearance efficacy of autoantibodies in double filtration plasmapheresis for pemphigus foliaceus. *Acta Derm Venereol.* (2013) 93:181–2. doi: 10.2340/00015555-1444
232. Higashihara T, Kawase M, Kobayashi M, Hara M, Matsuzaki H, Uni R, et al. Evaluating the efficacy of double-filtration plasmapheresis in treating five patients with drug-resistant pemphigus. *Ther Apher Dial.* (2017) 21:243–7. doi: 10.1111/1744-9987.12557
233. Lunardon L, Payne AS. Inhibitory human antichimeric antibodies to rituximab in a patient with pemphigus. *J Allergy Clin Immunol.* (2012) 130:800–3. doi: 10.1016/j.jaci.2012.03.022
234. Du FH, Mills EA, Mao-Draayer Y. Next-generation anti-CD20 monoclonal antibodies in autoimmune disease treatment. *Auto Immun Highlights.* (2017) 8:12. doi: 10.1007/s13317-017-0100-y
235. Karlin L, Coiffier B. Ofatumumab in the treatment of non-Hodgkin's lymphomas. *Expert Opin Biol Ther.* (2015) 15:1085–91. doi: 10.1517/14712598.2015.1055241
236. Rapp M, Pentland A, Richardson C. Successful treatment of pemphigus vulgaris with ofatumumab. *J Drugs Dermatol.* (2018) 17:1338–9.
237. Ellebrecht CT, Choi EJ, Allman DM, Tsai DE, Wegener WA, Goldenberg DM, et al. Subcutaneous veltuzumab, a humanized anti-CD20 antibody, in the treatment of refractory pemphigus vulgaris. *JAMA Dermatol.* (2014) 150:1331–5. doi: 10.1001/jamadermatol.2014.1939
238. Meyer S, Evers M, Jansen JHM, Buijs J, Broek B, Reitsma SE, et al. New insights in Type I and II CD20 antibody mechanisms-of-action with a panel of novel CD20 antibodies. *Br J Haematol.* (2018) 180:808–20. doi: 10.1111/bjh.15132
239. Reddy V, Dahal LN, Cragg MS, Leandro M. Optimising B-cell depletion in autoimmune disease: is obinutuzumab the answer? *Drug Discov Today.* (2016) 21:1330–8. doi: 10.1016/j.drudis.2016.06.009
240. Prica A, Crump M. Improving CD20 antibody therapy: obinutuzumab in lymphoproliferative disorders. *Leuk Lymphoma.* (2019) 60:573–82. doi: 10.1080/10428194.2018.1498490
241. Reddy V, Klein C, Isenberg DA, Glennie MJ, Cambridge G, Cragg MS, et al. Obinutuzumab induces superior B-cell cytotoxicity to rituximab in rheumatoid arthritis and systemic lupus erythematosus patient samples. *Rheumatology.* (2017) 56:1227–37. doi: 10.1093/rheumatology/kex067
242. Stohl W. Inhibition of B cell activating factor (BAFF) in the management of systemic lupus erythematosus (SLE). *Expert Rev Clin Immunol.* (2017) 13:623–33. doi: 10.1080/1744666X.2017.1291343
243. Kaul A, Gordon C, Crow MK, Touma Z, Urowitz MB, van Vollenhoven R, et al. Systemic lupus erythematosus. *Nat Rev Dis Primers.* (2016) 2:16039. doi: 10.1038/nrdp.2016.39
244. Crofford LJ, Nyhoff LE, Sheehan JH, Kendall PL. The role of Bruton's tyrosine kinase in autoimmunity and implications for therapy. *Expert Rev Clin Immunol.* (2016) 12:763–73. doi: 10.1586/1744666X.2016.1152888
245. Corneth OBJ, Klein Wolterink RGJ, Hendriks RW. BTK signaling in B cell differentiation and autoimmunity. *Curr Top Microbiol Immunol.* (2016) 393:67–105. doi: 10.1007/82_2015_478
246. Corneth OB, de Bruijn MJ, Rip J, Asmawidjaja PS, Kil LP, Hendriks RW. Enhanced expression of Bruton's tyrosine kinase in B cells drives systemic autoimmunity by disrupting T cell homeostasis. *J Immunol.* (2016) 197:58–67. doi: 10.4049/jimmunol.1600208
247. Ito Y, Makita S, Maeshima AM, Hatta S, Suzuki T, Yuda S, et al. Paraneoplastic pemphigus associated with B-cell chronic lymphocytic leukemia treated with ibrutinib and rituximab. *Intern Med.* (2018) 57:2395–8. doi: 10.2169/internalmedicine.0578-17
248. Vidal-Crespo A, Rodriguez V, Matas-Cespedes A, Lee E, Rivas-Delgado A, Gine E, et al. The Bruton tyrosine kinase inhibitor CC-292 shows activity in mantle cell lymphoma and synergizes with lenalidomide and NIK inhibitors depending on nuclear factor-kappaB mutational status. *Haematologica.* (2017) 102:e447-e51. doi: 10.3324/haematol.2017.168930
249. Haffenden GP, Blenkinsopp WK, Ring NP, Wojnarowska F, Fry L. The potassium iodide patch test in the dermatitis herpetiformis in relation to treatment with a gluten-free diet and dapsone. *Br J Dermatol.* (1980) 103:313–7. doi: 10.1111/j.1365-2133.1980.tb07250.x
250. Salter AI, Pont MJ, Riddell SR. Chimeric antigen receptor-modified T cells: CD19 and the road beyond. *Blood.* (2018) 131:2621–9. doi: 10.1182/blood-2018-01-785840
251. Bach PB, Giralt SA, Saltz LB. FDA approval of tisagenlecleucel: promise and complexities of a $475000 cancer drug. *JAMA.* (2017) 318:1861–2. doi: 10.1001/jama.2017.15218
252. McHayleh W, Bedi P, Sehgal R, Solh M. Chimeric antigen receptor T-cells: the future is now. *J Clin Med.* (2019) 8:E207. doi: 10.3390/jcm8020207
253. Chow VA, Shadman M, Gopal AK. Translating anti-CD19 CAR T-cell therapy into clinical practice for relapsed/refractory diffuse large B-cell lymphoma. *Blood.* (2018) 132:777–81. doi: 10.1182/blood-2018-04-839217
254. Neelapu SS, Locke FL, Bartlett NL, Lekakis LJ, Miklos DB, Jacobson CA, et al. Axicabtagene ciloleucel CAR T-cell therapy in refractory large B-cell lymphoma. *N Engl J Med.* (2017) 377:2531–44. doi: 10.1056/NEJMoa1707447
255. Chuntova P, Downey KM, Hegde B, Almeida ND, Okada H. Genetically engineered T-cells for malignant glioma: overcoming the barriers to effective immunotherapy. *Front Immunol.* (2018) 9:3062. doi: 10.3389/fimmu.2018.03062
256. Xu J, Wang Y, Shi J, Liu J, Li Q, Chen L. Combination therapy: a feasibility strategy for CAR-T cell therapy in the treatment of solid tumors. *Oncol Lett.* (2018) 16:2063–70. doi: 10.3892/ol.2018.8946
257. Simon B, Uslu U. CAR-T cell therapy in melanoma: a future success story? *Exp Dermatol.* (2018) 27:1315–21. doi: 10.1111/exd.13792
258. Flemming A. Autoimmune diseases: CAR-T cells take aim at autoimmunity. *Nat Rev Drug Discov.* (2016) 15:603. doi: 10.1038/nrd.2016.180
259. Wegner A. Chimeric antigen receptor T cells for the treatment of cancer and the future of preclinical models for predicting their toxicities. *Immunotherapy.* (2017) 9:669–80. doi: 10.2217/imt-2017-0028
260. Vafia K, Groth S, Beckmann T, Hirose M, Dworschak J, Recke A, et al. Pathogenicity of autoantibodies in anti-p200 pemphigoid. *PLoS ONE.* (2012) 7:e41769. doi: 10.1371/journal.pone.0041769

261. Eshhar Z, Waks T, Gross G, Schindler DG. Specific activation and targeting of cytotoxic lymphocytes through chimeric single chains consisting of antibody-binding domains and the gamma or zeta subunits of the immunoglobulin and T-cell receptors. *Proc Natl Acad Sci USA.* (1993) 90:720–4. doi: 10.1073/pnas.90.2.720
262. Dai H, Wang Y, Lu X, Han W. Chimeric antigen receptors modified T-cells for cancer therapy. *J Natl Cancer Inst.* (2016) 108:djv439. doi: 10.1093/jnci/djv439
263. Long KB, Young RM, Boesteanu AC, Davis MM, Melenhorst JJ, Lacey SF, et al. CAR T cell therapy of non-hematopoietic malignancies: detours on the road to clinical success. *Front Immunol.* (2018) 9:2740. doi: 10.3389/fimmu.2018.02740
264. Siddiqi HF, Staser KW, Nambudiri VE. Research techniques made simple: CAR T-cell therapy. *J Invest Dermatol.* (2018) 138:2501–4.e1. doi: 10.1016/j.jid.2018.09.002
265. Ellebrecht CT, Bhoj VG, Nace A, Choi EJ, Mao X, Cho MJ, et al. Reengineering chimeric antigen receptor T cells for targeted therapy of autoimmune disease. *Science.* (2016) 353:179–84. doi: 10.1126/science.aaf6756
266. Chatenoud L. Precision medicine for autoimmune disease. *Nat Biotechnol.* (2016) 34:930–2. doi: 10.1038/nbt.3670
267. Viaud S, Ma JSY, Hardy IR, Hampton EN, Benish B, Sherwood L, et al. Switchable control over *in vivo* CAR T expansion, B cell depletion, and induction of memory. *Proc Natl Acad Sci USA.* (2018) 115:E10898–906. doi: 10.1073/pnas.1810060115
268. Frey N, Porter D. Cytokine release syndrome with chimeric antigen receptor T cell therapy. *Biol Blood Marrow Transplant.* (2018) 25:e123–7. doi: 10.1016/j.bbmt.2018.12.756
269. Ito T, Moriuchi R, Kikuchi K, Shimizu S. Rapid transition from pemphigus vulgaris to pemphigus foliaceus. *J Eur Acad Dermatol Venereol.* (2016) 30:455–7. doi: 10.1111/jdv.12832
270. Pigozzi B, Peserico A, Schiesari L, Alaibac M. Pemphigus foliaceus evolving into pemphigus vulgaris: a probable example of 'intermolecular epitope spreading' confirmed by enzyme-linked immunosorbent assay study. *J Eur Acad Dermatol Venereol.* (2008) 22:242–4. doi: 10.1111/j.1468-3083.2007.02298.x
271. Zah E, Lin MY, Silva-Benedict A, Jensen MC, Chen YY. T Cells Expressing CD19/CD20 bispecific chimeric antigen receptors prevent antigen escape by malignant B cells. *Cancer Immunol Res.* (2016) 4:498–508. doi: 10.1158/2326-6066.CIR-15-0231
272. Wang Z, Wu Z, Liu Y, Han W. New development in CAR-T cell therapy. *J Hematol Oncol.* (2017) 10:53. doi: 10.1186/s13045-017-0423-1
273. Zhang Q, Lu W, Liang CL, Chen Y, Liu H, Qiu F, et al. Chimeric antigen receptor (CAR) treg: a promising approach to inducing immunological tolerance. *Front Immunol.* (2018) 9:2359. doi: 10.3389/fimmu.2018.02359
274. Schmidt T, Willenborg S, Hunig T, Deeg CA, Sonderstrup G, Hertl M, et al. Induction of T regulatory cells by the superagonistic anti-CD28 antibody D665 leads to decreased pathogenic IgG autoantibodies against desmoglein 3 in a HLA-transgenic mouse model of pemphigus vulgaris. *Exp Dermatol.* (2016) 25:293–8. doi: 10.1111/exd.12919
275. Fransson M, Piras E, Burman J, Nilsson B, Essand M, Lu B, et al. CAR/FoxP3-engineered T regulatory cells target the CNS and suppress EAE upon intranasal delivery. *J Neuroinflammation.* (2012) 9:112. doi: 10.1186/1742-2094-9-112
276. Hay AE, Cheung MC. CAR T-cells: costs, comparisons and commentary. *J Med Econ.* (2019) 2019:1582059. doi: 10.1080/13696998.2019.1582059
277. Junghans RP, Anderson CL. The protection receptor for IgG catabolism is the beta2-microglobulin-containing neonatal intestinal transport receptor. *Proc Natl Acad Sci USA.* (1996) 93:5512–6. doi: 10.1073/pnas.93.11.5512
278. Goebl NA, Babbey CM, Datta-Mannan A, Witcher DR, Wroblewski VJ, Dunn KW. Neonatal Fc receptor mediates internalization of Fc in transfected human endothelial cells. *Mol Biol Cell.* (2008) 19:5490–505. doi: 10.1091/mbc.e07-02-0101
279. Ward ES, Ober RJ. Targeting FcRn to generate antibody-based therapeutics. *Trends Pharmacol Sci.* (2018) 39:892–904. doi: 10.1016/j.tips.2018.07.007
280. Sesarman A, Vidarsson G, Sitaru C. The neonatal Fc receptor as therapeutic target in IgG-mediated autoimmune diseases. *Cell Mol Life Sci.* (2010) 67:2533–50. doi: 10.1007/s00018-010-0318-6
281. Cauza K, Hinterhuber G, Dingelmaier-Hovorka R, Brugger K, Klosner G, Horvat R, et al. Expression of FcRn, the MHC class I-related receptor for IgG, in human keratinocytes. *J Invest Dermatol.* (2005) 124:132–9. doi: 10.1111/j.0022-202X.2004.23542.x
282. Li N, Zhao M, Hilario-Vargas J, Prisayanh P, Warren S, Diaz LA, et al. Complete FcRn dependence for intravenous Ig therapy in autoimmune skin blistering diseases. *J Clin Invest.* (2005) 115:3440–50. doi: 10.1172/JCI24394
283. Arredondo J, Chernyavsky AI, Karaouni A, Grando SA. Novel mechanisms of target cell death and survival and of therapeutic action of IVIg in Pemphigus. *Am J Pathol.* (2005) 167:1531–44. doi: 10.1016/S0002-9440(10)61239-4
284. Chen Y, Chernyavsky A, Webber RJ, Grando SA, Wang PH. Critical role of the neonatal Fc receptor (FcRn) in the pathogenic action of antimitochondrial autoantibodies synergizing with anti-desmoglein autoantibodies in pemphigus vulgaris. *J Biol Chem.* (2015) 290:23826–37. doi: 10.1074/jbc.M115.668061
285. Recke A, Konitzer S, Lemcke S, Freitag M, Sommer NM, Abdelhady M, et al. The p.Arg435His variation of IgG3 with high affinity to FcRn is associated with susceptibility for pemphigus vulgaris-analysis of four different ethnic cohorts. *Front Immunol.* (2018) 9:1788. doi: 10.3389/fimmu.2018.01788
286. Ulrichts P, Guglietta A, Dreier T, van Bragt T, Hanssens V, Hofman E, et al. Neonatal Fc receptor antagonist efgartigimod safely and sustainably reduces IgGs in humans. *J Clin Invest.* (2018) 128:4372–86. doi: 10.1172/JCI97911
287. Sciurti M, Fornaroli F, Gaiani F, Bonaguri C, Leandro G, Di Mario F, et al. Genetic susceptibilty and celiac disease: what role do HLA haplotypes play? *Acta Biomed.* (2018) 89:17–21. doi: 10.23750/abm.v89i9-S.7953
288. Echigo T, Hasegawa M, Shimada Y, Inaoki M, Takehara K, Sato S. Both Th1 and Th2 chemokines are elevated in sera of patients with autoimmune blistering diseases. *Arch Dermatol Res.* (2006) 298:38–45. doi: 10.1007/s00403-006-0661-5
289. Amber KT, Staropoli P, Shiman MI, Elgart GW, Hertl M. Autoreactive T cells in the immune pathogenesis of pemphigus vulgaris. *Exp Dermatol.* (2013) 22:699–704. doi: 10.1111/exd.12229
290. Eming R, Hennerici T, Backlund J, Feliciani C, Visconti KC, Willenborg S, et al. Pathogenic IgG antibodies against desmoglein 3 in pemphigus vulgaris are regulated by HLA-DRB1*04:02-restricted T cells. *J Immunol.* (2014) 193:4391–9. doi: 10.4049/jimmunol.1401081
291. Schmidt T, Solimani F, Pollmann R, Stein R, Schmidt A, Stulberg I, et al. TH1/TH17 cell recognition of desmoglein 3 and bullous pemphigoid antigen 180 in patients with lichen planus. *J Allergy Clin Immunol.* (2018) 142:669–72.e7. doi: 10.1016/j.jaci.2018.02.044
292. Takahashi H, Amagai M, Nishikawa T, Fujii Y, Kawakami Y, Kuwana M. Novel system evaluating *in vivo* pathogenicity of desmoglein 3-reactive T cell clones using murine pemphigus vulgaris. *J Immunol.* (2008) 181:1526–35. doi: 10.4049/jimmunol.181.2.1526
293. Nagel A, Lang A, Engel D, Podstawa E, Hunzelmann N, de Pita O, et al. Clinical activity of pemphigus vulgaris relates to IgE autoantibodies against desmoglein 3. *Clin Immunol.* (2010) 134:320–30. doi: 10.1016/j.clim.2009.11.006
294. Maglie R, Hertl M. Pharmacological advances in pemphigoid. *Curr Opin Pharmacol.* (2019) 46:34–43. doi: 10.1016/j.coph.2018.12.007
295. Kaye A, Gordon SC, Deverapalli SC, Her MJ, Rosmarin D. Dupilumab for the treatment of recalcitrant bullous pemphigoid. *JAMA Dermatol.* (2018) 154:1225–6. doi: 10.1001/jamadermatol.2018.2526
296. Yokoyama T, Matsuda S, Takae Y, Wada N, Nishikawa T, Amagai M, et al. Antigen-independent development of Foxp3$^+$ regulatory T cells suppressing autoantibody production in experimental pemphigus vulgaris. *Int Immunol.* (2011) 23:365–73. doi: 10.1093/intimm/dxr020
297. Mao X, Payne AS. Seeking approval: present and future therapies for pemphigus vulgaris. *Curr Opin Investig Drugs.* (2008) 9:497–504.
298. Aoki-Ota M, Kinoshita M, Ota T, Tsunoda K, Iwasaki T, Tanaka S, et al. Tolerance induction by the blockade of CD40/CD154 interaction in pemphigus vulgaris mouse model. J *Invest Dermatol.* (2006) 126:105–13. doi: 10.1038/sj.jid.5700016
299. Liu Z, Li N, Diaz LA. Inhibition of pemphigus vulgaris by targeting of the CD40-CD154 co-stimulatory pathway: a step toward antigen-specific therapy? *J Invest Dermatol.* (2006) 126:11–3. doi: 10.1038/sj.jid.5700059

300. Vinay K, Kanwar AJ, Mittal A, Dogra S, Minz RW, Hashimoto T. Intralesional rituximab in the treatment of refractory oral pemphigus vulgaris. *JAMA Dermatol.* (2015) 151:878–82. doi: 10.1001/jamadermatol.2014.3674
301. Yuan H, Zhou S, Liu Z, Cong W, Fei X, Zeng W, et al. Pivotal role of lesional and perilesional T/B lymphocytes in pemphigus pathogenesis. *J Invest Dermatol.* (2017) 137:2362–70. doi: 10.1016/j.jid.2017.05.032
302. Tavakolpour S. Tofacitinib as the potent treatment for refractory pemphigus: a possible alternative treatment for pemphigus. *Dermatol Ther.* (2018) 31:e12696. doi: 10.1111/dth.12696
303. Banerjee S, Biehl A, Gadina M, Hasni S, Schwartz DM. JAK-STAT Signaling as a target for inflammatory and autoimmune diseases: current and future prospects. *Drugs.* (2017) 77:521–46. doi: 10.1007/s40265-017-0772-7
304. Gupta AK, Cernea M, Lynde CW. Tofacitinib in the treatment of rheumatoid arthritis and chronic plaque psoriasis. *Skin Therapy Lett.* (2017) 22:1–7.
305. Putterman E, Castelo-Soccio L. Topical 2% tofacitinib for children with alopecia areata, alopecia totalis, and alopecia universalis. *J Am Acad Dermatol.* (2018) 78:1207–9.e1. doi: 10.1016/j.jaad.2018.02.031
306. Egu DT, Walter E, Spindler V, Waschke J. Inhibition of p38MAPK signalling prevents epidermal blistering and alterations of desmosome structure induced by pemphigus autoantibodies in human epidermis. *Br J Dermatol.* (2017) 177:1612–8. doi: 10.1111/bjd.15721
307. Carter D, Warsen A, Mandell K, Cuschieri J, Maier RV, Arbabi S. Delayed topical p38 MAPK inhibition attenuates full-thickness burn wound inflammatory signaling. *J Burn Care Res.* (2014) 35:e83–92. doi: 10.1097/BCR.0b013e31828a8d6e
308. Mao X, Cho MJT, Ellebrecht CT, Mukherjee EM, Payne AS. Stat3 regulates desmoglein 3 transcription in epithelial keratinocytes. *JCI Insight.* (2017) 2:e92253. doi: 10.1172/jci.insight.92253
309. Grando SA, Laquer VT, Le HM. Sirolimus for acute pemphigus vulgaris: a case report and discussion of dualistic action providing for both immunosuppression and keratinocyte protection. *J Am Acad Dermatol.* (2011) 65:684–6. doi: 10.1016/j.jaad.2011.01.029
310. Poot AM, Jonkman MF. Topical sirolimus for oral pemphigus vulgaris: 3 unresponsive cases. *J Am Acad Dermatol.* (2012) 67:e228–9. doi: 10.1016/j.jaad.2012.04.032
311. Sen M, Thomas SM, Kim S, Yeh JI, Ferris RL, Johnson JT, et al. First-in-human trial of a STAT3 decoy oligonucleotide in head and neck tumors: implications for cancer therapy. *Cancer Discov.* (2012) 2:694–705. doi: 10.1158/2159-8290.CD-12-0191

13

Endocytosis of IgG, Desmoglein 1 and Plakoglobin in Pemphigus Foliaceus Patient Skin

Dyah A. M. Oktarina [1,2], Ena Sokol [1], Duco Kramer [1], Marcel F. Jonkman [1] and Hendri H. Pas [1]*

[1] Department of Dermatology, Centre for Blistering Diseases, University Medical Centre Groningen, University of Groningen, Groningen, Netherlands, [2] Department of Dermatology and Venereology, Faculty of Medicine, Public Health and Nursing, Universitas Gadjah Mada, Yogyakarta, Indonesia

***Correspondence:**
Hendri H. Pas
h.h.pas@umcg.nl

Pemphigus foliaceus (PF) is one of the two main forms of pemphigus and is characterized by circulating IgG to the desmosomal cadherin desmoglein 1 (DSG1) and by subcorneal blistering of the skin. The pathomechanism of blister formation in PF is unknown. Previously we have shown that PF IgG induces aggregation of DSG1, plakoglobin (PG), and IgG outside of desmosomes, what in immunofluorescence of PF patient skin visualizes as a granular IgG deposition pattern with a limited number of coarse IgG aggregates between cells. Here we have investigated the fate of these aggregates in skin and found that these are cleared by endocytosis. We performed double immunofluorescence staining on snap-frozen skin biopsies of six PF patients for the following molecules: IgG, the desmosomal proteins DSG1 and DSG3, desmocollins 1 and 3, PG, desmoplakin and plakophilin 3, and for the endosomal marker early endosomal antigen 1 and the lysosomal markers cathepsin D and lysosomal-associated membrane protein 1. Endosomes were present in all cells but did not make contact with the aggregates in the basal and suprabasal layers. In the higher layers they moored to the aggregates, often symmetrically from two adjacent cells, and IgG, DSG1, and PG were taken up. Finally these endosomes became localized perinuclear. Endocytosis was only observed in perilesional or lesional skin but not in non-lesional skin. Older immunoelectron microscopic studies have suggested that in PF skin endocytosis of detached desmosomes takes place but we found no other desmosomal proteins to be present in these endosomes. Double staining with cathepsin D and LAMP-1 revealed no overlap with IgG, DSG1, or PG suggesting that lysosomes have no role in the clearing process. Collectively, our results show that endocytosis is part of the pathogenic process in PF but that no detached desmosomes are taken up but instead the deposited IgG is taken up together with DSG1 and PG.

Keywords: pemphigus foliaceus, desmoglein 1, desmosomes, acantholysis, endocytosis

INTRODUCTION

Pemphigus is an autoimmune blistering disease of the skin and mucous membranes, which is characterized by a loss of cell-cell adhesion, known as acantholysis. Pemphigus foliaceus (PF) is one of the two major forms of pemphigus and it is characterized by blistering of the skin only and immunologically by circulating autoantibodies against desmoglein 1 (DSG1) (1, 2). DSG1 is a glycoprotein of desmosomes and is expressed through all the epidermal layers. Desmosomes are intercellular adhesion structures and are build-up of transmembrane desmosomal cadherins desmogleins and desmocollins (DSC), that by heterophilic interaction directly interconnect two opposite half-desmosomes, and intracellular desmosomal plaque proteins including plakoglobin (PG), desmoplakin (DP), and plakophilins (PKP) (3–6). The intracellular proteins connect the cytoplasmic tails of the desmosomal cadherins to the intermediate keratin filaments thereby providing strength to the tissue. The pathomechanism of the loss of cell-cell adhesion in PF is not exactly known and compared to PV only few studies have addressed it. It is clear that the anti-DSG1 IgG is the pathogenic factor that induces acantholysis as injection of PF IgG causes skin blistering in mice and in an *ex vivo* living human skin model (7–9). Injecting of PF IgG in mice also results in activation of p38MAPK and an inhibitor to p38MAPK abolishes this blistering (7). Waschke et al. showed that PF IgG reduces Rho A activity and in an *ex vivo* human skin model PF induced blistering could be abrogated by Rho A activation (10). Recent research by Walter et al. found that anti-DSG3 IgG and anti-DSG1 IgG led to activation of different signaling pathways. While both activated p38MAPK, anti-DSG3 activated Src while in contrast anti-DSG1 activated ERK, indicating that the pathomechanisms between PV and PF might differ (11). Steric hindrance i.e., obstruction of DSG transinteraction is also considered as a possible pathomechanism. Based on single molecule atomic force measurements and by laser trapping of surface- bound DSG1-coated microbeads Waschke et al. however found no evidence for this (12). We have shown that in the anti-DSG1 IgG induces a shift in distribution of DSG1 and PG in PF patient skin (8). In healthy human skin staining for DSG1 shows an evenly distributed signal over the cell membranes in line with a desmosomal distribution while instead in PF skin, especially in the lower epidermal layers, DSG1 is present in coarse clusters that also contain PG and IgG but no other desmosomal proteins. These clusters can be induced by bivalent PF IgG in the *ex vivo* living human skin model, but not by monovalent Fab fragments of this same IgG which suggest that crosslinking of DSG molecules underlies cluster formation (8, 9). Recently further evidence was provided that the polyvalence of bivalent PF IgG is responsible for clustering. A mixture of non-pathogenic PF monoclonal antibody (mAb) and pathogenic PF mAb is needed to induce clusters, but only pathogenic PF mAb is able to induce the loss of cell-cell adhesion (13). The clusters in PF skin contain DSG1 and PG, but no other desmosomal components which suggests that desmosomes

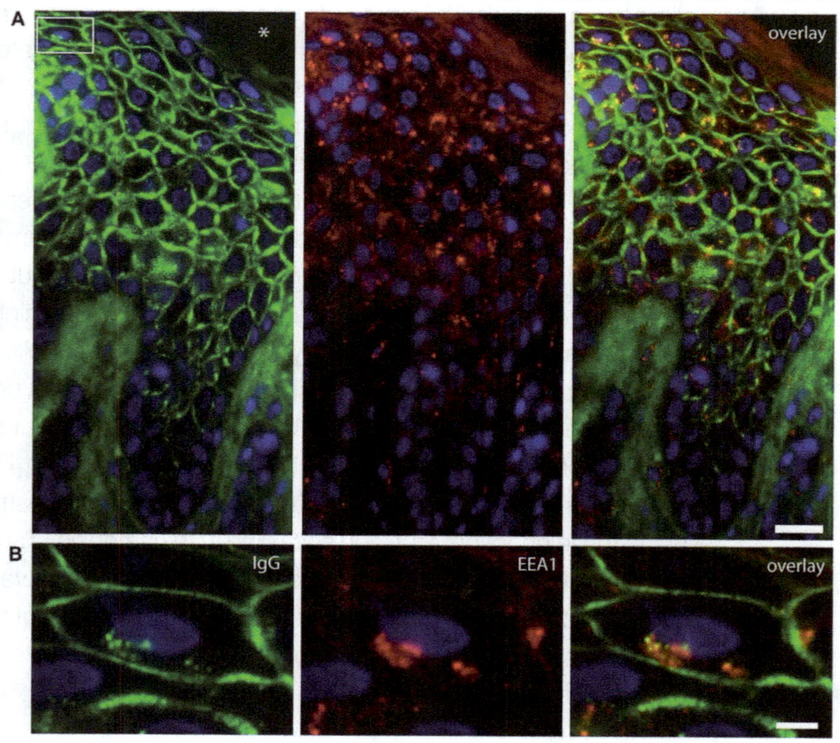

FIGURE 1 | Colocalization of IgG and endosomes in lesional PF patient skin. **(A)** IgG (green) and EEA1 (red) colocalize in the higher skin layers (right panel). The white box depicts the cell shown in **(B)**. The blister cavity is indicated by an asterix. White bar: 25 μm. **(B)** Detail showing the perinuclear localization of IgG. White bar: 5 μm.

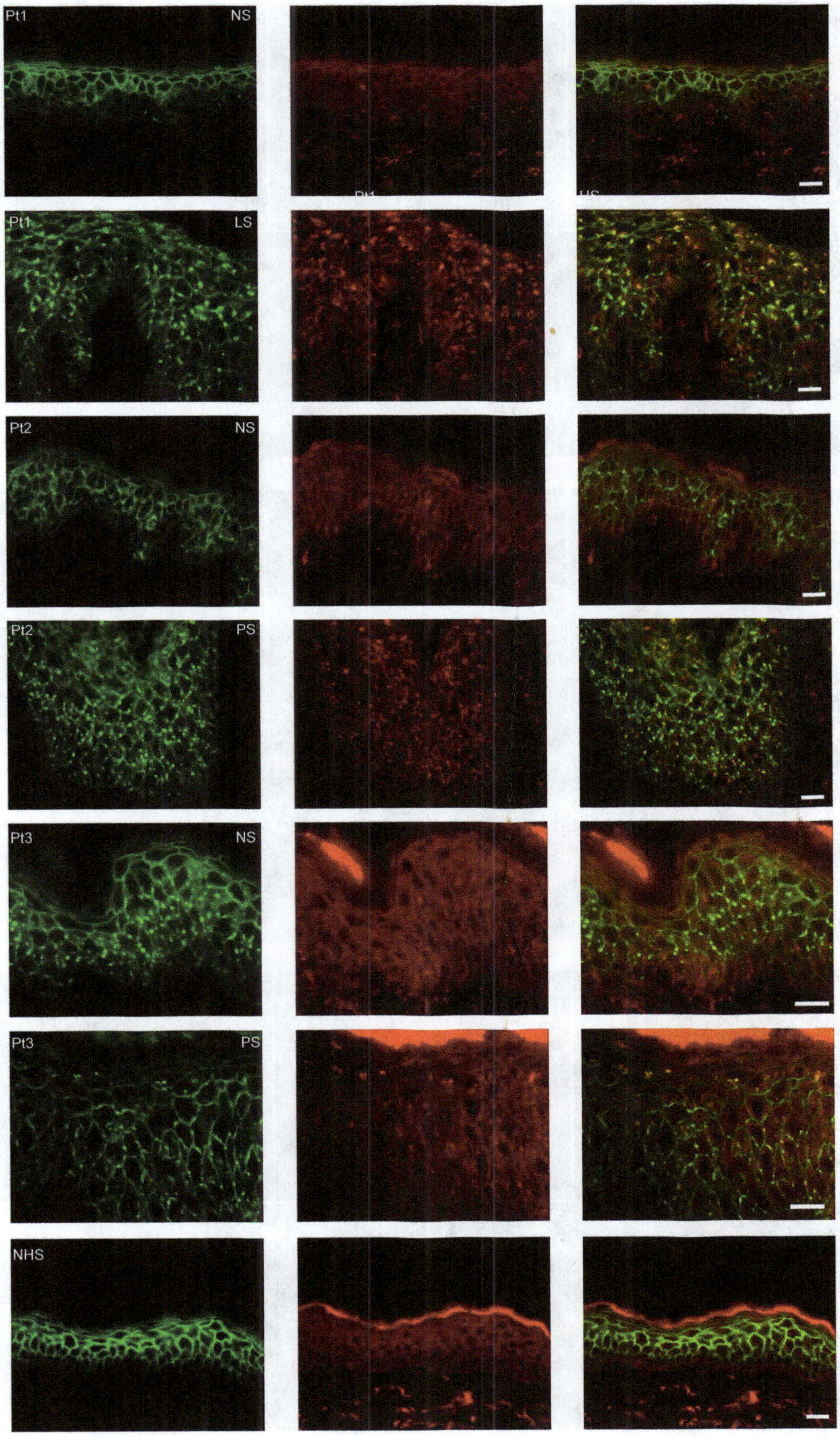

FIGURE 2 | Endocytosis from clusters is not present in non-lesional skin. The images are from three patients of whom we had biopsies of non-lesional skin next to biopsies of perilesional or lesional skin. As control healthy normal human skin is used. In green plakoglobin and in red early endosomal antigen. The panels to the right are overlays. Pt, patient; NS, non-lesional skin; PS, perilesional skin; LS, lesional skin; NHS, normal human skin. White bar is 20 μm.

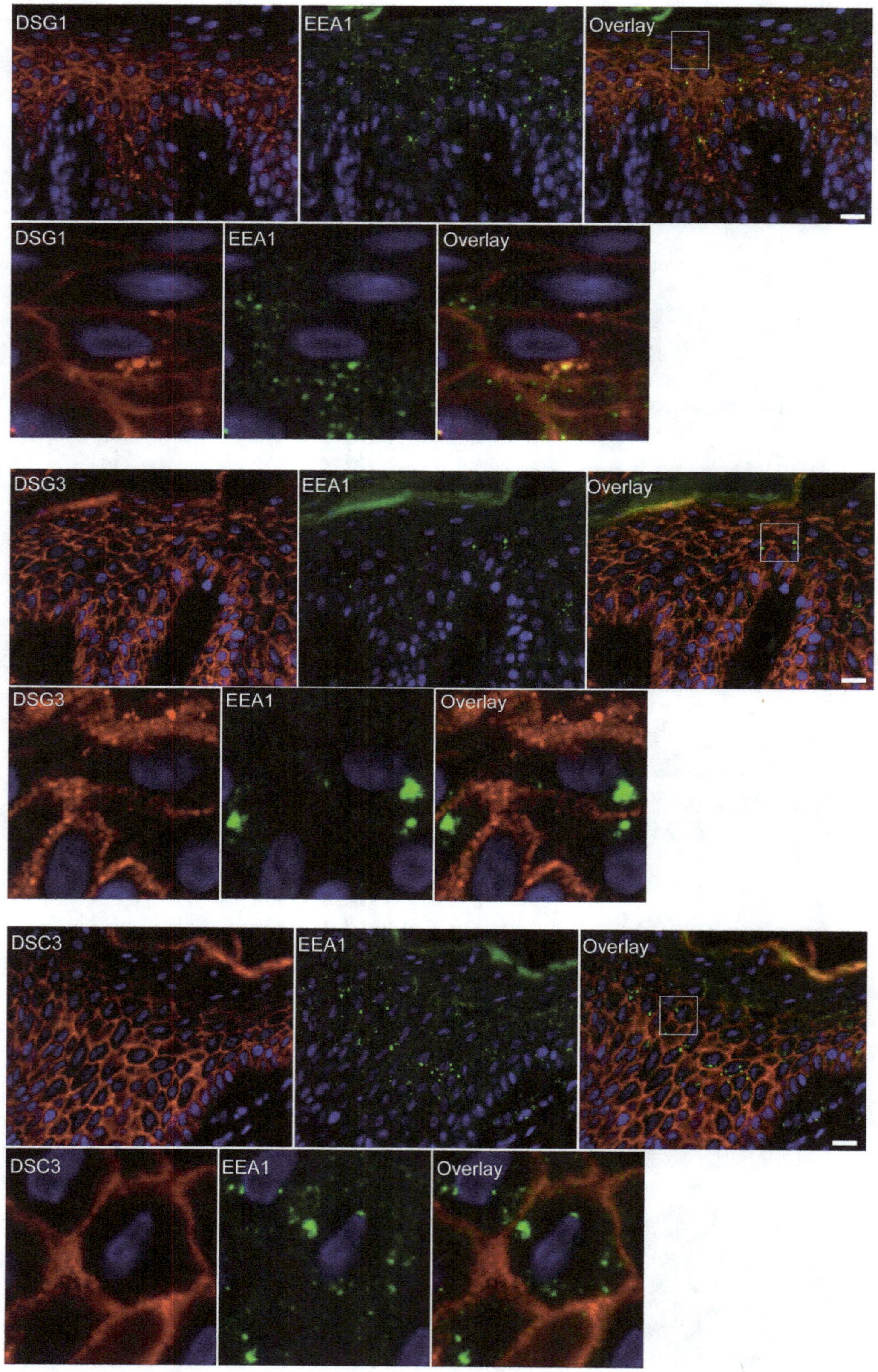

FIGURE 3 | Double staining shows colocalization of EEA1 with desmoglein 1 but not with desmoglein 3 and desmocollin 3. The upper panels show the overviews, the lower panels shows the details from the white boxes in the upper panels. White bar is 20 μm.

become depleted of DSG1 (8). In skin where IgG has induced clustering of DSG1 desmosomes become reduced in size and number (14). The reduction in size of the desmosomes can be induced in *ex vivo* living human skin by both pathogenic or non-pathogenic PF mAb, while their mixture enhances this effect (13).

Tada and Hashimoto (15) studied patient skin by immunoelectron microscopy and found what they called curvicircular cytoplasmic bodies in PF but not in PV skin. These were present in the higher, but not in the lower layers of the epidermis. These structures labeled positive for DSG1, PG, IgG, and connexin 43 (CNX43), and did not contain attachment plaques or inserted tonofilaments. These were hypothesized to be internalized IgG-bound desmosome-gap-junction complexes that transformed into curvicircular structures. In 1999, Iwatsuki et al. described cytoplasmic vesicles in acantholytic keratinocytes that labeled positive for DSG1 and seemed to contain detached desmosomes. We recently described the curvicircular structures to be double membrane structures, that may look intracellular but in fact seem the result of closely sealed (40 nm width) neighboring membranes (www.nanotomy.org). In perilesional skin they are present in the lower epidermal layers and they spread upwards to higher layers in lesional skin (16). We have speculated that these double membrane structures likely are the DSG1-PG-IgG clusters seen by light microscopy.

In order to further unravel the pathomechanism of PF we address in the present the faith of DSG1-PG-IgG clusters and investigate if endocytosis of DSG1 takes place in PF patient skin.

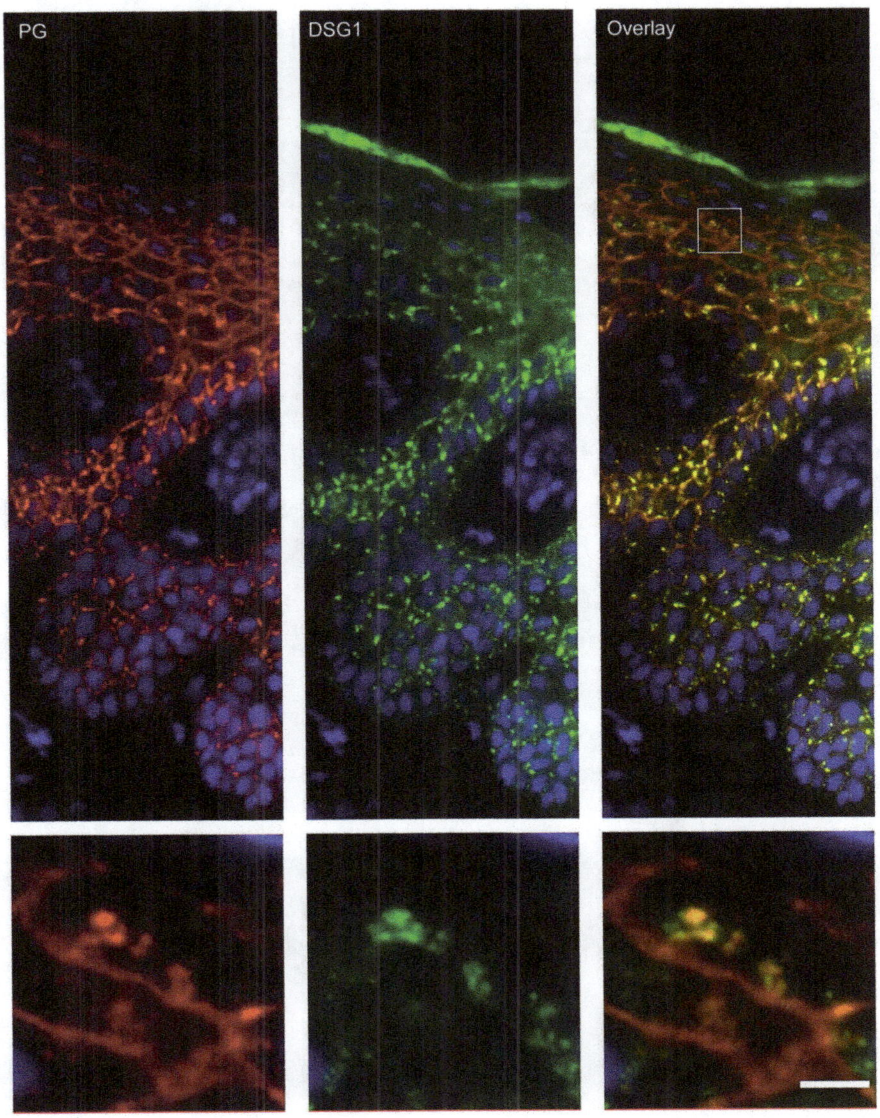

FIGURE 4 | Double staining of desmoglein 1 and plakoglobin 1 shows that these are both present in the endosomes. The upper panel shows the overview, the lower panel shows the detail from the white box in the upper panel. White bar is 5 μm.

MATERIALS AND METHODS

Patient Biopsies

We included 6 PF patients; from these 5 had a biopsy from lesional skin, 1 from perilesional skin, and from three patients we also had a concomitant biopsy from healthy skin.

The diagnosis in all six patients had been established on clinical criteria and laboratory investigation, including histology, positive immunofluorescence of skin (DIF), positive binding of serum IgG (1/40 dilution) to monkey esophagus in an epithelial cell surface (ECS) pattern, and serum anti-DSG1 antibodies by MESACUP-2 ELISA test for anti-DSG1 (MBL, Japan). The skin specimens had been immediately frozen in liquid nitrogen and stored at −80°C. Skin obtained from breast reduction was used as healthy control skin. According to national regulations this type of retrospective non-interventional study on leftover tissue from diagnostics does not need approval from the local medical ethical committee.

Immunofluorescence Microscopy

The procedure for immunofluorescence staining and image collection has been described in detail before (8). For visualization of adhesion molecules we used the following monoclonals: DSG1-P23 and DSG1-P124 (DSG1 ectodomain), 27B2, DG3.10, 18D4 and B-11 (DSG1 endodomain), DSG-G194 (DSG3), U100 (DSC1), U114 (DSC3), 15F11 (PG), DP2.15 (DP), and PKP3-270.6.2 (PKP3). Early endosomal antigen (EEA1) was stained with 14/EEA1, cathepsin D (CTS D) was stained with CTD-19, LAMP-1 with H4A3, and connexin 43 with 4E6.2. Double staining of IgG and adhesion molecules IgG was performed with fluoresceinthiocyanate (FITC)-conjugated Fcγ-specific goat F(ab')2 anti-human IgG (Protos Immunoresearch, Burlingame, CA, U.S.A) and Alexa 568-conjugated goat anti-mouse IgG (Molecular Probes Eugene, OR, U.S.A) as secondary steps. For double staining with two different mouse monoclonals we used

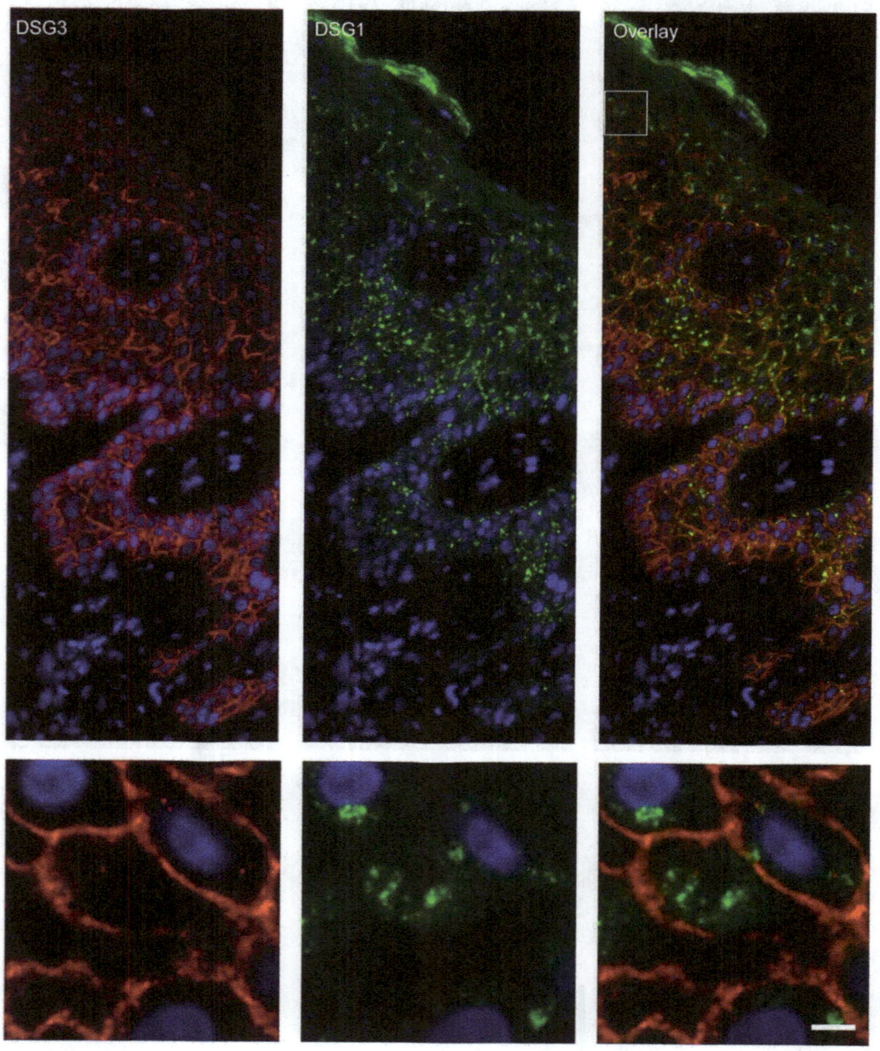

FIGURE 5 | Double staining of desmoglein 1 and desmoglein 3 shows no overlap in endosomes. The upper panel shows the overview, the lower panel shows the detail from the white box in the upper panel. White bar is 5 μm.

Zenon® Mouse IgG Labeling Kits Alexa Fluor®488 and Alexa Fluor®568 (Molecular Probes, Invitrogen, USA) by following technical protocols. **Supplementary Table 1** contains details on antibodies used.

RESULTS

Endosomal Uptake Takes Place in the Upper Layers of Lesional Pemphigus Foliaceus Skin

In order to examine the fate of DSG1, PG, and IgG clusters, we double stained the perilesional and lesional biopsies for EEA1 and IgG. In 4 of the 6 biopsies EEA1 colocalized with IgG demonstrating that IgG is taken up in endosomes. This is most prominent in the higher epidermal layers, next to and beneath the blister (**Figure 1A**). In more differentiated cells these endosomes are largely localized perinuclear (**Figure 1B**). In the 3 biopsies of non-lesional skin of our PF patients no endocytosis was observed. **Figure 2** compares endocytosis of PG in non-lesional skin with perilesional or lesional skin of the same patients. In normal healthy human skin no overlap of EEA1 and PG was observed (**Figure 2**).

Endosomes Contain Desmoglein 1 and Plakoglobin but No Other Desmosomal Proteins

Apart from IgG and PG also DSG1 is present in the same endosomes. In order to examine if other desmosomal components are also endocytosed we examined the localization of other desmosmal proteins in relation to the EEA1/DSG1/PG clusters. No overlap was found. **Figure 3** shows colocalization of EEA1 with DSG1 but not with DSG3 and DSC3. Where DSG1 and PG (**Figure 4**) colocalized in the intercellular

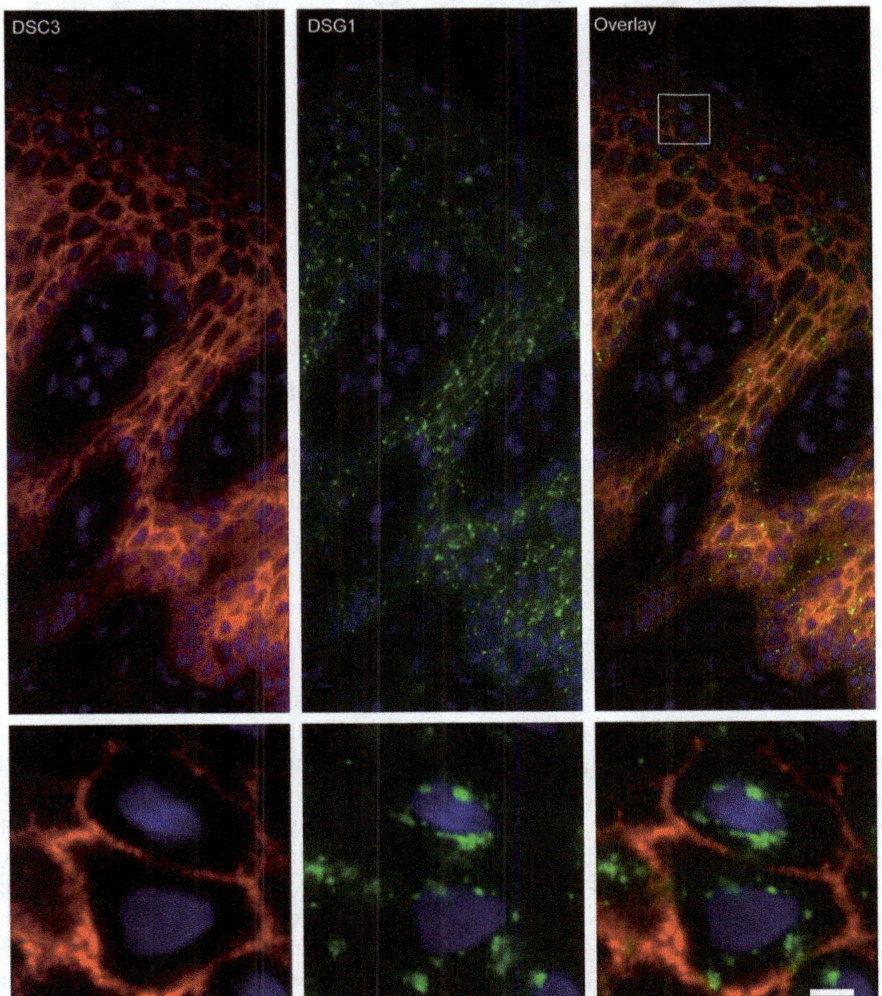

FIGURE 6 | Double staining of desmoglein 1 and desmocollin 3 shows no overlap in endosomes. The upper panel shows the overview, the lower panel shows the detail from the white box in the upper panel. White bar is 5 μm.

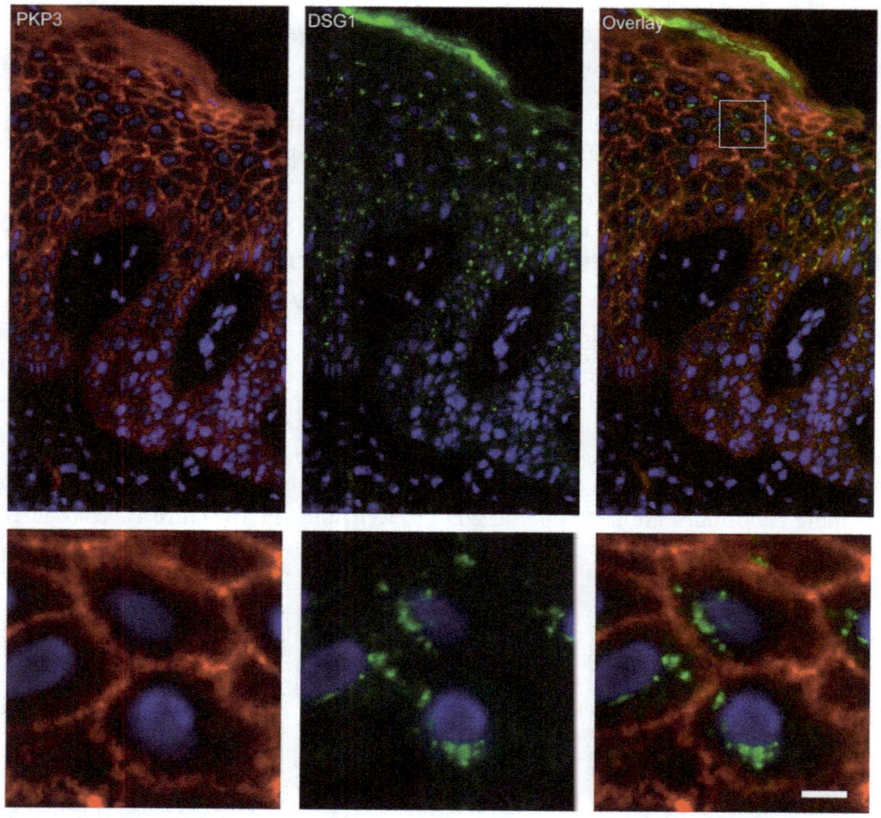

FIGURE 7 | Double staining of desmoglein 1 and plakophilin 3 shows no overlap in endosomes. The upper panel shows the overview, the lower panel shows the detail from the white box in the upper panel. White bar is 5 μm.

vesicles no co-localization of DSG1 with other desmosomal proteins was observed (**Figures 5–8**). The absence of desmosomal proteins as for instance DP in the clusters suggests that extra-desmosomal rather than desmosomal DSG1 is endocytosed.

Endosomal Uptake Starts From the IgG Clusters

In the basal layer endosomes do not contact the IgG clusters (**Figure 9C**). Upwards in the spinal layer endosomes moor on to the clusters and internalization starts to take place (**Figure 9B**). Then finally they become localized perinuclear (**Figure 9A**). Confocal microscopy shows that the endocytosis from the cluster takes place symmetrically in both cells that share the cluster (**Figure 9D**, white arrows).

Endosomes Do Not Contain Connexin 43 and Do Not Fuse With Lysosomes

Double staining of DSG1 and CNX43 showed that both were present in intracellular vesicles but these did not colocalize, implying they originate from different mechanisms (**Figure 10**). Surprisingly CTS D and LAMP-1 did also not colocalize with DSG1 indicating that lysosomes are not a destiny of the IgG-DSG1-PG clusters (**Figure 10**).

DISCUSSION

In this study we demonstrate that the clustered deposits of IgG in PF patient skin are cleared by endocytosis together with the co-clustered components DSG1 and PG (8). Although clusters are present in the basal epidermal layers active endocytosis starts in the spinous layer. Endocytosis is symmetrical in the way that in takes simultaneously place in both cells that share the cluster and progresses in more differentiated keratinocytes toward the cell nucleus.

Tada and Hashimoto suggested that binding of PF autoantibodies induce internalization of intact desmosomes and gap junctions in form of curvicircular structures that contained IgG, DSG1, PG, and CNX43 (15). Our double labeling results however show that CNX43 is present in separate organelles that are likely internalized annular gap junctions (17). Furthermore we did not find internalizations that contained other desmosomal components meaning that endocytosis of intact or half-desmosomes does not take place in PF skin as suggested before (18). Cirillo et al. demonstrated internalization of DSG1 upon incubation with PF patient sera in a monolayer of cultured cells (19). Cultured cells have characteristics of cells from the basal epidermal layer and no internalization of DSG1 was seen in the basal cells in any of PF biopsies. Therefore,

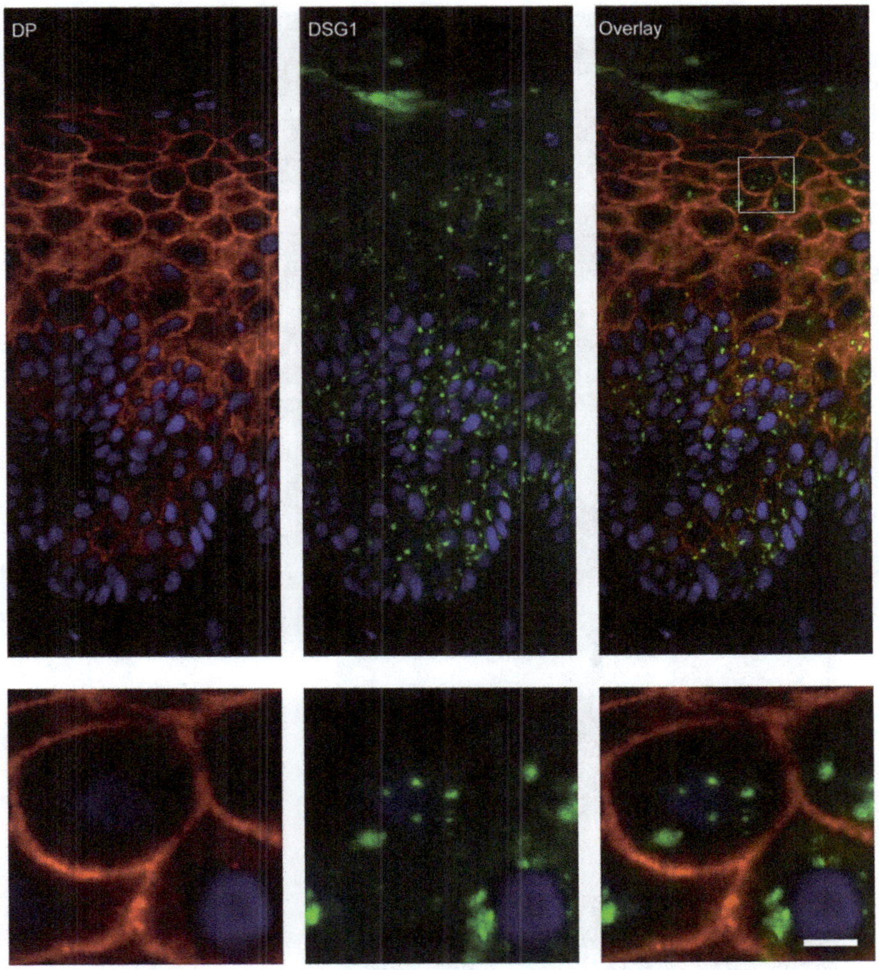

FIGURE 8 | Double staining of desmoglein 1 and desmoplakin shows no overlap in endosomes. The upper panel shows the overview, the lower panel shows the detail from the white box in the upper panel. White bar is 5 μm.

it seems that conclusions reached with cell models have to be interpreted with care.

In contrast with PF, PV was extensively studied in cultured cells and it is shown that PV IgG upon incubation is taken up by endocytosis together with DSG3 and PG (20–23). After 3 h the IgG-DSG3-PG complex colocalized with lysosomes which suggests that cultured cells degrade internalized IgG. However, in PF patient skin we could not find evidence for such a degradation pathway. This suggests that internalized PF-IgG containing endosomes remain in the cell and are finally lost by desquamation. Furthermore in cell monolayer experiments it was shown that upon incubation PV IgG rapidly depletes soluble DSG3 from the membrane followed later by disappearance of desmosomal DSG3 (20, 21). Jennings et al. showed that prior to its internalization insoluble DSG3 is reorganized together with other desmosomal proteins into structures that are perpendicular to the cell membranes that were named linear arrays (23). Stahley et al. by super resolution microscopy observed structures in mucocutaneous PV skin they believed to be the linear arrays from which endocytosis of insoluble DSG3 takes place (24). Although we used simple immunofluorescence microscopy our data do not in any way suggest that such arrays are present in PF skin. Therefore, PV and PF pathogenesis might differ in the way IgG and DSG1 are endocytosed. An indication for this is that in PV skin colocalization of IgG and EEA1 was present in multiple small puncta near the cell membranes while we observed in PF skin that colocalization of IgG and EEA1 is in very large endosomes and only in the upper epidermal layers (24). Furthermore unlike in PV skin endocytosis in PF skin is restricted to the clusters that are induced by the anti-DSG1 IgG only.

Taken together we propose the following sequence of the events in PF patient skin. PF IgG binding to non-desmosomal DSG1 induces clustering and reorganization of non-desmosomal DSG1 together with PG which is bound to the cytoplasmic tail of DSG1. As other molecules as DP are absent desmosomal DSG1 is likely not included in these clusters. This causes lack of DSG1 in desmosomal turnover resulting in depletion of DSG1 from desmosomes and reduction of their size. Reorganized DSG1-PG-IgG are trapped into clusters which are likely the double membrane structures seen by electron

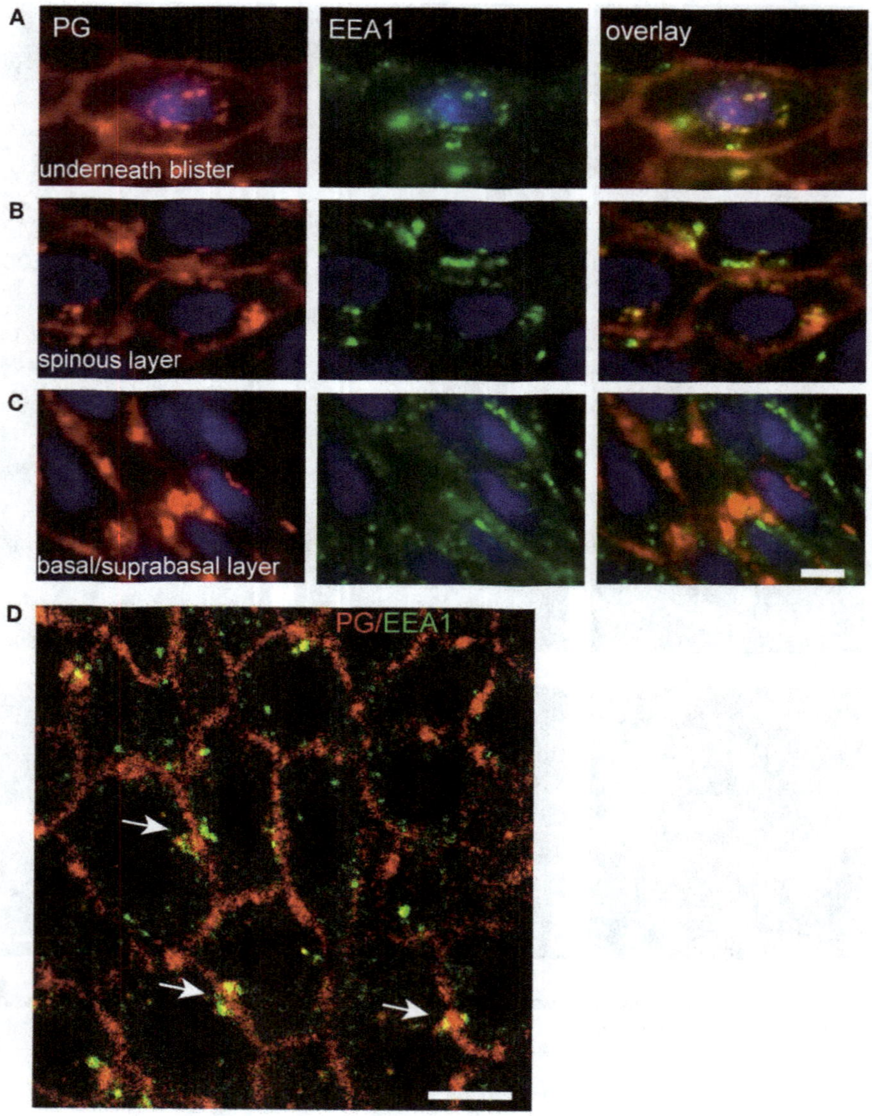

FIGURE 9 | Endocytosis of plakoglobin starts in the spinous layer. Lesional PF skin stained for PG (red) and EEA1 (green). **(A)** Below the blister cavity; **(B)** spinous layer; **(C)** basal/suprabasal layer. Note the colocalization of PG and EEA1 in the spinous layer and below the blister cavity. White bar: 5 μm. **(D)** Confocal microscopy of lesional PF skin stained for PG (red) and EEA1 (green). White arrows indicate symmetrical endocytosis into neighboring keratinocytes. White bar: 10 μm.

microscopy (16). Proteins from these clusters are taken up in endosomal compartments in the upper epidermal layers. This endosomes remain perinuclear until removed with desquamation of keratinocytes. Due to depletion of desmosomes from DSG1 and absence of compensatory DSG3 in the subcorneal layer desmosomes will weaken and finally "melt" away here what leads to blistering. Future research has to address how previous observations on effects of PF serum on signal transduction and the activation of signal transduction molecules are connected to the ultrastructural findings. What does emerge from this and previous studies is that many factors have to be taken into consideration, which complicates such research. For instance why acantholysis only occurs when DSG3 is absent, meaning that whatever is the primary cause of acantholysis, steric hindrance, signal transduction or DSG1 depletion, neither one of them is able to induce acantholysis when DSG3 is still present. It is possible that clustering is a main cause of DSG1 depletion of desmosomes, but PF blisters can also be induced in organ culture in the absence of clustering (8, 10). Then for endocytosis of DSG1 it is unclear why it is absent in the basal layer, although endosomes are present here. Clustering starts in the basal layer as this is the first layer that encounters the pathogenic PF IgG, so something must be missing to start endocytosis.

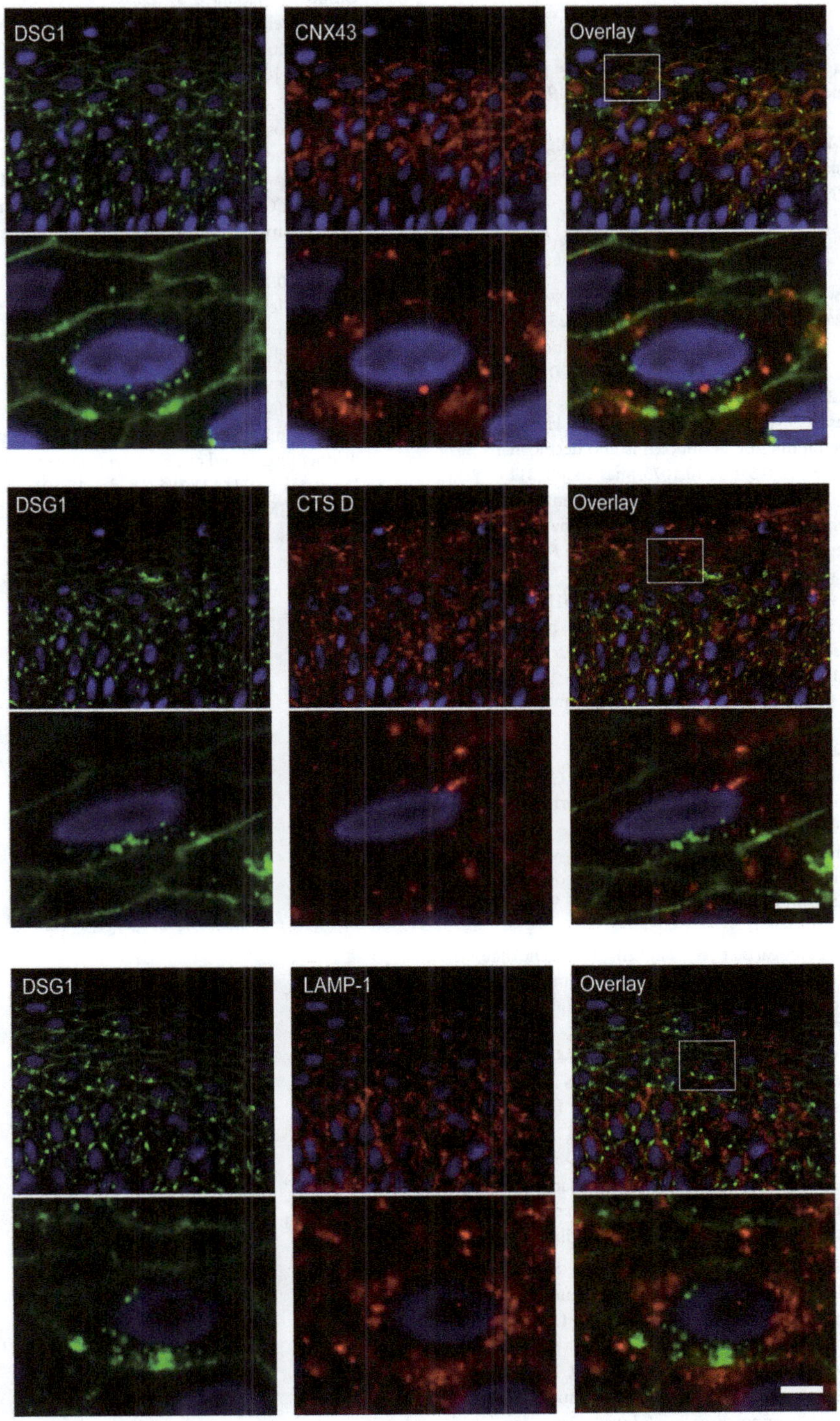

FIGURE 10 | No colocalization of endocytosed desmoglein 1 with connexin 43 and lysosomes in PF skin. Lesional PF patient skin stained for DSG1 and CNX43, upper panel overview with detail underneath, DSG1 and CTS D, middle panel overview with detail underneath, and DSG1 and LAMP-1, lower panel overview with detail underneath. The location of the detailed area is indicated by a white box in the overview. No colocalization is observed. White bar: 5 μm.

AUTHOR CONTRIBUTIONS

DO, HP, and MJ contributed to the design of the study. DO, DK, and ES performed the experiments. DO and ES wrote the manuscript. HP and MJ revised the manuscript.

REFERENCES

1. Stanley JR, Koulu L, Klaus-Kovtun V, Steinberg MS. A monoclonal antibody to the desmosomal glycoprotein desmoglein I binds the same polypeptide as human autoantibodies in pemphigus foliaceus. *J Immunol.* (1986) 136:1227–30.
2. Stanley JR, Amagai M. Pemphigus, bullous impetigo, and the staphylococcal scalded-skin syndrome. *N Engl J Med.* (2006) 355:1800–10. doi: 10.1056/NEJMra061111
3. Garrod D, Chidgey M. Desmosome structure, composition and function. *Biochim Biophys Acta.* (2008) 1778:572–87. doi: 10.1016/j.bbamem.2007.07.014
4. Delva E, Tucker DK, Kowalczyk AP. The desmosome. *Cold Spring Harb Perspect Biol.* (2009) 1:a002543. doi: 10.1101/cshperspect.a002543
5. Kowalczyk AP, Green KJ. Structure, function, and regulation of desmosomes. *Prog Mol Biol Transl Sci.* (2013) 116:95–118. doi: 10.1016/B978-0-12-394311-8.00005-4
6. Harrison OJ, Brasch J, Lasso G, Katsamba PS, Ahlsen G, Honig B, et al. Structural basis of adhesive binding by desmocollins and desmogleins. *Proc Natl Acad Sci USA.* (2016) 113:7160–5. doi: 10.1073/pnas.1606272113
7. Berkowitz P, Chua M, Liu Z, Diaz LA, Rubenstein DS. Autoantibodies in the autoimmune disease pemphigus foliaceus induce blistering via p38 mitogen-activated protein kinase-dependent signaling in the skin. *Am J Pathol.* (2008) 173:1628–36. doi: 10.2353/ajpath.2008.080391
8. Oktarina DA, van der Wier G, Diercks GF, Jonkman MF, Pas HH. IgG-induced clustering of desmogleins 1 and 3 in skin of patients with pemphigus fits with the desmoglein nonassembly depletion hypothesis. *Br J Dermatol.* (2011) 165:552–62. doi: 10.1111/j.1365-2133.2011.10463.x
9. van der Wier G, Pas HH, Jonkman MF. Experimental human cell and tissue models of pemphigus. *Dermatol Res Pract.* (2010) 2010:143871. doi: 10.1155/2010/143871
10. Waschke J, Spindler V, Bruggeman P, Zillikens D, Schmidt G, Drenckhahn D. Inhibition of Rho A activity causes pemphigus skin blistering. *J Cell Biol.* (2006) 175:721–7. doi: 10.1083/jcb.200605125
11. Walter E, Vielmuth F, Rotkopf L, Sardy M, Horvath ON, Goebeler M, et al. Different signaling patterns contribute to loss of keratinocyte cohesion dependent on autoantibody profile in pemphigus. *Sci Rep.* (2017) 7:3579. doi: 10.1038/s41598-017-03697-7
12. Waschke J, Bruggeman P, Baumgartner W, Zillikens D, Drenckhahn D. Pemphigus foliaceus IgG causes dissociation of desmoglein 1-containing junctions without blocking desmoglein 1 transinteraction. *J Clin Invest.* (2005) 115:3157–65. doi: 10.1172/JCI23475
13. Yoshida K, Ishii K, Shimizu A, Yokouchi M, Amagai M, Shiraishi K, et al. Non-pathogenic pemphigus foliaceus (PF) IgG acts synergistically with a directly pathogenic PF IgG to increase blistering by p38MAPK-dependent desmoglein 1 clustering. *J Dermatol Sci.* (2017) 85:197–207. doi: 10.1016/j.jdermsci.2016.12.010
14. van der Wier G, Pas HH, Kramer D, Diercks GFH, Jonkman MF. Smaller desmosomes are seen in the skin of pemphigus patients with anti-desmoglein 1 antibodies but not in patients with anti-desmoglein 3 antibodies. *J Invest Dermatol.* (2014) 134:2287–90. doi: 10.1038/jid.2014.140
15. Tada J, Hashimoto K. Curvicircular intracytoplasmic membranous structures in keratinocytes of pemphigus foliaceus. *J Cutan Pathol.* (1996) 23:511–7. doi: 10.1111/j.1600-0560.1996.tb01443.x
16. Sokol E, Kramer D, Diercks GFH, Kuipers J, Jonkman MF, Pas HH, et al. Large-scale electron microscopy maps of patient skin and mucosa provide insight into pathogenesis of blistering diseases. *J Invest Dermatol.* (2015) 135:1763–70. doi: 10.1038/jid.2015.109
17. Piehl M, Lehmann C, Gumpert A, Denizot JP, Segretain D, Falk MM. Internalization of large double-membrane intercellular vesicles by a clathrin-dependent endocytic process. *Mol Biol Cell.* (2007) 18:337–47. doi: 10.1091/mbc.e06-06-0487
18. Iwatsuki K, Han GW, Fukuti R, Ohtsuka M, Kikuchi S, Akiba H, et al. Internalization of constitutive desmogleins with the subsequent induction of desmoglein 2 in pemphigus lesions. *Br J Dermatol.* (1999) 140:35–43. doi: 10.1046/j.1365-2133.1999.02604.x
19. Cirillo N, Gombos F, Lanza A. Changes in desmoglein 1 expression and subcellular localization in cultured keratinocytes subjected to anti-desmoglein 1 pemphigus autoimmunity. *J Cell Physiol.* (2007) 210:411–6. doi: 10.1002/jcp.20856
20. Sato M, Aoyama Y, Kitajima Y. Assembly pathway of desmoglein 3 to desmosomes and its perturbation by pemphigus vulgaris-IgG in cultured keratinocytes, as revealed by time-lapsed labeling immunoelectron microscopy. *Lab Invest.* (2000) 80:1583–92. doi: 10.1038/labinvest.3780168
21. Calkins CC, Setzer SV, Jennings JM, Summers S, Tsunoda K, Amagai M, et al. Desmoglein endocytosis and desmosome disassembly are coordinated responses to pemphigus autoantibodies. *J Biol Chem.* (2006) 281:7623–34. doi: 10.1074/jbc.M512447200
22. Delva E, Jennings JM, Calkins CC, Kottke MD, Faundez V, Kowalczyk AP. Pemphigus vulgaris IgG-induced desmoglein-3 endocytosis and desmosomal disassembly are mediated by a clathrin- and dynamin-independent mechanism. *J Biol Chem.* (2008) 283:18303–13. doi: 10.1074/jbc.M710046200
23. Jennings JM, Tucker DK, Kottke MD, Saito M, Delva E, Hanakawa Y, et al. Desmosome disassembly in response to pemphigus vulgaris IgG occurs in distinct phases and can be reversed by expression of exogenous Dsg3. *J Invest Dermatol.* (2011) 131:706–18. doi: 10.1038/jid.2010.389
24. Stahley SN, Warren MF, Feldman RJ, Swerlick RA, Mattheyses AL, Kowalczyk AP. Super-resolution microscopy reveals altered desmosomal protein organization in tissue from patients with pemphigus vulgaris. *J Invest Dermatol.* (2016) 136:59–66. doi: 10.1038/JID.2015.353

14

Modifications of the Transcriptomic Profile of Autoreactive B Cells from Pemphigus Patients After Treatment with Rituximab or a Standard Corticosteroid Regimen

Vivien Hébert[1,2*], *Marie Petit*[1], *Maud Maho-Vaillant*[1,2], *Marie-Laure Golinski*[1,2], *Gaëtan Riou*[1], *Céline Derambure*[3], *Olivier Boyer*[1], *Pascal Joly*[1,2] and *Sébastien Calbo*[1]

[1] INSERM U1234, Normandie University, Rouen, France, [2] Department of Dermatology, Rouen University Hospital, Normandie University, Rouen, France, [3] INSERM U1245, Normandie University, Rouen, France

***Correspondence:**
Vivien Hébert
vivien.hebert@chu-rouen.fr

Pemphigus Vulgaris is an autoimmune disease of the skin and mucous membranes, which is due to the production of pathogenic autoantibodies targeting desmoglein (DSG) 1 and 3, which are adhesion proteins of the keratinocytes. Rituximab is an anti-CD20 mAb which induces a prolonged depletion of blood B cells. We recently showed that rituximab was more effective than a standard oral corticosteroid (CS) treatment, allowing 90% of patients to achieve complete remission (CR). Additionally, we showed that DSG-specific-B (DSG positive) cells were still detectable during the B cell recovery which follows the initial rituximab-induced B cell depletion, even in patients in CR. In order to characterize DSG positive B cells in patients in CR after rituximab or CS treatment relative to those detectable at baseline in patients with an active pemphigus, we studied the expression profile of 31 genes of interest related to inflammatory cytokines, TNF receptors and activation markers. Using quantitative Polymerase Chain Reaction performed on one cell with a microfluidic technique, we found that patients' autoreactive B cells collected at baseline had a significantly higher expression of genes encoding for IL-1β, IL-23p19, and IL-12p35 pro-inflammatory cytokines and the IRF5 transcription factor, than non-autoreactive B cells. Surprisingly, the gene expression profile of DSG positive B cells collected after rituximab treatment in patients in CR was close to that of DSG positive B cells at baseline in patients with active pemphigus, except for the IL-1β and the CD27 memory marker genes, which were under-expressed after rituximab compared to baseline. Conversely, we observed a decreased expression of genes encoding for IL-1β and IL-23p19 in patients treated with CS relative to baseline. This study showed that: (i) DSG positive autoreactive B cells have a different gene expression profile than non-autoreactive B cells; (ii) rituximab and CS have different effects on the genes' expression in autoreactive DSG positive B cells from pemphigus patients.

Keywords: pemphigus, rituximab, corticosteriods, autoreactive B cell, transcriptomic analysis

INTRODUCTION

Pemphigus is a rare life-threatening autoimmune blistering disease involving the skin and mucosa, leading to erosions and major weight loss, which severely impair patients' quality of life (1–5). It is characterized by the production of pathogenic autoantibodies directed against two desmosomal proteins involved in keratinocyte adhesion: desmoglein 1 (DSG1) and desmoglein 3 (DSG3) (1, 6). DSG3 is mainly found in deep skin epidermal layers and mucosa, while DSG1 is present throughout the epidermis. Anti-DSG3 antibodies (Abs) are observed in pemphigus vulgaris (PV) with mucosal involvement, and anti-DSG1 Abs are observed in patients with pemphigus foliaceus (PF) and those with PV and skin involvement. Binding of anti-DSG Abs to their target antigen results in a loss of keratinocyte adhesion, leading to the so called "acantholysis" phenomenon, which results in the formation of skin and mucosal blisters (7–9).

Until recently, high-dose of oral corticosteroids (CS) sometimes associated with immunosuppressive drugs (azathioprine, mycophenolate mofetil) were the mainstay of pemphigus treatment (10). A recent large randomized controlled study (RCT) from our group demonstrated the interest of the first line use of rituximab in pemphigus (11). A large difference was evidenced in the primary outcome: 89% of patients in the rituximab + short term CS arm were in complete remission off therapy after 2 years, compared with 34% of patients treated with prednisone alone ($p < 0001$).

Rituximab is a chimeric murine-human monoclonal antibody that binds to the CD20 antigen of B-lymphocytes (anti-CD20 mAb), which is expressed by pre-B-cell and pre-plasma cells. A stop in the renewal of the plasma cell pool is thought to be one of the main mechanisms of the short-term action of rituximab (12, 13). However, the long-term clinical course of pemphigus patients treated with rituximab has not been extensively assessed yet. In particular, apart from a reversal of the naïve/memory B-cell *ratio*, the long-term evolution of reappearing DSG1– and DSG3–specific B cells after rituximab treatment remains largely unknown (14). Furthermore, the effects of oral CS on DSG specific-B cells in pemphigus patients has not been studied yet.

In addition to producing antibodies, B cells secrete multiple cytokines with pro- or anti-inflammatory functions, which can either enhance or downregulate the immune response. Since understanding the long-term modifications of the DSG-specific autoimmune B cell response after rituximab treatment might improve the way we use this drug, we longitudinally analyzed the transcriptomic and phenotypic profiles of one-cell sorted autoreactive DSG-specific B cells from patients with a newly diagnosed pemphigus (during the active phase of disease) and after treatment with rituximab or a standard CS regimen, and compared these results with those observed from non-autoreactive B cells.

RESULTS

Baseline Analysis

Using quantitative polymerase chain reaction (qPCR), we analyzed the single cell mRNA expression of 33 genes encoding for membrane markers, cytokine receptors or transcription factors (**Table SI**) which are known to be expressed in B cells from 20 patients. Among them, nine pemphigus patients were treated by rituximab and assessed at baseline and at Month 36 (18 months after the last rituximab infusion); all of them were in complete remission at M36. Eleven pemphigus patients were treated by oral corticosteroids and assessed at baseline and Month 12, after tapering of CS doses; five of these 11 patients were in clinical complete remission at Month 12. The 20 patients had a pemphigus vulgaris with either isolated mucosal involvement or skin and mucosal involvement. Clinical, biological, and immunologic characteristics of patients are presented in **Tables 1**, **2**. Finally, we performed a transcriptomic analysis in seven out of 14 healthy donors (HD) who were studied with phenotypic analyses. Indeed, DSG1-positive (**Figure 1A**) and DSG3-positive (**Figure 1B**) B cells were detectable in HD, although at a lower frequency than in the 20 patients with active pemphigus (DSG1 positive 0.11 vs. 0.20%, $p < 0.001$; DSG3 positive 0.10% vs. 0.20%, $p < 0.001$).

We first compared the baseline gene expression between non-autoreactive DSG-negative B cells (201 single cells) and autoreactive DSG-positive B cells (191 single cells) from pemphigus patients. We observed that the mRNA of 11 genes (IL-2, IL-5, IL-9, IL-12p40, IL-13, IL-17F, IL-21, IL-27p28, IFNγ, TGF β2, and APRIL) was not detected at baseline neither in DSG-positive, nor in DSG negative B cells from pemphigus patients, whereas all housekeeping genes were detected. Therefore, these latter genes were not further analyzed. The 22 remaining genes detected were used to realize a heat map representing the ΔCT expression of these genes between autoreactive and non-autoreactive B cells at baseline (**Figure 1C**).

At baseline, autoreactive DSG-positive and non-autoreactive DSG-negative sorted B cells showed distinct mRNA expression profiles for the three pro-inflammatory cytokine genes IL-1β, IL-12p35, IL-23p19, and for the transcription factor IRF5 gene which were found to be overexpressed by the DSG-positive relative to the DSG-negative B cell populations (**Figure 1D**), whereas no difference of expression of these four genes was evidenced between DSG-positive (107 single cells) and DSG-negative (69 single cells) B cell populations from HD (data not shown).

Longitudinal Analyses in Patients Treated With Rituximab

We performed a longitudinal analysis by flow cytometry in the nine rituximab-treated pemphigus patients previously analyzed by qPCR. Frequency of DSG1-positive and DSG3-positive autoreactive B cells did not vary significantly between baseline and Month 36 when patients were in complete remission (DSG1 positive: 0.20% vs. 0.22%, $p = 0.67$; DSG3 positive 0.23% vs. 0.25, $p = 0.61$; **Figures 2A,B**).

We then analyzed the expression of selected genes in 306 single DSG-positive B cells from the nine rituximab-treated pemphigus patients, including 191 sorted-cells from blood samples collected at baseline and 115 sorted-cells from samples collected at Month 36 after RTX treatment. One hundred

TABLE 1 | Clinical and biological characteristics of patients from the rituximab group.

Age	Treatment	Type of pemphigus	Severity	ELISA anti-DSG1 Ab value at D0	ELISA anti-DSG3 Ab value at D0	Clinical status at M36	ELISA anti-DSG1 Ab value at M36	ELISA anti-DSG3 Ab value at M36
51	RTX	Mucosal	Moderate	30	750	Complete remission	<20	80
45	RTX	Mucosal	Severe	<20	360	Complete remission	<20	<20
63	RTX	Mucosal	Severe	<20	2,050	Complete remission	<20	111
28	RTX	PV skin + mucosa	Severe	330	120	Complete remission	<20	555
76	RTX	Mucosal	Severe	<20	530	Complete remission	<20	157
80	RTX	PV skin + mucosa	Severe	410	1,805	Complete remission	<20	<20
52	RTX	PV skin + mucosa	Severe	260	4,000	Complete remission	<20	<20
64	RTX	PV skin + mucosa	Severe	200	131	Complete remission	<20	<20
48	RTX	PV skin + mucosa	Severe	356	176	Complete remission	<20	<20

TABLE 2 | Clinical and biological characteristics of patients from the standard corticosteroids (CS) group.

Age	Type of pemphigus	Severity	ELISA anti-DSG1 Ab value at D0	ELISA anti-DSG3 Ab value at D0	Clinical status at M12	ELISA anti-DSG1 Ab value at M12	ELISA anti-DSG3 Ab value at M12
76	PV skin + mucosal	Severe	107	2,400	Complete remission	<20	<20
54	PV skin + mucosal	Severe	1,960	179	Complete remission	<20	<20
66	PV skin + Mucosal	Severe	27	3,350	Complete remission	<20	126
48	PV skin + mucosa	Severe	176	760	Complete remission	<20	<20
33	PV skin + mucosa	Severe	60	143	complete remission	<20	<20
79	PV skin + mucosa	Severe	1,110	553	Incomplete remission	<20	<20
45	PV skin + mucosa	Severe	156	5,217	Incomplete remission	30	1040
61	PV skin + mucosa	Severe	170	1,750	Incomplete remission	<20	550
71	PV skin + mucosa	Severe	665	225	Incomplete remission	77	<20
58	PV skin + mucosa	Severe	1,070	1,065	Incomplete remission	<20	<20
58	PV skin + mucosa	Severe	214	1,979	Incomplete remission	<20	128

and seven single DSG-positive B cells from the seven healthy individuals were used as controls (**Figure 3**).

Interestingly, the expression of the IL-1β gene in DSG-positive B cells, which was higher at baseline in pemphigus patients than in healthy individuals (12 vs. 6%, $p = 0.048$), returned to normal values after rituximab treatment (12 vs. 4%, $p = 0.039$). We also observed that, whereas the frequency of expression of the CD27 memory marker gene in desmoglein-positive B cells collected from pemphigus patients at baseline was close to that observed in healthy individuals (23 vs. 17%, $p = 0.24$), the CD27 gene expression decreased from baseline to Month 36 in pemphigus patients treated with rituximab (23 vs. 10%, $p = 0.03$).

Surprisingly, we did not observe any statistically significant variation in the frequency of the other genes studied between samples collected from pemphigus patients at baseline and after rituximab treatment.

In non-autoreactive desmoglein-negative B cells, rituximab treatment did not induce modification of gene expression for the pro-inflammatory cytokine IL-1β (2 vs. 4.1%, $p = 0.73$) whereas it induced a decreased frequency of expression of the CD27 memory marker gene (15.1 vs. 6.9%, $p = 0.04$; **Figure 4**).

Longitudinal Analyses in Patients Treated With Corticosteroids Alone

We performed a longitudinal flow cytometry analysis in the same 11 corticosteroids-treated pemphigus patients previously analyzed by qPCR. In these 11 CS-treated patients, 311 single DSG-positive cells were isolated including 191 sorted-cells from samples collected at baseline and 120 sorted-cells from samples collected at Month 12. This Month 12 evaluation was chosen because patients still received low doses of prednisone at this time point.

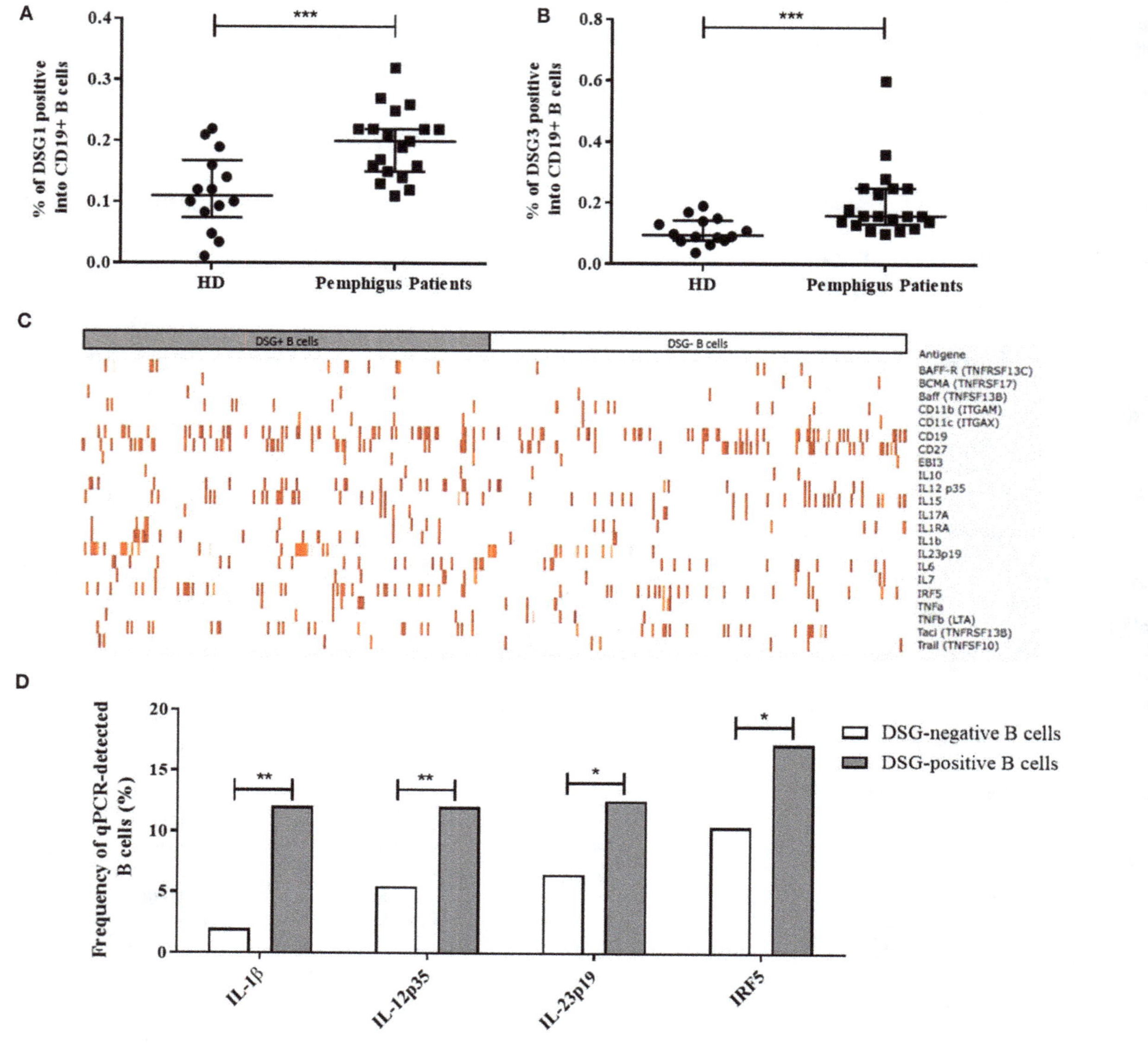

FIGURE 1 | (A,B) Percentage of autoreactive DSG1-positive (CD19+DSG1+) B cells **(A)** and DSG3-positive B cells (CD19+DSG3+) **(B)** among total B cells (CD19+) collected in 14 healthy donors and 20 pemphigus patients at baseline. Median with interquartile range were compared using the Mann-Whitney *t*-test. **(C)** Intensity of gene expression in one-cell sorted DSG-positive B cells (in gray $n = 191$ cells) and non-autoreactive DSG-negative B cells (in white, $n = 201$ cells) from pemphigus patients. The color intensity in each sorted cell depended on the ΔCT value relative to GAPDH house-keeping gene expression. Non-detected genes in one-cell qPCR were excluded from the map. **(D)** Comparison of the baseline frequencies of cells expressing the IL-1β, IL-12p35, IL-23p19 genes, and the transcription factor IRF5 gene between DSG-positive autoreactive B cells (gray columns, $n = 191$ cells) and non-autoreactive DSG-negative B cells (white columns, $n = 201$ cells) from pemphigus patients. Frequencies were compared using the Fisher's exact test.

After treatment with systemic corticosteroids (**Figure 5**), IL-1β gene was downregulated (12–1.7%, $p = 0.003$) allowing to return to values close to those observed in HD. Although the baseline gene expression of the pro-inflammatory cytokine IL-23p19 in desmoglein-positive B cells from patients was close to that detected in healthy individuals (12.5 vs. 15%, $p = 0.59$), we observed a downregulation of the gene after corticosteroids treatment (12.5 vs. 1.2%, $p < 0.005$). We did not observe significant variation in the expression of the other genes studied, including the CD27 memory marker gene (baseline: 23.5% vs. after CS treatment 26.6%, $p = 0.48$).

In non-autoreactive desmoglein-negative B cells (**Figure 6**), corticosteroids treatment induced non-significant variations of the IL-23p19, IL-1β, and CD27 genes, as other genes from the panel studied.

Assessment of the CD27 Memory Marker in Autoreactive B Cells After Rituximab

To extend the results of our transciptomic analysis, we studied the evolution of the CD27 expression on the cell surface of DSG-positive and DSG-negative B cells during treatment with rituximab or corticosteroids. According to the findings from

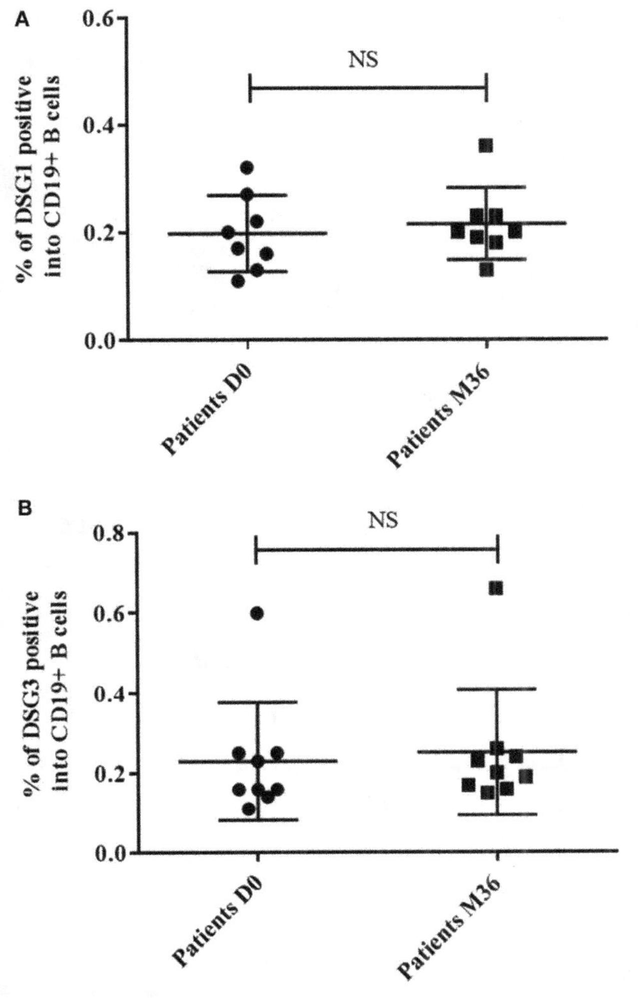

FIGURE 2 | Percentage of autoreactive DSG1-positive B cells (CD19+DSG1+) **(A)** and DSG3-positive B cells (CD19+DSG3+) **(B)** among total B cells (CD19+) collected in pemphigus patients at baseline and at Month 36 after rituximab treatment. Means ± standard deviations were compared using the Wilcoxon paired test.

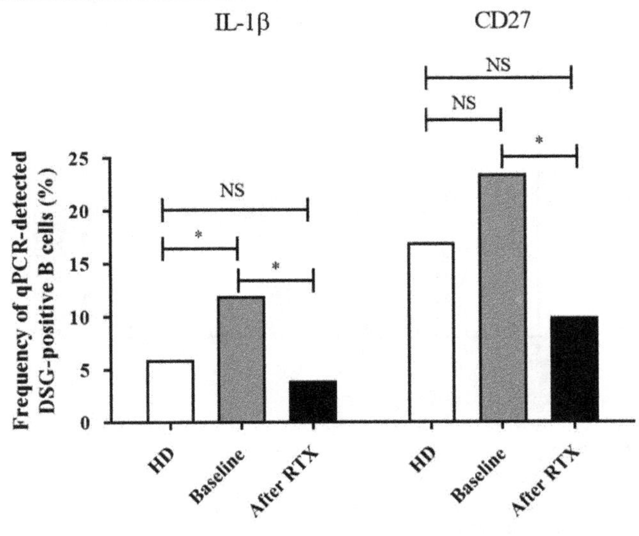

FIGURE 3 | Frequency of cells with detectable mRNA encoding for IL-1β and CD27 in one-cell sorted desmoglein-positive autoreactive B cells from healthy donors (white columns $n = 107$ cells) compared to pemphigus patients before treatment (gray columns, $n = 191$ cells) or after rituximab treatment (black columns, $n = 115$ cells). Frequencies were compared using the Fisher's exact test.

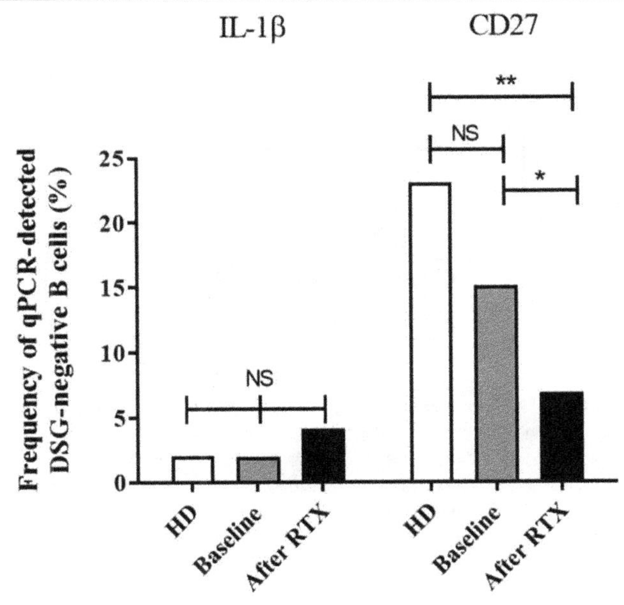

FIGURE 4 | Frequency of cells with detectable mRNA encoding for the IL-1β and CD27 genes in one-cell sorted desmoglein-negative B cells from healthy donors (white columns, $n = 69$ cells) and pemphigus patients at baseline (gray columns, $n = 201$ cells) and after rituximab treatment (black columns, $n = 106$ cells). Frequencies were compared using the Fisher's exact test.

transcriptomic analyses, we observed a significant decrease in the frequency of memory CD19+CD27+ autoreactive DSG-positive and DSG-negative B cells after rituximab treatment (**Figure 7A**), that were not observed in patients treated with CS alone without rituximab (**Figure 7B**).

ELISA Assays

In order to evaluate the consequences of the decreased IL-1β gene expression in DSG-positive B cells from pemphigus patients whether they were treated with corticosteroids or rituximab, we performed longitudinal dosages of serum IL-1β using ELISA assay.

We observed a non-significant decrease of serum IL-1β ELISA values in pemphigus patients during the first 3 months of treatment, that was secondarily followed by a re increase of serum levels to baseline values when corticosteroids doses were tapered during patients' follow-up (**Figure 8**).

Finally, the IL-23p19 cytokine, whose gene expression was downregulated after CS treatment in autoreactive B cells, was also analyzed by ELISA. No significant variation in the IL-23p19 serum level was detected in pemphigus patients whether they were treated with rituximab or CS alone (data not shown).

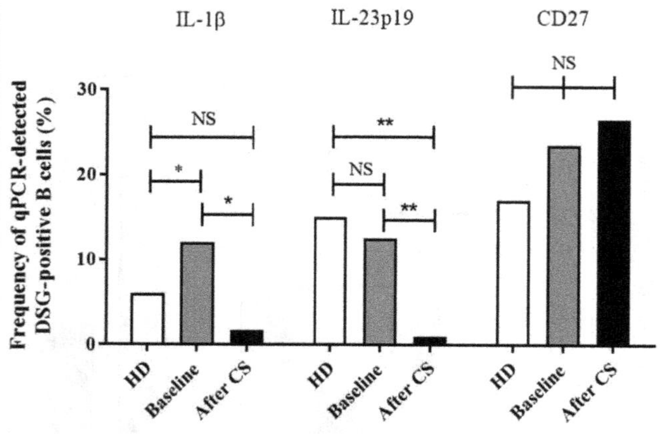

FIGURE 5 | Frequency of cells with detectable mRNA encoding for IL-1β, IL-23p19, and CD27 in one-cell sorted desmoglein-positive from healthy donors (white columns, $n = 107$ cells) compared to pemphigus patients before treatment before (gray columns, $n = 191$ cells) and after CS treatment (black columns, $n = 120$ cells). Frequencies were compared using the Fisher's exact test.

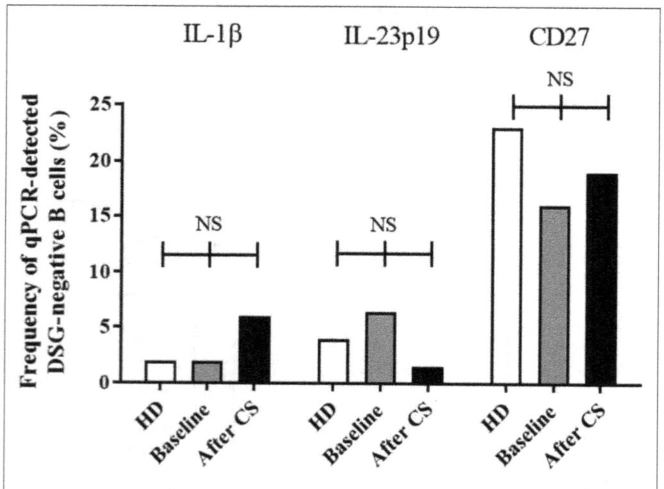

FIGURE 6 | Frequency of cells with detectable mRNA encoding for IL-1β, IL-23p19, and CD27 in one-cell sorted desmoglein-negative B cells from healthy donors (white columns, $n = 69$ cells), and pemphigus patients at baseline before treatment (gray columns, $n = 201$ cells) or after corticosteroids treatment (black columns, $n = 123$ cells). Frequencies were compared using the Fisher's exact test.

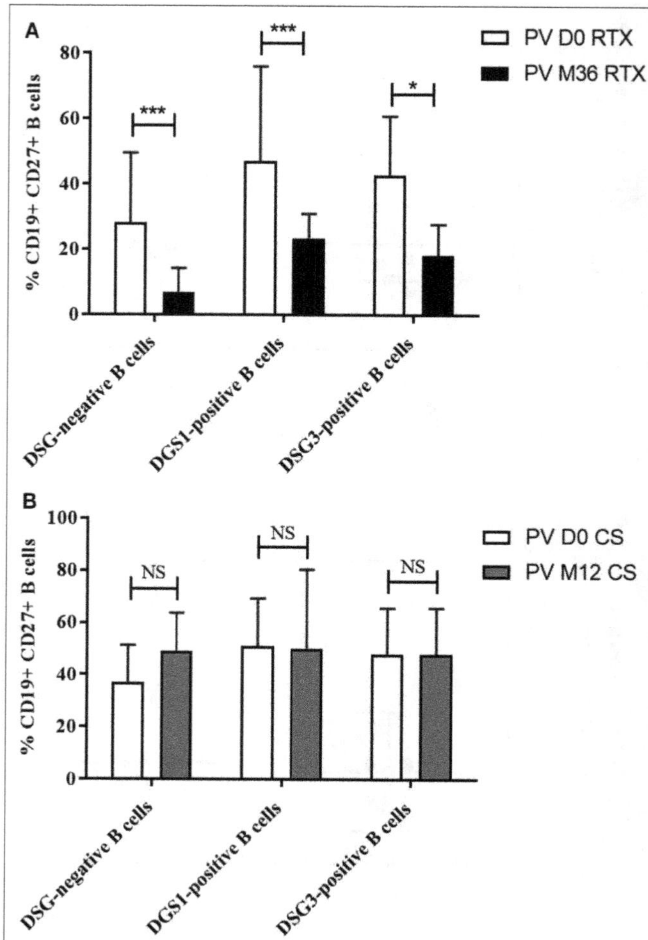

FIGURE 7 | (A) Percentage of memory B cells among non-desmoglein specific, desmoglein 1-specific (DSG1+), and desmogelin three-specific (DSG3+) B cells before (white columns) and after treatment with rituximab (black columns). **(B)** Percentage of memory B cells among non-desmoglein specific, desmoglein 1-specific (DSG1+), and desmogelin 3-specific (DSG3+) B cells before (white columns) and after treatment with corticosteroids (gray columns). Means ± standard deviations were compared using the Wilcoxon paired test.

DISCUSSION

In this study, we assessed the transcriptomic profiles of 33 genes of potential interest in pemphigus on one-cell sorted autoreactive B cells collected from pemphigus patients at different stages of their disease, in particular during the acute phase of the disease, and after two treatments (systemic corticosteroids alone or associated with rituximab) which were compared in a randomized controlled trial (11).

This methodology has several major interests. First, it allowed to study *ex vivo* autoreactive B-lymphocytes, since pemphigus is one of the rare autoimmune diseases in humans in which autoantibodies directed against DSG are pathogenic (15). Second, auto-reactive DSG positive B cells are the pre-stage of antibody-secreting plasma cells, which cannot be easily studied *ex vivo* in humans. Third, the one-cell sorting assays are likely relevant since a very low number of circulating autoreactive B cells in the peripheral blood are enough to trigger the disease, as we showed in the baseline analyses. To the best of our knowledge, this single-cell transcriptome analysis of autoreactive cells is the first one performed in patients with an auto immune disorder.

We first evidenced that the transcriptomic profiles of autoreactive and non-autoreactive B cells collected during the active phase of disease were different. Four out of the 31 genes studied (IL-1β, IL-12p35, IL-23p19, IRF5) were overexpressed in autoreactive relative to non-autoreactive B cells. The most surprising finding in this study was the observation that in addition to the fact that DSG-positive B cells are still detectable after rituximab treatment, arguing against a simple deletion mechanism, the gene expression profile of DSG-positive autoreactive B cells collected after rituximab treatment in patients

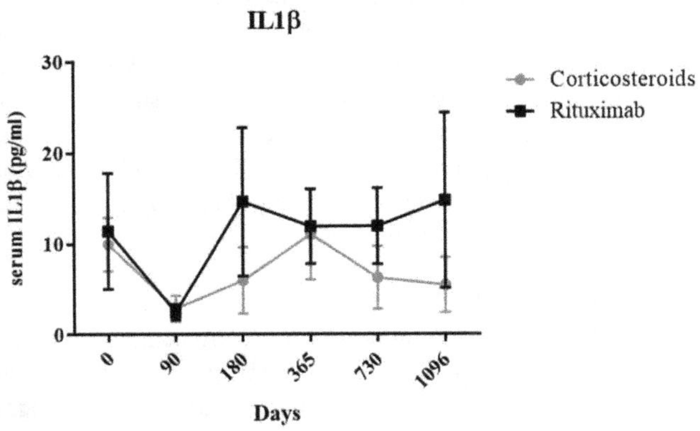

FIGURE 8 | Longitudinal analysis of mean serum IL-1β level in rituximab (black) and corticosteroids-treated (gray) patients. Means ± standard error of the mean were compared with baseline level in each group (RTX and CS) using one-way analysis of variance followed by Bonferroni *post-hoc* test.

in complete remission was actually pretty close to that of DSG-positive B cells collected at baseline in patients with active pemphigus, except for the IL-1β and the CD27 genes, which were downregulated after rituximab compared to baseline.

The downregulation of the CD27 memory marker gene observed in transcriptomic analysis was confirmed by flow cytometry, which showed a lower expression of the CD27 protein at the cell surface of autoreactive B cells after rituximab as well as in non-autoreactive B cells. Thus, the decreased expression of the CD27 gene after rituximab was not specific for DSG-positive B cells. However, the decreased expression of the CD27 marker reflects the blockage of B cell maturation, leading to a prolonged repopulation with naïve B cells, and a delayed reappearance of memory B cells. It has been suggested that autoantibodies are produced by a transitory subpopulation of autoreactive plasmablasts which are continuously refund from autoreactive switched memory B cells (CD20+IgG+CD27+) (13, 16). Thus, changes in CD27 expression which correlates with the disappearance of circulating DSG-positive IgG(+) B lymphocytes are likely responsible for the decreased production of anti-DSG autoantibodies, that contributes to the long lasting clinical remission of the disease after rituximab treatment (14). Another argument which supports this hypothesis is the fact that by using an ELISPOT assay, we showed that DSG3+CD27+ B cells but not DSG3+CD27− B cells are able to differentiate into antibody secreting cells after 72 h of stimulation by IL-2 and R848, a TLR7 and eight ligands (still unpublished data). This mechanism was specifically related to rituximab, since it was not observed in patients treated with CS alone, whether they were in complete or incomplete remission.

Conversely, changes in CD27 do not influence the production of alloreactive antibodies which are produced by long-lived plasma cells which do not express the CD20 marker, explaining the absence of modification of total serum IgG levels in after rituximab in most patients.

We also observed that the expression of the IL-1β gene in DSG specific B cells, which was higher in baseline samples from pemphigus patients than in healthy individuals, and returned to normal values after rituximab or oral CS treatment, whereas no modification was observed in non-autoreactive desmoglein-negative B cells. This observation might suggest the potential role of IL-1β in the pathogenicity of pemphigus, since the downregulation observed in autoreactive B cells paralleled disease remission, whether patients were treated with rituximab or oral CS. Indeed, IL-1β is a pro-inflammatory cytokine mainly produced by hematopoietic cells such as blood monocytes, tissue macrophages and skin dendritic cells in response to TLR ligand, activated complement components or other cytokines such as TNF-α and IL-1β itself (17, 18). In our work, we observed a slight decrease of serum IL-1β during the first 3 months of treatment in both CS- and RTX-treated groups, which was likely related to the effect of high doses of CS. It was then followed by a re-increase of serum levels to baseline values when corticosteroids doses were tapered. The role of IL-1β has previously been suggested by Feliciani et al. who demonstrated that an IL-1β KO mouse model was less susceptible to passive transfer of IgG isolated from the serum of a PV patient. Moreover, Increased concentrations of IL-1α and IL-1β were detected in the serum of untreated PV patients with active disease relative to healthy controls. Additionally, the *in vivo* and *in vitro* production of IL-1α and IL-1β decreased in patients in clinical remission after treatment with IVIG. Finally, IL-1β promotes Th17 polarization, which correlates with disease activity (19–24).

Since the frequency of autoreactive B cells in pemphigus patients was surprisingly only doubled compared to healthy donors, it is likely that the different gene expression profiles of IL-1β and CD27 play a major role in the onset of pemphigus by promoting the emergence/appearance of DSG + CD27+ IgG+ B memory cells, which were only detected in pemphigus patients but not in healthy individuals.

Despite the fact that we observed a difference in the baseline expression of the IL-12p35 between DSG-positive and DSG-negative B cells, we did not observe significant modification in RNA expression in patients in complete remission after rituximab, nor variation in the serum concentration of IL-12p35 during patients' follow-up, which does not support a major role for IL-12p35 in the healing of RTX-treated patients.

We did not analyse the serum concentration of cytokines relevant for B cell activation such as BAFF, APRIL, or IL-6, because we did not observe any modification of the gene expression of these cytokines by autoreactive DSG-positive B cells in our transcriptomic analyses.

Overall, this study showed that self-reactive and non-self-reactive B cell populations from pemphigus patients do not express the same genes during the acute phase of the disease, in particular genes encoding for IL-1β, IL-12p35, IL-23p19, and IRF5. Additionally, DSG-positive autoreactive B cells can still be observed in patients in complete remission, even in those treated with rituximab, when blood B-lymphocytes reappeared after the initial rituximab-induced depletion. Surprisingly, the gene expression of autoreactive DSG-positive B cells in remitted patients was close to that observed at baseline, except for the CD27 gene which was downregulated in patients treated with rituximab, and the IL-1β gene, which was down regulated in both treatment groups, likely related to the effect of oral CS.

METHODS

Clinical Study

In the randomized controlled trial, 90 newly-diagnosed pemphigus patients were randomly assigned to receive a standard regimen of CS vs. rituximab associated with a short-term CS regimen. Patients in the rituximab group were treated with the autoimmune regimen (two infusions of 1,000 mg of rituximab at day 0 and day 14) and a maintenance treatment corresponding to two infusions of 500 mg at Month 12 and Month 18. They also received an initial medium dose of prednisone, 0.5–1 mg/kg/day, depending on initial pemphigus severity (moderate vs. severe), which was rapidly tapered over 3–6 months. Patients assigned in the standard oral CS group were given a higher initial dose of prednisone, 1–1.5 mg/kg/day, with a progressive tapering over 12–18 months, depending on initial pemphigus severity. Patients who participated in the Ritux 3 clinical trial were included in the present study (ClinicalTrials.gov number, NCT00784589).

Patients

Blood samples from rituximab-treated patients were analyzed at baseline before treatment (Day 0) and after 36 months of follow-up, since we had to wait for the recovery of blood B-lymphocytes after the repeated infusions of rituximab at Day 1 and Month 12 and Month 18. Blood samples from CS-treated patients were analyzed before treatment and at Month 12 at which time patients in the standard CS group were still treated with oral CS.

Serum Auto-Antibody Titers and Cytokine Levels

Titers of IgG antibodies against DSG1 and three were measured by a DSG enzyme-linked immunosorbent assay test (ELISA) with 1:100 diluted serums (EUROIMMUN, Germany, Lübeck). Serum levels of IL-1β and Il-23p19 were quantified by ELISA (RD and ebioscience, respectively), according to the manufacturer's protocol.

Phenotyping of Desmoglein-Specific B Cells

In order to analyse DSG1 and DSG3 specific B cells, B cells were isolated using Dynabeads Untouched Human B-cells kit (Life Technologies) according to the manufacturer's instruction. Then, purified B cells were incubated for 30 min at 4°C with histidine-tagged recombinant DSG1 or DSG3 (30 ng/μl). After washing, B cells were stained with anti-human IgG antibodies (BD Biosciences). Cells were then incubated with Fc Block (eBioscience), LIVE/DEAD Fixable Aqua Dead Cell Stain (Life Technologies), anti-human antibodies directed against CD19, CD27, IgM (BD Biosciences). Anti-histidine coupled with phycoerythrin (R&D Systems) was used to identify desmoglein-specific B cells.

One-Cell Sorting and Pre-amplification

DSG-positive single B cells were sorted using FACS ARIA III into 96-well plates containing 10μL Platinum Taq polymerase and SuperScript III reverse transcriptase (Invitrogen), a mixture of Taqman primer-probes at 0.2× concentration specific for the transcripts of interest (**Table SI**) and CellsDirect qRT-PCR buffer (Invitrogen). Immediately after cell sorting, samples were centrifuged, incubated at 55°C for 10 min, and subjected to 30 cycles of PCR (50°C 15 min then 95°C for 15 s for the reverse transcription, followed by 30 cycles of 95°C 15 s, and 60°C 4 min for amplification). Subsequent pre-amplified single-cell cDNA was stored at −20°C until analysis.

Real-Time qPCR

After ¼ dilution in TE buffer, each cDNA sample was then separated into 48 separate reactions for further qPCR using the BioMark 48.48 dynamic array nanofluidic chip (Fluidigm, Inc.). Briefly, following hydraulic chip priming, 48 pre-amplified cDNA samples were mixed with a mild detergent loading solution to allow capillary flow. Samples were then added to a 48.48 nanofluidic chip (Fluidigm, Inc.) along with 38 individual Taqman primer-probe mixtures listed in **Table SI** (Applied Biosystems) specific for individual transcripts of interest, allowing a combination of each sample to mix with each probe in every possible combination (a total of 2,304 reactions). The chip was then thermocycled through 40 cycles and fluorescence in the FAM channel was detected using a CCD camera placed above the chip, normalized by ROX (6-carboxy-X-rhodamine) intensity. A well containing 100 CD19+ cells and a well without cell were used as positive and negative controls, respectively. To limit potentially biased measurement, cells with <2 expressed genes among the five control genes (HPRT1, B2M, GUSB, TUBB, and GAPDH) were excluded from the analysis. Data were analyzed using Real Time PCR Analysis software with or without normalization of the Ct value for each gene using GAPDH as calibrator gene. We considered that sorted cells expressed a gene if the Ct (threshold of detection) value was < 40 and if the detection curve was a sigmoid. Eleven genes were found to be unexpressed by single B cells including IL-2, IL-5, IL-9, IL-12p40, IL-13, IL-17F, IL-21, IL-27p28, IFNγ, TGFβ2, and APRIL. This absence of detection was due to a too low RNA amount since positive control wells containing 100 CD19+ cells showed detectable expression levels of all tested cytokine genes. We compared the frequency of cytokine gene expressing B cells using qPCR between treatment groups.

ΔCt Analysis

The ΔCt analysis allows to determine the intensity of the gene of interest expression in cells by comparing its threshold of detection (Ct) with the Ct of the housekeeping gene.

Statistical Analysis

Statistical comparison of the frequency of gene expressing cells was performed with Fisher's exact test. Statistical comparison of percentages of autoreactive B cells in flow cytometry were calculated using the Mann-Whitney *t*-test to compare healthy donors and pemphigus patients; and using the Wilcoxon *t*-test to compare patients before and after treatment. All analyses were performed using the GraphPad Prism Software. A p-value ≤ 0.05

was considered as significant. The *, **, *** refer to statistical values explained in the legends.

AUTHOR CONTRIBUTIONS

VH: transcriptomic, cytometric acquisitions, analyses, ELISA assays, and writer. MP: transcriptomic acquisitions. MM-V: transcriptomic, cytometric acquisitions, and ELISA assays. M-LG: cytometric acquisitions. GR: cytometric analyses. CD: transcriptomic analyses. OB: drafting and revision. SC and PJ: transcriptomic analyses, cytometric analyses, drafting, and revision.

REFERENCES

1. Amagai M, Klaus-Kovtun V, Stanley JR. Autoantibodies against a novel epithelial cadherin in pemphigus vulgaris, a disease of cell adhesion. *Cell.* (1991) 67:869–77. doi: 10.1016/0092-8674(91)90360-B
2. Stanley JR. Pemphigus and pemphigoid as paradigms of organ-specific, autoantibody-mediated diseases. *J Clin Invest.* (1989) 83:1443–8. doi: 10.1172/JCI114036
3. Anhalt GJ, Labib RS, Voorhees JJ, Beals TF, Diaz LA. Induction of pemphigus in neonatal mice by passive transfer of IgG from patients with the disease. *N Engl J Med.* (1982) 306:1189–96. doi: 10.1056/NEJM198205203062001
4. Langan SM, Smeeth L, Hubbard R, Fleming KM, Smith CJP, West J. Bullous pemphigoid and pemphigus vulgaris–incidence and mortality in the UK: population based cohort study. *BMJ.* (2008) 337:a180. doi: 10.1136/bmj.a180
5. Stanley JR, Amagai M. Pemphigus, bullous impetigo, and the staphylococcal scalded-skin syndrome. *N Engl J Med.* (2006) 355:1800–10. doi: 10.1056/NEJMra061111
6. Eyre RW, Stanley JR. Human autoantibodies against a desmosomal protein complex with a calcium-sensitive epitope are characteristic of pemphigus foliaceus patients. *J Exp Med.* (1987) 165:1719–24. doi: 10.1084/jem.165.6.1719
7. Hashimoto T, Amagai M, Garrod DR, Nishikawa T. Immunofluorescence and immunoblot studies on the reactivity of pemphigus vulgaris and pemphigus foliaceus sera with desmoglein 3 and desmoglein 1. *Epithelial Cell Biol.* (1995) 4:63–9.
8. Sekiguchi M, Futei Y, Fujii Y, Iwasaki T, Nishikawa T, Amagai M. Dominant autoimmune epitopes recognized by pemphigus antibodies map to the N-terminal adhesive region of desmogleins. *J Immunol Baltim Md 1950.* (2001) 167:5439–48. doi: 10.4049/jimmunol.167.9.5439
9. Amagai M, Tsunoda K, Zillikens D, Nagai T, Nishikawa T. The clinical phenotype of pemphigus is defined by the anti-desmoglein autoantibody profile. *J Am Acad Dermatol.* (1999) 40(2 Pt 1):167–70. doi: 10.1016/S0190-9622(99)70183-0
10. Zhao CY, Murrell DF. Pemphigus vulgaris: an evidence-based treatment update. *Drugs.* (2015) 75:271–84. doi: 10.1007/s40265-015-0353-6
11. Joly P, Maho-Vaillant M, Prost-Squarcioni C, Hebert V, Houivet E, Calbo S, et al. First-line rituximab combined with short-term prednisone versus prednisone alone for the treatment of pemphigus (Ritux 3): a prospective, multicentre, parallel-group, open-label randomised trial. *Lancet Lond Engl.* (2017) 389:2031–40. doi: 10.1016/S0140-6736(17)30070-3
12. Zambruno G, Borradori L. Rituximab immunotherapy in pemphigus: therapeutic effects beyond B-cell depletion. *J Invest Dermatol.* (2008) 128:2745–7. doi: 10.1038/jid.2008.330
13. Mouquet H, Musette P, Gougeon M-L, Jacquot S, Lemercier B, Lim A, et al. B-cell depletion immunotherapy in pemphigus: effects on cellular and humoral immune responses. *J Invest Dermatol.* (2008) 128:2859–69. doi: 10.1038/jid.2008.178
14. Colliou N, Picard D, Caillot F, Calbo S, Le Corre S, Lim A, et al. Long-term remissions of severe pemphigus after rituximab therapy are associated with prolonged failure of desmoglein B cell response. *Sci Transl Med.* (2013) 5:175ra30. doi: 10.1126/scitranslmed.3005166
15. Futamura S, Martins C, Rivitti EA, Labib RS, Diaz LA, Anhalt GJ. Ultrastructural studies of acantholysis induced *in vivo* by passive transfer of IgG from endemic pemphigus foliaceus (Fogo Selvagem). *J Invest Dermatol.* (1989) 93:480–5. doi: 10.1111/1523-1747.ep12284041
16. Ellebrecht CT, Payne AS. Setting the target for pemphigus vulgaris therapy. *JCI Insight.* (2017) 2:e92021. doi: 10.1172/jci.insight.92021
17. Dinarello CA. Interleukin-1 in the pathogenesis and treatment of inflammatory diseases. *Blood.* (2011) 117:3720–32. doi: 10.1182/blood-2010-07-273417
18. Garlanda C, Dinarello CA, Mantovani A. The interleukin-1 family: back to the future. *Immunity.* (2013) 39:1003–18. doi: 10.1016/j.immuni.2013.11.010
19. Feliciani C, Toto P, Amerio P, Pour SM, Coscione G, Shivji G, et al. *In vitro* and *in vivo* expression of interleukin-1alpha and tumor necrosis factor-alpha mRNA in pemphigus vulgaris: interleukin-1alpha and tumor necrosis factor-alpha are involved in acantholysis. *J Invest Dermatol.* (2000) 114:71–7. doi: 10.1046/j.1523-1747.2000.00835.x
20. Bhol KC, Desai A, Kumari S, Colon JE, Ahmed AR. Pemphigus vulgaris: the role of IL-1 and IL-1 receptor antagonist in pathogenesis and effects of intravenous immunoglobulin on their production. *Clin Immunol Orlando Fla.* (2001) 100:172–80. doi: 10.1006/clim.2001.5061
21. Santarlasci V, Cosmi L, Maggi L, Liotta F, Annunziato F. IL-1 and T helper immune responses. *Front Immunol.* (2013) 4:182. doi: 10.3389/fimmu.2013.00182
22. Asothai R, Anand V, Das D, Antil PS, Khandpur S, Sharma VK, et al. Distinctive Treg associated CCR4-CCL22 expression profile with altered frequency of Th17/Treg cell in the immunopathogenesis of Pemphigus Vulgaris. *Immunobiology.* (2015) 220:1129–35. doi: 10.1016/j.imbio.2015.06.008
23. Xu R-C, Zhu H-Q, Li W-P, Zhao X-Q, Yuan H-J, Zheng J, et al. The imbalance of Th17 and regulatory T cells in pemphigus patients. *Eur J Dermatol EJD.* (2013) 23:795–802. doi: 10.1684/ejd.2013.2177
24. Hennerici T, Pollmann R, Schmidt T, Seipelt M, Tackenberg B, Möbs C, et al. Increased frequency of T follicular helper cells and elevated interleukin-27 plasma levels in patients with pemphigus. *PLoS ONE.* (2016) 11:e0148919. doi: 10.1371/journal.pone.0148919

15

Junctional Epidermolysis Bullosa: Allelic Heterogeneity and Mutation Stratification for Precision Medicine

Irina Condrat[1,2], *Yinghong He*[1], *Rodica Cosgarea*[2] *and Cristina Has*[1*]

[1] *Department of Dermatology and Venerology, Medical Center - University of Freiburg, Faculty of Medicine, University of Freiburg, Freiburg, Germany,* [2] *Department of Dermatology, Iuliu Hatieganu University of Medicine and Pharmacy, Cluj Napoca, Romania*

Correspondence:
Cristina Has
cristina.has@uniklinik-freiburg.de

Junctional epidermolysis bullosa (JEB) is a hereditary blistering disease caused by reduced dermal-epidermal adhesion due to deficiencies of one of the proteins, laminin-332, type XVII collagen, integrin $\alpha6\beta4$ or integrin $\alpha3$. Significant progress has been achieved in the development of therapies for EB, such as bone-marrow transplantation, local or systemic injections with fibroblasts or mesenchymal stromal cells, readthrough of premature termination codons, or exon skipping. These were tailored in particular for dystrophic EB, which is caused by type VII collagen deficiency and have not yet reached broad clinical practice. Recently, pioneering combined gene and stem cell therapy was successful in treating one boy with junctional EB. Beside these exclusive approaches, no specific therapy to amend the major clinical features, skin and mucosal blistering and non-healing wounds is available to date. Here we extend the mutational spectrum of junctional EB, provide a stratification of *COL17A1* mutations and discuss potential molecular therapeutic approaches.

Keywords: junctional epidermolysis bullosa, collagen XVII, *COL17A1*, mutation, premature termination codon, therapy

INTRODUCTION

Inherited epidermolysis bullosa (EB) is a group of genetic diseases characterized by skin fragility and is caused by mutations in the genes encoding different proteins with roles in cell adhesion. Junctional EB (JEB) is a subtype of EB in which dermal-epidermal adhesion is reduced, due to deficiencies in one of the proteins laminin-332, type XVII collagen, integrin $\alpha6\beta4$ or integrin $\alpha3$ (1).

Type XVII collagen (also known as ERED, BP180, BPA-2, BPAG2, LAD-1, BA16H23.2) is expressed by basal epidermal keratinocytes and plays an important role in cell-matrix interactions as a transmembrane component of the hemidesmosomes. Structurally, type XVII collagen is a homotrimer, consisting of three collagen alpha-1(XVII) chains, each with a molecular weight of 180-kDa. It is a type II protein, which spans the cell membrane with two domains, an endodomain toward the cytosol and an ectodomain toward the lamina densa of the basement membrane. It links, together with integrin $\alpha6\beta4$ and CD151, the inner hemidesmosomal plaque consisting of plectin and BPAG1 to the anchoring filaments buildup of laminin-332 (2). The primary, secondary and tertiary structures, post-translational modifications, as well as interactions and functions of type XVII collagen have been recently extensively reviewed (3, 4).

The main function of type XVII collagen as an adhesion molecule is assured by tight, but dynamic incorporation into hemidesmosomal multiprotein complexes in stratified, pseudostratified and transitional epithelia (e.g., skin, oral mucosa, ocular conjunctiva, epithelial basement membrane of the cornea, upper esophagus, transitional epithelium of the bladder). Besides this role in cell-matrix adhesion, type XVII collagen is responsible for maintenance of follicular stem cells, cell polarity, and migration.

Against this dogma, recent studies provide evidence for the presence of type XVII collagen between the basal keratinocytes, this type being known as the non-hemidesmosomal collagen XVII (4). Non-hemidesmosomal collagen XVII is not a part of the dermal-epidermal adhesion and after its discovery, questions emerged regarding its role. Molecular interactions and cross-talk with focal adhesions and the actin cytoskeleton may be implicated (5, 6). Watanabe and colleagues reported that reduction of non-hemidesmosomal collagen XVII in the interfollicular epidermis is involved in physiological aging, but further work is required in order to decode the exact mechanism (4, 5). Besides these findings, type XVII collagen is also found in the hair follicles stem cells and its proteolytic degradation grounds for age-related hair loss, making it a potential targeted candidate for age-related alopecia, explaining definitive hair loss in patients with JEB (7, 8).

Type XVII collagen is encoded by *COL17A1* which spans 52 kb of the genome and is located on the long arm of chromosome 10 (10q24.3). *COL17A1* consists of 56 exons and short introns. Mutations in this gene lead to a complete or partial loss-of-function of type XVII collagen in tissues and cause generalized or localized skin blistering, amelogenesis imperfecta, epithelial recurrent erosion dystrophy, alopecia and nail dystrophy (3). Although life expectancy is not reduced, patients with JEB due to *COL17A1* pathogenic variants experience extensive trauma-induced blistering resulting in multiple wounds that tend to heal slower with time, excessive caries, diffuse progressive irreversible alopecia, and have impaired quality of life (**Figure 1**).

Currently, EB research is focused on elucidating the disease mechanisms and development of therapies (9). Experimental therapeutic approaches include *ex vivo* gene therapy to correct *LAMB3* and *COL7A1* mutations in epidermal stem cells (10, 11), cell therapies for dystrophic EB, repurposed drugs with anti-inflammatory effects for dystrophic EB and EB simplex and topical agents aiming at improving wound healing. There is an urgent need for new treatments for JEB with *COL17A1* mutations for which no experimental therapies are presently available.

Extensive genetic testing and research has provided a comprehensive database (Human Gene Mutation Database® Professional 2018.2) with over 100 distinct mutations encountered in *COL17A1*, but the database constant development is an ongoing task. The need for such mutational and patients databases is crucial for patients' counseling and prognosis. Development of therapies and selection of patients for clinical trials also depends on their individual mutations.

Abbreviations: EB, epidermolysis bullosa; JEB, junctional epidermolysis bullosa; PTC, premature termination codon; NMD, nonsense mediated decay.

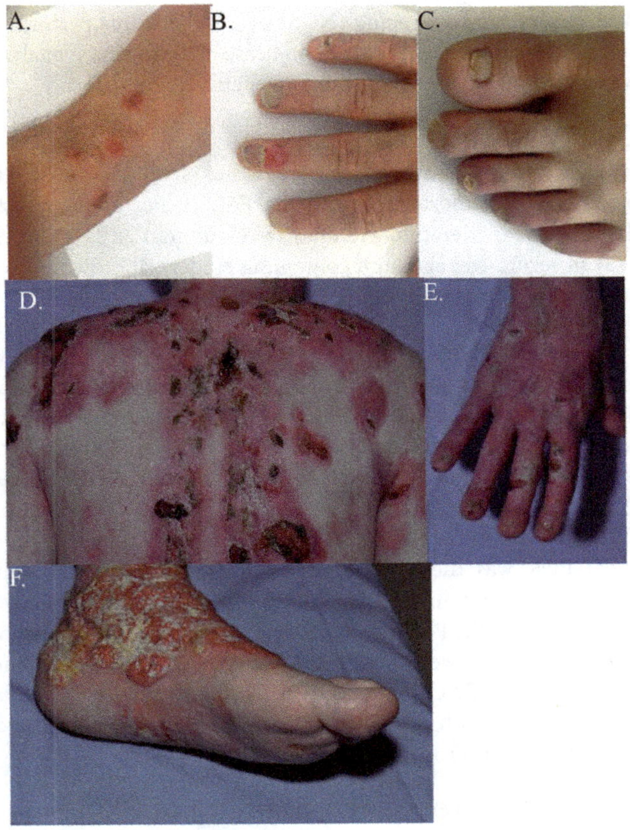

FIGURE 1 | Clinical presentation and different phenotypes in JEB. The clinical manifestations of two JEB patients, both with *COL17A1* mutations. **(A–C)** Case 66, compound heterozygous with a missense mutation c.3908G > A and a deletion c.4100_4101delTT, mildly affected. **(A)** discrete erosions and blisters on upper hand; **(B)** nail dystrophy and crusts on the hand; **(C)** toe-nail dystrophy. **(D–F)** Case 68, a 45 y-old male compound heterozygous with a missense mutation c.2T > A and a deletion c.3164delT, severely affected. **(D)** Extensive crusts and scarring on the upper posterior thorax. **(E)** Nail dystrophy, erosions and crusts on the right hand. **(F)** Squamous cell carcinoma on the lower left leg.

Here, we review our cohort comprising of 68 JEB patients with *COL17A1* mutations diagnosed over the past 15 years, report novel mutations, genotype-phenotype correlations and finally, discuss potential experimental therapies for these patients.

METHODS

The study was conducted according to the Principles of Helsinki and was approved by the Ethics Committee of the University of Freiburg. Written informed consent was obtained from the participants for the publication of the case reports and identifiable images included in this article.

Mutation Detection

After informed consent genomic DNA was extracted from EDTA-blood using the Qiagen blood minikit (Qiagen, Hilden Germany). In most cases, mutation analysis was performed by bidirectional Sanger sequencing as reported before (12). Targeted next generation sequencing (NGS) of EB genes was performed since 2016 as described (13). In one case clinical exome analysis was performed (http://www.humangenetik-freiburg.de/).

Cell Culture

Human primary keratinocytes were isolated from the skin of the patients and immortalized with the E6E7 genes as previously described (14). Keratinocyte lines were cultured at 37°C in 5% CO_2 in serum-free medium containing epidermal growth factor and bovine pituitary extract (Invitrogen).

RNA Isolation and RT-PCR

Isolation of total RNA from confluent cell monolayers was performed using the RNeasy Plus Kit (Qiagen, Hilden, Germany) according to the manufacturer's instructions. One Microgram of isolated RNA was used for cDNA synthesis with the First Strand cDNA Synthesis Kit (Thermo Fisher Scientific, Wilmington, USA) in a volume of 100 μl.

RT-PCR was then performed with 5 μl of the cDNA in a 50 μl mix containing 10x Puffer, nucleoside diphosphatase (dNTP), Taq DNA Polymerase (Sigma) and primers. Primers for *COL17A1* cDNA were F: TACCATGTACGTGTCAGGCC and R: TGATGCTGGACCACACATTG. The annealing temperature was calculated with UCSC *in-silico* PCR (https://genome.ucsc.edu/cgi-bin/hgPcr).

Immunofluorescence Staining of Skin Sections

Biopsy technique, tissue processions, antigen-antibody interaction, and afterwards visualization were previously described (15).

Protein Isolation and Immunoblotting

For protein extraction, cells were lysed on ice for 20 min in lysis buffer, proteinase inhibitors and phosphatase inhibitors and centrifuged for 20 min at 14,000 rpm. Extracts were subsequently heated to 95°C for 5 min. Bradford assay (BioRad) was used to determine the protein concentration. For collagen XVII immunodetection (case 61), 35 μg protein was run on a 8% SDS Page for 1.5 h and transferred to a nitrocellulose membrane at 300 mA for 1.5 h. For detection, collagen XVII-specific antibodies were used: NC16A, against epitope within the NC16A region, at a dilution of 1:1000 (16).

RESULTS

The results of the genetic and molecular analysis of the cohort are described below. Also, novel mutations, genotype-phenotype correlations, and immunofluorescence mapping are reported in **Table 1**.

Novel *COL17A1* Mutations and Genotype-Phenotype Correlations

This study contributes to the *COL17A1* mutational database with 9 mutations that, to the best of our knowledge, have not been reported before (**Table 1**, **Figure 2**). These include two nonsense mutations c.1750C > T, p.R584* and c.4153C > T, p.Q1385*, five frameshift mutations, one mutation of the translation initiation codon, and one splice site mutation. Several of these cases demonstrated interesting genotype-phenotype correlations or clinical course of the disease and will be highlighted here.

Case 61 was a female patient suffering from mild skin blistering since birth. Epidermolysis bullosa simplex was suspected and several candidate genes analyzed, but no mutations were found. Clinically, skin blisters and erosions were present on the face, upper posterior thorax, and lower limbs (**Figure 3**). As the girl grew older, nails became dystrophic and were progressively lost, suggesting the diagnosis of JEB. She was found to be compound heterozygous for the *COL17A1* mutations c.1750C > T, p.R584* and c.3509-1G > C. To the best of our knowledge both mutations were previously unreported. The mutation c.3509-1G > C is located in intron 49 of *COL17A1* and alters the conserved acceptor splice site. RT-PCR and sequencing of the RNA extracted from keratinocytes of the patient revealed that an alternative splice site was used, 33 nucleotides downstream in the middle of exon 50, thus restoring the reading frame and allowing the synthesis of an eleven amino acids shorter truncated polypeptide. Intriguingly, in immunofluorescence mapping, the immunoreactivity for collagen XVII with the commercial monoclonal antibody NC16A3 (Abcam) was comparable to the control skin (**Figure 3B**). The polyclonal sera NC16A (17) demonstrated reduced immunoreactivity in the skin of the patient and a decreased amount of collagen XVII in lysates from patient's keratinocytes as compared to the controls (**Figure 3B**), explaining the mild phenotype.

Case 66 was a 22-year-old male who presented with acral blistering that had started at the age of 16 and was induced by sport activities. Additionally, he displayed nail dystrophy (**Figures 1A–C**). Immunofluorescence microscopy demonstrated a broadened staining pattern of type XVII collagen and no skin split. Clinical exome sequencing demonstrated that he was compound heterozygous for the *COL17A1* mutations c.3908G>A, and the frame shift deletion c.4100_4101delTT, p.F1367Cfs*8, that truncates the last 130 amino acids in the C-terminus of the α1(XVII)-chain.

The severe clinical picture of generalized intermediate JEB is illustrated in case 68 from our cohort, a 45-year-old male, compound heterozygous for the previously unpublished mutation in the translation initiation codon, c.2T>A, p.?, and the also novel frame-shift deletion c.3164delT, p.F1055Sfs*11. Generalized blistering resulted in multiple chronic non-healing wounds at sites of permanent trauma (**Figures 1D,E**); on such a wound on the lower left leg, he developed a squamous cell carcinoma at the age of 44 (**Figure 1F**). Although initially the histological aspect was that of a verrucous carcinoma, recurrence occurred rapidly with local invasion, necessitating amputation. This is the only patient of this cohort who developed squamous cell carcinoma during the observation period. Squamous cell carcinoma has been reported in JEB patients from The Netherlands (18), but the precise risk for developing this complication in JEB remains unknown.

TABLE 1 | Mutational analysis, immunofluorescence mapping and genotype-phenotype correlations of the patients previously unpublished.

Case	Mutations c.DNA level	Mutation Protein level	Immunofluorescence	Clinical phenotype (age)
44	**c.4153C>T**	**p.Q1385***	Not available	Not available
45	c.2861delG	p.G954Afs*112	Not available	Not available
49	c.2062C>T	p.R688*	Negative staining for collagen XVII	Severely affected with generalized blistering, nail dystrophy (age 1)
50	c.2407G>T	p.G803*	Reduced immunoreactivity for collagen XVII	Multiple blisters and erosions, nail loss, dental abnormalities (age 3)
51	c.[3487G>T;4319dup]	p.[E1163*;G1441Wfs*14]	Reduced immunoreactivity for collagen XVII	Mildly affected, nail dystrophy (age 1)
52	c.2237del	p.G746Afs*53	Reduced immunoreactivity for collagen XVII, almost negative	Severely affected, extensive blisters and erosion, nail loss (1 week old)
58	c.418_419delAG	p.S140*	Reduced immunoreactivity for collagen XVII, almost negative	Not available
59	c.[2237delG;3198C>T]	p.[G746Afs*53;S1066S]	Strongly reduced immunoreactivity for collagen XVII at the blister roof	Mildly affected
60	c.2062C>T	R688*	Negative staining for collagen XVII	Not available
61	**c.[1750C>T;3509-1G>C]**	**p.[R584*;?]**	Reduced immunoreactivity for collagen XVII at blister floor (**Figure 3**)	Mildly affected, nail dystrophy and loss (age 2) (**Figure 3**)
62	**c.2282_2283delGG**	**p.G761Dfs*40**	Reduced immunoreactivity for collagen XVII, almost negative	Not available
64	**c.[779delC;3569dupG]**	**p.[P260Qfs*32;N1191Qfs*51]**	Reduced immunoreactivity for collagen XVII at blister roof	Skin blisters, alopecia, nail loss
65	c.2062C>T	p.R688*	Negative staining for collagen XVII	Flaccid serous and hemorrhagic blisters, alopecia, poikiloderma, multiple hypopigmented scarred areas, mucosal involvement, generalized enamel defects
66	c.[3908G>A;**4100_4101delTT]**	p.[R1303Q;F1367Cfs*8]	Collagen XVII is present at blister roof	Mildly affected (see **Figure 1**)
68	**c.[2T>A;3164delT]**	p.[?;F1055Sfs*11]	Not available	Severely affected (see **Figure 1**) and squamous cell carcinoma

*Mutations in bold have not been reported before. *if only one mutation mentioned, then homozygous.*

Stratification of *COL17A1* Mutations

Stratified medicine, and in particular stratification of mutations, focuses on establishing a therapeutic approach tailored to the specific needs of a patient. Therefore, determining the most prevalent mutations and addressing their consequences is a practical and feasible concept, with previous work in cystic fibrosis supporting this aim (19).Currently, no international database of patients with JEB and *COL17A1* mutations is available, although many countries have established registries with clinical, molecular and follow up data for EB patients. Over 100 distinct *COL17A1* mutations have been reported in the literature (HGMD professional as of 1/15/2018) including 24 nonsense mutations, 14 missense mutations, 24 splicing mutations, 27 small deletions, 20 small insertions, one small indel, one gross deletion, and one gross insertion. Even though *COL17A1* is the only gene involved, phenotypes may differ in severity, so that mutations leading to complete loss of type XVII collagen will result in a more severe phenotype as compared to mutations that allow some degree of protein synthesis and function.

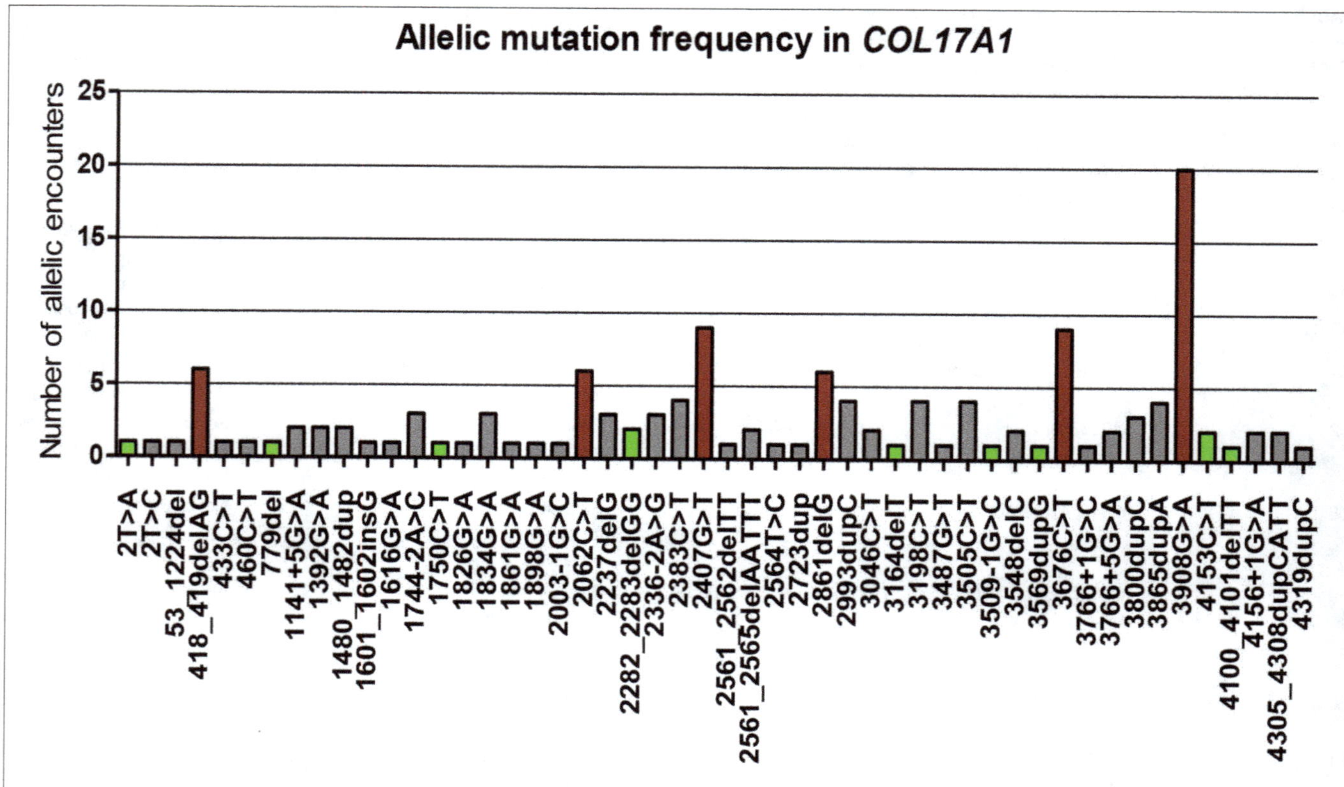

FIGURE 2 | Illustration of all 50 distinct mutations (both previously published and not) and their allelic mutation frequency, included in the article. The mutations have been sorted based on their position on the *COL17A1* gene. Mutations are at cDNA levels. Novel mutations are highlighted in green squares and the most frequent are shown in dark red squares. The Y axis represents numbers of allelic encounters in our cohort.

In the past 15 years we have systematically performed molecular diagnostics for EB employing immunofluorescence mapping and mutation detection (13, 15). Altogether, we identified 68 patients with JEB with *COL17A1* mutations, with a mean of about 5 new cases per year.

Fifty distinct *COL17A1* mutations were identified (**Table 2**). Evaluation and stratification of these mutations was performed based on the number of allelic encounters and mutation type (**Figure 2**). As shown in **Figure 2**, most mutations are unique, occurring in single cases / families and only few are recurrent. Approximately 33% of *COL17A1* mutant alleles are nonsense mutations, and another 33% are frame shift mutations leading to formation of premature termination codons (PTC). Splice site mutations account for 10% of mutant alleles.

In this cohort, the most frequent recurrent mutation was c.3908G > A, p.R1303Q detected in 16.17% of cases and 14.70% of the mutant alleles (in 9 patients in a homozygous state and in 2 patients in heterozygous manner), respectively. This missense mutation changes the amino acid arginine with glutamine and is located in the fourth non-collagenous domain (NC4) of the α1(XVII)-chain, which is part of the putative laminin-332 binding region in type XVII collagen (20). Secondary protein structure analysis and predicted changes in the structural integrity within this binding region suggested that these modifications result in abnormal laminin-332 binding (21). This mutation also appears to hamper the physiological C-terminal cleavage of type XVII collagen. Consequently, non-cleaved type XVII collagen ectodomain remnants induce the aberrant deposition of laminin-332 in the extracellular matrix (12, 22). Clinically, p.R1303Q is associated with a mild, Kindler-syndrome-like phenotype, manifesting with late onset skin blistering, progressive skin atrophy and sclerosis, loss of dermatoglyphics, scarring, and nail anomalies. Typically, type XVII collagen is deposited at the dermal-epidermal junction in a broad irregular pattern (13, 16).

Second most common mutation was c.2407G > T, representing 6.61% of the mutant alleles in 10.29% of cases (in 5 patients in a heterozygous state and in 2 homozygous patients). This mutation located in exon 34, where it converts a glycine residue to a premature termination codon (PTC), p.G803*,was also frequent in patients with Austrian (18) and Finish background (23). With the same allele frequency there was also c. 3676C > T, found in 11.76% of patients. It also translates into a PTC, p.R1226*. This recurrent mutation has also been previously reported in Dutch population (24) and leads to nonsense mediated mRNA decay, demonstrated by absence of full length collagen XVII (12, 25). Next, we found c.2062C > T, p.R688*, c.2861delG, p.G954Afs*112 and 418_419delAG, p.S140* to represent 4.41% of the mutant alleles in 4.31% of our patients. All these null-mutations lead to absence of type XVII collagen and generalized intermediate JEB (previously known as generalized atrophic benign epidermolysis bullosa (GABEB) and

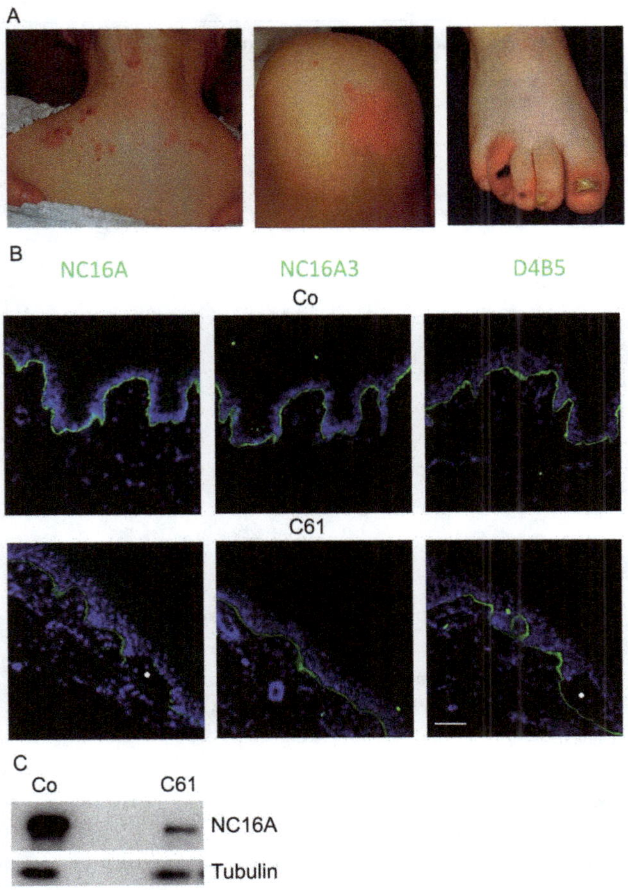

FIGURE 3 | Case 61, a 2 y-old female JEB patient, mildly affected. **(A)** Clinical manifestations include skin blisters on the upper posterior thorax, erosions on the lower limb and nail dystrophy on lower limbs. **(B)** Immunofluorescence antigen mapping performed with domain-specific antibodies against collagen XVII (NC16A, NC16A3) and collagen IV (D4B5) on normal control human skin (Co, upper pictures) and case 61 (C61, lower pictures) with JEB. The antibodies used were NC16A rabbit polyclonal (Abcam), NC16A3 mouse monoclonal (Medimabs), and D4B5 mouse monoclonal for collagen IV (Abcam). Collagen XVII and collagen IV appear in green and nuclei appear in blue. Blisters are marked with circles. **(C)** Immunoblot analysis with lysates from control normal keratinocytes and from Case 61 with NC16A and antibodies to tubulin, as a loading control. Scale bar for all panels 100 μm.

later as non-Herlitz JEB). This most severe *COL17A1*-associated phenotype was the first to be recognized (12, 17, 22). The main clinical manifestation is represented by mechanically induced skin blistering that starts at birth, is generalized and persists lifelong, without spontaneous improvement. Repeated wound and healing episodes result in skin scarring and atrophy. Nails become dystrophic and are progressively lost, as are scalp and body hairs. Teeth exhibit amelogenesis imperfecta which leads to excessive and premature caries and loss of dentition.

Such stratification of mutations endorses the high frequency of nonsense mutations or frame-shift leading to premature termination codons and the need for therapy of JEB patients. Moreover, the recurrence rates gives perspective to the possible similarities between different cultural backgrounds or to the extent in which external factors may impact this disease.

DISCUSSIONS

Consequences of *COL17A1* Mutations and Potential Therapeutic Strategies

Potential therapeutic strategies emerge from analysis of the mutations, their consequences and from the resulting phenotypes (**Table 2**). Patients with acral or late onset JEB, like our cases 61 and 66, have limited disease burden and can be treated symptomatically. In contrast, severely affected patients, like our case 68 require effective therapeutic strategies for their chronic wounds. There is also no existing treatment for other disease manifestations, such as: (i) hair loss, which is definitive; (ii) nail dystrophy or loss, which are regarded as cosmetic problems; (iii) amelogenesis imperfecta leading to increased caries and premature destruction of teeth, which require careful and sustained dental care and treatment. The analysis of genotype-phenotype correlations in patients the JEB suggests that 12–25% of the normal type XVII collagen levels are sufficient to provide a certain degree of skin stability and consequently ameliorate the phenotype (3).

Taking into account the large number of *COL17A1* PTC-mutations, therapies to restore the mutant gene seem to be appropriate in this EB subtype. In our study 33% of mutations are nonsense mutations. These relatively high figures render the thoroughfare for an efficient therapeutic approach directed against these particular types of mutations. *Ex-vivo* gene therapy, where the defective gene is corrected, transduced in cells and later grafted to the patient is highly complex and expensive. As an alternative approach, RNA trans-splicing was developed and showed expression of the replaced exon 52 in up to 61% assayed cells *in vitro* (26).

Revertant mosaicism is frequent in patients with JEB-*COL17A1* (18), but GMP-cultivation and expansion of revertant epidermal stem cells is not yet broadly available. Because type XVII is solely synthetized by keratinocytes and must be correctly assembled as a transmembrane protein in a supramolecular complex, fibroblast / mesenchymal stem cell therapies and protein therapy are not feasible.

Type XVII collagen has a modular collagenous structure, and *COL17A1* has 54 out of 56 exons in-frame, except of the first and last. In-frame truncations seem to be tolerated, and account for the presence of molecules which are stable and partially functional, such in our case 61 and in other cases reported in the literature (27, 28). Thus, antisense-mediated skipping of exons with PTCs might also be an alternative strategy for *COL17A1* mutations (29).

Nevertheless, drug-based therapeutic strategies that aim to modify either the synthesis of protein by inducing readthrough or the mechanisms that lay the ground for RNA translation might be easier available. Suppression of stop codons and enabling readthrough in translation can be effective for several genetic disorders, including EB (24, 27, 30, 31).

Readthrough therapy modifies the response of the translational ribosome to nonsense mutations, by allowing a near-cognate aminoacyl tRNA to step into the spot on the stop codon and thus proceeding toward protein synthesis and allowing a functional protein to be produced. In order to restore

TABLE 2 | Cohort description with position of mutations on *COL17A1* gene and proposed treatment based on the type of mutation.

COL17A1 mutations cDNA	Location	Mutation protein	Proposed treatment	Comment
2T>A	2	?	Gene therapy	
2T>C	2	?	Gene therapy	
53_1224del	3	?	Gene therapy	
418_419delAG	8	S140*	Readthrough	
433C>T	8	R145*	Readthrough	
460C>T	8	R154*	Readthrough	
779del	11	P260Qfs*32	Gene therapy	
1141+5G>A	IVS14	Residual expression of full-length collagen XVII due to leaky splice site	Symptom reliefing therapies	Moderate disease severity
1392G>A	17	W464*	Readthrough	
1480_1482dup	18	K494dup	Symptom reliefing therapies	Moderate disease severity
1601_1602insG	18	S534Efs*10	Exon 18 in frame skipping	
1616G>A	18	G539E	Symptom reliefing therapies	Moderate disease severity
1744-2A>C	IVS20	In frame skipping of exons 21 and 22 or partial skipping of exon 21 leading to residual expression of collagen XVII	Symptom reliefing therapies	Moderate disease severity
1750C>T	21	R584*	Readthrough	
1826G>A	22	G609D	Symptom reliefing therapies	Moderate disease severity
1834G>A	22	G612R	Symptom reliefing therapies	Moderate disease severity
1861G>A	23	G621S	Symptom reliefing therapies	Moderate disease severity
1898G>A	23	G633D	Symptom reliefing therapies	Moderate disease severity
2003-1G>C	IVS24	?	Gene therapy	
2062C>T	26	R688*	Readthrough	
2237delG	30	G746Afs*53	Exon 30 in frame skipping	
2282_2283delGG	31	G761Dfs*40	Exon 31 in frameskipping	
2336-2A>G	IVS31	In frame skipping of exon 32 leading to expression of truncated protein	Symptom reliefing therapies	Moderate disease severity
2383C>T	33	R795*	Readthrough	
2407G>T	34	G803*	Readthrough	
2561_2565delAATTT	37	N854Tfs*109	Exon 37 in frame skipping	
2561_2562delTT	37	N854Ifs*110	Exon 37 in frame skipping	
2564T>G	37	L855*	Readthrough	
2723dup	40	G909Rfs*56	Exon 40 in frame skipping	
2861delG	43	G954Afs*112	Exon 43 in frame skipping	
2993dupC	44	G999Wfs*22	Exon 44 in frame skipping	
3046C>T	45	Q1016*	Readthrough	
3164delT	46	F1055Sfs*11	Exon 46 in frame skipping	
3198C>T	46	Residual expression of full-length collagen XVII due to leaky splice site	Symptom reliefing therapies	Moderate disease severity
3487G>T	49	E1163*	Readthrough	
3505C>T	49	R1169*	Readthrough	
3509-1G>C	IVS49	In frame skipping of part of exon 50 leading to truncated protein expression	Symptom reliefing therapies	Moderate disease severity
3548delC	50	P1183Rfs*68	Exon 50 in frame skipping	
3569dupG	50	N1191Qfs*51	Exon 50 in frame skipping	
3676C>T	51	R1226*	Readthrough	Recurrent mutation
3766+1G>C	IVS51	Out of frame and absence of collagen XVII	Gene therapy	
3766+5G>A	IVS51	Absence of collagen XVII	Gene therapy	
3800dupC	52	G1268Rfs*25	Exon 52 in frame skipping	
3865dupA	52	S1289Kfs*4	Exon 52 in frame skipping	

(Continued)

TABLE 2 | Continued

COL17A1 mutations cDNA	Location	Mutation protein	Proposed treatment	Comment
3908G>A	52	R1303Q	Symptom reliefing therapies	Late onset and moderate disease severity
4153C>T	52	Q1385*	Readthrough	
4100_4101delTT	52	F1367Cfs*8	Exon 52 in frame skipping	
4156+1G>A	IVS52	In frame skipping of exon 52	Symptom reliefing therapies	Moderate disease severity
4305_4308dupCATT	54	Q1437Hfs*19	Symptom reliefing therapies	Moderate disease severity
4319dupC	54	G1441Wfs*14	Symptom reliefing therapies	Moderate disease severity

stands for a premature termination codon.

the function of nonsense mutations carrying genes several compounds have been identified in the last decades. The PTCs are normally recognized by a mechanism called nonsense-mediated mRNA decay (NMD), which tries to eliminate them in order to reduce errors in the expression of a particular gene. NMD efficiency can influence the response of readthrough by several factors (32). Particularly, when some key factors in NMD pathway are inhibited, such as ATP dependent RNA helicase upframeshift 1 (UPF1) and upframeshift 2 (UPF2), a better function of the gene implicated in the pathology of cystic fibrosis was noticed (32). On the contrary, in recessive dystrophic epidermolysis bullosa, it has been shown that a better response to readthrough was associated with an increase in the factor UPF1 in all cells treated, results which support that the more stable this UPF1 factor is, the more inhibited NMD pathway is (33). Another factor that can be limiting in the response of readthrough could be the PTC bearing transcripts of patients. These may vary among individuals and could be beneficial to assess before treatment (32).

CONCLUSIONS

We report here nine previously unpublished mutations, which will enhance the already established database with *COL17A1* mutations. The additionally reported genotype-phenotype correlations will help in diagnosis and genetic counseling, thus providing advantage in the clinical setting. The stratification of the mutations and their consequences should also provide insights for mutation analysis strategies and potential therapies.

As far as therapeutic strategies are regarded for *COL17A1* PTC-mutations, readthrough compounds and exon skipping-approaches seem to be reliable and aim at increasing stability of the skin, wound healing and improving the quality of life. Progress still needs to be made for the other cutting-edge therapeutic possibilities.

AUTHOR CONTRIBUTIONS

CH has molecularly characterized the cohort of patients and has written the final version of the manuscript. IC has analyzed the data, performed the molecular analyses in patient 61, the characterization of the cell lines and has drafted the manuscript and figures. YH has analyzed data. RC has contributed with the phenotypes analysis. All authors have read and corrected the manuscript.

ACKNOWLEDGMENTS

We thank Dr. Julie Christiansen for sending samples and providing clinical pictures of patient 61. We thank Prof. Jürgen Kohlhase and his team for the collaboration. We thank all patients and their families and our physician colleagues. The excellent technical assistance of Juna Leppert, Vera Morand, Gabriele Grüninger, Käthe Thoma, and Ioannis Athanasiou is acknowledged. We thank also Kirstyn Crossley for proofing the manuscript language-wise. We thank all our clinician colleagues and the EB center Freiburg.

REFERENCES

1. Fine J-D, Bruckner-Tuderman L, Eady RAJ, Bauer EA, Bauer JW, Has C, et al. Inherited epidermolysis bullosa: updated recommendations on diagnosis and classification. *J Am Acad Dermatol.* (2014) 70:1103–26. doi: 10.1016/j.jaad.2014.01.903
2. Walko G, Castañón MJ, Wiche G. Molecular architecture and function of the hemidesmosome. *Cell Tissue Res.* (2015) 360:529–44. doi: 10.1007/s00441-015-2216-6
3. Has C, Nyström A, Saeidian AH, Bruckner-Tuderman L, Uitto J. Epidermolysis bullosa: Molecular pathology of connective tissue components in the cutaneous basement membrane zone. *Matrix Biol.* (2018) 71–72:313–29. doi: 10.1016/j.matbio.2018.04.001
4. Natsuga K, Watanabe M, Nishie W, Shimizu H. Life before and beyond blistering: the role of collagen XVII in epidermal physiology. *Exp Dermatol.* (2018) doi: 10.1111/exd.13550. [Epub ahead of print].

5. Watanabe M, Natsuga K, Nishie W, Kobayashi Y, Donati G, Suzuki S, et al. Type XVII collagen coordinates proliferation in the interfollicular epidermis. *eLife* (2017) 6:e26635. doi: 10.7554/eLife.26635
6. Hiroyasu S, Colburn ZT, Jones JCR. A hemidesmosomal protein regulates actin dynamics and traction forces in motile keratinocytes. *FASEB J.* (2016) 30:2298–310. doi: 10.1096/fj.201500160R
7. Matsumura H, Mohri Y, Binh NT, Morinaga H, Fukuda M, Ito M, et al. Hair follicle aging is driven by transepidermal elimination of stem cells via COL17A1 proteolysis. *Science* (2016) 351:aad4395. doi: 10.1126/science.aad4395
8. Tanimura S, Tadokoro Y, Inomata K, Binh NT, Nishie W, Yamazaki S, et al. Hair follicle stem cells provide a functional niche for melanocyte stem cells. *Cell Stem Cell* (2011) 8:177–87. doi: 10.1016/j.stem.2010.11.029
9. Uitto J, McGrath JA, Rodeck U, Bruckner-Tuderman L, Robinson EC. Progress in epidermolysis bullosa research: toward treatment and cure. *J Invest Dermatol.* (2010) 130:1778–84. doi: 10.1038/jid.2010.90
10. Hirsch T, Rothoeft T, Teig N, Bauer JW, Pellegrini G, De Rosa L, et al. Regeneration of the entire human epidermis using transgenic stem cells. *Nature* (2017) 551:327–32. doi: 10.1038/nature24487
11. Siprashvili Z, Nguyen NT, Gorell ES, Loutit K, Khuu P, Furukawa LK, et al. Safety and wound outcomes following genetically corrected autologous epidermal grafts in patients with recessive dystrophic epidermolysis bullosa. *JAMA* (2016) 316:1808–17. doi: 10.1001/jama.2016.15588
12. Kroeger J, Hoppe E, Galiger C, Has C, Franzke C-W. Amino acid substitution in the C-terminal domain of collagen XVII reduces laminin-332 interaction causing mild skin fragility with atrophic scarring. *Matrix Biol J Int Soc Matrix Biol.* (2018). doi: 10.1016/j.matbio.2018.10.003
13. Has C, Küsel J, Reimer A, Hoffmann J, Schauer F, Zimmer A, et al. The position of targeted next-generation sequencing in epidermolysis bullosa diagnosis. *Acta Derm Venereol.* (2018) 98:437–40. doi: 10.2340/00015555-2863
14. Maier K, He Y, Esser PR, Thriene K, Sarca D, Kohlhase J, et al. Single amino acid deletion in kindlin-1 results in partial protein degradation which can be rescued by chaperone treatment. *J Invest Dermatol.* (2016) 136:920–9. doi: 10.1016/j.jid.2015.12.039
15. Has C, He Y. Research techniques made simple: immunofluorescence antigen mapping in epidermolysis bullosa. *J Invest Dermatol.* (2016) 136:e65–71. doi: 10.1016/j.jid.2016.05.093
16. Schäcke H, Schumann H, Hammami-Hauasli N, Raghunath M, Bruckner-Tuderman L. Two forms of collagen XVII in keratinocytes. A full-length transmembrane protein and a soluble ectodomain. *J Biol Chem.* (1998) 273:25937–43. doi: 10.1074/jbc.273.40.25937
17. Yuen WY, Pas HH, Sinke RJ, Jonkman MF. Junctional epidermolysis bullosa of late onset explained by mutations in COL17A1. *Br J Dermatol.* (2011) 164:1280–4. doi: 10.1111/j.1365-2133.2011.10359.x
18. Darling TN, McGrath JA, Yee C, Gatalica B, Hametner R, Bauer JW, et al. Premature termination codons are present on both alleles of the bullous pemphigoid antigen 2/type XVII collagen gene in five Austrian families with generalized atrophic benign epidermolysis bullosa. *J Invest Dermatol.* (1997) 108:463–8. doi: 10.1111/1523-1747.ep12289718
19. Bobadilla JL, Macek M, Fine JP, Farrell PM. Cystic fibrosis: a worldwide analysis of CFTR mutations–correlation with incidence data and application to screening. *Hum Mutat.* (2002) 19:575–606. doi: 10.1002/humu.10041
20. Tasanen K, Tunggal L, Chometon G, Bruckner-Tuderman L, Aumailley M. Keratinocytes from patients lacking collagen XVII display a migratory phenotype. *Am J Pathol.* (2004) 164:2027–38. doi: 10.1016/S0002-9440(10)63762-5
21. Has C, Kiritsi D, Mellerio JE, Franzke C-W, Wedgeworth E, Tantcheva-Poor I, et al. The missense mutation p.R1303Q in type XVII collagen underlies junctional epidermolysis bullosa resembling Kindler syndrome. *J Invest Dermatol.* (2014) 134:845–9. doi: 10.1038/jid.2013.367
22. Nishimura M, Nishie W, Shirafuji Y, Shinkuma S, Natsuga K, Nakamura H, et al. Extracellular cleavage of collagen XVII is essential for correct cutaneous basement membrane formation. *Hum Mol Genet.* (2016) 25:328–39. doi: 10.1093/hmg/ddv478
23. Gatalica B, Pulkkinen L, Li K, Kuokkanen K, Ryynänen M, McGrath JA, et al. Cloning of the human type XVII collagen gene (COL17A1), and detection of novel mutations in generalized atrophic benign epidermolysis bullosa. *Am J Hum Genet.* (1997) 60:352–65.
24. Pasmooij AMG, Pas HH, Jansen GHL, Lemmink HH, Jonkman MF. Localized and generalized forms of blistering in junctional epidermolysis bullosa due to COL17A1 mutations in the Netherlanhds. *Br J Dermatol.* (2007) 156:861–70. doi: 10.1111/j.1365-2133.2006.07730.x
25. McGrath JA, Gatalica B, Christiano AM, Li K, Owaribe K, McMillan JR, et al. Mutations in the 180-kD bullous pemphigoid antigen (BPAG2), a hemidesmosomal transmembrane collagen (COL17A1), in generalized atrophic benign epidermolysis bullosa. *Nat Genet.* (1995) 11:83–6. doi: 10.1038/ng0995-83
26. Koller U, Wally V, Mitchell LG, Klausegger A, Murauer EM, Mayr E, et al. A novel screening system improves genetic correction by internal exon replacement. *Nucleic Acids Res.* (2011) 39:e108. doi: 10.1093/nar/gkr465
27. Yancey KB, Hintner H. Non-herlitz junctional epidermolysis bullosa. *Dermatol Clin.* (2010) 28:67–77. doi: 10.1016/j.det.2009.10.008
28. Hintner H, Wolff K. Generalized atrophic benign epidermolysis bullosa. *Arch Dermatol.* (1982) 118:375–84. doi: 10.1001/archderm.1982.01650180009008
29. Lincoln V, Cogan J, Hou Y, Hirsch M, Hao M, Alexeev V, et al. Gentamicin induces LAMB3 nonsense mutation readthrough and restores functional laminin 332 in junctional epidermolysis bullosa. *Proc Natl Acad Sci USA.* (2018) 115:E6536–45. doi: 10.1073/pnas.1803154115
30. Huber M, Floeth M, Borradori L, Schäcke H, Rugg EL, Lane EB, et al. Deletion of the cytoplasmatic domain of BP180/collagen XVII causes a phenotype with predominant features of epidermolysis bullosa simplex. *J Invest Dermatol.* (2002) 118:185–92. doi: 10.1046/j.0022-202x.2001.01617.x
31. Bruckner-Tuderman L, Has C. Disorders of the cutaneous basement membrane zone–the paradigm of epidermolysis bullosa. *Matrix Biol J Int Soc Matrix Biol.* (2014) 33:29–34. doi: 10.1016/j.matbio.2013.07.007
32. Linde L, Kerem B. Introducing sense into nonsense in treatments of human genetic diseases. *Trends Genet TIG* (2008) 24:552–63. doi: 10.1016/j.tig.2008.08.010
33. Kurosaki T, Li W, Hoque M, Popp MW-L, Ermolenko DN, Tian B, et al. A post-translational regulatory switch on UPF1 controls targeted mRNA degradation. *Genes Dev.* (2014) 28:1900–16. doi: 10.1101/gad.245506.114

16

Current Clinical Trials in Pemphigus and Pemphigoid

Kentaro Izumi[1,2], Katja Bieber[2] and Ralf J. Ludwig[2*]

[1] Department of Dermatology, Hokkaido University Graduate School of Medicine, Sapporo, Japan, [2] Lübeck Institute of Experimental Dermatology, Center for Research on Inflammation of the Skin, University of Lübeck, Lübeck, Germany

***Correspondence:**
Ralf J. Ludwig
ralf.ludwig@uksh.de

Autoimmune bullous dermatoses (AIBDs) are a group of rare chronic inflammatory skin diseases, which clinically manifest as blisters and erosions of the skin and/or mucosa. Immunologically, AIBDs are characterized and caused by autoantibodies targeting adhesion molecules in the skin and mucosa. According to the histological location of the blistering, AIBDs are classified into the following two main subtypes: pemphigus (intraepidermal blistering) and pemphigoid (subepidermal blistering). Most AIBDs were potentially life-threatening diseases before the advent of immunosuppressive drugs, especially systemic steroid therapies, which suppress pathogenic immunological activity. Although there have been recent advancements in the understanding of the pathogenesis of AIBDs, glucocorticosteroids and/or adjuvant immunosuppressive drugs are still needed to control disease activity. However, the long-term use of systemic immunosuppression is associated with major adverse events, including death. Based on the growing understanding of AIBD pathogenesis, novel treatment targets have emerged, some of which are currently being evaluated in clinical trials. Within this article, we review the current clinical trials involving pemphigus and pemphigoid and discuss the rationale that lead to these trials. Overall, we aim to foster insights into translational research in AIBDs to improve patient care.

Keywords: autoimmune blistering skin disease, pemphigus, pemphigoid, clinical trial, treatment

INTRODUCTION

Autoimmune bullous dermatoses (AIBDs) are a heterogeneous group of skin diseases that are characterized and caused by autoantibodies targeting adhesion molecules in the skin and/or mucous membranes. Depending on the targeted adhesion molecules and the location of the blistering, AIBDs are classified into the following two major types: pemphigus diseases with autoantibodies targeting desmosomal proteins (1) and pemphigoid diseases with autoantibodies targeting the structural proteins of dermal-epidermal junction (2). In pemphigus diseases, including pemphigus vulgaris (PV) and pemphigus foliaceus (PF), autoantibody binding leads to the disruption of epidermal adhesion, resulting in the clinical finding of flaccid blisters and the histological finding of intraepidermal blistering (1). In pemphigoid diseases, the linear deposition of autoantibodies along the dermal-epidermal junction causes subepidermal blistering, resulting in tense blisters. Based on the target molecules of the autoantibodies and the clinical manifestations, pemphigoid diseases are classified as bullous pemphigoid (BP), mucous membrane pemphigoid (MMP), epidermolysis bullosa acquisita (EBA), anti-laminin-γ1/p200 pemphigoid (p200), pemphigoid gestationis (PG), lichen planus pemphigoides (LPP), linear IgA bullous dermatosis (LAD), and dermatitis herpetiformis (DH), which is associated with gluten-sensitive enteropathy and characteristic granular IgA deposits in the upper dermis (3–5).

Although the advent of systemic steroid therapy significantly improved the prognosis of AIBDs, these groups of diseases are still potentially life-threatening, now mainly due to adverse events resulting from corticosteroid treatment (6). Due to the chronicity of AIBDs, the prolonged administration of systemic steroids is often needed to induce and maintain clinical remission, leading to various adverse effects such as cytopenia, diabetes mellitus, osteoporosis, hypertension, gastrointestinal ulcers, and infections due to immunosuppression (7). Furthermore, severe infection induced by an immunocompromised state is one of the most important causes of death during AIBD treatment (8, 9). Thus, the development of alternative treatment modalities that have fewer adverse events is urgently needed for the treatment of AIBD patients.

Based on the growing understanding of AIBD pathogenesis (1, 10, 11), novel therapeutic targets and/or treatment modalities have been identified (12–15). Some of those new treatments are currently being evaluated in clinical trials. To foster translational AIBD research, in this article, we summarize the current clinical trials involving pemphigus and pemphigoid diseases. For this purpose, we searched clinicaltrials.gov[1] and the EU clinical trials register[2] through December 2018 and selected clinical trials on pemphigus or pemphigoid disease with the status "recruiting (the study is currently recruiting participants)," "active, not recruiting (the study is ongoing, and participants are receiving an intervention or being examined, but not currently being recruited or enrolled)," and "completed (the study has ended normally, and participants are no longer being examined or treated)," and an initiation in 2013 or later (**Tables 1, 2, Figure 1**). To provide a more comprehensive overview, we list the trials before this time frame in **Supplementary Tables 1, 2**. In addition, we included one clinical trial that is registered with the Australia and New Zealand Clinical Trials Registry, which was recently presented at the 5th International Pemphigus and Pemphigoid Foundation Scientific Conference in Orlando (16).

PEMPHIGUS

Anti-CD20 in Pemphigus (Rituximab or Ofatumumab)

Rituximab is a human chimeric IgG1 monoclonal antibody targeting CD20, which is a cell surface marker expressed by B cells (17). Rituximab exerts its treatment effects via the depletion of B-cells following its binding to CD20. Regarding the treatment of pemphigus with rituximab, case reports have suggested the efficacy of rituximab as a second- or third-line therapy (18–20). There are two main rituximab regimens for pemphigus; one regimen, which is based on the lymphoma protocol, is composed of a total of 4 doses of 375 mg/m^2 weekly infusions (21), while the other regimen, which is based on the rheumatoid arthritis protocol, consists of a total of two doses of 1,000 mg (or 500 mg) biweekly intravenous infusions (22). Prior to evaluating the efficacy of a single cycle regimen of rituximab in refractory pemphigus cases, a multicenter, single arm, phase 2/3 clinical trial was conducted in France (23). At 3 months after rituximab treatment, 18 (86%) of 21 cases achieved complete remission (CR). Furthermore, 18 (86%) of 21 cases maintained CR after a median follow-up of 34 months. In addition, 8 of these 18 cases did not receive systemic corticosteroid therapy. To evaluate the safety and efficacy of rituximab in a controlled clinical trial, a prospective, parallel-group, open-label, randomized, phase 3 clinical trial of rituximab as a first-line treatment for moderate to severe cases of pemphigus (**NCT00784589**) was initiated (**Table 1**). Patients with PV or PF were randomized to receive either oral prednisolone at 1.0 to 1.5 mg/kg/day that was tapered over 12–18 months or oral prednisolone at 0.5–1.0 mg/kg/day that was tapered over 3–6 months plus rituximab 1 g on days 0 and 14 and 0.5 g at months 12 and 18. The primary endpoint was the proportion of patients who achieved CR off-therapy at month 24. The results of this clinical trial were recently reported (24). Regarding the primary endpoint, 34% of patients in the prednisolone arm achieved CR at month 24. In the rituximab plus prednisolone arm, CR was reached by 89% of the patients; the difference was significant. Furthermore, fewer grade 3–4 adverse events were observed in the rituximab plus prednisone group than in the prednisone alone group (27 events in 16 out of 46 patients; mean 0.59 [SD 1.15] vs. 53 events in 29 out of 44 patients; mean 1.20 [1.25]). Overall, this trial demonstrated that the first-line treatment of pemphigus with rituximab and lower doses of prednisolone is more effective and safer compared to high-dose prednisolone treatment. Based on the results of this clinical trial, the Food and Drug Administration approved the expansion of health insurance coverage of rituximab for pemphigus vulgaris in the United States.

In addition to rituximab, ofatumumab, a fully human anti-CD20 monoclonal antibody, has been demonstrated to be safe and effective for the treatment of autoimmune disorders other than pemphigus or pemphigoid (25). Preclinical studies suggested that ofatumumab shows a high affinity for CD20 and activates complement-dependent cytotoxicity (26). A double-blind, randomized, placebo-controlled, phase 3 clinical trial evaluating the efficacy of ofatumumab in pemphigus was completed in January 2018 (**NCT01920477**). This clinical trial enrolled moderate

[1]https://clinicaltrials.gov/

[2]https://www.clinicaltrialsregister.eu/

Abbreviations: AIBDs, autoimmune bullous dermatoses; PV, pemphigus vulgaris; PF, pemphigus foliaceus; BP, bullous pemphigoid; EBA, epidermolysis acquisita; p200, anti-laminin-γ1/p200 pemphigoid; PG, pemphigoid gestationis; LPP, lichen planus pemphigoides; LAD, linear IgA bullous dermatosis; DH, dermatitis herpetiformis; RA, rheumatoid arthritis; MS, multiple sclerosis; CR, complete remission; MMF, mycophenolate mofetil; BAFF, B cell activating factor of the tumor necrosis factor family; BAFF-R, B cell activating factor of the tumor necrosis factor family receptor; BCR, B cell receptor; PDAI, Pemphigus Disease Area Index; FcRn, neonatal Fc receptor; IVIg, intravenous immunoglobulin; BTK, Bruton's tyrosine kinase; Tregs, regulatory T cells; GVHD, graft vs. host disease; Dsg, desmoglein; PRP, Platelet-rich plasma; CAR, chimeric antigen receptor; Dsg3-CAART, Dsg3 chimeric autoantibody receptor T cell; IL, interleukin; EAE, experimental autoimmune encephalomyelitis; DAS, disease activity score; NLRP3, nucleotide-binding domain, leucine-rich repeat family, pyrin domain-containing 3; BPDAI, bullous pemphigoid disease area index; ECP, eosinophil cationic protein; SYK, spleen tyrosine kinase; FcγR, Fc gamma receptor; LTB4, leukotriene B4.

TABLE 1 | Current clinical trials in pemphigus.

NCT number	Disease	Interventions	Target	Allocation	Masking	Phase	Status
NCT01930175	PV	VAY736	BAFF-R	Randomized	Double blind	2	Active, not recruiting
NCT01920477	PV	Ofatumumab	CD20	Randomized	Double blind	3	Completed
NCT03334058	PV	ARGX-113	FcRn	Single group	None	2	Recruiting
NCT02704429	PV or PF	PRN1008	BTK	Single group	None	2	Recruiting
NCT03762265	PV or PF	PRN1008	BTK	Randomized	Quadruple blind	3	Recruiting
NCT02383589	PV	Rituximab MMF	CD20 IMPDH	Randomized	Double blind	3	Active, not recruiting
NCT03239470	PV or PF	Poly Tregs	Immune tolerance	Non- randomized	None	1	Recruiting
NCT02828163	PV	PRP	Wound healing	Randomized	Double blind	3	Recruiting
NCT00784589	PV or PF	Rituximab	CD20	Randomized	None	3	Completed
NCT03075904	PV or PF	SYNT001	FcRn	Non-randomized	None	1/2	Completed

PV, pemphigus vulgaris; PF, pemphigus foliaceus; BAFF-R, B cell activating factor of the tumor necrosis factor family receptor; FcRn, neonatal Fc receptor; BTK, Bruton's tyrosine kinase; MMF, mycophenolate mofetil; IMPDH, inosine 5′-monophosphate dehydrogenase; Tregs, regulatory T cells; PRP, Platelet rich plasma.

TABLE 2 | Current clinical trials in bullous pemphigoid.

NCT number	Interventions	Target	Allocation	Masking	Phase	Status
NCT03099538	Ixekizumab	IL-17	Single group	None	2	Recruiting
NCT01408550	NPB-1	FcRn	Randomized	Double blind	3	Completed
NCT03286582	AC-203	Inflammasome	Randomized	None	2	Recruiting
NCT02226146	Bertilimumab	eotaxin	Single group	None	2	Completed
NCT00525616	Rituximab	CD20	Single group	None	3	Completed

No clinical trials are being performed for any other pemphigoid diseases. FcRn, neonatal Fc receptor.

to severe PV patients with a history of at least failure of tapered steroid therapy. Participants received a stable dose of prednisone/prednisolone from a minimum of 20 mg/day up to a maximum of 120 mg/day or 1.5 mg/kg/day for 2 weeks prior to randomization. Thirty-five patients with PV were randomized to receive either ofatumumab or a placebo. Ofatumumab at 40 mg was subcutaneously injected at week 0 and week 4. From week 8, subjects were subcutaneously administered ofatumumab 20 mg every 4 weeks through week 56. The primary endpoints were the time to sustained CR on minimal steroid therapy (prednisone/prednisolone dose to <10 mg/day) and the duration of CR on minimal steroid therapy. The results of this study have thus far not been reported.

Similar to these two trials, another double-blind, randomized, phase 3 clinical trial of adjuvant rituximab vs. mycophenolate mofetil (MMF) as a therapy for pemphigus is ongoing (**NCT02383589**). In that study, 135 PV patients who are receiving standard systemic steroid treatment (oral prednisone 60–120 mg/day or equivalent) will randomly receive either (i) MMF and a rituximab-matched placebo or (ii) an MMF-matched placebo and rituximab. MMF is orally administered twice daily from day 1 to week 56. The initial dose of MMF is 500 mg, and the dose will be titrated to achieve a goal of 1,000 mg. Rituximab is administered at a dose of 1,000 mg intravenously on days 1, 15, 168, and 182. The primary endpoint is the proportion of patients who achieve sustained CR.

VAY736 in Pemphigus

B cell activating factor of the tumor necrosis factor family (BAFF) is a crucial cytokine for regulating B cell development in mice and humans (27, 28). BAFF functions by binding to the BAFF receptor (BAFF-R), B cell maturation antigen, and tumor necrosis factor receptor superfamily member (29). Although at physiological concentrations BAFF cannot rescue B cell apoptosis due to a strong B cell death signal, which is transduced via the B cell receptor (BCR) stimulated by autoantigens, at higher concentrations, BAFF causes the survival of autoreactive B cells, which contributes to the pathogenesis of autoimmune diseases (27, 30, 31). For example, elevated BAFF serum levels have been detected in various autoimmune diseases such as RA, systemic lupus erythematosus, Sjögren's syndrome, and systemic sclerosis (32–34). Taken together, BAFF is a likely therapeutic target for the treatment of autoimmune diseases. Regarding clinical translation, the anti-BAFF antibody belimumab was licensed for the treatment of systemic lupus erythematosus in 2011 (35). However, clinical trials of belimumab have not been conducted in pemphigus thus far. Alternatively, with regard to the inhibition of BAFF, its receptor can be blocked to achieve similar results. BAFF-R signaling drives B cell differentiation, proliferation and survival (36). VAY736 is a novel, defucosylated, human IgG1 monoclonal antibody targeting BAFF-R, providing both enhanced antibody-dependent cellular cytotoxicity-mediated depletion of B cells and the blockade of BAFF. To investigate the safety, tolerability and efficacy of VAY736 in PV, a randomized, placebo-controlled, double-blind,

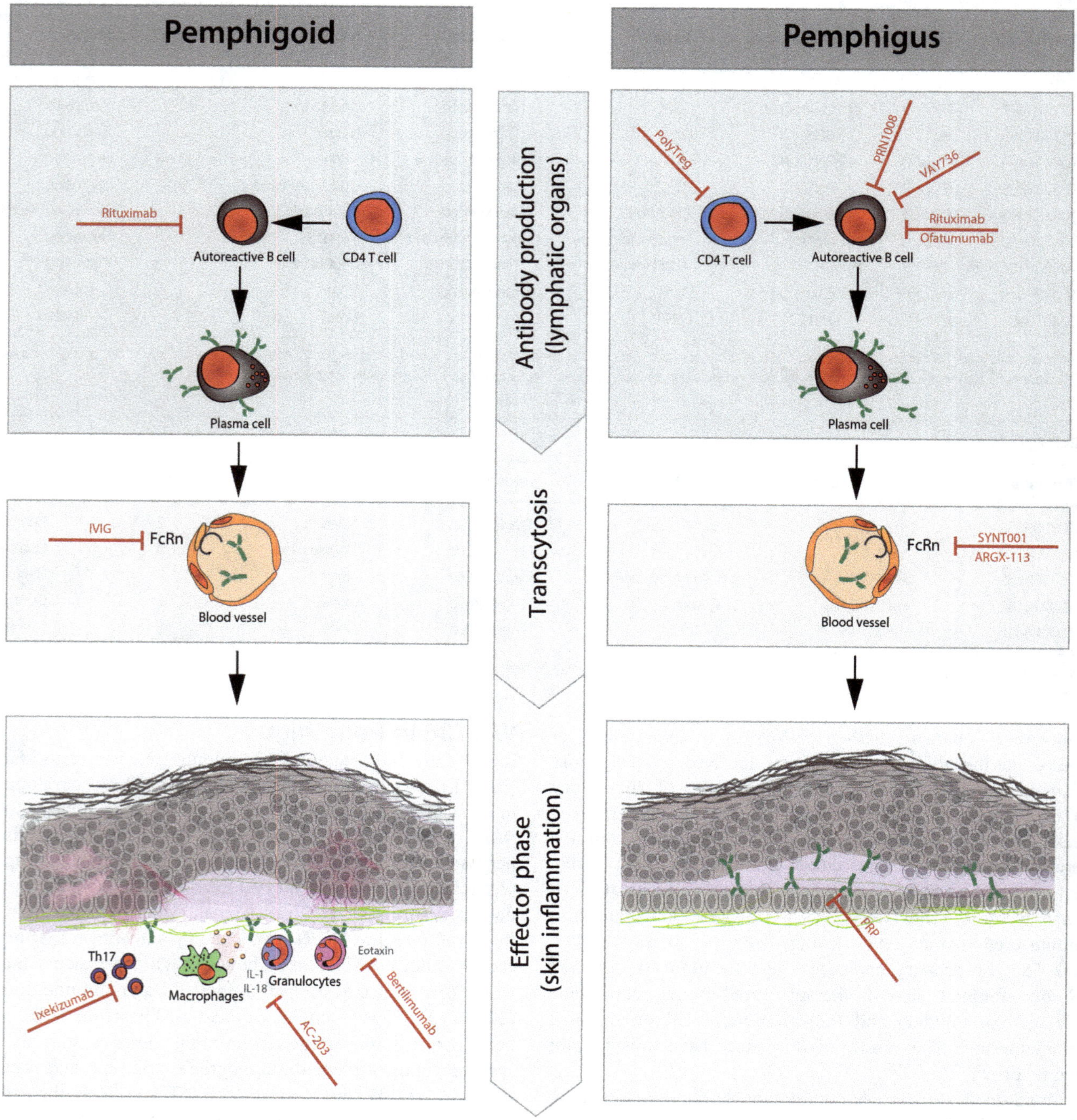

FIGURE 1 | Schematic representation of the pathophysiology and new therapeutic targets of pemphigus and pemphigoid diseases. The pathophysiology of pemphigus and pemphigoid diseases consists of the following three phases: (1) CD4+T cells promote autoreactive B cell activation, proliferation, and differentiation to plasma cells that produce pathogenic autoantibodies. (2) Circulating pathogenic antibodies are transferred to the dermal epidermal junction or intracellular space of the epidermis. Neonatal Fc receptor (FcRn) plays a role in prolonging the half-life of IgG antibodies during this phase. (3) After the binding of pathogenic autoantibodies to target molecules, pro-inflammatory cells such as granulocytes and macrophages are recruited to the immune complex in lesional skin by chemokines (e.g., eotaxin). Then, granulocytes elicit reactive oxygen species (ROS), elastases, and proteases, resulting in tissue damage such as blisters and/or erythema, which are clinical symptoms in pemphigoid diseases but not in pemphigus diseases. Cytokines [e.g., interleukin (IL)-1beta and IL-18] and Th17 polarization are thought to enhance local inflammation. During the antibody production phase, rituximab and ofatumumab deplete autoreactive B cells to prevent their differentiation to plasma cells. PolyTregs act on CD4+ T cells, and VAY736 and PRN1008 act on autoreactive B cells, resulting in less activation of autoreactive B cells. In the transcytosis phase, intravenous immunoglobulin (IVIg), SYNT001, and ARGX-113 saturate FcRn, contributing to the shortened half-life of pathogenic autoantibodies. In the effector phase, ixekizumab restores Th17 polarization and suppresses inflammatory augmentation. AC-203 modulates cytokines such as IL-1beta and IL-18, contributing to decreased inflammation. The inhibition of eotaxin with bertilimumab ameliorates the recruitment of eosinophils to local inflammation sites in pemphigoid disease, especially bullous pemphigoid. Platelet-rich plasma (PRP) is thought to promote wound healing in erosions.

phase 2 clinical trial is currently ongoing (**NCT01930175**). In this trial, 16 mild-moderate PV patients will randomly receive either intravenous VAY736 or a placebo once. The primary endpoint is the efficacy of single cycle VAY736 administration in reducing Pemphigus Disease Area Index (PDAI) scores at week 12 compared to at the baseline. No results of this trial are currently available.

Anti-neonatal Fc Receptor (FcRn) in Pemphigus (SYNT001, ARGX-113)

FcRn plays an essential role in regulating host circulating IgG levels (37). FcRn protects IgG from intracellular digestion, leading to the prolongation of its half-life. This "IgG recycling system" is essential for host defense. However, it also maintains the concentration of circulating pathogenic IgG in various autoimmune diseases, including AIBD. Specifically, FcRn-deficient mice do not (or to a lesser extent) develop experimental AIBD after the injection of AIBD-inducing antibodies (10). Interestingly, saturation of the FcRn by the administration of high-dose human IgG (IVIg) reduces the pathogenic effects in antibody-transfer AIBD models. Thus, FcRn inhibition is one possible mode of action of IVIg therapy in AIBD (38, 39). Based on these observations, anti-FcRn targeting treatments have been developed. Currently, the following 2 clinical trials targeting FcRn are being conducted in pemphigus: SYNT001 (**NCT03075904**) and ARGX-113 (**NCT03334058**). SYNT001 is a humanized, deimmunized IgG4 monoclonal antibody that blocks the binding of FcRn to the Fc portion of IgG (40). ARGX-113 is a human IgG1-derived Fc-modified fragment with increased affinity for FcRn that reduces the circulating IgG concentration (41). In addition, both SYNT001 and ARGX-113 do not alter serum levels of albumin. As both trials are ongoing, no results have been published so far. Regarding **NCT03075904**, 16 PV or PF patients will be sequentially assigned to receive three different doses of intravenous SYNT001 weekly for either 5 or 14 weeks, and the primary endpoint is the count and percentage of adverse events (time frame; days 0–112 or days 0–175). At the 2018 pre-International Investigative Dermatology meeting in Orlando, the first results were reported for SYNT001. The infusion of SYNT001 in human subjects resulted in a rapid lowering of the circulating levels of IgG (mean total IgG reduction of 56% by day 30) with good safety and tolerability. Furthermore, 5 of the 7 subjects showed a reduction in disease activity by day 42 (42). Regarding **NCT03334058**, 12 newly diagnosed or relapsed PV patients will receive ARGX-113 intravenously. The primary endpoints are safety and tolerability up to 17 weeks.

PRN1008 in Pemphigus

B cell receptor signaling is a key player in B cell development and function. Bruton's tyrosine kinase (BTK) belongs to the Tec family of nonreceptor tyrosine kinases, and it is a vital component of B cell receptor signaling (43). BTK is predominantly expressed by B-lymphocytes from the pre-B cell stage to the mature B cell stage (44, 45). Based on the crucial role of BTK in B cell function, it has been identified as a potential target for the treatment of autoimmune disorders. Several studies have shown that ibrutinib, which is one of the BTK inhibitors under development, binds to BTK with high affinity, leading to the inhibition of B cell receptor signaling and resulting in the reduction of B cell activation involved in autoimmunity (46). In pemphigus treatment, a previous case report showed that ibrutinib improved clinical cutaneous lesions of paraneoplastic pemphigus complicated with chronic lymphocytic leukemia (47). However, there have been no case reports or series investigating the effects of this BTK inhibitor in PNP, PV and/or PF. PRN1008 is another BTK inhibitor that was evaluated in a phase 1 clinical trial that enrolled 80 healthy volunteers (Australian New Zealand Clinical Trials Registry No. **ACTRN12614000359639**). In that study, PRN1008 was considered safe. Regarding the pharmacokinetics and pharmacodynamics, BTK occupancy of more than 90% was observed within 4 h after dosing in both the single and multiple dose regimens and was closely correlated with the maximum plasma concentration (48). Based on the promising results from the phase 1 trial, an open-label, single-armed, phase 2 clinical trial of PRN1008 for PV treatment has been conducted (**NCT02704429**). In this trial, 27 pemphigus patients (including PV and PF) received PRN1008 orally for 12 weeks with a 12-week follow-up period. The primary efficacy endpoint was the initial control of disease activity during the first 4 weeks of therapy, during which new lesions cease to form and existing lesions begin to heal, without the need for prednisone-equivalent corticosteroid doses >0.5 mg/kg/day. More than 50% of patients have achieved control of disease activity within 4 weeks of starting PRN1008 thus far[3]. Furthermore, Principia has recently initiated a global, randomized, double-blind, placebo-controlled, pivotal phase 3 clinical trial (**NCT03762265**) in approximately 120 PV or PF patients to evaluate PRN1008 vs. a placebo. The primary endpoint is the proportion of participants who are in CR from week $\leq$ 29 to 37 with a prednisone dose of $\leq$5 mg/day.

Polyclonal Regulatory T Cells (PolyTregs) in Pemphigus

Among the T cell subtypes, regulatory T cells (Tregs) play an important role in regulating the immune system and preventing autoimmune disease development. Based on findings in animal models, including AIBD (49, 50), it is hypothesized that naturally occurring Tregs may be utilized for the treatment of autoimmune diseases and potentially replace the use of chronic immunosuppressive therapies that are associated with multiple adverse effects. A clinical trial of Treg adoptive therapy was started by treating graft vs. host diseases (GVHD) with expanded allogeneic Tregs (51). There has been a small study demonstrating the safe administration of autologous Tregs with decreased disease activity in patients with insulin-dependent diabetes (52). Subsequently, Brunstein et al. reported that HLA-matched umbilical cord blood-derived Tregs decreased the incidence of GVHD after double umbilical cord blood transplantation (53), indicating the potential efficacy and safety profile of the passive transfer of autologous Tregs in humans. The application of Tregs for lupus, cancer and organ transplantation

[3]https://ir.principiabio.com/news-releases/news-release-details/principia-biopharma-reports-positive-prn1008-phase-2-top-line

has been addressed (54). The suppressive effects of Tregs have been reported by studies using an active PV mouse model (55). A recent study indicated that Treg induction via the anti-CD28 antibody reduces pathogenic IgG directing desmoglein (Dsg) 3 in the HLA-DRB1*04:02- transgenic PV mouse model (56). Although Tregs are expected to improve PV symptoms, there are no case reports or case series of autologous Treg injections in patients with PV to date. To evaluate the effects of Tregs on the manifestation of PV, a nonrandomized, open-label, phase 1 clinical trial is ongoing (**NCT03239470**). In this trial, 12 PV or PF patients will receive one infusion of autologous expanded Tregs (CD4+CD127lo/negCD25+) at one of the following doses: either 2.5 x 10^8 poly Tregs or 10 × 10^8 poly Tregs. The primary endpoint is the number of significant grade 3 or higher adverse events by week 52. The results from this study have thus far not been reported.

Comparison of Injections of Steroids to Autologous Platelet-Rich Plasma (PRP) in Oral Erosions in PV

Oral erosive lesions are a major hallmark of PV. These oral lesions cause severe pain, resulting in problems with eating and drinking (57). To improve oral lesions in PV, adjuvant topical or intralesional steroids are used, and based on evidence from case reports, the treatment is effective (58, 59). To date, however, no controlled clinical trial of the treatment of oral lesions in PV has been performed. PRP, which is concentrated plasma derived from autologous whole blood, is believed to promote wound healing (60). In a case report series, El-Komy et al. reported that six of seven PV patients showed improvement of their oral PDAI scores after PRP intralesional injection (61). To evaluate the effects of PRP in PV, an open-label, dose-escalation, multicenter phase 1 trial using autologous PRP has been conducted in adults with active PV (**NCT02828163**). This clinical trial was designed to compare the effects of PRP to those of intralesional steroid injection. Eleven PV patients received a 10 mg/mL triamcinolone injection on one side of the oral mucosa and a 1-mL PRP injection on the other side every 2 weeks for 3 months. The primary endpoint was the improvement of oral PV lesions in 3 months. Nine out of 11 participants completed the protocol, and 7 (78%) of those 9 patients showed improvement in oral PDAI and/or pain scores at the PRP injection sites. Although PRP resulted in clinical improvement, as in the previous study, there were no significant differences between PRP and intralesional steroid injections (62). Thus, autologous PRP might be used for the treatment of resistant oral erosions in pemphigus patients when intralesional steroid injection is contraindicated.

Future Potential Clinical Trials in Pemphigus

B cell depletion therapy using an anti-CD20 monoclonal antibody leads to short-term remission in the majority of pemphigus patients; however, we often observe relapsing disease after treatment. Although disease remission is related to the depletion of circulating Dsg3-specific B cells, the expansion of the same pathogenic B cell clone is observed during relapsing disease (63). Therefore, to maintain complete remission in PV, targeted removal of anti-Dsg3 memory B cells is essential. Recently, chimeric antigen receptor (CAR) technology was developed and resulted in novel treatments that led to the prolonged remission of refractory B cell leukemia and lymphoma. Adapted from that strategy, Dsg3 chimeric autoantibody receptor T cell (Dsg3-CAART) therapy has been reported to result in serological and histological improvements in experimental pemphigus mice without detectable off-target toxicity (15). A phase 1 clinical trial of Dsg3-CAART in PV patients is planned to investigate its safety and therapeutic potential.

PEMPHIGOID

Ixekizumab in BP

Th17 cells were first identified by their production of interleukin (IL)-17 (64, 65). A previous study indicated that the transfer of IL-17-producing Th17 cells into healthy SJL/J mice induced experimental autoimmune encephalomyelitis an animal model of MS (66). The prominent role of the Th17 polarization of T cells, as well as that of IL-17, in inflammation and autoimmunity was recognized after this observation. In addition to EAE, the Th17-IL-17 axis is also important in the pathogenesis of RA (67–69). Notably, neutralizing anti-IL-17 antibodies significantly decreased joint inflammation, cartilage destruction, and bone erosion in a collagen-immunized arthritis mouse model. Several recent studies suggest that Th17 cells and their cytokines also play roles in the pathogenesis of AIBD, including BP (70). More specifically, Le Jan et al. reported that IL-17A expression was significantly higher in both serum and lesional skin in BP patients than in normal healthy individuals (71). Furthermore, Chakievska et al. reported that IL-17A -/- mice were protected from the development of experimental BP induced by the transfer of anti-COL17 IgG (72). Taken together, these results indicate that IL-17A is a potential target for the treatment of BP. Ixekizumab is a recombinant fully humanized monoclonal antibody targeting IL-17 and is used for the treatment of psoriasis (73). However, there are neither case reports nor clinical studies reporting the effect of ixekizumab or other IL-17-targeting compounds on BP. To determine the efficacy of ixekizumab for the treatment of BP, an open-label, single-group phase 2 clinical trial is currently ongoing (**NCT03099538**). In this trial, twelve BP patients will receive subcutaneous injections of 160 mg ixekizumab on day 0, and then they will receive 80 mg of ixekizumab every 2 weeks until week 12. The primary endpoint is the median time from the start of treatment to the cessation of blister formation during the 12 weeks of therapy. There is no available report of the results of this trial to date.

NPB-01 in BP Unresponsive to Corticosteroids

With regard to pemphigus, the efficacy and safety of IVIg in refractory BP patients has been suggested by case reports and case report series (74–76). Based on these observations, several guidelines and consensus statements recommend the use of IVIg for refractory BP (77–79). Recently, Sasaoka et al. reported that IVIg reduced serum IL-6 concentrations, circulating pathogenic IgG levels, and skin inflammation disease activity in an active BP mouse model (80). Kamaguchi et al. reported that an anti-idiotypic antibody in IVIg significantly reduced the BP180 depletion of cultured keratinocytes stimulated with BP pathogenic IgG (81). To evaluate the effectiveness of IVIg in BP, a multicenter, randomized, double-blind, placebo-controlled, phase 3 clinical trial was conducted (**NCT01408550**). In this trial, 56 BP patients were parallelly assigned to receive either IVIg or a placebo. The IVIg group received an intravenous drip infusion of human IgG at 400 mg/kg/day for 5 consecutive days. The primary endpoint was the disease activity score (DAS) of skin lesions on day 15. The results of that study have recently been published (82). The DAS on day 15 was evaluated as the primary endpoint. Although the DAS on day 15 in the IVIg group (19.8 ± 22.2) was 12.5 points lower than that in the placebo group (32.3 ± 31.5), the difference between the groups was not significant ($p = 0.089$). However, a *post hoc* analysis of covariance using the DAS on day 1 as a covariate showed a significant difference between the IVIg and placebo groups ($p = 0.041$). Regarding the safety of IVIg in BP, the incidence of adverse drug reactions was 37.9% ($n = 11/29$) in the IVIg group vs. 18.5% ($n = 5/27$) in the placebo group. No significant difference in the incidence of adverse drug reactions was observed between the IVIg and placebo groups ($p = 0.143$). No patients in either group experienced any severe adverse drug reactions. Therefore, this report suggested that IVIg is a beneficial treatment modality for refractory BP cases treated with a moderate dose of systemic steroids.

Topical AC-203 in BP

The nucleotide-binding domain, leucine-rich repeat family, pyrin domain-containing 3 (NLRP3) inflammasome regulates the activation of caspase-1 and the release of pro-inflammatory cytokines such as IL-1β and IL-18 in macrophages (83–87). It is an essential innate immune sensor that is activated in response to various damage-associated molecular patterns (83, 84). Previous reports have suggested that dysregulation of the inflammasome attenuates several chronic diseases, including autoimmune diseases such as EAE (88) and systemic lupus erythematosus (89, 90). In addition, polymorphisms in both NLRP3 and caspase-1 recruitment domain-8 genes led to increased IL-1β production and are related to disease susceptibility and severity in RA (91). A recent study demonstrated that the expression levels of NLRP3 and inflammasome components are significantly higher in peripheral blood mononuclear cells from BP patients than in those from healthy donors (92). Furthermore, higher NLRP3 levels were positively correlated with BP disease activity. Although the precise mechanism by which NLRP3 contributes to pathogenesis in BP is still unclear, pharmacological modulation of the inflammasome pathway could be a novel therapeutic strategy in BP. However, in a mouse model of inflammatory EBA, caspase-1/11-deficient mice developed clinical disease manifestations identical to those of the wild-type controls after the injection of autoantibodies against type VII collagen (93).

To evaluate the therapeutic efficacy of caspase-1 inhibition in BP, AC-203, which is a topical ointment formulation of a modulator of the inflammasome and IL-1β pathways, was developed. To investigate the effects of AC-203 on BP, a randomized, open-label phase 2 clinical trial is currently conducted (**NCT03286582**). Forty BP patients received either topical AC-203 or clobetasol 0.05% topical ointment twice a day (time frame is 10 weeks). The primary endpoint is the incidence of adverse effects during the treatment period. No results of this trial are currently available.

Bertilimumab in BP

While the presence of eosinophils in the dermal infiltrate is one of the histological hallmarks of BP, their contribution to the pathogenesis of BP remains to be determined (94–97). Recent data, however, support the notion that eosinophils promote subepidermal blistering in BP (98). In line with the presence of eosinophils in the dermal infiltrate in BP, elevated expression levels of IL-5, eotaxin, and eosinophil colony-stimulating factor were detected in BP blister fluids (99). Furthermore, matrix metallopeptidase 9 is secreted by eosinophils in BP lesional skin (100), eosinophil cationic protein (ECP) is detected at the dermal-epidermal junction of lesional skin, and serum concentrations of ECP correlate with BP disease activity (101, 102). Based on these findings, eotaxin, which is released upon eosinophil activation (103), has emerged as a therapeutic target for the treatment of BP.

Bertilimumab is a fully human monoclonal antibody targeting eotaxin-1 (104). Therefore, the administration of bertilimumab is expected to impair eosinophil infiltration into the skin in BP. This hypothesis has been recently tested in an open-label, single arm, phase 2 clinical trial (**NCT02226146**). Eleven moderate to severe BP patients received 10 mg/kg of bertilimumab intravenously on days 0, 14, and 28 with approximately 13 weeks of follow-up. The primary endpoint was safety, including the incidence of adverse effects. The results of the study were presented at the 2018 American Academy of Dermatology annual meeting. Of the 11 subjects enrolled, 2 patients withdrew consent and 9 received bertilimumab. Bertilimumab was well tolerated in all 9 subjects, and no drug-associated serious adverse events were reported[4] Preliminary analyses indicated that the subjects had an 81% decline in their Bullous Pemphigoid Disease Area Index (BPDAI) scores. Based on these results, bertilimumab has been granted fast track designation for the treatment of BP[5].

Rituximab in BP

Rituximab has a well-documented efficacy in treating pemphigus (24). However, controlled clinical trials in pemphigoid diseases, including BP, are missing. Several case reports and case report series reported good outcomes of rituximab treatment for BP. Although the efficiency of rituximab for the treatment of BP varied among the studies, the overall CR rates were

[4]https://www.immunepharma.com/what-we-do/bertilimumab

[5]https://ir.immunepharma.com/press-releases/detail/168/bertilimumab-granted-fast-track-designation-for-the

60–70% and the relapse rates were approximately 20% in BP patients receiving rituximab therapy (105, 106). To evaluate the efficacy and safety of rituximab for the treatment of BP, an open-label, prospective, phase 3 clinical trial was conducted (**NCT00525616**). Eighteen BP patients received two intravenous injections of 1,000 mg of rituximab at 15-day intervals. The primary endpoint was clinical and biological disease control for up to 2 years. To date, no results of this trial are available.

Future Potential Clinical Trials in Pemphigoid

Spleen tyrosine kinase (SYK) is a nonreceptor cytoplasmic enzyme that is mainly expressed in hematopoietic cells and plays a pivotal role in regulating cellular responses to extracellular pathogens or antigen-immunoglobulin complexes (107). Because SYK acts downstream of activating Fc gamma receptor (FcγR), it has been considered a candidate drug target for antibody-induced diseases, such as pemphigoid diseases. In fact, a previous study has shown that SYK inhibition led to less activation of neutrophils stimulated with immune complexes and prevented the development of skin lesions in a preclinical EBA mouse model (108). In lesional skin in pemphigoid diseases, both eicosanoid leukotriene B4 (LTB4) and complement factor C5, the precursor of anaphylatoxin C5a, are found; however, their significance in the pathogenesis of pemphigoid diseases still needs to be elucidated. A previous preclinical mouse model of pemphigoid disease indicated a critical role of LTB4 in the recruitment of polymorph nuclear cells to the dermal epidermal junction (109). It is suggested that LTB4 may closely interact with C5a in the regulation of skin inflammation. Thus, inhibiting these two factors individually or in parallel might be effective for the treatment of pemphigoid diseases. These newly identified therapeutic targets should be addressed in future clinical trials.

CONCLUSIONS

The clinical trials discussed here, which include several trials investigating novel therapeutic targets, demonstrate that translational research in pemphigus and pemphigoid is a fast-growing field. We thus expect that several novel treatments will be shortly available for the treatment of pemphigus and pemphigoid patients. Given the high, and thus far unmet, medical need in this field (110), this is highly encouraging and will hopefully improve the quality of life of the affected patients. In addition to the compounds and targets described here, several new targets have been recently identified in preclinical model systems, such as PDE4 or PI3Kδ inhibitors (111, 112). Hence, the preclinical pipeline is well developed and will contribute to the growing number of clinical trials in pemphigus and pemphigoid.

AUTHOR CONTRIBUTIONS

KI and RL wrote the manuscript. KB prepared the figure. All authors read, commented on, and approved the final version of the manuscript.

REFERENCES

1. Kasperkiewicz M, Ellebrecht CT, Takahashi H, Yamagami J, Zillikens D, Payne AS, et al. Pemphigus. *Nat Rev Dis Primers.* (2017) 3:17026. doi: 10.1038/nrdp.2017.26
2. Schmidt E, Zillikens D. Pemphigoid diseases. *Lancet.* (2013) 381:320–32. doi: 10.1016/S0140-6736(12)61140-4
3. van Beek N, Zillikens D, Schmidt E. Diagnosis of autoimmune bullous diseases. *J Dtsch Dermatol Ges.* (2018) 16:1077–91. doi: 10.1111/ddg.13637
4. Kasperkiewicz M, Zillikens D, Schmidt E. Pemphigoid diseases: pathogenesis, diagnosis, and treatment. *Autoimmunity.* (2012) 45:55–70. doi: 10.3109/08916934.2011.606447
5. Otten JV, Hashimoto T, Hertl M, Payne AS, Sitaru C. Molecular diagnosis in autoimmune skin blistering conditions. *Curr Mol Med.* (2014) 14:69–95. doi: 10.2174/15665240113136660079
6. Joly P, Roujeau JC, Benichou J, Picard C, Dreno B, Delaporte E, et al. A comparison of oral and topical corticosteroids in patients with bullous pemphigoid. *N Engl J Med.* (2002) 346:321–7. doi: 10.1056/NEJMoa011592
7. Buchman AL. Side effects of corticosteroid therapy. *J Clin Gastroenterol.* (2001) 33:289–94.
8. Kridin K, Sagi SZ, Bergman R. Mortality and cause of death in patients with pemphigus. *Acta Derm Venereol.* (2017) 97:607–11. doi: 10.2340/00015555-2611
9. Cai SC, Allen JC, Lim YL, Chua SH, Tan SH, Tang MB. Mortality of bullous pemphigoid in Singapore: risk factors and causes of death in 359 patients seen at the National Skin Centre. *Br J Dermatol.* (2014) 170:1319–26. doi: 10.1111/bjd.12806
10. Ludwig RJ, Vanhoorelbeke K, Leypoldt F, Kaya Z, Bieber K, McLachlan SM, et al. Mechanisms of autoantibody-induced pathology. *Front Immunol.* (2017) 8:603. doi: 10.3389/fimmu.2017.00603
11. Liu Y, Li L, Xia Y. BP180 is critical in the autoimmunity of bullous pemphigoid. *Front Immunol.* (2017) 8:1752. doi: 10.3389/fimmu.2017.01752
12. Spindler V, Rotzer V, Dehner C, Kempf B, Gliem M, Radeva M, et al. Peptide-mediated desmoglein 3 crosslinking prevents pemphigus vulgaris autoantibody-induced skin blistering. *J Clin Invest.* (2013) 123:800–11. doi: 10.1172/JCI60139
13. Dehner C, Rotzer V, Waschke J, Spindler V. A desmoplakin point mutation with enhanced keratin association ameliorates pemphigus vulgaris autoantibody-mediated loss of cell cohesion. *Am J Pathol.* (2014) 184:2528–36. doi: 10.1016/j.ajpath.2014.05.016
14. Mao X, Cho MJT, Ellebrecht CT, Mukherjee EM, Payne AS. Stat3 regulates desmoglein 3 transcription in epithelial keratinocytes. *JCI Insight.* (2017) 2:92253. doi: 10.1172/jci.insight.92253
15. Ellebrecht CT, Bhoj VG, Nace A, Choi EJ, Mao X, Cho MJ, et al. Reengineering chimeric antigen receptor T cells for targeted

therapy of autoimmune disease. *Science.* (2016) 353:179–84. doi: 10.1126/science.aaf6756

16. Lee J, Werth VP, Hall RP 3rd, Eming R, Fairley JA, Fajgenbaum DC, et al. Perspective from the 5th international pemphigus and pemphigoid foundation scientific conference. *Front Med.* (2018) 5:306. doi: 10.3389/fmed.2018.00306
17. Coiffier B, Haioun C, Ketterer N, Engert A, Tilly H, Ma D, et al. Rituximab (anti-CD20 monoclonal antibody) for the treatment of patients with relapsing or refractory aggressive lymphoma: a multicenter phase II study. *Blood.* (1998) 92:1927–32.
18. Herrmann G, Hunzelmann N, Engert A. Treatment of pemphigus vulgaris with anti-CD20 monoclonal antibody (rituximab). *Br J Dermatol.* (2003) 148:602–3. doi: 10.1046/j.1365-2133.2003.05209_10.x
19. Cooper HL, Healy E, Theaker JM, Friedmann PS. Treatment of resistant pemphigus vulgaris with an anti-CD20 monoclonal antibody (Rituximab). *Clin Exp Dermatol.* (2003) 28:366–8. doi: 10.1046/j.1365-2230.2003.01283.x
20. Goebeler M, Herzog S, Brocker EB, Zillikens D. Rapid response of treatment-resistant pemphigus foliaceus to the anti-CD20 antibody rituximab. *Br J Dermatol.* (2003) 149:899–901. doi: 10.1046/j.1365-2133.2003.05580.x
21. Salopek TG, Logsetty S, Tredget EE. Anti-CD20 chimeric monoclonal antibody (rituximab) for the treatment of recalcitrant, life-threatening pemphigus vulgaris with implications in the pathogenesis of the disorder. *J Am Acad Dermatol.* (2002) 47:785–8. doi: 10.1067/mjd.2002.126273
22. Leshem YA, Hodak E, David M, Anhalt GJ, Mimouni D. Successful treatment of pemphigus with biweekly 1-g infusions of rituximab: a retrospective study of 47 patients. *J Am Acad Dermatol.* (2013) 68:404–11. doi: 10.1016/j.jaad.2012.08.010
23. Joly P, Mouquet H, Roujeau JC, D'Incan M, Gilbert D, Jacquot S, et al. A single cycle of rituximab for the treatment of severe pemphigus. *N Engl J Med.* (2007) 357:545–52. doi: 10.1056/NEJMoa067752
24. Joly P, Maho-Vaillant M, Prost-Squarcioni C, Hebert V, Houivet E, Calbo S, et al. First-line rituximab combined with short-term prednisone versus prednisone alone for the treatment of pemphigus (Ritux 3): a prospective, multicentre, parallel-group, open-label randomised trial. *Lancet.* (2017) 389:2031–40. doi: 10.1016/S0140-6736(17)30070-3
25. Castillo J, Milani C, Mendez-Allwood D. Ofatumumab, a second-generation anti-CD20 monoclonal antibody, for the treatment of lymphoproliferative and autoimmune disorders. *Expert Opin Investig Drugs.* (2009) 18:491–500. doi: 10.1517/13543780902832679
26. Lin TS. Ofatumumab: a novel monoclonal anti-CD20 antibody. *Pharmgenomics Pers Med.* (2010) 3:51–9.
27. Mackay F, Browning JL. BAFF: a fundamental survival factor for B cells. *Nat Rev Immunol.* (2002) 2:465–75. doi: 10.1038/nri844
28. Ng LG, Sutherland AP, Newton R, Qian F, Cachero TG, Scott ML, et al. B cell-activating factor belonging to the TNF family (BAFF)-R is the principal BAFF receptor facilitating BAFF costimulation of circulating T and B cells. *J Immunol.* (2004) 173:807–17. doi: 10.4049/jimmunol.173.2.807
29. Salzer U, Jennings S, Grimbacher B. To switch or not to switch–the opposing roles of TACI in terminal B cell differentiation. *Eur J Immunol.* (2007) 37:17–20. doi: 10.1002/eji.200636914
30. Lesley R, Xu Y, Kalled SL, Hess DM, Schwab SR, Shu HB, et al. Reduced competitiveness of autoantigen-engaged B cells due to increased dependence on BAFF. *Immunity.* (2004) 20:441–453. doi: 10.1016/S1074-7613(04)00079-2
31. Mackay F, Woodcock SA, Lawton P, Ambrose C, Baetscher M, Schneider P, et al. Mice transgenic for BAFF develop lymphocytic disorders along with autoimmune manifestations. *J Exp Med.* (1999) 190:1697–710.
32. Matsushita T, Hasegawa M, Matsushita Y, Echigo T, Wayaku T, Horikawa M, et al. Elevated serum BAFF levels in patients with localized scleroderma in contrast to other organ-specific autoimmune diseases. *Exp Dermatol.* (2007) 16:87–93. doi: 10.1111/j.1600-0625.2006.00485.x
33. Groom J, Kalled SL, Cutler AH, Olson C, Woodcock SA, Schneider P, et al. Association of BAFF/BLyS overexpression and altered B cell differentiation with Sjogren's syndrome. *J Clin Invest.* (2002) 109:59–68. doi: 10.1172/JCI14121
34. Cheema GS, Roschke V, Hilbert DM, Stohl W. Elevated serum B lymphocyte stimulator levels in patients with systemicimmune-based rheumatic diseases. *Arthritis Rheum.* (2001) 44:1313–9. doi: 10.1002/1529-0131(200106)44:6<1313::AID-ART223>3.0.CO;2-S
35. Navarra SV, Guzman RM, Gallacher AE, Hall S, Levy RA, Jimenez RE, et al. Efficacy and safety of belimumab in patients with active systemic lupus erythematosus: a randomised, placebo-controlled, phase 3 trial. *Lancet.* (2011) 377:721–31. doi: 10.1016/S0140-6736(10)61354-2
36. Dörner T, Posch M, Wagner F, Hüser A, Fischer T, Mooney L, et al. THU0313 Double-blind, randomized study of VAY736 single dose treatment in patients with primary sjögren's syndrome (PSS). *Ann Rheumatic Dis.* (2016) 75(Suppl. 2):300–1. doi: 10.1136/annrheumdis-2016-eular.5840
37. Yoshida M, Kobayashi K, Kuo TT, Bry L, Glickman JN, Claypool SM, et al. Neonatal Fc receptor for IgG regulates mucosal immune responses to luminal bacteria. *J Clin Invest.* (2006) 116:2142–2151. doi: 10.1172/JCI27821
38. Iwata H, Vorobyev A, Koga H, Recke A, Zillikens D, Prost-Squarcioni C, et al. Meta-analysis of the clinical and immunopathological characteristics and treatment outcomes in epidermolysis bullosa acquisita patients. *Orphanet J Rare Dis.* (2018) 13:153. doi: 10.1186/s13023-018-0896-1
39. Ishii N, Hashimoto T, Zillikens D, Ludwig RJ. High-dose intravenous immunoglobulin (IVIG) therapy in autoimmune skin blistering diseases. *Clin Rev Allergy Immunol.* (2010) 38:186–195. doi: 10.1007/s12016-009-8153-y
40. Blumberg L, Jumphries JE, Lasseter KC, Blumberg RS. SYNT001: a humanized IgG4 monoclonal antibody that disrupts the interaction of FcRn and IgG for the treatment of IgG-mediated autoimmune diseases. *Blood.* (2017) 130(Suppl. 1):3483.
41. Ulrichts P, Guglietta A, Dreier T, van Bragt T, Hanssens V, Hofman E, et al. Neonatal Fc receptor antagonist efgartigimod safely and sustainably reduces IgGs in humans. *J Clin Invest.* (2018) 128:4372–86. doi: 10.1172/JCI97911
42. Werth VP CD, Blumberg L, Humphries J, Blumberg R, Hall R. FcRn blockade with SYNT001 for the treatment of pemphigus. *J Invest Dermatol.* (2018) 138:S92. doi: 10.1016/j.jid.2018.03.546
43. Satterthwaite AB, Li Z, Witte ON. Btk function in B cell development and response. *Semin Immunol.* (1998) 10:309–16. doi: 10.1006/smim.1998.0123
44. de Weers M, Verschuren MC, Kraakman ME, Mensink RG, Schuurman RK, van Dongen JJ, et al. The Bruton's tyrosine kinase gene is expressed throughout B cell differentiation, from early precursor B cell stages preceding immunoglobulin gene rearrangement up to mature B cell stages. *Eur J Immunol.* (1993) 23:3109–14. doi: 10.1002/eji.1830231210
45. Smith CI, Islam TC, Mattsson PT, Mohamed AJ, Nore BF, Vihinen M. The Tec family of cytoplasmic tyrosine kinases: mammalian Btk, Bmx, Itk, Tec, Txk and homologs in other species. *Bioessays.* (2001) 23:436–46. doi: 10.1002/bies.1062
46. Hutcheson J, Vanarsa K, Bashmakov A, Grewal S, Sajitharan D, Chang BY, et al. Modulating proximal cell signaling by targeting Btk ameliorates humoral autoimmunity and end-organ disease in murine lupus. *Arthritis Res Ther.* (2012) 14:R243. doi: 10.1186/ar4086
47. Lee A, Sandhu S, Imlay-Gillespie L, Mulligan S, Shumack S. Successful use of Bruton's kinase inhibitor, ibrutinib, to control paraneoplastic pemphigus in a patient with paraneoplastic autoimmune multiorgan syndrome and chronic lymphocytic leukaemia. *Australas J Dermatol.* (2017) 58:e240–2. doi: 10.1111/ajd.12615
48. Smith PF, Krishnarajah J, Nunn PA, Hill RJ, Karr D, Tam D, et al. A phase I trial of PRN1008, a novel reversible covalent inhibitor of Bruton's tyrosine kinase, in healthy volunteers. *Br J Clin Pharmacol.* (2017) 83:2367–76. doi: 10.1111/bcp.13351
49. Haeberle S, Wei X, Bieber K, Goletz S, Ludwig RJ, Schmidt E, et al. Regulatory T-cell deficiency leads to pathogenic bullous pemphigoid antigen 230 autoantibody and autoimmune bullous disease. *J Allergy Clin Immunol.* (2018) 142:1831–42.e1837. doi: 10.1016/j.jaci.2018.04.006
50. Bieber K, Sun S, Witte M, Kasprick A, Beltsiou F, Behnen M, et al. Regulatory T cells suppress inflammation and blistering in pemphigoid diseases. *Front Immunol.* (2017) 8:1628. doi: 10.3389/fimmu.2017.01628
51. Trzonkowski P, Bieniaszewska M, Juscinska J, Dobyszuk A, Krzystyniak A, Marek N, et al. First-in-man clinical results of the treatment of patients with graft versus host disease with human *ex vivo* expanded CD4+CD25+CD127- T regulatory cells. *Clin Immunol.* (2009) 133:22–6. doi: 10.1016/j.clim.2009.06.001

52. Bluestone JA, Buckner JH, Fitch M, Gitelman SE, Gupta S, Hellerstein MK, et al. Type 1 diabetes immunotherapy using polyclonal regulatory T cells. *Sci Transl Med.* (2015) 7:315ra189. doi: 10.1126/scitranslmed.aad4134
53. Brunstein CG, Miller JS, Cao Q, McKenna DH, Hippen KL, Curtsinger J, et al. Infusion of *ex vivo* expanded T regulatory cells in adults transplanted with umbilical cord blood: safety profile and detection kinetics. *Blood.* (2011) 117:1061–70. doi: 10.1182/blood-2010-07-293795
54. Zwang NA, Leventhal JR. Cell therapy in kidney transplantation: focus on regulatory T cells. *J Am Soc Nephrol.* (2017) 28:1960–72. doi: 10.1681/ASN.2016111206
55. Yokoyama T, Matsuda S, Takae Y, Wada N, Nishikawa T, Amagai M, et al. Antigen-independent development of Foxp3+ regulatory T cells suppressing autoantibody production in experimental pemphigus vulgaris. *Int Immunol.* (2011) 23:365–73. doi: 10.1093/intimm/dxr020
56. Schmidt T, Willenborg S, Hunig T, Deeg CA, Sonderstrup G, Hertl M, et al. Induction of T regulatory cells by the superagonistic anti-CD28 antibody D665 leads to decreased pathogenic IgG autoantibodies against desmoglein 3 in a HLA-transgenic mouse model of pemphigus vulgaris. *Exp Dermatol.* (2016) 25:293–8. doi: 10.1111/exd.12919
57. Zand N, Mansouri P, Fateh M, Ataie-Fashtami L, Rezaee Khiabanloo S, Safar F, et al. Relieving pain in oral lesions of pemphigus vulgaris using the non-ablative, non-thermal, CO2 laser therapy (NTCLT): preliminary results of a novel approach. *J Lasers Med Sci.* (2017) 8:7–12. doi: 10.15171/jlms.2017.02
58. Mignogna MD, Fortuna G, Leuci S, Adamo D, Dell'Aversana Orabona G, Ruoppo E. Adjuvant triamcinolone acetonide injections in oro-pharyngeal pemphigus vulgaris. *J Eur Acad Dermatol Venereol.* (2010) 24:1157–65. doi: 10.1111/j.1468-3083.2010.03610.x
59. Bystryn JC, Rudolph JL. Pemphigus. *Lancet.* (2005) 366:61–73. doi: 10.1016/S0140-6736(05)66829-8
60. Chicharro-Alcantara D, Rubio-Zaragoza M, Damia-Gimenez E, Carrillo-Poveda JM, Cuervo-Serrato B, Pelaez-Gorrea P, et al. Platelet rich plasma: new insights for cutaneous wound healing management. *J Funct Biomater.* (2018) 9:10. doi: 10.3390/jfb9010010
61. EL-Komy MH, Hassan AS, Abdel Raheem HM, Doss SS, EL-Kaliouby M, Saleh NA, et al. Platelet-rich plasma for resistant oral erosions of pemphigus vulgaris: a pilot study. *Wound Repair Regen.* (2015) 23:953–5. doi: 10.1111/wrr.12363
62. El-Komy MHM, Saleh NA, Saleh MA. Autologous platelet-rich plasma and triamcinolone acetonide intralesional injection in the treatment of oral erosions of pemphigus vulgaris: a pilot study. *Arch Dermatol Res.* (2018) 310:375–81. doi: 10.1007/s00403-018-1824-x
63. Hammers CM, Chen J, Lin C, Kacir S, Siegel DL, Payne AS, et al. Persistence of anti-desmoglein 3 IgG(+) B-cell clones in pemphigus patients over years. *J Invest Dermatol.* (2015) 135:742–9. doi: 10.1038/jid.2014.291
64. Miossec P, Korn T, Kuchroo VK. Interleukin-17 and type 17 helper T cells. *N Engl J Med.* (2009) 361:888–98. doi: 10.1056/NEJMra0707449
65. Volpe E, Servant N, Zollinger R, Bogiatzi SI, Hupe P, Barillot E, et al. A critical function for transforming growth factor-beta, interleukin 23 and proinflammatory cytokines in driving and modulating human T(H)-17 responses. *Nat Immunol.* (2008) 9:650–7. doi: 10.1038/ni.1613
66. Langrish CL, Chen Y, Blumenschein WM, Mattson J, Basham B, Sedgwick JD, et al. IL-23 drives a pathogenic T cell population that induces autoimmune inflammation. *J Exp Med.* (2005) 201:233–40. doi: 10.1084/jem.20041257
67. Yang J, Sundrud MS, Skepner J, Yamagata T. Targeting Th17 cells in autoimmune diseases. *Trends Pharmacol Sci.* (2014) 35:493–500. doi: 10.1016/j.tips.2014.07.006
68. Takahashi H, Tsuji H, Hashimoto Y, Ishida-Yamamoto A, Iizuka H. Serum cytokines and growth factor levels in Japanese patients with psoriasis. *Clin Exp Dermatol.* (2010) 35:645–9. doi: 10.1111/j.1365-2230.2009.03704.x
69. Lubberts E, Joosten LA, van de Loo FA, Schwarzenberger P, Kolls J, van den Berg WB. Overexpression of IL-17 in the knee joint of collagen type II immunized mice promotes collagen arthritis and aggravates joint destruction. *Inflamm Res.* (2002) 51:102–4. doi: 10.1007/BF02684010
70. Toosi S, Bystryn JC. Potential role of interleukin-17 in the pathogenesis of bullous pemphigoid. *Med Hypotheses.* (2010) 74:727–8. doi: 10.1016/j.mehy.2009.10.038
71. Le Jan S, Plee J, Vallerand D, Dupont A, Delanez E, Durlach A, et al. Innate immune cell-produced IL-17 sustains inflammation in bullous pemphigoid. *J Invest Dermatol.* (2014) 134:2908–17. doi: 10.1038/jid.2014.263
72. Chakievska L, Holtsche MM, Kunstner A, Goletz S, Petersen BS, Thaci D, et al. IL-17A is functionally relevant and a potential therapeutic target in bullous pemphigoid. *J Autoimmun.* (2018) 96:104–12. doi: 10.1016/j.jaut.2018.09.003
73. Gordon KB, Blauvelt A, Papp KA, Langley RG, Luger T, Ohtsuki M, et al. Phase 3 trials of ixekizumab in moderate-to-severe plaque psoriasis. *N Engl J Med.* (2016) 375:345–56. doi: 10.1056/NEJMoa1512711
74. Engineer L, Ahmed AR. Role of intravenous immunoglobulin in the treatment of bullous pemphigoid: analysis of current data. *J Am Acad Dermatol.* (2001) 44:83–8. doi: 10.1067/mjd.2000.112288
75. Jolles S. A review of high-dose intravenous immunoglobulin (hdIVIg) in the treatment of the autoimmune blistering disorders. *Clin Exp Dermatol.* (2001) 26:127–31. doi: 10.1046/j.1365-2230.2001.00779.x
76. Ahmed AR. Intravenous immunoglobulin therapy for patients with bullous pemphigoid unresponsive to conventional immunosuppressive treatment. *J Am Acad Dermatol.* (2001) 45:825–35. doi: 10.1067/mjd.2001.116337
77. Venning VA, Taghipour K, Mohd Mustapa MF, Highet AS, Kirtschig G. British association of dermatologists' guidelines for the management of bullous pemphigoid 2012. *Br J Dermatol.* (2012) 167:1200–14. doi: 10.1111/bjd.12072
78. Mydlarski PR, Ho V, Shear NH. Canadian consensus statement on the use of intravenous immunoglobulin therapy in dermatology. *J Cutan Med Surg.* (2006) 10:205–21. doi: 10.2310/7750.2006.00048
79. Ahmed AR, Dahl MV. Consensus statement on the use of intravenous immunoglobulin therapy in the treatment of autoimmune mucocutaneous blistering diseases. *Arch Dermatol.* (2003) 139:1051–9. doi: 10.1001/archderm.139.8.1051
80. Sasaoka T, Ujiie H, Nishie W, Iwata H, Ishikawa M, Higashino H, et al. Intravenous IgG reduces pathogenic autoantibodies, serum IL-6 levels, and disease severity in experimental bullous pemphigoid models. *J Invest Dermatol.* (2018) 138:1260–7. doi: 10.1016/j.jid.2018.01.005
81. Kamaguchi M, Iwata H, Mori Y, Toyonaga E, Ujiie H, Kitagawa Y, et al. Anti-idiotypic antibodies against BP-IgG prevent type XVII collagen depletion. *Front Immunol.* (2017) 8:1669. doi: 10.3389/fimmu.2017.01669
82. Amagai M, Ikeda S, Hashimoto T, Mizuashi M, Fujisawa A, Ihn H, et al. A randomized double-blind trial of intravenous immunoglobulin for bullous pemphigoid. *J Dermatol Sci.* (2017) 85:77–84. doi: 10.1016/j.jdermsci.2016.11.003
83. Martinon F, Mayor A, Tschopp J. The inflammasomes: guardians of the body. *Annu Rev Immunol.* (2009) 27:229–65. doi: 10.1146/annurev.immunol.021908.132715
84. Lamkanfi M, Dixit VM. Mechanisms and functions of inflammasomes. *Cell.* (2014) 157:1013–22. doi: 10.1016/j.cell.2014.04.007
85. Wen H, Miao EA, Ting JP. Mechanisms of NOD-like receptor-associated inflammasome activation. *Immunity.* (2013) 39:432–41. doi: 10.1016/j.immuni.2013.08.037
86. Latz E, Xiao TS, Stutz A. Activation and regulation of the inflammasomes. *Nat Rev Immunol.* (2013) 13:397–411. doi: 10.1038/nri3452
87. Franchi L, Eigenbrod T, Munoz-Planillo R, Nunez G. The inflammasome: a caspase-1-activation platform that regulates immune responses and disease pathogenesis. *Nat Immunol.* (2009) 10:241–7. doi: 10.1038/ni.1703
88. Shaw PJ, Lukens JR, Burns S, Chi H, McGargill MA, Kanneganti TD. Cutting edge: critical role for PYCARD/ASC in the development of experimental autoimmune encephalomyelitis. *J Immunol.* (2010) 184:4610–4. doi: 10.4049/jimmunol.1000217
89. Kahlenberg JM, Kaplan MJ. The inflammasome and lupus: another innate immune mechanism contributing to disease pathogenesis? *Curr Opin Rheumatol.* (2014) 26:475–81. doi: 10.1097/BOR.0000000000000088
90. Duan Z, Zhang Y, Zeng Z, Pan F. Comment on "Inflammasome activation of IL-18 results in endothelial progenitor cell dysfunction in systemic lupus erythematosus". *J Immunol.* (2012) 189:499; author reply 499–500. doi: 10.4049/jimmunol.1290031

91. Kastbom A, Verma D, Eriksson P, Skogh T, Wingren G, Soderkvist P. Genetic variation in proteins of the cryopyrin inflammasome influences susceptibility and severity of rheumatoid arthritis (the Swedish TIRA project). *Rheumatology.* (2008) 47:415–7. doi: 10.1093/rheumatology/kem372
92. Fang H, Shao S, Cao T, Lei J, Dang E, Zhang J, et al. Increased expression of NLRP3 inflammasome components and interleukin-18 in patients with bullous pemphigoid. *J Dermatol Sci.* (2016) 83:116–23. doi: 10.1016/j.jdermsci.2016.04.009
93. Sadeghi H, Lockmann A, Hund AC, Samavedam UK, Pipi E, Vafia K, et al. Caspase-1-independent IL-1 release mediates blister formation in autoantibody-induced tissue injury through modulation of endothelial adhesion molecules. *J Immunol.* (2015) 194:3656–63. doi: 10.4049/jimmunol.1402688
94. Amber KT, Murrell DF, Schmidt E, Joly P, Borradori L. Autoimmune subepidermal bullous diseases of the skin and mucosae: clinical features, diagnosis, and management. *Clin Rev Allergy Immunol.* (2018) 54:26–51. doi: 10.1007/s12016-017-8633-4
95. Hashimoto T, Ohzono A, Teye K, Numata S, Hiroyasu S, Tsuruta D, et al. Detection of IgE autoantibodies to BP180 and BP230 and their relationship to clinical features in bullous pemphigoid. *Br J Dermatol.* (2017) 177:141–51. doi: 10.1111/bjd.15114
96. van Beek N, Luttmann N, Huebner F, Recke A, Karl I, Schulze FS, et al. Correlation of serum levels of IgE autoantibodies against BP180 with bullous pemphigoid disease activity. *JAMA Dermatol.* (2017) 153:30–8. doi: 10.1001/jamadermatol.2016.3357
97. Amber KT, Valdebran M, Kridin K, Grando SA. The role of eosinophils in bullous pemphigoid: a developing model of eosinophil pathogenicity in mucocutaneous disease. *Front Med.* (2018) 5:201. doi: 10.3389/fmed.2018.00201
98. Lin L, Hwang BJ, Culton DA, Li N, Burette S, Koller BH, et al. Eosinophils mediate tissue injury in the autoimmune skin disease bullous pemphigoid. *J Invest Dermatol.* (2018) 138:1032–43. doi: 10.1016/j.jid.2017.11.031
99. Wakugawa M, Nakamura K, Hino H, Toyama K, Hattori N, Okochi H, et al. Elevated levels of eotaxin and interleukin-5 in blister fluid of bullous pemphigoid: correlation with tissue eosinophilia. *Br J Dermatol.* (2000) 143:112–6. doi: 10.1046/j.1365-2133.2000.03599.x
100. Stahle-Backdahl M, Inoue M, Guidice GJ, Parks WC. 92-kD gelatinase is produced by eosinophils at the site of blister formation in bullous pemphigoid and cleaves the extracellular domain of recombinant 180-kD bullous pemphigoid autoantigen. *J Clin Invest.* (1994) 93:2022–30. doi: 10.1172/JCI117196
101. Borrego L, Maynard B, Peterson EA, George T, Iglesias L, Peters MS, et al. Deposition of eosinophil granule proteins precedes blister formation in bullous pemphigoid. Comparison with neutrophil and mast cell granule proteins. *Am J Pathol.* (1996) 148:897–909.
102. Bieber K, Ernst AL, Tukaj S, Holtsche MM, Schmidt E, Zillikens D, et al. Analysis of serum markers of cellular immune activation in patients with bullous pemphigoid. *Exp Dermatol.* (2017) 26:1248–52. doi: 10.1111/exd.13382
103. Honda K, Chihara J. Eosinophil activation by eotaxin–eotaxin primes the production of reactive oxygen species from eosinophils. *Allergy.* (1999) 54:1262–9.
104. Ding C, Li J, Zhang X. Bertilimumab Cambridge antibody technology group. *Curr Opin Investig Drugs.* (2004) 5:1213–8.
105. Amber KT, Maglie R, Solimani F, Eming R, Hertl M. Targeted therapies for autoimmune bullous diseases: current status. *Drugs.* (2018) 78:1527–48. doi: 10.1007/s40265-018-0976-5
106. Lamberts A, Euverman HI, Terra JB, Jonkman MF, Horvath B. Effectiveness and safety of rituximab in recalcitrant pemphigoid diseases. *Front Immunol.* (2018) 9:248. doi: 10.3389/fimmu.2018.00248
107. Geahlen RL. Getting Syk: spleen tyrosine kinase as a therapeutic target. *Trends Pharmacol Sci.* (2014) 35:414–22. doi: 10.1016/j.tips.2014.05.007
108. Samavedam UK, Mitschker N, Kasprick A, Bieber K, Schmidt E, Laskay T, et al. Whole-genome expression profiling in skin reveals SYK as a key regulator of inflammation in experimental epidermolysis bullosa acquisita. *Front Immunol.* (2018) 9:249. doi: 10.3389/fimmu.2018.00249
109. Sezin T, Krajewski M, Wutkowski A, Mousavi S, Chakievska L, Bieber K, et al. The leukotriene B4 and its receptor BLT1 act as critical drivers of neutrophil recruitment in murine bullous pemphigoid-like epidermolysis bullosa acquisita. *J Invest Dermatol.* (2017) 137:1104–13. doi: 10.1016/j.jid.2016.12.021
110. Lamberts A, Yale M, Grando SA, Horvath B, Zillikens D, Jonkman MF. Unmet needs in pemphigoid diseases: an international survey amongst patients, clinicians and researchers. *Acta Derm Venereol.* (2018) 99:224–5. doi: 10.2340/00015555-3052
111. Koga H, Kasprick A, Lopez R, Auli M, Pont M, Godessart N, et al. Therapeutic effect of a novel phosphatidylinositol-3-kinase delta inhibitor in experimental epidermolysis bullosa acquisita. *Front Immunol.* (2018) 9:1558. doi: 10.3389/fimmu.2018.01558
112. Koga H, Recke A, Vidarsson G, Pas HH, Jonkman MF, Hashimoto T, et al. PDE4 inhibition as potential treatment of epidermolysis bullosa acquisita. *J Invest Dermatol.* (2016) 136:2211–20. doi: 10.1016/j.jid.2016.06.619

17

Preferential Reactivity of Dipeptidyl Peptidase-IV Inhibitor-Associated Bullous Pemphigoid Autoantibodies to the Processed Extracellular Domains of BP180

Yosuke Mai, Wataru Nishie, Kentaro Izumi and Hiroshi Shimizu*

Department of Dermatology, Hokkaido University Graduate School of Medicine, Sapporo, Japan

Correspondence:
Wataru Nishie
nishie@med.hokudai.ac.jp

Bullous pemphigoid (BP) is a common autoimmune blistering disease in which autoantibodies target the hemidesmosomal components BP180 and/or BP230 in basal keratinocytes. In BP, 80 to 90% of autoantibodies target the juxtamembranous extracellular non-collagenous 16th A (NC16A) domain of BP180. Recently, the administration of dipeptidyl peptidase-IV inhibitors (DPP4i), which are widely used as antihyperglycemic drugs, has been recognized to be a causative factor for BP. DPP4i-associated BP (DPP4i-BP) autoantibodies tend to target epitopes on non-NC16A regions of BP180, and the pathomechanism for the development of the unique autoantibodies remains unknown. To address the characteristics of DPP4i-BP autoantibodies in detail, we performed epitope analysis of 18 DPP4i-BP autoantibodies targeting the non-NC16A domains of BP180 using various domain-specific as well as plasmin-digested polypeptides derived from recombinant BP180. Firstly, Western blotting showed that only one DPP4i-BP serum reacted with the epitopes on the intracellular domain of BP180, and no sera reacted with the C-terminal domain of the molecule. In addition, only 2 DPP4i-BP sera reacted with BP230 as determined by enzyme-linked immunosorbent assay. Thus, DPP4i-BP autoantibodies were found to mainly target the non-NC16A mid-portion of the extracellular domain of BP. Interestingly, Western blotting using plasmin-digested BP180 as a substrate revealed that all of the DPP4i-BP sera reacted more intensively with the 97-kDa processed extracellular domain of BP180, which is known as the LABD97 autoantigen, than full-length BP180 did. All of the DPP4i-BP autoantibodies targeting the LABD97 autoantigen were IgG1, and IgG4 was observed to react with the molecule in only 7 cases (38.9%). In summary, the present study suggests that IgG1-class autoantibodies targeting epitopes on the processed extracellular domain of BP180, i.e., LABD97, are the major autoantibodies in DPP4i-BP.

Keywords: bullous pemphigoid, dipeptidyl peptidase-IV inhibitor, dipeptidyl peptidase-IV inhibitor-associated bullous pemphigoid, autoantibodies, IgG subclass, BP180, BP230, autoimmune disease

INTRODUCTION

Bullous pemphigoid (BP) is a common autoimmune blistering disease in which autoantibodies target the hemidesmosomal components BP180 and/or BP230 in basal keratinocytes (1). In BP, almost 90% of autoantibodies target the juxtamembranous extracellular non-collagenous 16th A (NC16A) domain of BP180 (2). Recently, the administration of dipeptidyl peptidase-IV inhibitors (DPP4i), which are widely used as antihyperglycemic drugs, is recognized to be a causative factor for BP (3). In 2016, a strong relationship between the onset of BP under DPP4i exposure was reported from the France Pharmacovigilance Database (4). Thereafter, retrospective case-control studies from Finland, (5) Switzerland, (6) France, (6) Israel (7), and Japan (the Japanese Adverse Drug Event Report Database) (8) also confirmed that the administration of DPP4i, especially vildagliptin, was associated with increased risk of BP development. In addition, based on the National Healthcare Insurance Agency of France, the observed frequencies of DPP4i intake in the BP population are higher than those in the general population (9). Although the increased risk of BP development after the use of DPP4i has been intensively studied, the mechanisms whereby DPP4i administration causes BP development remains to be elucidated.

We and other groups have recently reported that Japanese patients with DPP4i-associated BP (DPP4i-BP) may show unique clinical and immunological characteristics (10–14). Clinically, DPP4i-BP patients tend to show a less severe erythematous phenotype than typical non-DPP4i BP patients show. In terms of the Bullous Pemphigoid Disease Area Index (BPDAI) (15) a commonly used disease severity score for BP, patients with typical BP do not differ significantly from patients with DPP4i-BP in terms of erosion/blister scores, whereas patients with DPP4i-BP have significantly less severe erythema/urticaria than patients with typical BP have. Immunologically, DPP4i-BP autoantibodies preferentially target the mid-portion of the extracellular region of BP180 without reactivity toward the NC16A domain (10). Interestingly anti-BP180 NC16A autoantibodies may be produced during the clinical course of DPP4i-BP as a result of epitope spreading (13, 14). After the production of anti-BP180 NC16A autoantibodies, clinical manifestations of DPP4i-BP may resemble those of typical non-DPP4i-BP (13, 14). Thus, anti-BP180 NC16A autoantibodies may be observed also in DPP4i-BP.

In this study, we collected 18 cases of "pure" DPP4i-BP in which autoantibodies did not target the NC16A domain of BP180. As a result, it has been revealed that DPP4i-BP autoantibodies are IgG1-class autoantibodies which target epitopes on the non-NC16A processed extracellular domains of BP180.

Abbreviations: BP, bullous pemphigoid; NC16A, the 16th non-collagenous domain; DPP4i, dipeptidyl peptidase-IV inhibitor(s); DPP4i-BP, dipeptidyl peptidase-IV inhibitor-associated bullous pemphigoid; ELISA, enzyme-linked immunosorbent assay; BPDAI, bullous pemphigoid disease area index.

MATERIALS AND METHODS

Patient Characteristics

BP was diagnosed based on clinical, histopathological, and immunological findings (1). The clinical and immunological characteristics of the DPP4i-BP cases in this study are listed in **Table 1** and summarized in **Table 2**. Direct immunofluorescence study showed positive results for IgG and/or C3 deposition at the basement membrane zone in all cases. The mean age was 78.8 and ranged from 57 to 93. The female/male ratio was 6:12. The mean index value of full-length BP180 ELISA was 108.2 and ranged from 60.9 to 171.7 (cutoff < 4.64). None of our cases was positive for BP180 NC16A by chemiluminescent enzyme immunoassay. BPDAI scores for blister/erosion, urticaria/erythema, and total mucosa are summarized in **Table 1**. Vildagliptin was the most common DPP4i (38.9%), followed by teneligliptin (33.3%), and Sitagliptin (27.8%) (**Table 3**).

Preparation of Recombinant Proteins

Full-length human BP180 recombinant protein (Met^{1} – Pro^{1497}) and polypeptides corresponding to the intracellular domain (Met^{1} to Trp^{467}) and the C-terminus region (Leu^{1281} – Pro^{1497}) of BP180 were produced using the Flp-In 293 system (Invitrogen, CA) as previously reported (10). Processed BP180 extracellular fragments of 120-kDa and 97-kDa forms, which are known as LAD-1 and LABD97, respectively, were generated by limited plasmin digestion of the full-length recombinant BP180 protein (10). Schematics of the recombinant proteins and the plasmin-digested proteins are given in **Figure 1A**. Mixture substrate samples of full-length BP180, LAD-1, and LABD97 were used for Western blotting, of which even doses were confirmed by Coomassie Blue staining (**Figure 1B**).

Immunofluorescence Study

For indirect immunofluorescence study using 1 M NaCl-split skin, normal human skin was incubated in 1 M NaCl solution for 48 h at 4°C. Thereafter, the skin was mounted and snap-frozen in OCT compound (Thermo Fisher Scientific, MA), and 5-μm cryosections were prepared. The sections were then incubated with patients' sera (dilution 1:10–20) for 40 min at 37°C. After washing with PBS 3 times, the sections were incubated with FITC-conjugated antibodies to human IgG (dilution 1:100) (Dako Cytomation, Denmark) for 30 min at 37°C.

Western Blotting

Protein samples were separated by SDS-PAGE electrophoresis using 7 or 10% SDS-polyacrylamide gel. The gels were transferred to nitrocellulose membranes (Bio Rad, CA). The membranes were blocked for 30 min at room temperature with 2% skimmed milk in TBS. After incubation with 1:200 diluted patient serum with 2% skimmed milk in TBS for 1 h at room temperature, horseradish peroxidase-conjugated secondary anti-human IgG (1:1,000) (Dako Cytomation, Denmark), IgG1 (1:500) (Thermo Fisher Scientific, MA), or IgG4 (1:500) (Thermo Fisher Scientific, MA) antibodies in the same buffer were reacted at room temperature for 1 h. Signals were visualized with Clarity Western ECL Substrate (Bio Rad, CA). Each protein band was quantified using Fiji (16). Relative intensities were calculated for each band

TABLE 1 | List of DPP4i-BP cases.

No	Age	Sex	Full-length BP180	BP180 NC16A	BP230	DPP4i	DIF	ssIIF	Delay after BP onset	BPDAI
1	55–60	Male	94.4	(–)	2.3	Teneligliptin	IgG, C3	roof side	–	–
2	75–80	Male	86.6	(–)	1.5	Vildagliptin, Teneligliptin, Sitagliptin	IgG, C3	roof side	7 months	–
3	90–95	Male	150.6	(–)	2.3	Anagliptin	IgG, IgA, IgM, C3	roof side	7 months	52–7–0
4	90–95	Female	130.6	(–)	3.4	Vildagliptin	IgG, C3	roof side	2 months	36–NA–5
5	70–75	Male	103.8	(–)	1.7	Teneligliptin, Vildagliptin	IgG, C3	roof side	6 months	–
6	80–85	Male	102.3	(–)	4.7	Vildagliptin	IgG, C3	roof side	2 months	–
7	65–70	Male	60.93	(–)	0.4	Sitagliptin	IgG, C3	roof side	3 months	–
8	85–90	Female	109.9	(–)	1.7	Teneligliptin	IgG, IgM, C3	roof side	2 months	total 30
9	80–85	Female	171.7	(–)	1.1	Omarigliptin	C3	roof side	2 months	–
10	90–95	Female	98.9	(–)	20.3	Alogliptin, Sitagliptin	IgG, C3	roof side	2 months	–
11	85–90	Male	113.2	(–)	1.9	Teneligliptin	IgG, C3	roof side	1 month	7–6–0
12	55–60	Female	139	(–)	2.6	Vildagliptin	IgG, C3	roof side	2 months	9–7–15
13	70–75	Male	81.7	(–)	4.1	Vildagliptin, Sitagliptin	IgG, IgA, C3	roof side	–	13–0–0
14	85–90	Male	111.2	(–)	3.3	Alogliptin, Linagliptin	IgG, IgA, IgM, C3	roof side	2 months	38–0–0
15	70–74	Male	103.7	(–)	14.3	Vildagliptin	IgG, C3	roof side	3 months	46–3–0
16	75–80	Male	84.5	(–)	2.5	Teneligliptin	IgG C3	roof side	2 weeks	–
17	50–60	Female	79.5	(–)	2.3	Anagliptin, Linagliptin	IgG, C3	roof side	8 months	–
18	90–95	Male	125.4	(–)	3.7	Sitagliptin, Linagliptin	IgG, C3	roof side	2 weeks	–

Full-length BP180 ELISA: Index values, cutoff<4.64. BP230ELISA: Index values, cutoff < 9.0. NA, means not available.

TABLE 2 | Summary of patient attributes.

Age, mean (range), years	78.8 (57–93)
Female/male, *n*; sex ratio	6/12
Full-length BP180 ELISA, mean (range), index values	108.2 (60.9–171)
BP180 NC16a, positive rate, *n* (%)	0 (0%)
BP230 ELISA, mean (range), index values	4.2 (1.1–20.3)
BP230 ELISA, positive rate, *n* (%)	2 (11.1%)

TABLE 3 | DPP4i use.

Vildagliptin	7 (38.9%)
Teneligliptin	6 (33.3%)
Sitagliptin	5 (27.8%)
Linagliptin	3 (16.7%)
Alogliptin	2 (11.1%)
Anagliptin	2 (111%)
Omarigliptin	1 (5.6%)

based on the intensity of the 180-kDa bands. Case No.11 was excluded since the intensity of the 180-kDa band was faint.

Enzyme-Linked Immunosorbent Assay (ELISA)

ELISA using full-length BP180 recombinant proteins was performed as previously described, with a minor modification (10). Briefly, 96-well plates (Thermo Fisher Scientific, MA) were coated with 1 μg/well of the recombinant proteins in 50 mM carbonate buffer pH 9.5 and then blocked with Blocking Reagent for ELISA (Roche, Swiss) for 2 h at room temperature. Patient sera were diluted to 1:100 and incubated for 1 h at room temperature. After washing, the plates were incubated with 1:500 diluted horseradish peroxidase-conjugated anti-human IgG antibody for 1 h at room temperature. Subsequently, the plates were reacted with a substrate solution, 3, 3′, 5, 5′tetramthylbenzidine dihydrochloride single solution (Thermo Fisher Scientific, MA). After color development, the reaction was stopped with the addition of 0.12 N hydrochloric acid, and absorbance was measured at 450 nm by a microplate reader with the correlation wavelength set at 620 nm (Tecan Austria GmbH, Austria). To detect anti-BP230 autoantibodies, BP230 ELISA (MESACUP BP230 ELISA kit, MBL, Japan) was performed according to the manufacturer's instructions.

Statistical Analysis

Statistical analysis was performed using GraphPad Prism 6 (GraphPad Software, USA). Data were analyzed using two-way analysis of variance, followed by Tukey's multiple comparison test. p-values are indicated as $^{*}0.01 < p < 0.05$, $^{**}0.001 < p < 0.01$, and $^{****}p < 0.0001$.

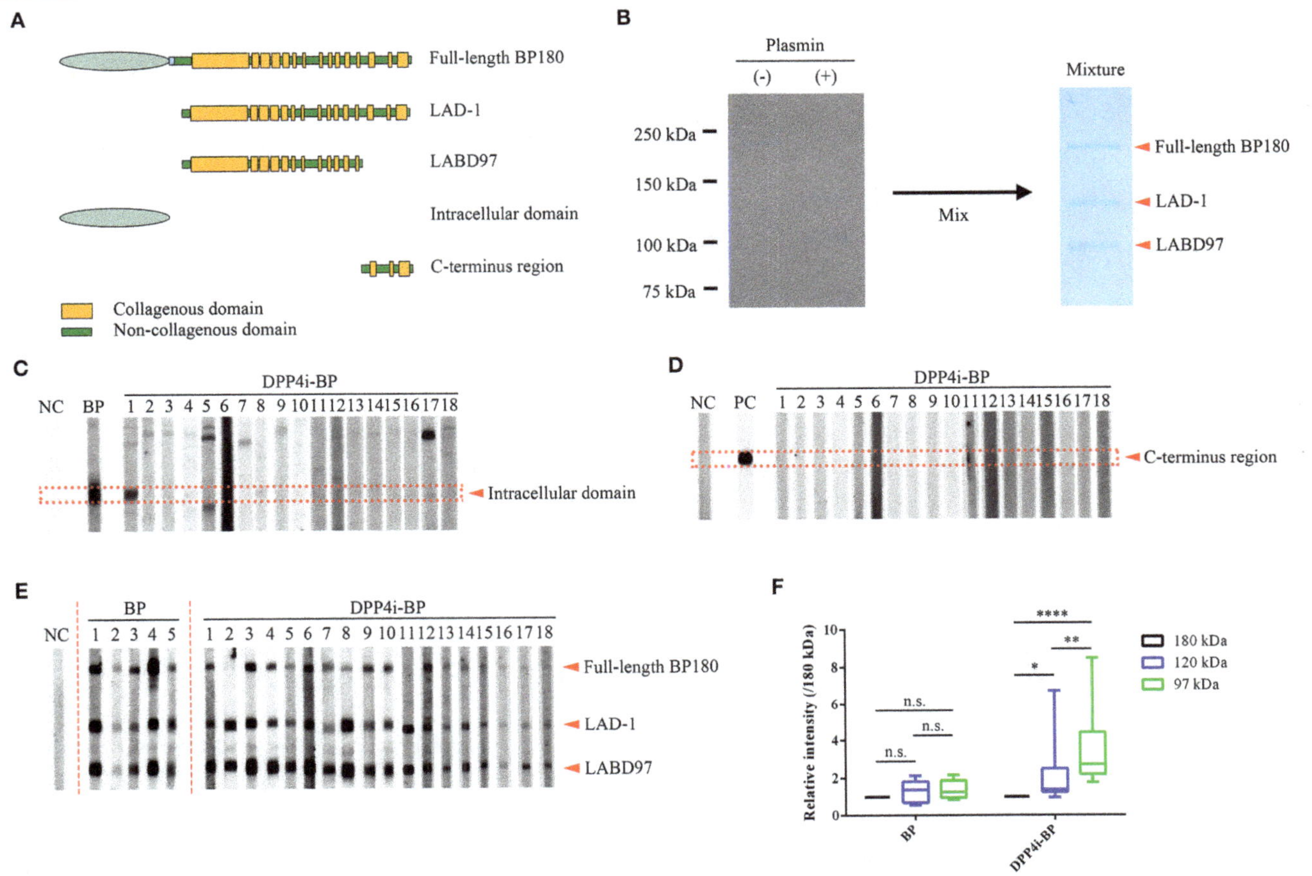

FIGURE 1 | Epitope mapping of DPP4i-BP autoantibodies. **(A)** Schematic of recombinant proteins. **(B)** Coomassie Blue staining using a mixture of substrates including the full-length recombinant BP180 and plasmin-digested BP180 proteins. **(C–E)** Western blots using the intracellular domain of BP180 **(C)**, C-terminal regions of BP180 **(D)**, and a mixture of full-length recombinant BP180 and plasmin-digested BP180 proteins **(E)**. Relative intensities of 180-kDa, 120-kDa, and 97-kDa bands in BP and DPP4i-BP **(F)**. Data were analyzed using two-way analysis of variance, followed by Tukey's multiple comparison test. p-values are indicated as $^{*}0.01 < p < 0.05$, $^{**}0.001 < p < 0.01$, and $^{****}p < 0.0001$. n.s., Not significant; NC, Negative control using healthy individual sera; PC, Positive control using anti-FLAG antibody.

RESULTS

Preferential Reactivity of DPP4i-BP Autoantibodies to the Processed Extracellular Domain of BP180

Firstly, we performed Western blotting using the recombinant intracellular and C-terminal proteins of BP180 (**Figures 1C,D**). Only one case had autoantibodies targeting the intracellular region of BP180, and no cases had autoantibodies targeting both fragments (**Figures 1C,D**). In addition, autoantibodies targeting BP230 were only detected in two cases (11.1%) by BP230 ELISA (cutoff < 9.0) (**Tables 1, 2**). We also confirmed that there were no IgG autoantibodies targeting the dermal side of the artificial blisters in 1 M NaCl-split skin indirect immunofluorescence (**Supplemental Figure 1**).

To identify the epitopes of IgG autoantibodies in DPP4i-BP, we performed Western blotting using mixture samples of full-length BP180 and plasmin-digested 120-kDa (LAD-1) and 97-kDa (LABD97) fragments (**Figure 1E**). IgG autoantibodies of all cases except for case No.11 reacted to the full-length BP180 (**Figure 1E**), which is mostly consistent with the result of full-length BP180 ELISA (**Table 1**). Interestingly, IgG autoantibodies showed more intense reactivity to LABD97 than to LAD-1 or full-length BP180 (**Figures 1E,F**). In contrast, the autoantibodies in typical non-DPP4i BP reacted almost equally to each band (**Figures 1E,F**). Since none of the cases reacted with the NC16A domain of BP180, all of the DPP4i-BP autoantibodies tested in this study showed preferential reactivities toward the processed extracellular domain of BP180.

IgG1 Autoantibodies to LABD97 Are Major Autoantibodies in DPP4I-BP

It is known that both IgG1 and IgG4 are the predominant autoantibodies in BP (17). Therefore, we evaluated IgG1 and IgG4 autoantibody reactivities to the full-length BP180 and the plasmin-digested LAD-1 and LABD97 fragments of BP180. Although all cases had IgG1 autoantibodies targeting each form of BP180, it should be noted that significant reactivities to LABD97 were observed (**Figure 2**). In contrast, 7 of 18 cases (38.9%) had IgG4 autoantibodies targeting

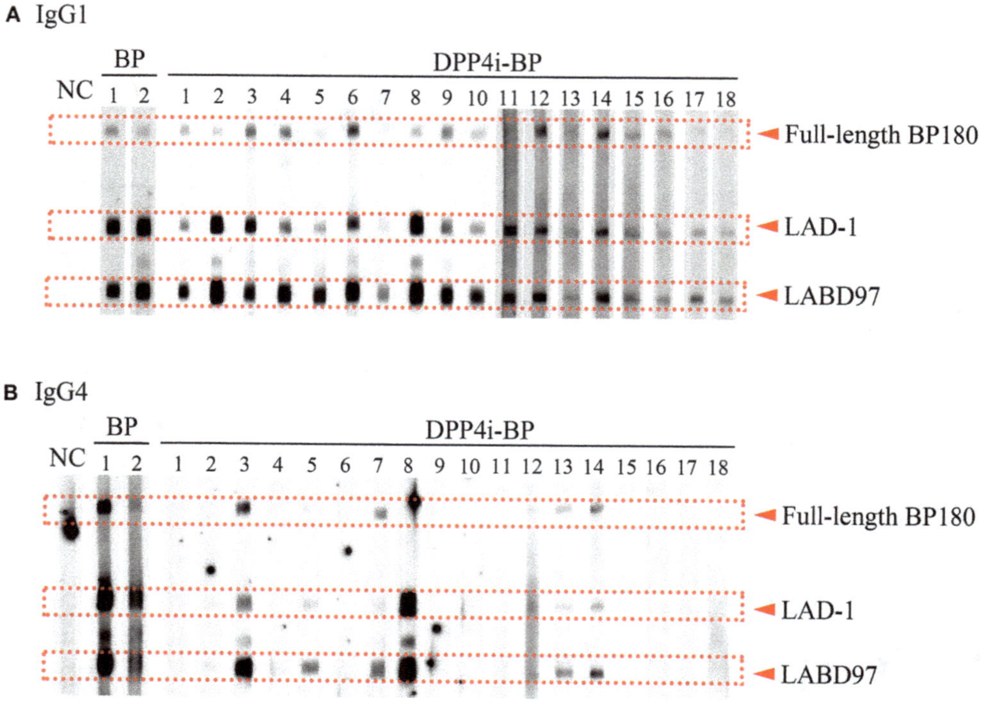

FIGURE 2 | IgG subclass analysis of DPP4i-BP. Detection of IgG1 **(A)** and IgG4 **(B)** autoantibodies by Western blot using a mixture of full-length recombinant BP180 and plasmin-digested BP180 proteins.

various forms of BP180 (**Figure 2**). These findings suggest that IgG1 autoantibodies to LABD97 are major autoantibodies in DPP4i-BP.

DISCUSSION

In this study, we analyzed autoantibodies of 18 DPP4i-BP cases without reactivity to the NC16A domain of BP180. Consistent with our previous study using small numbers of DPP4i-BP cases, (10) all of the autoantibodies showed positive reactivity to the processed extracellular domain of BP180. Interestingly, all of the DPP4i-BP autoantibodies tested in this study showed preferential reactivity to LABD97. A similar characteristic of autoantibodies can be found in another autoimmune blistering skin disease, linear IgA bullous dermatosis. In linear IgA bullous dermatosis, autoantibodies preferentially react with neoepitopes that selectively develop on LAD-1 and LABD97, and they do not react with full-length BP180 (18, 19). BP180 can be processed by several proteases under physiological or pathological conditions, Franzke et al. (20), Hofmann et al. (21) and the N-terminal deletion resulting from cleavage within the NC16A domain of BP180 results in the production of LAD-1 (20). In addition, further C-terminal deletion produces LABD97 (21). This processing of BP180 may induce conformational changes on the molecule, which also may induce new epitopes distinct from those on the native full-length form of BP180 (22–25). Several studies have shown that antibodies targeting the 15th collagenous domain or its neighboring regions in BP180 preferentially react with LAD-1 and LABD97 (22, 23). In addition, our previous study revealed that the C-terminus processing of BP180 induces neoepitopes on the 15th collagenous domain of BP180 (24). Thus, not only does cleavage within the NC16A domain cause neoepitopes to develop on the 15th collagenous domain of BP180, but so does C-terminal processing (25). Although fine epitope mapping of DPP4i-BP autoantibodies will be necessary in future studies, the preferential reactivity of DPP4i-BP autoantibodies to LABD97 may suggest the possibility that putative epitopes may exit on the 15th collagenous domain or in its neighboring regions.

The present study also revealed that all of the DPP4i-BP autoantibodies which preferentially targeted the LABD97 fragment of BP180 were IgG1. In contrast, IgG4-subclass autoantibodies were only observed in 38.9% of our cases. These results indicate that IgG1 autoantibodies targeting epitopes on LABD97 are the main autoantibodies in DPP4i-BP. This finding was unexpected, because it is well-known that IgG1 BP autoantibodies are able to activate the complement pathway associated with the development of inflammation, (26) whereas DPP4i-BP tends to show a non-inflammatory phenotype associated with scant urticarial erythema and fewer infiltrating eosinophils than those of non-DPP4i BP, despite activating the complement at dermal-epidermal junctions (10–14). Thus, the predominance of IgG1 autoantibodies in DPP4i-BP stands in contrast to the previous concept of BP pathogenesis (26). Although further studies are necessary to resolve this issue, the present study indicates that complement activation is insufficient to induce inflammation in DPP4i-BP.

The pathogenicity of IgG4 is controversial. An experimental mouse model showed that IgG4 plays a protective role against the development of BP (27). In contrast, it is experimentally shown that IgG4 BP autoantibodies have the capacity to induce leucocyte-dependent dermal-epidermal separation (28). In addition, BP cases with only IgG4 autoantibodies have been reported (29). As this IgG4-type BP shows a non-inflammatory phenotype, IgG4 autoantibodies are assumed to play complement-independent roles in BP development, such as a role in BP180 depletion in keratinocytes, the Fc-dependent activation of neutrophils, or leucocyte-dependent dermal-epidermal separation (26, 28, 30). In our subclass analysis of DPP4i-BP, IgG4 autoantibodies preferentially reacted to LABD97, similar to IgG1 autoantibodies. However, the positive rates for IgG4 autoantibodies to LABD97 and full-length BP180 were lower than those of IgG1 autoantibodies, especially to full-length BP180. This discrepancy may suggest that the development of IgG1 autoantibodies might precede IgG4 autoantibody development in DPP4i-BP, although other possibilities cannot be ruled out.

CONCLUDING REMARKS

In conclusion, major epitopes of DPP4i-BP were located in the mid-portion of the extracellular domain, and these epitopes can be presented on LABD97. All such autoantibodies were in the IgG1 class. The unique immunological characteristics of DPP4i-BP autoantibodies may help us understand the pathological mechanism behind the development of the disease.

ETHICS STATEMENT

This report on a single patient complies with the Declaration of Helsinki. The patient gave written informed consent for publication. This study was approved by the institutional review board of Hokkaido University (institutional review board number: 016-0061).

AUTHOR CONTRIBUTIONS

YM, WN, and KI drafted the paper and collected the clinical data. HS supervised the writing of the manuscript.

ACKNOWLEDGMENTS

The authors thank the patient and express their appreciation to Nami Ikeshita for her technical assistance.

REFERENCES

1. Schmidt E, Zillikens D. Pemphigoid diseases. *Lancet.* (2013) 26:320–32. doi: 10.1016/S0140-6736(12)61140-4
2. Kobayashi M, Amagai M, Kuroda-Kinoshita K, Hashimoto T, Shirakata Y, Hashimoto K, et al. BP180 ELISA using bacterial recombinant NC16a protein as a diagnostic and monitoring tool for bullous pemphigoid. *J Dermatol Sci.* (2002) 30:224–32. doi: 10.1016/S0923-1811(02)00109-3
3. Skandalis K, Spirova M, Gaitanis G, Tsartsarakis A, Bassukas ID. Drug-induced bullous pemphigoid in diabetes mellitus patients receiving dipeptidyl peptidase-IV inhibitors plus metformin. *J Eur Acad Dermatol Venereol.* (2012) 26:249–53. doi: 10.1111/j.1468-3083.2011.04062.x
4. Béné J, Moulis G, Bennani I, Auffret M, Coupe P, Babai S, et al. Bullous pemphigoid and dipeptidyl peptidase IV inhibitors: a case-noncase study in the French Pharmacovigilance Database. *Br J Dermatol.* (2016) 175:296–301. doi: 10.1111/bjd.14601
5. Varpuluoma O, Försti AK, Jokelainen J, Turpeinen M, Timonen M, Huilaja L, et al. Vildagliptin significantly increases the risk of bullous pemphigoid: a finnish nationwide registry study. *J Invest Dermatol.* (2018) 138:1659–61. doi: 10.1016/j.jid.2018.01.027
6. Benzaquen M, Borradori L, Berbis P, Cazzaniga S, Valero R, Richard MA, et al. Dipeptidyl pepidase IV inhibitors, a risk factor for bullous pemphigoid: retrospective multicenter case-control study from France and Switzerland. *J Am Acad Dermatol.* (2018) 78:1090–6. doi: 10.1016/j.jaad.2017.12.038
7. Kridin K, Bergman R. Association of bullous pemphigoid with dipeptidyl-peptidase 4 inhibitors in patients with diabetes: estimating the risk of the new agents and characterizing the patients *JAMA Dermatol.* (2018) 154:1152–8. doi: 10.1001/jamadermatol.2018.2352
8. Arai M, Shirakawa J, Konishi H, Sagawa N, Terauchi Y. Bullous pemphigoid and dipeptidyl peptidase 4 inhibitors: a disproportionality analysis based on the japanese adverse drug event report database. *Diabetes Care.* (2018) 41:e130–2. doi: 10.2337/dc18-0210
9. Plaquevent M, Tétart F, Fardet L, Ingen-Housz-Oro S, Valeyrie-Allanore L, Bernard P, et al. Higher frequency of dipeptidyl peptidase IV inhibitor intake in bullous pemphigoid patients than in the French general population. *J Invest Dermatol.* (2019) 139:835–41. doi: 10.1016/j.jid.2018.10.045
10. Izumi K, Nishie W, Mai Y, Wada M, Natsuga K, Ujiie H, et al. Autoantibody profile differentiates between inflammatory and noninflammatory bullous pemphigoid. *J Invest Dermatol.* (2016) 136:2201–10. doi: 10.1016/j.jid.2016.06.622
11. Ujiie H, Muramatsu K, Mushiroda T, Ozeki T, Miyoshi H, Iwata H, et al. HLA-DQB1*03:01 as a biomarker for genetic susceptibility to bullous pemphigoid induced by DPP-4 inhibitors. *J Invest Dermatol.* (2018) 138:1201–4. doi: 10.1016/j.jid.2017.11.023
12. Horikawa H, Kurihara Y, Funakoshi T, Umegaki-Arao N, Takahashi H, Kubo A, et al. Unique clinical and serological features of bullous pemphigoid associated with dipeptidyl peptidase-4 inhibitors. *Br J Dermatol.* (2018) 178:1462–3. doi: 10.1111/bjd.16479
13. Mai Y, Nishie W, Izumi K, Yoshimoto N, Morita Y, Watanabe M, et al. Detection of anti-BP180 NC16A autoantibodies after the onset of dipeptidyl peptidase-IV inhibitor-associated bullous pemphigoid: a report of three patients. *Br J Dermatol.* (2018) 179:790–1. doi: 10.1111/bjd.16656
14. Takama H, Yoshida M, Izumi K, Yanagishita T, Muto J, Ohshima Y, et al. Dipeptidyl peptidase-4 inhibitor-associated bullous pemphigoid: recurrence with epitope spreading. *Acta Derm Venereol.* (2018) 98:983–4. doi: 10.2340/00015555-3010

15. Murrell DF, Daniel BS, Joly P, Borradori L, Amagai M, Hashimoto T, et al. Definitions and outcome measures for bullous pemphigoid: recommendations by an international panel of experts. *J Am Acad Dermatol.* (2012) 66:479–85. doi: 10.1016/j.jaad.2011.06.032
16. Schindelin J, Arganda-Carreras I, Frise E, Kaynig V, Longair M, Pietzsch T, et al. Fiji: an open-source platform for biological- image analysis. *Nat Method.* (2012) 28:676–82. doi: 10.1038/nmeth.2019
17. Sitaru C, Mihai S, Zillikens D. The relevance of the IgG subclass of autoantibodies for blister induction in autoimmune bullous skin disease. *Arch Dermatol Res.* (2007) 299:1–8. doi: 10.1007/s00403-007-0734-0
18. Zone JJ, Taylor TB, Kadunce DP, Meyer LJ. Identification of the cutaneous basement membrane zone antigen and isolation of antibody in linear immunoglobulin A bullous dermatosis. *J Clin Invest.* (1990) 85:812–20. doi: 10.1172/JCI114508
19. Marinkovich MP, Taylor TB, Keene DR, Burgeson RE, Zone JJ. LAD-1, the linear IgA bullous dermatosis autoantigen, is a novel 120-kDa anchoring filament protein synthesized by epidermal cells. *J Invest Dermatol.* (1996) 106:734–8. doi: 10.1111/1523-1747.ep12345782
20. Franzke CW, Tasanen K, Schäcke H, Zhou Z, Tryggvason K, Mauch C, et al. Transmembrane collagen XVII, an epithelial adhesion protein, is shed from the cell surface by ADAMs. *EMBO J.* (2002) 21:5026–35. doi: 10.1093/emboj/cdf532
21. Hofmann SC, Voith U, Schönau V, Sorokin L, Bruckner-Tuderman L, Franzke CW. Plasmin plays a role in the *in vitro* generation of the linear IgA dermatosis antigen LADB97. *J Invest Dermatol.* (2009) 129:1730–9. doi: 10.1038/jid.2008.424
22. Nie Z, Nagata Y, Joubeh S, Hirako Y, Owaribe K, Kitajima Y, et al. IgA antibodies of linear IgA bullous dermatosis recognize the 15th collagenous domain of BP180. *J Invest Dermatol.* (2000) 115:1164–6. doi: 10.1046/j.1523-1747.2000.0202a-7.x
23. Yamauchi T, Matsushita S, Hashimoto T, Hirako Y. Major cleavage-dependent epitopes for linear IgA bullous dermatosis are formed at the boundary between the non-collagenous 16A and collagenous 15 domains of BP180. *J Dermatol Sci.* (2014) 76:25–33. doi: 10.1016/j.jdermsci.2014.07.008
24. Toyonaga E, Nishie W, Izumi K, Natsuga K, Ujiie H, Iwata H, et al. C-termial processing of collagen XVII induces neoepitopes for linear IgA dermatosis. *J Invest Dermatol.* (2017) 137:2552–9. doi: 10.1016/j.jid.2017.07.831
25. Hashimoto T, Ishii N, Tsuruta D. Production of neoepitopes by dnamic structural changes on BP180/type XVII collagen. *J Invest Dermatol.* (2017) 137:2462–4. doi: 10.1016/j.jid.2017.09.001
26. Dainichi T, Chow Z, Kabashima K. IgG4, complement, and the mechanisms of blister formation in pemphigus and bullous pemphigoid. *J Dermatol Sci.* (2017) 88:265–70. doi: 10.1016/j.jdermsci.2017.07.012
27. Zuo Y, Evangelista F, Culton D, Guilabert A, Lin L, Li N, et al. IgG4 autoantibodies are inhibitory in the autoimmune disease bullous pemphigoid. *J Autoimmun.* (2016) 73:111–9. doi: 10.1016/j.jaut.2016.06.019
28. Mihai S, Chiriac MT, Herrero-González JE, Goodall M, Jefferis R, Savage CO, et al. IgG4 autoantibodies induce dermal-epidermal separation. *J Cell Mol Med.* (2007) 11:1117–28. doi: 10.1111/j.1582-4934.2007.00081.x
29. Dainichi T, Nishie W, Yamagami Y, Sonobe H, Ujiie H, Kaku Y, et al. Bullous pemphigoid suggestive of complement-independent blister formation with anti-BP180 IgG4 autoantibodies. *Br J Dermatol.* (2016) 175:187–90. doi: 10.1111/bjd.14411
30. Zhao M, Trimbeger ME, Li N, Diaz LA, Shapiro SD, Liu Z. Role of FcRs in animal model of autoimmune bullous pemphigoid. *J Immunol.* (2006) 177:3398–405. doi: 10.4049/jimmunol.177.5.3398

18

Radiation-Associated Pemphigus Vulgaris in a Patient with Preceding Malignancy: Treatment with Rituximab as a Valuable Option

*Franziska Schauer[1], Norito Ishii[2,3], Maja Mockenhaupt[1], Leena Bruckner-Tuderman[1], Takashi Hashimoto[4] and Dimitra Kiritsi[1]**

[1] Department of Dermatology, Medical Center - University of Freiburg, Faculty of Medicine, University of Freiburg, Freiburg, Germany, [2] Department of Dermatology, Kurume University School of Medicine, Kurume, Japan, [3] Institute of Cutaneous Cell Biology, Kurume University, Kurume, Japan, [4] Department of Dermatology, Osaka City University Graduate School of Medicine, Osaka, Japan

***Correspondence:**
Dimitra Kiritsi
dimitra.kiritsi@uniklinik-freiburg.de

Pemphigus is a chronic autoimmune blistering disorder, characterized by (muco-)cutaneous erosions due to autoantibodies against desmoglein 3 and/or 1. Pemphigus induction might be associated with drugs, malignancy or radiation therapy (RT); the latter being only rarely described. A rigorous literature review revealed around 30 cases of RT-associated pemphigus, which had been primarily treated with topical and/or systemic steroids, in some cases also dapsone or few other immunosuppressive agents were given. The most common underlying cancer type was breast cancer. We here present a 63-year-old male patient, who was pre-treated with adjuvant RT for larynx carcinoma 3 months before admission. He developed extensive cutaneous, ocular, and oral erosions. Despite the clinical picture comparable to a paraneoplastic pemphigus, the diagnosis of pemphigus vulgaris of mucocutaneous type was established based on the direct immunofluorescence, showing positive cell surface IgG and discrete C3 deposits, with matching cell surface IgG pattern on monkey esophagus. Serum autoantibodies to desmoglein 1 and 3 were highly positive. No further autoantibodies were found, thus paraneoplastic pemphigus was excluded. The patient was treated with high dose prednisolone, partially given intravenously up to 2 mg/kg per day, as well as topical disinfectants and class IV steroid cream. To stabilize the disease rituximab 2 × 1,000 mg was given, leading to clinical and serological remission for up to 2 years now. We show that rituximab represents a good treatment option for the frequently treatment-refractory RT-associated pemphigus, a clinically and immunologically specific RT-induced skin disorder, resulting in long-term clinical, and serological remission.

Keywords: autoimmune blistering disorder, desmoglein, desmosome, desmosomal adhesion, radiation therapy

INTRODUCTION

The incidence of pemphigus has been estimated to be between 0.5 and 34 cases/million inhabitants/year (1), thus the disease is considered to be rare. As factors related to the induction of pemphigus, specific drugs and malignancy, but also radiation therapy (RT) have been proposed. Malignancy-associated pemphigus has an incidence of 5–11%, while malignancy-associated bullous pemphigoid has a reported incidence of 5.8–10.2% in retrospective studies (2, 3). As the underlying malignancy, lung cancer was most common in pemphigus, and gastric cancer in bullous pemphigoid (3). Cases of RT-associated pemphigus have only rarely been described in the literature (**Table 1**). In this study, we report the development of pemphigus vulgaris (PV) in a patient who received RT for cancer treatment and review the literature on RT-associated pemphigus. Search terms included irradiation, radiation, radiotherapy, and cobalt therapy. The data provided include age, gender, underlying malignancy, dosage of RT, time intervals between RT and the onset of pemphigus, immunofluorescence data, and the treatment regime. In our patient we show that treatment with rituximab induces long-term clinical and serological remission for over two and a half years.

METHODS

Immunofluorescence (IF) Studies

Direct immunofluorescence (DIF) and indirect immunofluorescence (IIF) were performed in the Department of Dermatology, Medical Center—University of Freiburg. The FITC-labeled antibodies were anti-human IgG, IgA, IgM, and C3c (Dako, Hamburg, Germany) at a dilution of 1:200, 1:50, 1:50 and 1:500, respectively. For IIF on monkey esophagus, patients' sera were diluted 1:10; secondary antibodies used were FITC-labeled anti-human IgG (Dako, Hamburg, Germany) at a dilution of 1:100.

Immunoblotting Studies

Immunoblotting of normal human epidermal extracts (31, 32), the BP180 NC16a domain recombinant protein (33), the BP180 C-terminal domain recombinant protein (34), the concentrated culture supernatant of HaCaT cells (35), normal human dermal extract (36), and purified human laminin-332 for both IgG and/or IgA antibodies (37) were performed at the Kurume University and Osaka City University as previously described.

Enzyme-Linked Immunosorbent Assays (ELISA) Studies

Commercially available IgG ELISAs of Dsg1 and Dsg3 (MESACUP, MBL, Nagoya, Japan) were conducted according to the manufacturer's instructions and measured by ELISA reader.

RESULTS

We present a 63-year-old male patient, who was referred to our department due to extensive cutaneous (**Figures 1A–C**) and mucosal erosions (eyes, nose, lips, mouth, and esophagus). No paronychia-like or lichen planus-like lesions were observed. Until 3 months prior to admission, the patient had received adjuvant RT, following surgical reconstruction and bilateral neck lymph node dissection to treat larynx carcinoma. At that time point, the patient had received 54 Gy (single dose 1.8 Gy each) for his cervical right (level II-IV) and left region (III-IV), as well as a single boost at the tumor bed and additional 63.9 Gy (single dose 2.13 Gy each) for the left cervical lymph nodes (level II). The tumor appeared to be in remission. Histopathology of a skin specimen showed an intraepidermal split with the characteristic tombstone pattern of the basal keratinocytes (not shown). DIF of a skin specimen from the thigh revealed cell surface deposition of IgG (**Figure 2A**) and C3 in the entire epidermis. IIF with normal human skin and monkey esophagus (**Figure 2B**) revealed circulating cell surface IgG autoantibodies at a titer of 1:160. No reaction to the basement membrane zone or transitional epithelium of rat bladder was observed.

Immunoblotting of normal human epidermal extracts demonstrated IgG autoantibodies against the 130-kDa Dsg3 (**Figure 2C**, lane 4) (32), but no reactivity with Dsg1, envoplakin, periplakin, BP230, BP180, LAD-1 antigen, collagen VII, or laminin-332. Other immunoblotting methods did not detect any other autoantigens, including BP180, LAD-1 antigen, collagen VII, laminin gamma-1, and laminin-332. ELISA results were positive for both anti-Dsg1 (191 units; positive index $\geqq$ 20), and anti-Dsg3 antibodies (144 units; positive index $\geqq$ 20). ELISAs for recombinant eukaryotic desmocollin 1-3 proteins were negative (38). The discrepancy between immunoblotting and ELISA for anti-Dsg1 antibodies can be explained by that the PV sera tend to react with non-conformational epitopes, which are destroyed during the procedure of immunoblot, but not ELISA. The higher sensitivity in ELISA diagnostics has been well-established by previous studies (39). In fact it has been shown that in immunoblot with normal epidermal extracts most PV sera react with Dsg3, while only about two-thirds or PF sera react with Dsg1 (32). PV with underlying malignancy and PNP are sometimes difficult to distinguish. However, although our case had severe oral and ocular mucosal paraneoplastic pemphigus-like lesions, immunoblotting showed reactivity neither with envoplakin nor periplakin, excluding the diagnosis of PNP.

Initially, the patient was treated with high dose prednisolone, first given intravenously up to 2 mg/kg per day, topical disinfectants, and class IV steroid creams, combined with meticulous wound care for several weeks. Administration of rituximab 2 × 1,000 mg led to quick stabilization of the disease and to clinical and serological remission. Currently, the follow-up-time is two and a half years (**Figure 1D**), showing that rituximab is a valuable treatment for this rare pemphigus subtype; it improved the patient's quality of life tremendously.

A rigorous literature search for RT-associated pemphigus revealed 29 reported cases (**Table 1**). Of these, 23 represented PV and eight pemphigus foliaceus (PF). The age of the patients ranged from 37 to 92 years, with a median of 62 years. In 11 cases, the disease onset was within <1 month, in 12 cases skin lesions developed within the first 3 months after therapy initiation. Twenty-seven of 30 (90%) cases initially presented with lesions at the irradiated side with the majority of these patients (24/30 cases, corresponding to 80%) having a progression to the non-irradiated skin (11/24 cases, corresponding to 46%) or even to a generalized distribution (13/24 cases, corresponding to 54%).

Abbreviations: DIF, direct immunofluorescence; HMGB1, High mobility group box 1; IIF, indirect immunofluorescence; ELISA, Enzyme-linked immunosorbent assay; PF, pemphigus foliaceus; PNP, paraneoplastic pemphigus; PV, pemphigus vulgaris; RAGE, receptor for advanced glycation endproduct; RT, radiation therapy.

TABLE 1 | Patients with radiation-associated pemphigus described in the literature.

No	Age	Diagnosis	Time from radiation to start of eruption	DIF (cell surface)	IIF (cell surface)	Neoplasm	Radiation characteristics	Localization (irradiated area, non-irradiated area, generalized)	Treatment	References
1	63	PV	1 month	IgG	IgG	Hypopharynx carcinoma	LN cervical R II-IV, L III-IV 54 Gy, tumor bed, and LN cervical II 63,9 Gy	Irradiated area with generalized progression	Prednisolone 2 mg/kg/day, topical clobetasol propionate 0.05% ointment (body), followed by rituximab 2 × 1,000 mg	Current case
2	48	PV	3 months	+	na	Medullary breast cancer	100 Gy	Irradiated area with progression to non-irradiated area	Prednisone 150 mg/day	(4)
3	56	PV	1 year	na	na	Epidermoid bladder carcinoma	65 Gy	Generalized mucocutaneous type	Prednisone 60 mg/day	(5)
4	65	PV	<1 month	na	na	Breast cancer	n.a	Irradiated area with generalized progression	Prednisone 80 mg/day, later 120 mg/day, methotrexate 25 mg, then azathioprine 100 mg/day	(5)
5	70	PV	14 days	IgG, C3	+	Gastric lymphosarcoma	40 Gy	Irradiated area with generalized progression	Prednisone 120 mg/day	(6)
6	70	PV	4 months	+	+	Solar keratosis on the forehead	48 Gy	Irradiated area to non- irradiated area	Prednisone 100 mg/day	(7)
7	52	PV	3 weeks	na	na	Bronchial squamous cell carcinoma	40 Gy	Irradiated area with generalized progression	Methylprednisolone intravenously 1,250 mg 6 days, then 1 mg/kg BW and tapering 45 days	(8)
8	73	PV	3 months	+	+	Breast cancer	55 Gy	Irradiated area with generalized progression	Prednisone 50 mg/day	(9)
9	70	PF	1 month	+	+	Laryngeal squamous cell carcinoma	60 Gy	Irradiated area with progression to non-irradiated area	Prednisone 2 mg/kg/day, azathioprine 50 mg/day	(9)
10	54	PV	3 weeks	+	IgG	Lymphoma	38 Gy	Irradiated area with generalized progression	Prednisone 2 mg/kg/ day	(10)
11	77	PV	na	+	+	Basal cell carcinoma	60 Gy	Irradiated area with progression to non-irradiated	Prednisone 100 mg/day, dapsone 100 mg/day	(11)
12	45	PV	1 week	+	na	Breast cancer	68 Gy	Irradiated area	Prednisone 80 mg/day	(12)
13	61	PV	2 months	+	na	SCC of the lower lip	70 Gy	Irradiated area with progression to non-irradiated	Prednisone 1 mg/kg/day	(13)
14	54	PV	1 month	IgG, C3	IgG	SCC of the lung	59.4 Gy	Irradiated area with progression to non-irradiated	Methylprednisolone intravenously, then oral prednisone	(14)
15	73	PV	3 weeks	+	na	Epidermoid carcinoma	66 Gy	Irradiated area with progression to non-irradiated	Prednisone 1.5 mg/day, followed by rituximab 6 x 375 mg/m^2	(15)
16	49	PV	4 weeks	+	na	Breast cancer	50 Gy	Non-irradiated area (mouth and esophagus)	Prednisone 60 mg/day, methotrexate 15 mg weekly	(16)

(Continued)

TABLE 1 | Continued

No	Age	Diagnosis	Time from radiation to start of eruption	DIF (cell surface)	IIF (cell surface)	Neoplasm	Radiation characteristics	Localization (irradiated area, non-irradiated area, generalized)	Treatment AIBD	References
17	48	PV	6 months	na	+	Breast cancer (ductal carcinoma *in situ*)	Megavoltage radiation therapy–50 Gy	Irradiated area	Prednisone 100 mg/day, topical steroids	(17)
18	61	PV	1 month	IgG, C3	IgG (rabbit tongue)	Epidermoid carcinoma of the piriform sinus	70 Gy tumor bed, 54 Gy cercical area	Irradiated area with generalized progression	Methylprednisolone 1 g, followed by oral prednisolone 1.5 mg/kg/day	(18)
19	47	PV	Within days (face), 6 months body	C4	IgG	Acinic cell carcinoma of the parotid gland	39, 6 Gy (cheek and chin)	Irradiated area with generalized progression	Prednisolone 1 mg/kg/day, azathioprine 150 mg/day and rituximab 2 × 375 mg/m^2	(19)
20	58	PV	21 days	IgG, C3	+	Low grade infiltrating ductal carcinoma	Tumor area 65 Gy, subclavicular area (46 Gy), right internal mammary node chain (50 Gy)	Irradiated area with progression to non-irradiated area	Prednisone 2 mg/kg/day, MMF 2 g/day	(20)
21	84	PV	8 months	IgG	IgG	Breast cancer	60 Gy	Non-irradiated area (mouth)	Topical clobetasol propionate ointment, oral prednisolone 1 mg/kg/day, azathioprine 2.5 mg/kg/day	(21)
22	58	PV	14 months	IgG	+	Breast cancer (*in situ* ductal)	na	Irradiated area with progression to non-irradiated	Prednisone 60 mg/day, azathioprine 50 mg/day	(22)
23	68	PV	< 1 month	+	na	Breast cancer	40 Gy	Irradiated area with generalized progression	Prednisolone, MMF	(23)
24	37	PF	<1 month	+	+	Malignant thymoma	30 Gy	Irradiated area with generalized progression (after sun exposure)	Methylprednisolone 12 mg, azathioprine 50 mg/day, dapsone 100 mg/day	(24)
25	92	PF	3 months	+	na	Breast cancer (*in situ* intraductal)	50,4 Gy	Irradiated area with generalized progression	na	(25)
26	70	PF	12 months	IgG, C3	IgG	Breast cancer	60 Gy	Irradiated area with progression to non-irradiated	Dapsone 100 mg/ day, topical clobetasol propionate ointment	(26)
27	59	PF	1 month	IgG, C3	na	Extramammary Paget disease	52.5 Gy	Irradiated area with progression to non-irradiated	Prednisolone 0.5 mg/kg/day	(27)
28	65	PF	2 months	IgG, C3	na	Breast cancer	50 Gy	Irradiated area	Prednisolone 30 mg/day	(28)
39	44	PF	< 2 months	IgG and C3, focal staining C3d, and C4d	na	Breast cancer	na	Irradiated area with generalized progression	Oral prednisolone 1 mg/kg/day, topical hydrocortisone 2.5% ointment (face), clobetasol propionate 0.05% ointment (body), oral dapsone	(29)
30	66	PF	1 month	IgG, C3	na	Breast cancer (ductal carcinoma *in situ*)	50 Gy	Irradiated area with generalized progression	Oral triamcinolone 40 mg/day	(30)

BW, body weight; C3, complement 3; C4, complement 4; CS, cell surface; PF, pemphigus foliaceus; PV, pemphigus vulgaris; MMF, mycophenolate mofetil; na, not available; +, positive (fluorescence pattern not described).

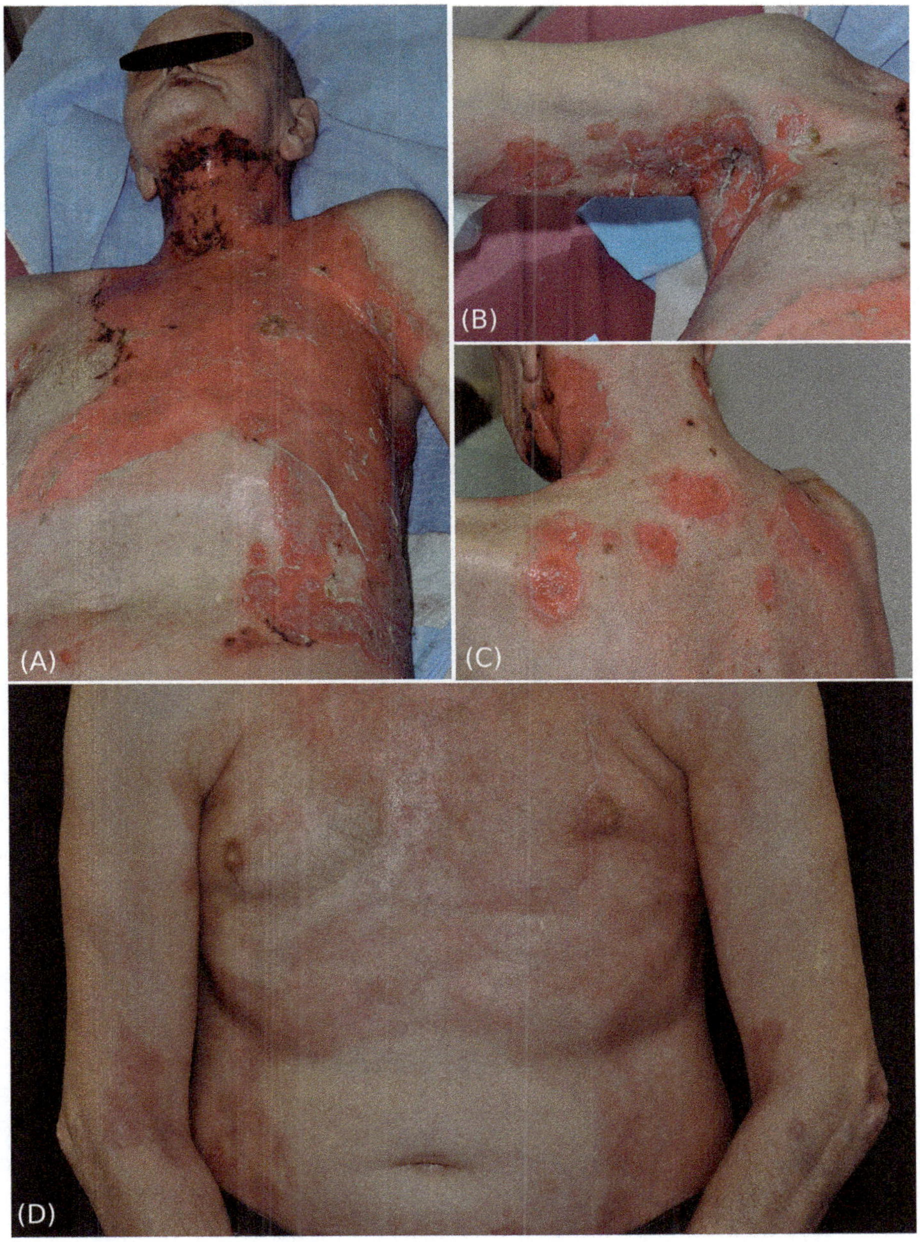

FIGURE 1 | Clinical pictures of the patient at initial presentation and after treatment. Extensive erosive skin detachment of the frontal trunk and neck **(A)**, right axillary fold **(B),** and shoulders and neck **(C)**. Three months after systemic treatment with rituximab and ongoing low dose glucocorticosteroids, intact skin with postinflammatory hyperpigmentations was observed **(D)**.

The skin lesions stayed at the irradiation side in only three patients (3/30 cases, corresponding 10%). Two patients developed erosions in the non-irradiated area at their first presentation, while one patient showed a generalized distribution pattern of PV. At least three cases (including ours) clinically imitated PNP. The pemphigus diagnosis was made in 20 cases by DIF, and in 14 of these cases additionally by IIF. ELISA was performed in only four cases. Fifteen patients ($n = 9$ PV, $n = 6$ PF) were treated for breast cancer. Others received radiotherapy for miscellaneous forms of cancer, for example lymphoma, gastric lymphosarcoma, squamous cell carcinoma of the skin or the lung, and bladder carcinoma. The RT dose varied from 38 to 100 Gy, conducted in fractional application. All published patients, but one, have received oral, or intravenous glucocorticosteroids (prednisolone or methylprednisolone) in a medium to high dose. Ten individuals, representing one third of the reported, needed additional agents like dapsone, azathioprine or mycophenolate mofetil, at least temporarily. In two previously published cases

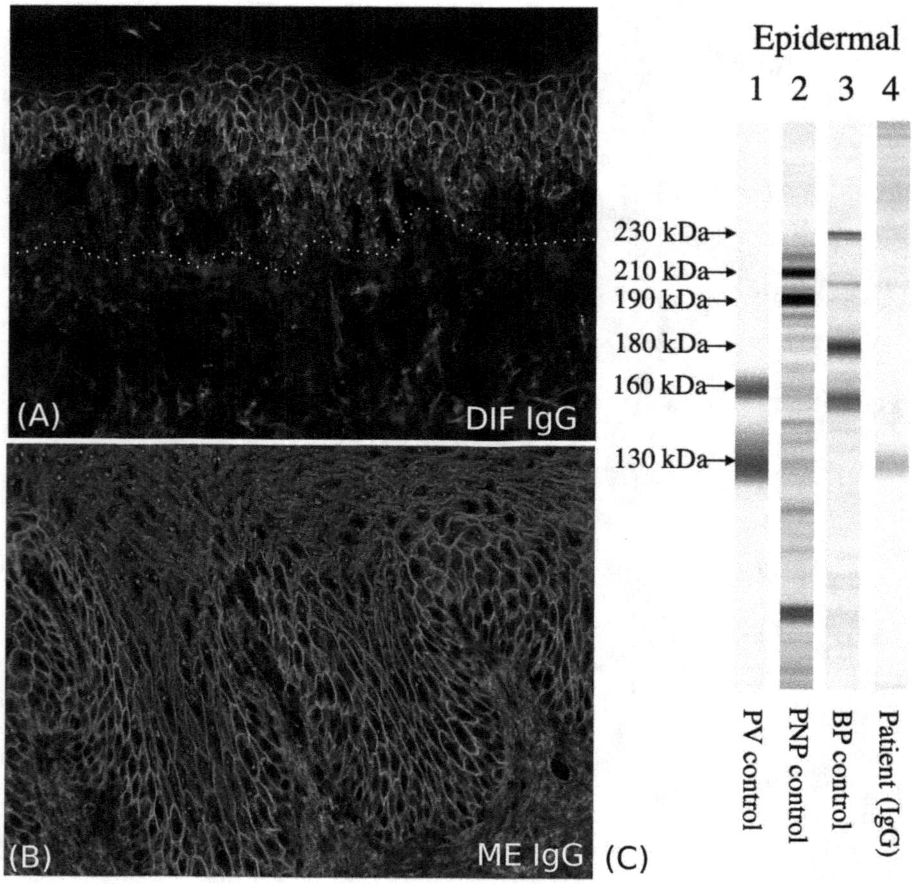

FIGURE 2 | Immunological characterization of the patient. **(A)** The direct immunofluorescence (DIF) shows cell surface IgG deposition on the keratinocytes of the entire epidermis. **(B)** Indirect immunofluorescence (IIF) with monkey esophagus (ME) shows circulating cell surface IgG autoantibodies. **(C)** Immunoblotting with normal human epidermal extracts shows IgG antibodies reactive with 130-kDa Dsg3 (lane 4).

rituximab had been given in different dosages (2 × 375 and 6 × 375 mg/m^2) and resulted in remission with a follow up of up to 6 months (15, 19). Three patients had a pre-existing PF (27–29) that aggravated during radiotherapy; suggesting that in patients with a history of an autoimmune blistering skin disorder, RT should be cautiously considered. Nevertheless, it is not an absolute contraindication, since patients with PV have tolerated radiation without exacerbation of the disease (40).

DISCUSSION

Here we report a severely affected patient with PV in whom RT for larynx cancer triggered the onset of the disease. So far, 29 cases RT-associated pemphigus have been reported in the literature with the majority of cases having lesions first at the RT site, soon followed by generalized erosions (**Table 1**). This clinical sign facilitates differentiation from a classical RT-induced dermatitis. In our case, high dose prednisolone and B-cell depletion by rituximab was required to induce clinical and serological remission for more than two and a half years, without need for further immunosuppression. Since this is the third case of RT-associated PV treated with rituximab, showing a quick response and resulting in clear remission in all three cases, we propose that rituximab should be considered early, when treating such patients. Rituximab selectively binds to CD20 and leads to B-cell depletion due to antibody- and complement-dependent cytotoxicity, as well as induction of apoptosis. The use of immunosuppression in patients with malignancies should be avoided, whenever possible. However, in around one third of the already reported RT-associated pemphigus cases such drugs had to be given to control disease (**Table 1**). Thus, especially for the most severely affected patients, requiring additional immunosuppression than steroids, rituximab given at the already published regimen for PV (41) (1,000 mg rituximab on days 1 and 15) would be probably the most advantageous treatment option.

Another autoimmune skin blistering disorder that is pathogenetically often connected to malignancy or RT is bullous pemphigoid (BP). The so far published cases comprise similarly to RT-associated pemphigus more than 30 (42), including a stage IV melanoma patient with dual exposure to PD-1 checkpoint inhibition and RT therapy (43). Nguyen et al. have summarized 29 patients with BP following radiation for malignancy treatment. BP was localized on the irradiated area in 25 of them, in two it was localized in non-irradiated sites and in another two it was generalized (44). All cases had a rather benign course, with corticosteroids being sufficient to control the disease. RT-associated pemphigus appears to have a more severe disease course, since it tends to spread to non-irradiated skin and in one third of cases further treatment with other immunosuppressants was required to control disease.

Several hypotheses have been proposed about the role of RT in induction of autoimmune skin blistering disorders. The efficacy and role of RT in anti-tumor therapy is believed to be due to the RT-induced DNA damage to malignant cells, but recent evidence demonstrates that RT also activates the innate immune system, promoting specific danger signals like complement, calreticulin, and high mobility group box 1 protein (HMGB1), as well as a variety of cytokines and chemokines (45). Beside a few patients who may have circulating autoantibodies before RT, the substantial role of complement in activation of BP is well-established, while the role of complement in pemphigus has a controversial standing (46). HMGB1, released by damaged cells can stimulate macrophages and dendritic cells, thus resulting in an activation of T cells. Increased serological concentration, paired with plentiful cytoplasmic overexpression of HMGB1 and its receptor RAGE has been observed in the epidermis of pemphigus patients (47). This results in tissue destruction and unmasking of epidermal structures, thus promoting auto-reactivity in the irritated, immunocompromised area (48, 49). Furthermore, there are no sufficient data about the effects of RT damage and recovery of the thymus, which is in anatomical proximity to the tumor region in our patient. Post-RT effects in total body RT mouse model comprised reduced thymocyte numbers and long-term suppression of thymopoesis (50), supporting a hypothesis of impaired T-cell education and disturbed selection processes inducing autoimmunity. Finally, RT-associated pemphigus appears to have a similar incidence as pemphigoid. This contrasts the situation in the non-radiated population, where BP is more common. That is another argument for the direct induction of autoantibodies by the tumor in the RT-associated pemphigus. Additional studies to characterize the pathogenesis of RT-associated pemphigus are required to gain a better understanding of the disease.

Taken together, we show that rituximab represents a good treatment option for the frequently treatment-refractory RT-associated pemphigus, resulting in long-term clinical, and serological remission.

ETHICS STATEMENT

The study has been approved by the Ethics committee in Freiburg (Number 235/15). All analyzes were performed with written informed consent of the patient, after ethics approval and in accordance to the Declaration of Helsinki.

AUTHOR CONTRIBUTIONS

FS and DK contributed conception and design of the study, they also wrote the initial manuscript draft. NI and TH performed part of the diagnostics and wrote sections of the manuscript. FS, MM, and DK cared for the patient, performed part of the diagnostics, and interpreted the results. LB-T interpreted the data and revised the manuscript critically for important intellectual content. All authors contributed to manuscript revision, read and approved the submitted version.

ACKNOWLEDGMENTS

We thank the patient. In addition, the excellent technical support by Kaethe Thoma, Ioannis Athanasiou, and Annegret Bedorf is gratefully acknowledged.

REFERENCES

1. Jelti L, Cordel N, Gillibert A, Lacour J-P, Uthurriague C, Doutre M-S, et al. Incidence and mortality of pemphigus in France. *J Invest Dermatol.* (2019) 139:469–73. doi: 10.1016/j.jid.2018.07.042
2. Iwashita K, Matsuyama T, Akasaka E, Mizutani K, Yamamoto K, Kondoh A, et al. The incidence of internal malignancies in autoimmune bullous diseases. *Tokai J Exp Clin Med.* (2007) 32:42–7.
3. Ogawa H, Sakuma M, Morioka S, Kitamura K, Sasai Y, Imamura S, Inaba Y. The incidence of internal malignancies in pemphigus and bullous pemphigoid in Japan. *J Dermatol Sci.* (1995) 9:136–41. doi: 10.1016/0923-1811(94)00371-K
4. Lunder M. Una rara combinazione del pemfigo con cancro della mamella. *Minerva Dermatol.* (1973) 108:576–7.
5. Krain LS, Bierman SM. Pemphigus vulgaris and internal malignancy. *Cancer.* (1974) 33:1091–9. doi: 10.1002/1097-0142(197404)33:4<1091::AID-CNCR2820330430>3.0.CO;2-Y
6. David M, Feuerman EJ. Induction of pemphigus by X-ray irradiation. *Clin Exp Dermatol.* (1987) 12:197–9. doi: 10.1111/j.1365-2230.1987.tb01894.x
7. Hunziker T, Zala L, Krebs A. [Roentgen ray-induced pemphigus vulgaris]. *Hautarzt Z Dermatol Venerol Verwandte Geb.* (1988) 39:308–10.
8. Girolomoni G, Mazzone E, Zambruno G. Pemphigus vulgaris following cobalt therapy for bronchial carcinoma. *Dermatologica.* (1989) 178:37–8. doi: 10.1159/000248384
9. Low GJ, Keeling JH. Ionizing radiation-induced pemphigus. Case presentations and literature review. *Arch Dermatol.* (1990) 126:1319–23. doi: 10.1001/archderm.126.10.1319

10. Delaporte E, Piette F, Bergoend H. [Pemphigus vulgaris induced by radiotherapy]. *Ann Dermatol Venereol.* (1991) 118:447–51.
11. Krauze E, Wygledowska-Kania M, Kaminska-Budzinska G, Lis A, Brzezinska-Wcislo L. [Radiotherapy induced pemphigus vulgaris]. *Ann Dermatol Venereol.* (2003) 130:549–50.
12. Orion E, Matz H, Wolf R. Pemphigus vulgaris induced by radiotherapy. *J Eur Acad Dermatol Venereol.* (2004) 18:508–9. doi: 10.1111/j.1468-3083.2004.00952.x
13. Mseddi M, Bouassida S, Khemakhem M, Marrekchi S, Abdelmaksoud W, Hadjtaieb H, et al. [Radiotherapy-induced pemphigus: a case report]. *Cancer Radiother J Soc Francaise Radiother Oncol.* (2005) 9:96–8. doi: 10.1016/j.canrad.2004.10.007
14. Robbins AC, Lazarova Z, Janson MM, Fairley JA. Pemphigus vulgaris presenting in a radiation portal. *J Am Acad Dermatol.* (2007) 56:S82–85. doi: 10.1016/j.jaad.2006.10.956
15. Saint-Jean M, Quéreux G, Peuvrel P, Dréno B. [Post-radiotherapy erosive lesion]. *Ann Dermatol Venereol.* (2008) 135:780–2. doi: 10.1016/j.annder.2008.03.009
16. Bar-Sela G, Baum S, Trau H, Kuten A. Pemphigus vulgaris of the larynx and upper gastro-intestinal tract induced by radiotherapy. *Acta Oncol Stockh Swed.* (2008) 47:324–326. doi: 10.1080/02841860701558831
17. Vigna-Taglianti R, Russi EG, Denaro N, Numico G, Brizio R. Radiation-induced pemphigus vulgaris of the breast. *Cancer/Radiothér.* (2011) 15:334–7. doi: 10.1016/j.canrad.2011.01.006
18. Badri T, Hammami H, Lachkham A, Benmously-Mlika R, Mokhtar I, Fenniche S. Radiotherapy-induced pemphigus vulgaris with autoantibodies targeting a 110 kDa epidermal antigen. *Int J Dermatol.* (2011) 50:1475–9. doi: 10.1111/j.1365-4632.2011.04889.x
19. Jang HW, Chun SH, Lee JM, Jeon J, Hashimoto T, Kim I-H. Radiotherapy-induced pemphigus vulgaris. *J Dermatol.* (2014) 41:851–2. doi: 10.1111/1346-8138.12582
20. Thimon S, Machet L, Machet M-C, Samimi M, Maruani A. Pemphigus induced by radiotherapy for breast cancer: clinical, immunological and histological features of one case with antidesmoglein immunostaining. *Eur J Dermatol.* (2014) 24:119–20. doi: 10.1684/ejd.2013.2239
21. Tang HKC, Lee DYH, Thompson I, Ingram JR, Stone N, Patel GK. Delayed and localized pemphigus vulgaris after breast cancer radiotherapy. *Breast J.* (2017) 23:747–9. doi: 10.1111/tbj.12910
22. Shon W, Wada DA, Kalaaji AN. Radiation-induced pemphigus or pemphigoid disease in 3 patients with distinct underlying malignancies. *Cutis.* (2016) 97:219–22.
23. O'Leary B, Alarcon L, Mallon E, Kirby A. Radiotherapy-associated pemphigus – a rare cause of grade 4 skin toxicity. *Clin Oncol.* (2017) 29:e50. doi: 10.1016/j.clon.2016.08.013
24. Tagami H, Imamura S, Noguchi S, Nishitani H. Coexistence of peculiar pemphigus, myasthenia gravis and malignant thymoma. *Dermatologica.* (1976) 152:181–90. doi: 10.1159/000251246
25. Ambay A, Stratman E. Ionizing radiation-induced pemphigus foliaceus. *J Am Acad Dermatol.* (2006) 54:251–2. doi: 10.1016/j.jaad.2005.12.024
26. Cianchini G, Lembo L, Colonna L, Puddu P. Pemphigus foliaceus induced by radiotherapy and responsive to dapsone. *J Dermatol Treat.* (2006) 17:244–6. doi: 10.1080/09546630600921197
27. Kikuchi K, Inokuma D, Moriuchi R, Koguchi-Yoshioka H, Yasui C, Shimizu S. Exacerbation of pemphigus foliaceus after electron-beam radiation. *Acta Derm Venereol.* (2014) 94:729–30. doi: 10.2340/00015555-1811
28. Inadomi T. A case of pemphigus foliaceus aggravated in an irradiated area by radiotherapy against breast cancer. *Indian J Dermatol.* (2015) 60:93–4. doi: 10.4103/0019-5154.147818
29. Liebman TN, Lieberman MR, Burris K. Pemphigus foliaceus exacerbated by radiation, in association with myasthenia gravis. *Dermatol Online J.* (2016) 22:13030/qt50p1246h.
30. Criado PR, Apparecida CD, Criado RFJ, Etcheverria ICR, Umeda LM, Landman G. Radiotherapy-induced Pemphigus Foliaceous: a rare adverse effect of breast cancer therapy. *Int J Dermatol.* (2018) 57:e165–7. doi: 10.1111/ijd.14248
31. Sugi T, Hashimoto T, Hibi T, Nishikawa T. Production of human monoclonal anti-basement membrane zone. (BMZ) antibodies from a patient with bullous pemphigoid. (BP) by Epstein-Barr virus transformation. Analyses of the heterogeneity of anti-BMZ antibodies in BP sera using them. *J Clin Invest.* (1989) 84:1050–5. doi: 10.1172/JCI114266
32. Hashimoto T, Ogawa MM, Konohana A, Nishikawa T. Detection of pemphigus vulgaris and pemphigus foliaceus antigens by immunoblot analysis using different antigen sources. *J Invest Dermatol.* (1990) 94:327–31. doi: 10.1111/1523-1747.ep12874456
33. Matsumura K, Amagai M, Nishikawa T, Hashimoto T. The majority of bullous pemphigoid and herpes gestationis serum samples react with the NC16a domain of the 180-kDa bullous pemphigoid antigen. *Arch Dermatol Res.* (1996) 288:507–9. doi: 10.1007/BF02505245
34. Nie Z, Hashimoto T. IgA antibodies of cicatricial pemphigoid sera specifically react with C-terminus of BP180. *J Invest Dermatol.* (1999) 112:254–5. doi: 10.1046/j.1523-1747.1999.00501.x
35. Ishii N, Ohyama B, Yamaguchi Z, Hashimoto T. IgA autoantibodies against the NC16a domain of BP180 but not 120-kDa LAD-1 detected in a patient with linear IgA disease. *Br J Dermatol.* (2008) 158:1151–3. doi: 10.1111/j.1365-2133.2008.08492.x
36. Ishii N, Yoshida M, Hisamatsu Y, Ishida-Yamamoto A, Nakane H, Iizuka H, et al. Epidermolysis bullosa acquisita sera react with distinct epitopes on the NC1 and NC2 domains of type VII collagen: study using immunoblotting of domain-specific recombinant proteins and postembedding immunoelectron microscopy. *Br J Dermatol.* (2004) 150:843–51. doi: 10.1111/j.1365-2133.2004.05933.x
37. Hisamatsu Y, Nishiyama T, Amano S, Matsui C, Ghohestani R, Hashimoto T. Usefulness of immunoblotting using purified laminin 5 in the diagnosis of anti-laminin 5 cicatricial pemphigoid. *J Dermatol Sci.* (2003) 33:113–9. doi: 10.1016/S0923-1811(03)00158-0
38. Ishii N, Teye K, Fukuda S, Uehara R, Hachiya T, Koga H, et al. Anti-desmocollin autoantibodies in nonclassical pemphigus. *Br J Dermatol.* (2015) 173:59–68. doi: 10.1111/bjd.13711
39. Amagai M, Komai A, Hashimoto T, Shirakata Y, Hashimoto K, Yamada T, et al. Usefulness of enzyme-linked immunosorbent assay using recombinant desmogleins 1 and 3 for serodiagnosis of pemphigus. *Br J Dermatol.* (1999) 140:351–7. doi: 10.1046/j.1365-2133.1999.02752.x
40. De Cicco L, Bracelli S. Pemphigus Vulgaris and Radiotherapy. *Clin Oncol R Coll Radiol G B.* (2018) 30:e38. doi: 10.1016/j.clon.2017.10.011
41. Chen DM, Odueyungbo A, Csinady E, Gearhart L, Lehane P, Cheu M, et al. Rituximab is an effective treatment in patients with pemphigus vulgaris and demonstrates a steroid-sparing effect. *Br J Dermatol.* (2019). doi: 10.1111/bjd.18482. [Epub ahead of print].
42. Mai Y, Nishie W, Sato K, Hotta M, Izumi K, Ito K, et al. Bullous pemphigoid triggered by thermal burn under medication with a dipeptidyl peptidase-IV inhibitor: a case report and review of the literature. *Front Immunol.* (2018) 9:542. doi: 10.3389/fimmu.2018.00542
43. Hirotsu K, Chiou AS, Chiang A, Kim J, Kwong BY, Pugliese S. Localized bullous pemphigoid in a melanoma patient with dual exposure to PD-1 checkpoint inhibition and radiation therapy. *JAAD Case Rep.* (2017) 3:404–6. doi: 10.1016/j.jdcr.2017.06.004
44. Nguyen T, Kwan JM, Ahmed AR. Relationship between radiation therapy and bullous pemphigoid. *Dermatol Basel Switz.* (2014) 229:88–96. doi: 10.1159/000362208
45. Dar TB, Henson RM, Shiao SL. Targeting innate immunity to enhance the efficacy of radiation therapy. *Front Immunol.* (2018) 9:3077. doi: 10.3389/fimmu.2018.03077
46. Hammers CM, Stanley JR. Mechanisms of disease: pemphigus and bullous pemphigoid. *Annu Rev Pathol.* (2016) 11:175–97. doi: 10.1146/annurev-pathol-012615-044313
47. Li J-Y, Lu Y-H, Zhang L-W, Zhou P-M, Chen T. Increased serum high mobility group box 1. (HMGB1) concentration and the altered expression of HMGB1 and its receptor advanced glycation endproducts in pemphigus. *Ann Dermatol.* (2017) 29:121–3. doi: 10.5021/ad.2017.29.1.121

48. Lehmann PV, Forsthuber T, Miller A, Sercarz EE. Spreading of T-cell autoimmunity to cryptic determinants of an autoantigen. *Nature.* (1992) 358:155–7. doi: 10.1038/358155a0
49. Ruocco V, Brunetti G, Puca RV, Ruocco E. The immunocompromised district: a unifying concept for lymphoedematous, herpes-infected and otherwise damaged sites. *J Eur Acad Dermatol Venereol.* (2009) 23:1364–73. doi: 10.1111/j.1468-3083.2009.03345.x
50. Xiao S, Shterev ID, Zhang W, Young L, Shieh J-H, Moore M, van den Brink M, et al. Sublethal total body irradiation causes long-term deficits in thymus function by reducing lymphoid progenitors. *J Immunol Baltim Md 1950.* (2017) 199:2701–12. doi: 10.4049/jimmunol.1600934

19

Interaction of Psoriasis and Bullous Diseases

Teruki Dainichi[1*] *and Kenji Kabashima*[1,2]

[1] *Department of Dermatology, Kyoto University Graduate School of Medicine, Kyoto, Japan,* [2] *Singapore Immunology Network and Institute of Medical Biology, Agency for Science, Technology and Research (A*STAR), Singapore, Singapore*

Correspondence:
Teruki Dainichi
dainichi@kuhp.kyoto-u.ac.jp

Patients with psoriasis are frequently complicated with autoimmune bullous diseases, especially, pemphigoid diseases. It has been known that one-third cases of anti-laminin gamma1 pemphigoid, formerly anti-p200 pemphigoid, are associated with psoriasis whereas bullous pemphigoid is the most frequently associated bullous disease in psoriasis cases regardless of the lack of detectable levels of the accompanying anti-laminin gamma1 autoantibodies. Despite several suggestions, however, the definitive reason of the striking association of psoriasis and these autoimmune bullous diseases remains elusive. In this review, we look over the epidemiological evidence of the association of psoriasis and autoimmune bullous diseases and the information of genetic susceptibilities of each disease, and discuss the possible mechanisms of their complication with reference to the recent understandings of each pathogenesis.

Keywords: autoimmunity, Th2, Th17, psoriasis, pemphigoid, laminin, MMP, senescence

INTRODUCTION

Autoimmune bullous diseases, as well as psoriasis, are skin disorders affecting the epidermis. In both diseases, immune reactions target the epidermis, and induce the development of the skin lesions following the failures in epithelial cell contacts or the defects in epithelial cell proliferation and differentiation. There is remarkable progress in the understandings of their pathogenesis in these decades, respectively. Nevertheless, (1) what triggers the pathogenic immune reactions, (2) which cells by which molecules respond to the internal or external changes and direct the subsequent immune reactions, and (3) which step is critical for the decision of the immune type, have not yet been fully elucidated.

Physicians and dermatologists have long time been aware that psoriasis patients are frequently complicated with autoimmune bullous diseases. Indeed, epidemiological evidence indicates that the incidence of some pemphigoid diseases in psoriasis patients is significantly higher than that in the control individuals without psoriasis. Moreover, recent investigations have suggested that there are in part similarities and shared players in their pathogenesis.

In this review, first we look over the epidemiological evidence of the association of psoriasis and autoimmune bullous diseases. Second, we compare their genetic susceptibilities. And third, we discuss the possible mechanisms of their association with reference to the current understandings on each pathogenesis.

EPIDEMIOLOGICAL EVIDENCE

Psoriasis and Pemphigus

Most reported cases of pemphigus developed in psoriasis patients were pemphigus foliaceus including pemphigus erythematosus. A case series of 145 patients with concomitant psoriasis and autoimmune blistering diseases from Japan reported that all four (2.8%) pemphigus cases with psoriasis were pemphigus foliaceus (124). The first case-control study of 51,800 psoriasis patients from Taiwan demonstrated the significantly higher prevalence rate of pemphigus in the patients than that in the control subjects (odds ratio (OR), 41.8; 95% confidence interval (CI), 12.4–140.9; $P < 0.0001$) (125).

There is another study evaluating their association in an inverse direction: a case-control study of 1985 pemphigus patients from Israel demonstrated that the prevalence rate of psoriasis in pemphigus patients was also higher than that in the controls (OR, 2.84; 95% CI, 2.09–3.85, $P < 0.001$) (126).

Psoriasis and Pemphigoid Diseases Including Epidermolysis Bullosa Acquisita

Complication of psoriasis cases with pemphigoid diseases are much more commonly experienced than those with pemphigus whereas the number of the report of the psoriasis cases with pemphigoid is only about three times as many as those with pemphigus (**Figure 1**). Indeed, in the case series of 145 patients with psoriasis and autoimmune blistering diseases from Japan, almost all the cases are complicated with bullous pemphigoid (63%), anti-laminin γ1 pemphigoid (formerly anti-p200 pemphigoid) (37%), or their combination (8%) (**Figure 2**). Psoriasis including pustular psoriasis precedes the development of pemphigoid in most cases. Of note, 111 (78.7%) cases had no history of any phototherapies in this case series (124).

The case-control study of 51,800 psoriasis patients from Taiwan also demonstrated the higher prevalence rate of pemphigoid in the patients than that in the control subjects (OR, 14.8; 95% CI, 5.00–43.50, $P < 0.0001$) (125).

Inversely, early case-controlled study has shown that 7 out of 62 (11%) pemphigoid cases are complicated with psoriasis and the prevalence was significantly higher than expected in the controls ($P < 0.01$) (40). Following studies also confirmed that psoriasis cases are significantly associated with bullous pemphigoid: A study of 3,485 bullous pemphigoid cases from Taiwan (OR 2.02; 95% CI 1.54–2.66, $P < 0.003$) (127), and another of 287 bullous pemphigoid cases from Israel (OR 4.39; 95% CI 2.17–8.92, $P < 0.0001$) (128), respectively.

Anti-laminin γ1 pemphigoid is originally reported as pemphigoid developed in psoriasis patients with circulating autoantibodies against unknown autoantigen. Around one-third of the following cases have also been associated with psoriasis (129).

There are only a few reported cases of psoriasis associated with other pemphigoid diseases. The case series of 145 patients with psoriasis and autoimmune blistering diseases from Japan included three cases with linear IgA bullous dermatosis and two cases with epidermolysis bullosa acquisita (124). There are few independent reports of a case with epidermolysis bullosa acquisita (51, 112), or with anti-laminin 332 mucous membrane pemphigoid (109).

Psoriasis and Other Blistering Diseases

Intriguingly, as far as we looked up, there is no reported case of psoriasis in any type of epidermolysis bullosa: simplex, junctional, or dystrophic type, except for one case report of the dystrophic type without confirmation by DNA sequencing analysis (116). There are seven reports of a case with psoriasis in Hailey-Hailey disease since the first reported case (117).

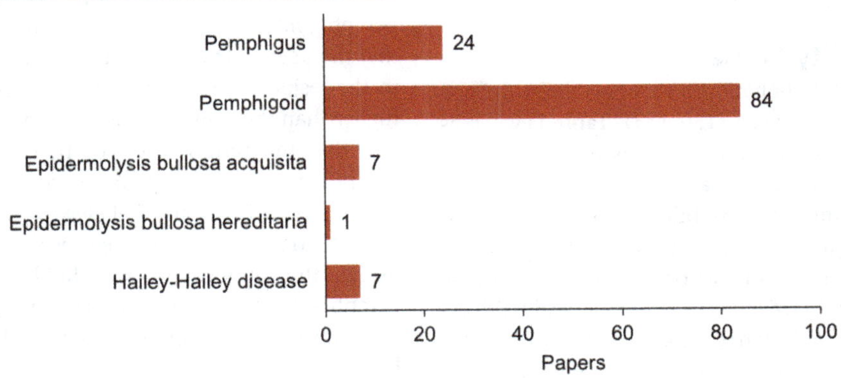

FIGURE 1 | Publication of the report of cases with association of psoriasis and bullous diseases until the end of 2017. All the publications were searched in PubMed database, and case reports and case series were selected manually with exclusion of redundancy. Cases with coexistence of two or more autoimmune blistering diseases were counted in each category: (psoriasis[tiab] AND pemphigoid[tiab]) for pemphigoid diseases; (psoriasis[tiab] AND pemphigus[tiab] NOT pemphigoid[tiab]) for pemphigus; psoriasis[tiab] AND (epidermolysis bullosa acquisita[tiab]) for epidermolysis bullosa acquisita; psoriasis AND (epidermolysis bullosa hereditaria OR epidermolysis bullosa simplex OR junctional epidermolysis bullosa OR dystrophic epidermolysis bullosa OR kindler's syndrome OR kindler syndrome) for epidermolysis bullosa hereditaria; psoriasis[tiab] AND (hailey-hailey OR familial pemphigus OR familial benign chronic pemphigus) for Hailey-Hailey disease. References are as follows. Pemphigus (24): 1990 or earlier (5) (1–5); 1991–2000 (5) (6–10); 2001–2010 (6) (11–16); 2011 or later (8) (17–25). Pemphigoid (84): 1980 or earlier (7) (26–32); 1981–1990 (16) (3, 33–47); 1991–2000 (10) (48–57); 2001–2010 (21) (58–78); 2011 or later (30) (79–109). Epidermolysis bullosa acquisita (7) (51, 110–115). Epidermolysis bullosa hereditaria (1) (116). Hailey-Hailey disease (7) (117–123).

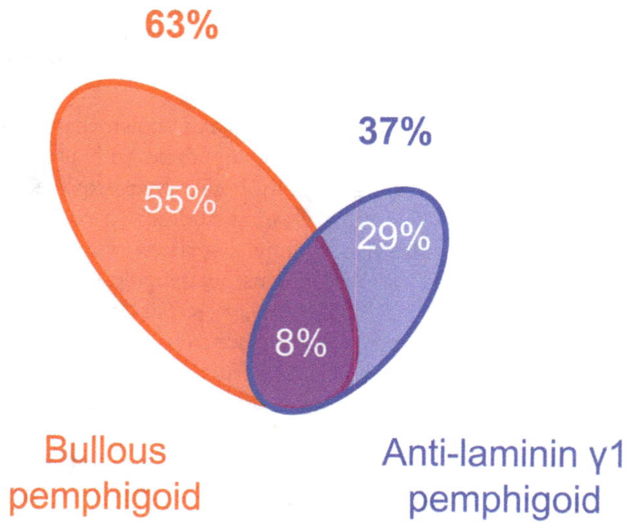

FIGURE 2 | Component of pemphigoid diseases associated with psoriasis (124).

SUSCEPTIBILITIES OF PSORIASIS AND BULLOUS DISEASES

HLA

No shared susceptibility human leukocyte antigen (HLA) alleles have been reported between psoriasis and bullous diseases that can be associated with psoriasis: HLA-Cw*0602 allele has been identified in psoriasis susceptibility 1 (*PSORS1*), a major psoriasis susceptibility locus (130). On the other hand, HLA-DRB1 alleles, such as DRB1*1401, DRB1*0402, and DRB1*08 alleles are associated with pemphigus vulgaris (131). HLA-DQB1*0301 allele has been identified as a susceptibility gene for bullous pemphigoid. Epidermolysis bullosa acquisita is associated with DRB1*15:03 allele (132).

Other Susceptibility Genes

Studies for single nucleotide polymorphisms have been defined several psoriasis susceptibility genes (130, 133) (**Table 1**) whereas it has been challenging to identify the susceptibility genes of pemphigus or pemphigoid diseases and there is much less information about their susceptibility genes. As for two major bullous diseases that can be associated with psoriasis, following genes are suggested to be associated with the disease susceptibility:, *IL1B* (135), *CD16* (136), *ATP8* (137), and *CYP2D6* (138) in bullous pemphigoid; and *CD40L*, *CD40*, *BLYS* (139), *CTLA4* (140), and *CD59* (141) in pemphigus foliaceus. However, they are not included in the major psoriasis susceptibility genes except for the risk loci at *IL1B* in late onset psoriasis (142). Susceptible SNPs in mucous membrane pemphigoid were recently reported (143) whereas mucous membrane pemphigoid rarely accompanied with psoriasis.

Transcriptomic Studies

Whereas transcriptomic analyses are preferentially demonstrated to investigate the pathogenesis of psoriasis, it is not in the case of autoimmune bullous diseases. The increased expression levels of *CD1D* (4.0) and *LILRB2* (4.7) were reported in pemphigus foliaceus (144), neither of them were included in the upregulated genes in psoriasis lesions (134) (**Table 2**).

Consequently, these results suggest that the complication of psoriasis with bullous pemphigoid or pemphigus foliaceus are not attributed to the shared susceptibility. Therefore, it would be more reasonable to consider that the epigenetic events in psoriasis lesions give rise to the increased rate of the complication with autoimmune bullous diseases.

POTENTIAL MECHANISMS OF THE ASSOCIATION OF PSORIASIS AND PEMPHIGOID DISEASES

Local Inflammation

Psoriasis plaques are the frequently affected sites for the blister formation of associated autoimmune bullous diseases, such as bullous pemphigoid (58), anti-laminin γ1 pemphigoid (49), and pemphigus foliaceus (7). It would be reasonable to consider that epigenetic changes altered by psoriasis lesion may trigger or accelerate autoreactive response to specific antigens resulting in autoantibody production, blistering formation, and further positive loop of organ-specific autoimmunity (145). Whereas detailed speculations in this context are described below, it is of not that local inflammation exacerbates cutaneous manifestations in a murine autoimmune pemphigus model (146), suggesting effective recruitment of autoantibodies into psoriasis lesions and further autoimmune loop.

Th17

There are much more psoriasis cases complicated with bullous pemphigoid than those with pemphigus. We have demonstrated that the percentages of interleukin (IL)-17+ cells in CD4+ cells in the lesional skin from bullous pemphigoid are significantly higher than those in the lesional skin from pemphigus foliaceus, and that the serum levels of IL-17 in patients with bullous pemphigoid is higher than those in healthy controls (147). Although IL-17 from T helper type 17 (Th17) cells have an essential role in pathogenesis of psoriasis, it does not explain the common order of the disease development: bullous pemphigoid following psoriasis despite the existence of a rare, inverse case: psoriasis following bullous pemphigoid (77). However, one may speculate that pathological events around the epidermis shared between psoriasis and bullous pemphigoid is related to the activation of Th17 in these diseases, and incidental switch of the immune response from Th1 to Th2 induce the production of the IgG autoantibodies resulting the complication of psoriasis with bullous pemphigoid (77) (**Figure 3**). Because, animal studies have demonstrated that single helper T cell clone specific for desmoglein 3 is sufficient to recapitulate autoimmune blister formation whereas the Th17-deviated T cell clone specific for desmoglein 3 induces

TABLE 1 | SNPs in psoriasis and the related bullous diseases (130, 133).

Disease	Category	Symbols
Psoriasis	HLA	*HLA-C*12:03, HLA-B, HLA-A, HLA-DQA1*
	MHC class-I processing	*ERAP1*
	NF-κB signaling	*REL, TNIP1, NFKBIA, CARD14*
	IFN signaling	*IL28RA, TYK2*
	T-cell regulation	*RUNX3, IL13, TAGAP, ETS1, MBD2, PTPN22*
	Antiviral signaling	*IFIH1, DDX58, RNF114*
	IL-23/IL-17 axis	*TNFAIP3, IL23R, IL12B, TRAF3IP2, IL23A, STAT3*
	Th2	*IL4, IL13*
	Late cornified envelope	*LCE3B, LCE3C, LCE3D*
	Ubiquitin pathway	*ZNF313*
	Unknown	*CDKAL1*
Bullous pemphigoid		*IL1B, CD16, ATP8, CYP2D6*
multicolumn1lPemphigus foliaceus		*CD40L, CD40, BLYS, CTLA4, CD59*

TABLE 2 | Top 25 upregulated genes in the psoriasis lesions relative to the non-lesional skin (134).

#	Symbol	Description	Fold change
1	*SERPINB4*	serpin peptidase inhibitor, clade B (ovalbumin), member 4	661
2	*S100A12*	S100 calcium binding protein A12	328
3	*TCN1*	transcobalamin I (vitamin B12 binding protein, R binder family)	309
4	*S100A7A*	S100 calcium binding protein A7A	260
5	*SPRR2C*	small proline-rich protein 2C (pseudogene)	167
6	*DEFB4A*	defensin, beta 4A	138
7	*AKR1B10*	aldo-keto reductase family 1, member B10 (aldose reductase)	89
8	*PI3*	peptidase inhibitor 3, skin-derived	80
9	*IL8*	interleukin 8	66
10	*TMPRSS11D*	transmembrane protease, serine 11D	63
11	*SERPINB3*	serpin peptidase inhibitor, clade B (ovalbumin), member 3	62
12	*S100A9*	S100 calcium binding protein A9	60
13	*OASL*	29-59-oligoadenylate synthetase-like	56
14	*ATP12A*	ATPase, H+/K+ transporting, nongastric, alpha polypeptide	54
15	*LCN2*	lipocalin 2	53
16	*RHCG*	Rh family, C glycoprotein	52
17	*IGFL1*	IGF-like family member 1	48
18	*KYNU*	kynureninase (L-kynurenine hydrolase)	48
19	*IL1F9*	interleukin 1 family, member 9	43
20	*KLK6*	kallikrein-related peptidase 6	43
21	*LTF*	lactotransferrin	36
22	*CCL20*	chemokine (C-C motif) ligand 20	35
23	*C10orf99*	chromosome 10 open reading frame 99	34
24	*HPSE*	heparanase	33
25	*ADAMDEC1*	ADAM-like, decysin 1	33

psoriasiform dermatitis (148, 149). Occasional production of autoantibodies against BP180 and desmogleins in lichen planus cases has been reported regardless of accompanying blister formation, probably because of the consequence of interface dermatitis, suggesting Th1/Th2 dichotomy among lichen planus vs. pemphigus or pemphigoid diseases (150). In psoriasis, however, production of neither autoantibodies against BP180 nor desmogleins, but α6 integrin (151), in psoriasis has been reported without complication with blistering diseases. It is therefore unlikely that psoriasis and bullous pemphigoid or pemphigus diseases are sharing their primary effector memory T cells.

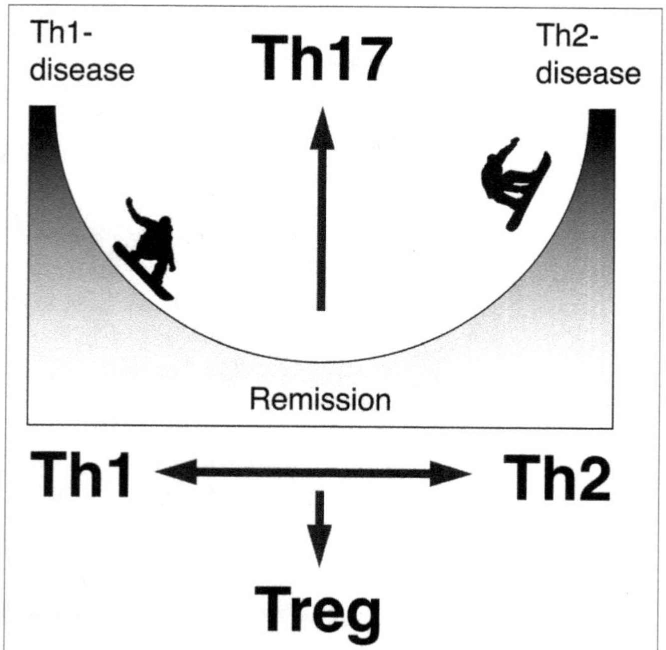

FIGURE 3 | A mechanistic model to produce autoantibodies in psoriasis. Can switch from the Th1/Th17-dominant to Th2/Th17-dominant state be involved?.

Neutrophils and MMP

Keratinocytes in both psoriasis and bullous pemphigoid produce neutrophil chemoattractants, such as IL-8, and infiltration of neutrophil is a common histologic feature in these diseases (130, 131). Consequently, neutrophils release a series of metalloproteases, and it might be related to the substantial degradation of matrix proteins and the subsequent exposure of the antigenic epitopes from matrix autoantigens composing the dermal-epidermal junction. Specifically, a disintegrin and metalloprotease (ADAM) 9, ADAM10, and ADAM17/ tumor necrosis factor-alpha converting enzyme (TACE) degrade BP180/type XVII collagen (152), which is a major autoantigen in bullous pemphigoid while matrix metalloprotease (MMP) 2, 7, 8, 12, 14, 15, and 19 degrades laminins (153), of which trimers are targeted in anti-laminin γ1 pemphigoid (154) and anti-laminin 332 mucous membrane pemphigoid (155).

Laminins

One may be tempted by the following idea: very high prevalence of psoriasis in anti-laminin γ1 pemphigoid can be explained by a positive loop of laminin degradation in psoriasis (129). In psoriasis, as well as in trauma or staphylococcal infections, degradation of laminin is accelerated through the increased expression levels of α5β1 integrin, fibronectin, and plasminogen activators (156). The laminin degradation is also stimulated by MMP9 released from neutrophils. Furthermore, laminin fragments stimulate the MMP9 expression. This laminin degradation loop may be contributed to decrease the threshold of spontaneous production of autoantibodies against laminin γ1 in the development of anti-laminin γ1 pemphigoid in psoriasis patients.

Senescence

The median age of the development of bullous pemphigoid is around 80 years of age. Cell cycle and turnover of the epidermal keratinocytes are extremely accelerated in psoriasis whereas keratinocytes in psoriasis are not immortalized like carcinoma cells. Therefore, it is a plausible idea that the extracellular matrix in psoriatic skin simulates the senescent extracellular matrix and contribute to the development of bullous pemphigoid if the development of bullous pemphigoid is triggered by the senescence of the extracellular matrix produced by senescent keratinocytes. The shortened telomere lengths in psoriasis have not yet determined in keratinocytes or dermal fibroblasts, but in lymphocytes (157). In terms of senescence, type XVII collagen (BP180) changes its distribution (158) and the protein amount due to proteolysis (159) by aging. Despite several suggestions, however, the definitive reason of the predilection of bullous pemphigoid in an extremely old age remains to be elucidated.

CONCLUDING REMARKS

Epidemiological studies have confirmed that psoriasis is highly complicated by the subsequent development of autoimmune bullous diseases. The order of the disease development and the lack of shared susceptibility genes ask whether epigenetic events and molecular circumstances in psoriasis lesions raise the susceptibility to the organ-specific autoimmunity in the skin. The high prevalence of bullous pemphigoid and anti-laminin γ1 pemphigoid in patients with psoriasis promotes following investigations on the pathogenesis of each disease, especially about their unique types of immune responses, as well as the involvement of the degradation and senescence of extracellular proteins around the dermal-epidermal junctions.

AUTHOR CONTRIBUTIONS

All authors listed have made a substantial, direct and intellectual contribution to the work, and approved it for publication.

REFERENCES

1. Leoni A. [Pemphigus foliaceus during the course of psoriasis]. *Minerva Dermatol.* (1952) 27:238–40.
2. Chowaniec O, Blichowska T. [Case of generalized pustular psoriasis caused by corticosteroid treatment of simple psoriasis and pemphigus]. *Przegl Dermatol.* (1979) 66:541–4.
3. Grunwald MH, David M, Feuerman EJ. Coexistence of psoriasis vulgaris and bullous diseases. *J Am Acad Dermatol.* (1985) 13:224–8. doi: 10.1016/S0190-9622(85)70163-6
4. Lee CW, Ro YS, Kim JH, Kim JH. Concurrent development of pemphigus foliaceus and psoriasis. *Int J Dermatol.* (1985) 24:316–7. doi: 10.1111/j.1365-4362.1985.tb05483.x

5. Yokoo M, Oka D, Ueki H. Coexistence of psoriasis vulgaris and pemphigus foliaceus. *Dermatologica* (1989) 179:222–3. doi: 10.1159/000248369
6. Fryer EJ, Lebwohl M. Pemphigus vulgaris after initiation of psoralen and UVA therapy for psoriasis. *J Am Acad Dermatol.* (1994) 30:651–3. doi: 10.1016/S0190-9622(09)80116-3
7. Lee CW, Ro YS. Pemphigus developed on preexisting dermatoses. *J Dermatol.* (1994) 21:213–5. doi: 10.1111/j.1346-8138.1994.tb01724.x
8. Perez GL, Agger WA, Abellera RM, Dahlberg P. Pemphigus foliaceus coexisting with IgA nephropathy in a patient with psoriasis vulgaris. *Int J Dermatol.* (1995) 34:794–6. doi: 10.1111/j.1365-4362.1995.tb04400.x
9. Panzarella K, Camisa C. Coexistence of superficial pemphigus and psoriasis. *Cutis* (1996) 57:414–8.
10. Morita E, Amagai M, Tanaka T, Horiuchi K, Yamamoto S. A case of herpetiform pemphigus coexisting with psoriasis vulgaris. *Br J Dermatol.* (1999) 141:754–5. doi: 10.1046/j.1365-2133.1999.03129.x
11. Stavropoulos PG, Kostakis PG, Papakonstantinou AM, Panagiotopoulos A, Petridis AD. Coexistence of psoriasis and pemphigus after enalapril intake. *Dermatology* (2003) 207:336–7. doi: 10.1159/000073106
12. Giomi B, Cardinali C, Pestelli E, Caproni M, Fabbri P. Pemphigus foliaceus developing on pre-existing psoriasis: a supposed pathogenetic linkage. *Acta Derm Venereol.* (2004) 84:82–3. doi: 10.1080/00015550310020567
13. Sanchez-Palacios C, Chan LS. Development of pemphigus herpetiformis in a patient with psoriasis receiving UV-light treatment. *J Cutan Pathol.* (2004) 31:346–9. doi: 10.1111/j.0303-6987.2004.0188.x
14. Hasse-Cieslinska M, Dmochowski M, Bowszyc-Dmochowska M, Silny W, Danczak-Pazdrowska A. [A case of sporadic pemphigus foliaceus in teenage girl with psoriasis vulgaris]. *Pol Merkur Lekarski* (2005) 18:568–70.
15. Masmoudi A, Hadj Taieb H, Ben Ayed M, Abida O, Makni H, Turki H, et al. [Tunisian erythematosus pemphigus associated with psoriasis in two sisters]. *Ann Dermatol Venereol.* (2006) 133:184–5. doi: 10.1016/S0151-9638(06)77553-6
16. Caldarola G, Carbone A, De Simone C, Pellicano R. Development of pemphigus vulgaris in a patient with psoriasis treated with cyclosporine. *J Am Acad Dermatol.* (2010) 63:356–7. doi: 10.1016/j.jaad.2009.05.032
17. Rallis E, Stavropoulos P, Christofidou E, Rigopoulos D, Koumantaki-Mathioudaki E. Pemphigus vulgaris with plaque-type psoriasis successfully treated with cyclosporine monotherapy. *Am J Clin Dermatol.* (2011) 12:283–4. doi: 10.2165/11586680-000000000-00000
18. Rosmaninho A, Oliveira A, Sanches M, Velho G, Amorim I, Selores M. IgA pemphigus and pustular psoriasis: a possible relation. *Eur J Dermatol.* (2011) 21:100–1. doi: 10.1684/ejd.2011.1159
19. Grekin SJ, Fox MC, Gudjonsson JE, Fullen DR. Psoriasiform pemphigus foliaceus: a report of two cases. *J Cutan Pathol.* (2012) 39:549–53. doi: 10.1111/j.1600-0560.2012.01866.x
20. Kato K, Hanafusa T, Igawa K, Tatsumi M, Takahashi Y, Yamanaka T, et al. A rare case of annular pustular psoriasis associated with pemphigus foliaceus. *Ann Dermatol.* (2014) 26:260–1. doi: 10.5021/ad.2014.26.2.260
21. Kurtzman DJ, Christopher M, Lian F, Sligh JE. A blistering response: concurrent psoriasis and pemphigus foliaceus. *Am J Med.* (2015) 128:24–6. doi: 10.1016/j.amjmed.2014.09.003
22. Claus S, Ziemer M, Simon JC, Treudler R. Coincidence of annular pustular psoriasis, pemphigus foliaceus, and leukocytoclastic vasculitis associated with chronic cholecystitis. *J Dtsch Dermatol Ges.* (2016) 14:830–1. doi: 10.1111/ddg.12619
23. Sanz-Bueno J, Gallo E, Caro-Gutierrez D, Sanchez-Gilo A, Gutierrez Pascual M, Rojas-Scheffer L, et al. Penfigo foliaceo agravado por farmacos en un paciente con psoriasis, con buena respuesta a adalimumab. *Dermatol Online J.* 23:13030/qt8tr4j1f2.
24. Sousa VB, Santana C, Pereira DDN, Gripp AC. Pemphigus foliaceus with pustular presentation in a patient with psoriasis. *An Bras Dermatol.* (2017) 92:115–7. doi: 10.1590/abd1806-4841.20175709
25. Fujimoto N, Matsuo S, Satoh T. Psoriasis vulgaris in a patient with pemphigus vulgaris on corticosteroid therapy. *J Dtsch Dermatol Ges.* (2018) 16:606–8. doi: 10.1111/ddg.13505
26. Person JR, Rogers RS III. Bullous pemphigoid and psoriasis: does subclinical bullous pemphigoid exist? *Br. J. Dermatol.* (1976) 95, 535–540.
27. Ahmed AR, Winkler NW. Psoriasis and bullous pemphigoid. *Arch Dermatol.* (1977) 113:845. doi: 10.1001/archderm.1977.01640060141023
28. Robledo, A., Pais, T., Nine, C., Fonseca T. [Bullous pemphigoid and psoriasis]. *Actas Dermosifiliogr.* (1977) 68:409–416.
29. Koerber WAJr, Price NM, Watson W. Coexistent psoriasis and bullous pemphigoid: a report of six cases. *Arch Dermatol.* (1978) 114:1643–6. doi: 10.1001/archderm.1978.01640230017005
30. Stuttgen G, Bockendahl H, Remy W, Lewicki D. [Psoriasis and bullous dermatoses]. *Hautarzt* (1978) 29:134–40.
31. Abel EA, Bennett A. Bullous pemphigoid. Occurrence in psoriasis treated with psoralens plus long-wave ultraviolet radiation. *Arch Dermatol.* (1979) 115:988–9. doi: 10.1001/archderm.1979.04010080052026
32. Stuttgen G, Kentsch V. Psoriasis and pemphigoid positive correlation. *Acta Derm Venereol Suppl.* (1979) 87:99–101.
33. Olmos L, De Diego V. [Psoriasis and pemphigoid (author's transl)]. *Dermatologica* (1981) 163:105–12. doi: 10.1159/000250146
34. Albergo RP, Gilgor RS. Delayed onset of bullous pemphigoid after PUVA and sunlight treatment of psoriasis. *Cutis* (1982) 30:621–4.
35. Brun P, Baran R. [Bullous pemphigoid induced by photochemotherapy of psoriasis. Apropos of 2 cases, with a review of the literature]. *Ann. Dermatol. Venereol.* (1982) 109:461–468.
36. Wallach D, Cottenot F. Erythrodermic bullous pemphigoid or erythrodermic psoriasis and bullous pemphigoid? *J Am Acad Dermatol.* (1982) 7:800.
37. Mashkilleison AL, Golousenko I, Reznikova MM. [Bullous pemphigoid associated with psoriasis]. *Vestn Dermatol Venerol.* (1983) 37–8.
38. Weltfriend S, David M, Feuerman EJ. [Bullous pemphigoid in a patient with psoriasis]. *Harefuah* (1983) 105:218–9.
39. Barba A, Leoni A, Peroni A. [Psoriasis and pemphigoid]. *G Ital Dermatol Venereol.* (1985) 120:75–7.
40. Grattan CE. Evidence of an association between bullous pemphigoid and psoriasis. *Br J Dermatol.* (1985) 113:281–3. doi: 10.1111/j.1365-2133.1985.tb02079.x
41. Mozzanica N, Tadini GL, Pigatto P, Altomare GF. [Psoriasis and bullous pemphigoid. Presentation of 2 cases]. *G. Ital. Dermatol. Venereol.* (1985) 120:189–92.
42. Bork K. [Psoriasis and bullous pemphigoid]. *Hautarzt* (1987) 38:348–51.
43. Wollina U, Roth H. [Psoriasis vulgaris partim inversa and bullous pemphigoid. Case report and short review of the literature] *Dermatol Monatsschr.* (1987) 173:29–32.
44. Rotoli M, Rossi GF, Bono R, Rusciani L. [Association of psoriasis and bullous pemphigoid. Clinical case] *G Ital Dermatol Venereol.* (1988) 123:161–2.
45. Di Silverio A, Vignini M, Gabba P, Bellosta M, Brandozzi G. [Psoriasis-pemphigoid association. Description of a case] *G Ital Dermatol Venereol.* (1989) 124:359–61.
46. Nicoletti A, Riva MI, Crippa D, Sala GP, Albanese G, Beneggi M. [Psoriasis and bullous pemphigoid. Description of 3 clinical cases]. *G. Ital. Dermatol. Venereol.* (1989) 124:277–9.
47. Weber PJ, Salazar JE. Bullous eruption in a psoriatic patient. Bullous pemphigoid and psoriasis. *Arch Dermatol.* (1989) 125:691–2.
48. Bianchi L, Gatti S, Nini G. Bullous pemphigoid and severe erythrodermic psoriasis: combined low-dose treatment with cyclosporine and systemic steroids. *J Am Acad Dermatol.* (1992) 27:278. doi: 10.1016/S0190-9622(08)80749-9
49. Chen KR, Shimizu S, Miyakawa S, Ishiko A, Shimizu H, Hashimoto T. Coexistence of psoriasis and an unusual IgG-mediated subepidermal bullous dermatosis: identification of a novel 200-kDa lower lamina lucida target antigen. *Br J Dermatol.* (1996) 134:340–6. doi: 10.1111/j.1365-2133.1996.tb07625.x
50. George PM. Bullous pemphigoid possibly induced by psoralen plus ultraviolet A therapy. *Photodermatol Photoimmunol Photomed.* (1996) 11:185–7. doi: 10.1111/j.1600-0781.1995.tb00166.x
51. Kirtschig G, Chow ET, Venning VA, Wojnarowska FT. Acquired subepidermal bullous diseases associated with psoriasis: a clinical, immunopathological and immunogenetic study. *Br J Dermatol.* (1996) 135:738–45. doi: 10.1111/j.1365-2133.1996.tb03883.x
52. Perl S, Rappersberger K, Fodinger D, Anegg B, Honigsmann H, Ortel B. Bullous pemphigoid induced by PUVA therapy. *Dermatology* (1996) 193:245–7. doi: 10.1159/000246255

53. Rotstein H. Psoriasis: changing clinical patterns. *Australas J Dermatol.* (1996) 37 (Suppl. 1):S27–9. doi: 10.1111/j.1440-0960.1996.tb01075.x
54. Saeki H, Hayashi N, Komine M, Soma Y, Shimada S, Watanabe K, et al. A case of generalized pustular psoriasis followed by bullous disease: an atypical case of bullous pemphigoid or a novel bullous disease? *Br J Dermatol.* (1996) 134:152–5.
55. Primka EJ III, Camisa C. Psoriasis and bullous pemphigoid treated with azathioprine. *J. Am. Acad. Dermatol.* (1998) 39:121–123. doi: 10.1016/S0190-9622(98)70414-1
56. Roeder C, Driesch PV. Psoriatic erythroderma and bullous pemphigoid treated successfully with acitretin and azathioprine. *Eur J Dermatol.* (1999) 9:537–9.
57. Kawahara Y, Zillikens D, Yancey KB, Marinkovich MP, Nie Z, Hashimoto T, et al. Subepidermal blistering disease with autoantibodies against a novel dermal 200-kDa antigen. *J Dermatol Sci.* (2000) 23:93–102. doi: 10.1016/S0923-1811(99)00093-6
58. Kobayashi TT, Elston DM, Libow LF, David-Bajar K. A case of bullous pemphigoid limited to psoriatic plaques. *Cutis* (2002) 70:283–7.
59. Pasic A, Ljubojevic S, Lipozencic J, Marinovic B, Loncaric D. Coexistence of psoriasis vulgaris, bullous pemphigoid and vitiligo: a case report. *J Eur Acad Dermatol Venereol.* (2002) 16:426–7. doi: 10.1046/j.1468-3083.2002.00570_12.x
60. Burnett PE. Bullous pemphigoid and psoriasis vulgaris. *Dermatol Online J.* (2003) 9:19.
61. Paul J. Bullous pemphigoid in a patient with psoriasis and possible drug reaction: a case report. *Conn Med.* (2004) 68:611–5.
62. Yasuda H, Tomita Y, Shibaki A, Hashimoto T. Two cases of subepidermal blistering disease with anti-p200 or 180-kD bullous pemphigoid antigen associated with psoriasis. *Dermatology* (2004) 209:149–55. doi: 10.1159/000079602
63. Bourdon-Lanoy E, Roujeau JC, Joly P, Guillaume JC, Bernard P, Prost C, et al. [Bullous pemphigoid in young patients: a retrospective study of 74 cases]. *Ann Dermatol Venereol.* (2005) 132:115–22. doi: 10.1016/S0151-9638(05)79220-6
64. Washio H, Hara H, Suzuki H, Yoshida M, Hashimoto T. Bullous pemphigoid on psoriasis lesions after UVA radiation. *Acta Derm Venereol.* (2005) 85:561–3. doi: 10.1080/00015550510035677
65. Arregui MA, Soloeta R, Gonzalez R, Garcia I, Trebol I, Tamayo C. [Bullous pemphigoid related to PUVA therapy: two further cases]. *Actas Dermosifiliogr.* (2006) 97:444–7. doi: 10.1016/S0001-7310(06)73437-8
66. Barnadas MA, Gilaberte M, Pujol R, Agusti M, Gelpi C, Alomar A. Bullous pemphigoid in a patient with psoriasis during the course of PUVA therapy: study by ELISA test. *Int J Dermatol.* (2006) 45:1089–92. doi: 10.1111/j.1365-4632.2004.02517.x
67. Lazarczyk M, Wozniak K, Ishii N, Gorkiewicz-Petkov A, Hashimoto T, Schwarz R, et al. Coexistence of psoriasis and pemphigoid–only a coincidence? *Int J Mol Med.* (2006) 18:619–23. doi :10.3892/ijmm.18.4.619
68. Wilczek A, Sticherling M. Concomitant psoriasis and bullous pemphigoid: coincidence or pathogenic relationship? *Int J Dermatol.* (2006) 45:1353–7. doi: 10.1111/j.1365-4632.2006.02861.x
69. Yamauchi PS, Lowe NJ, Gindi V. Treatment of coexisting bullous pemphigoid and psoriasis with the tumor necrosis factor antagonist etanercept. *J Am Acad Dermatol.* (2006) 54:S121–2. doi: 10.1016/j.jaad.2005.10.055
70. Sugita K, Kabashima K, Nishio D, Hashimoto T, Tokura Y. Th2 cell fluctuation in association with reciprocal occurrence of bullous pemphigoid and psoriasis vulgaris. *J Eur Acad Dermatol Venereol.* (2007) 21:569–70. doi: 10.1111/j.1468-3083.2006.01966.x
71. Miyakura T, Yamamoto T, Tashiro A, Okubo Y, Oyama B, Ishii N, et al. Anti-p200 pemphigoid associated with annular pustular psoriasis. *Eur J Dermatol.* (2008) 18:481–2. doi: 10.1684/ejd.2008.0465
72. Rallis E, Anyfantakis V. Coexistent psoriasis and bullous pemphigoid responding to mycophenolate mofetil monotherapy. *Skinmed* (2008) 7:101–2. doi: 10.1111/j.1751-7125.2008.07318.x
73. Saraceno R, Citarella L, Spallone G, Chimenti S. A biological approach in a patient with psoriasis and bullous pemphigoid associated with losartan therapy. *Clin Exp Dermatol.* (2008) 33:154–5. doi: 10.1111/j.1365-2230.2007.02603.x
74. Inokuma D, Kodama K, Natsuga K, Kasai M, Abe M, Nishie W, et al. Autoantibodies against type XVII collagen C-terminal domain in a patient with bullous pemphigoid associated with psoriasis vulgaris. *Br J Dermatol.* (2009) 160:451–4. doi: 10.1111/j.1365-2133.2008.08961.x
75. Monnier-Murina K, Du Thanh A, Merlet-Albran S, Guillot B, Dereure O. Bullous pemphigoid occurring during efalizumab treatment for psoriasis: a paradoxical auto-immune reaction? *Dermatology* (2009) 219:89–90. doi: 10.1159/000207792
76. Stausbol-Gron B, Deleuran M, Sommer Hansen E, Kragballe K. Development of bullous pemphigoid during treatment of psoriasis with adalimumab. *Clin Exp Dermatol.* (2009) 34:e285–6. doi: 10.1111/j.1365-2230.2008.03204.x
77. Yasukawa S, Dainichi T, Kokuba H, Moroi Y, Urabe K, Hashimoto T, et al. Bullous pemphigoid followed by pustular psoriasis showing Th1, Th2, Treg and Th17 immunological changes. *Eur J Dermatol.* (2009) 19:69–71. doi: 10.1684/ejd.2008.0572
78. Cusano F, Iannazzone SS, Riccio G, Piccirillo F. Coexisting bullous pemphigoid and psoriasis successfully treated with etanercept. *Eur J Dermatol.* (2010) 20:520. doi: 10.1684/ejd.2010.0970
79. Kluk J, Goulding JM, Bhat J, Finch TM. Drug-induced bullous pemphigoid: cases triggered by intravenous iodine and etanercept. *Clin Exp Dermatol.* (2011) 36:871–3. doi: 10.1111/j.1365-2230.2011.04102.x
80. Kwon HH, Kwon IH, Chung JH, Youn JI. Pemphigus foliaceus associated with psoriasis during the course of narrow-band UVB therapy: a simple coincidence? *Ann Dermatol.* (2011) 23:S281–4. doi: 10.5021/ad.2011.23.S3.S281
81. Rao R, Gupta A, Yunis F, Handettu S, Chandrashekar B. Coexistence of psoriasis with bullous pemphigoid. *Indian Dermatol Online J.* (2012) 3:119–21. doi: 10.4103/2229-5178.96707
82. Gunay U, Gunduz K, Ermertcan AT, Kandiloglu AR. Coexistence of psoriasis and bullous pemphigoid: remission with low-dose methotrexate. *Cutan Ocul Toxicol.* (2013) 32:168–9. doi: 10.3109/15569527.2012.667030
83. Majima Y, Yagi H, Tateishi C, Groth S, Schmidt E, Zillikens D, et al. A successful treatment with ustekinumab in a case of antilaminin-gamma1 pemphigoid associated with psoriasis. *Br J Dermatol.* (2013) 168:1367–9. doi: 10.1111/bjd.12163
84. Ohata C, Fukuda S, Ishii N, Koga H, Hamada T, Furumura M, et al. Refractory anti-laminin gamma1 pemphigoid with psoriasis vulgaris successfully treated by double-filtration plasmapheresis. *Eur J Dermatol.* (2013) 23:715–6. doi: 10.1684/ejd.2013.2138
85. Ansai S, Hashizume S, Kawana S, Tateishi C, Koga H, Hashimoto T. Case of anti-laminin gamma-1 pemphigoid with antibody against C-terminal domain of BP180 in a patient with psoriasis vulgaris. *J Dermatol.* (2014) 41:1031–3. doi: 10.1111/1346-8138.12625
86. Igarashi M, Tsunemi Y, Koga H, Hashimoto T, Tateishi C, Tsuruta D, et al. Anti-laminin gamma1 pemphigoid associated with pustular psoriasis. *Eur J Dermatol.* (2014) 24:629–30. doi: 10.1684/ejd.2014.2419
87. Jankowski M, Czajkowski R, Scibior K, Schwartz RA. Coexistence of psoriasis vulgaris and vitiligo with bullous pemphigoid: a case report. *Int J Dermatol.* (2014) 53:e359–61. doi: 10.1111/ijd.12349
88. Li Z, Jin P, Feng S, Wang B. Treatment of coexisting bullous pemphigoid and psoriasis with tripterygium wilfordii. *Chin Med J.* (2014) 127:3037.
89. Marek-Jozefowicz L, Scibior K, Czajkowski R. PUVA induced bullous pemphigoid in a patient with psoriasis. *Acta Dermatovenerol Croat.* (2014) 22:301–4.
90. Si X, Ge L, Xin H, Cao W, Sun X, Li W. Erythrodermic psoriasis with bullous pemphigoid: combination treatment with methotrexate and compound glycyrrhizin. *Diagn Pathol.* (2014) 9:102. doi: 10.1186/1746-1596-9-102
91. Stoica LE, Patrascu V, Dascalu RC, Ciurea ME. Bullous pemphigoid associated with psoriasis, breast cancer and Parkinson's disease. *Curr Health Sci J.* (2014) 40:62–6. doi: 10.12865/CHSJ.40.01.12
92. Wang TS, Tsai TF. Remission of bullous pemphigoid after rituximab treatment in a psoriasis patient on regular low-dose methotrexate. *Acta Derm Venereol.* (2014) 94:108–9. doi: 10.2340/00015555-1619
93. Akasaka E, Nakano H, Korekawa A, Fukui T, Kaneko T, Koga H, et al. Anti-laminin gamma1 pemphigoid associated with ulcerative colitis and psoriasis vulgaris showing autoantibodies to laminin gamma1, type XVII collagen and laminin-332. *Eur J Dermatol.* (2015) 25:198–9. doi: 10.1684/ejd.2014.2499

94. Garrido Colmenero C, Arias Santiago S, Blasco Morente G, Perez Lopez I, Aneiros Fernandez J. Photoletter to the editor: Psoriatic erythroderma associated with bullous pemphigoid: clinical appearance and histopathology. *J Dermatol Case Rep.* (2015) 9:23–4. doi: 10.3315/jdcr.2015.1194
95. Iino Y, Kano T, Adachi F, Suzuki M, Nishikawa R, Ishii N, et al. A case of bullous pemphigoid associated with psoriasis vulgaris showing Hailey-Hailey disease-like histopathological changes in regenerated epidermis without genomic mutation in ATP2C1 or ATP2A2 gene. *J Eur Acad Dermatol Venereol.* (2015) 29:1646–8. doi: 10.1111/jdv.12521
96. Imanishi A, Tateishi C, Imanishi H, Sowa-Osako J, Koga H, Tsuruta D, et al. Pemphigoid with antibodies to laminin gamma1, BP180 and BP230, associated with psoriasis vulgaris: successful disease control with cyclosporin. *J Dermatol.* (2015) 42:394–7. doi: 10.1111/1346-8138.12798
97. Ishida S, Takahashi K, Kanaoka M, Okawa T, Tateishi C, Yasukochi A, et al. Case of subepidermal autoimmune bullous disease with psoriasis vulgaris reacting to both BP180 C-terminal domain and laminin gamma-1. *J Dermatol.* (2015) 42:391–3. doi: 10.1111/1346-8138.12801
98. Iskandarli M, Gerceker Turk B, Yaman B, Ozturk G. Pemphigoid diseases as a sign of active psoriasis: a case report and brief review. *Dermatology* (2015) 231:319–21. doi: 10.1159/000435912
99. Nakayama C, Fujita Y, Watanabe M, Shimizu H. Development of bullous pemphigoid during treatment of psoriatic onycho-pachydermo periostitis with ustekinumab. *J Dermatol.* (2015a) 42:996–8. doi: 10.1111/1346-8138.12943
100. Nakayama C, Iwata H, Haga N, Hamade Y, Mizuno O, Nishie W, et al. The different intensity of autoantibody deposits in bullous pemphigoid associated with psoriasis vulgaris. *Eur J Dermatol.* (2015b) 25:70–1. doi: 10.1684/ejd.2014.2444
101. Okahashi K, Oiso N, Ishii N, Uchida S, Matsuda H, Hashimoto T, et al. Bullous pemphigoid associated with psoriasis: a possible example of an inverse intramolecular epitope-spreading phenomenon. *J Dermatol.* (2015) 42:758–9. doi: 10.1111/1346-8138.12891
102. Caca-Biljanovska N, Arsovska-Bezhoska I, V'lckova-Laskoska M. PUVA-induced bullous pemphigoid in psoriasis. *Acta Dermatovenerol. Croat.* (2016) 24:214–7.
103. Commin MH, Schmidt E, Duvert-Lehembre S, Lasek A, Morice C, Estival JL, et al. Clinical and immunological features and outcome of anti-p200 pemphigoid. *Br J Dermatol.* (2016) 175:776–81. doi: 10.1111/bjd.14629
104. Fujimura Y, Natsuga K, Hamade Y, Nomura Y, Kaku Y, Muramatsu R, et al. Anti-laminin-gamma 1 pemphigoid with generalized pustular psoriasis and psoriasis vulgaris. *Acta Derm Venereol.* (2016) 96:120–1. doi: 10.2340/00015555-2168
105. Lesniewska A, Kalinska-Bienias A, Kowalewski C, Schwartz R, Wozniak K. Development of bullous pemphigoid in a patient with psoriasis and metabolic syndrome. *Cutis* (2016) 98:E19–23.
106. Maki N, Demitsu T, Umemoto N, Nagashima K, Nakamura T, Kakurai M, et al. Possible paraneoplastic syndrome case of bullous pemphigoid with immunoglobulin G anti-BP180 C-terminal domain antibodies associated with psoriasis and primary macroglobulinemia. *J Dermatol.* (2016) 43:571–4. doi: 10.1111/1346-8138.13170
107. Ho PH, Tsai TF. Development of bullous pemphigoid during secukinumab treatment for psoriasis. *J Dermatol.* (2017) 44:e220–1. doi: 10.1111/1346-8138.13909
108. Loget J, Plee J, Antonicelli F, Bernard P. A successful treatment with ustekinumab in a case of relapsing bullous pemphigoid associated with psoriasis. *J Eur Acad Dermatol Venereol.* (2017) 31:e228–30. doi: 10.1111/jdv.14002
109. Ohashi M, Takagi H, Mizutani Y, Seishima M, Koga H, Hashimoto T. Bullous pemphigoid with IgG autoantibodies to the alpha3 subunit of laminin 332 associated with psoriasis vulgaris. *Eur J Dermatol.* (2017) 27:306–7. doi: 10.1684/ejd.2017.2980
110. Endo Y, Tamura A, Ishikawa O, Miyachi Y, Hashimoto T. Psoriasis vulgaris coexistent with epidermolysis bullosa acquisita. *Br J Dermatol.* (1997) 137:783–6. doi: 10.1111/j.1365-2133.1997.tb01119.x
111. Morris SD, Mallipeddi R, Oyama N, Gratian MJ, Harman KE, Bhogal BS, et al. Psoriasis bullosa acquisita. *Clin Exp Dermatol.* (2002) 27:665–9. doi: 10.1046/j.1365-2230.2002.01100.x
112. Hoshina D, Sawamura D, Nomura T, Tanimura S, Abe M, Onozuka T, et al. Epidermolysis bullosa acquisita associated with psoriasis vulgaris. *Clin Exp Dermatol.* (2007) 32:516–8. doi: 10.1111/j.1365-2230.2007.02430.x
113. Kabashima R, Hino R, Bito T, Kabashima K, Nakamura M, Bungo O, et al. Epidermolysis bullosa acquisita associated with psoriasis. *Acta Derm Venereol.* (2010) 90:314–6. doi: 10.2340/00015555-0832
114. Min L, Kensuke M, Takashi H, Naoyuki H. Epidermolysis bullosa acquisita in a patient with psoriasis vulgaris. *Eur J Dermatol.* (2015) 25:499–500. doi: 10.1684/ejd.2015.2623
115. Moon SY, Eun DH, Jung HJ, Kim JY, Park TI, Lee WJ, et al. Coexistence of psoriasis and epidermolysis bullosa acquisita: evaluation of the integrity of the basement membrane. *J Cutan Pathol.* (2017) 44:602–3. doi: 10.1111/cup.12940
116. Gubinelli E, Angelo C, Pacifico V. A case of dystrophic epidermolysis bullosa improved with etanercept for concomitant psoriatic arthritis. *Am J Clin Dermatol* (2010) 11 (Suppl. 1):53–4. doi: 10.2165/1153427-S0-000000000-00000
117. Heaphy MR, Winkelmann RK. Coexistence of benign familial pemphigus and psoriasis vulgaris. *Arch Dermatol.* (1976) 112:1571–4. doi: 10.1001/archderm.1976.01630350047013
118. Boxley JD, Byrne JP, Summerly R. Bi-directional isomorphism: coexistence of psoriasis vulgaris and familial benign chronic pemphigus. *Arch Dermatol.* (1977) 113:846–7. doi: 10.1001/archderm.1977.01640060142025
119. Kochergin NG, Shkrebets SV. [Combination of psoriasis and Hailey-Hailey disease]. *Vestn Dermatol Venerol.* (1987) 68–70.
120. Mallen JK. Psoriasis, chronic benign familial pemphigus, and dysplastic naevus syndrome in a family. *Australas J Dermatol.* (1992) 33:55. doi: 10.1111/j.1440-0960.1992.tb00059.x
121. Hayakawa K, Shiohara T. Coexistence of psoriasis and familial benign chronic pemphigus: efficacy of ultraviolet B treatment. *Br J Dermatol.* (1999) 140:374–5. doi: 10.1046/j.1365-2133.1999.02690.x
122. Santos-Juanes J, Coto-Segura P, Saavedra J, Laviano S, Galache C. Development of familial benign chronic pemphigus in a patient undergoing treatment with efalizumab for psoriasis. *J Eur Acad Dermatol Venereol.* (2009) 23:605–6. doi: 10.1111/j.1468-3083.2008.02979.x
123. Chao SC, Lee JY, Wu MC, Hsu MM. A novel splice mutation in the ATP2C1 gene in a woman with concomitant psoriasis vulgaris and disseminated Hailey-Hailey disease. *Int J Dermatol.* (2012) 51:947–51. doi: 10.1111/j.1365-4632.2010.04800.x
124. Ohata C, Ishii N, Koga H, Fukuda S, Tateishi C, Tsuruta D, et al. Coexistence of autoimmune bullous diseases (AIBDs) and psoriasis: a series of 145 cases. *J Am Acad Dermatol.* (2015) 73:50–5. doi: 10.1016/j.jaad.2015.03.016
125. Tsai TF, Wang TS, Hung ST, Tsai PI, Schenkel B, Zhang M, et al. Epidemiology and comorbidities of psoriasis patients in a national database in Taiwan. *J Dermatol Sci.* (2011) 63:40–6. doi: 10.1016/j.jdermsci.2011.03.002
126. Kridin K, Zelber-Sagi S, Comaneshter D, Cohen AD. Association between pemphigus and psoriasis: a population-based large-scale study. *J Am Acad Dermatol.* (2017) 77:1174–5. doi: 10.1016/j.jaad.2017.07.007
127. Chen YJ, Wu CY, Lin MW, Chen TJ, Liao KK, Chen YC, et al. Comorbidity profiles among patients with bullous pemphigoid: a nationwide population-based study. *Br J Dermatol.* (2011) 165:593–9. doi: 10.1111/j.1365-2133.2011.10386.x
128. Kridin K, Bergman R. Association between bullous pemphigoid and psoriasis: a case-control study. *J Am Acad Dermatol.* (2017) 77:370–2. doi: 10.1016/j.jaad.2017.02.057
129. Dainichi T, Koga H, Tsuji T, Ishii N, Ohyama B, Ueda A, et al. From anti-p200 pemphigoid to anti-laminin gamma1 pemphigoid. *J Dermatol.* (2010) 37:231–8. doi: 10.1111/j.1346-8138.2009.00793.x
130. Perera GK, Di Meglio P, Nestle FO. Psoriasis. *Annu Rev Pathol.* (2012) 7:385–422. doi: 10.1146/annurev-pathol-011811-132448
131. Hammers CM, Stanley JR. Mechanisms of Disease: Pemphigus and Bullous Pemphigoid. *Annu Rev Pathol.* (2016) 11:175–97. doi: 10.1146/annurev-pathol-012615-044313
132. Schmidt E, Zillikens D. Pemphigoid diseases. *Lancet* (2013) 381:320–32. doi: 10.1016/S0140-6736(12)61140-4

133. Ray-Jones H, Eyre S, Barton A, Warren RB. One SNP at a Time: Moving beyond GWAS in Psoriasis. *J Invest Dermatol.* (2016) 136:567–73. doi: 10.1016/j.jid.2015.11.025
134. Tian S, Krueger JG, Li K, Jabbari A, Brodmerkel C, Lowes MA, et al. Meta-analysis derived (MAD) transcriptome of psoriasis defines the "core" pathogenesis of disease. *PLoS ONE* (2012) 7:e44274. doi: 10.1371/journal.pone.0044274
135. Chang YT, Liu HN, Yu CW, Lin MW, Huang CH, Chen CC, et al. Cytokine gene polymorphisms in bullous pemphigoid in a Chinese population. *Br J Dermatol.* (2006) 154:79–84. doi: 10.1111/j.1365-2133.2005.06938.x
136. Weisenseel P, Martin S, Partscht K, Messer G, Prinz JC. Relevance of the low-affinity type of the Fcgamma-receptor IIIa-polymorphism in bullous pemphigoid. *Arch Dermatol Res.* (2007) 299:163–4. doi: 10.1007/s00403-007-0755-8
137. Hirose M, Schilf P, Benoit S, Eming R, Glaser R, Homey B, et al. Polymorphisms in the mitochondrially encoded ATP synthase 8 gene are associated with susceptibility to bullous pemphigoid in the German population. *Exp Dermatol.* (2015) 24:715–7. doi: 10.1111/exd.12732
138. Rychlik-Sych M, Baranska M, Wojtczak A, Skretkowicz J, Zebrowska A, Waszczykowska E. The impact of the CYP2D6 gene polymorphism on the risk of pemphigoid. *Int J Dermatol.* (2015) 54:1396–401. doi: 10.1111/ijd.12967
139. Malheiros D, Petzl-Erler ML. Individual and epistatic effects of genetic polymorphisms of B-cell co-stimulatory molecules on susceptibility to pemphigus foliaceus. *Genes Immun.* (2009) 10:547–58. doi: 10.1038/gene.2009.36
140. Tanasilovic S, Popadic S, Medenica L, Popadic D. Pemphigus vulgaris and pemphigus foliaceus determined by CD86 and CTLA4 polymorphisms. *Clin Dermatol.* (2017) 35:236–41. doi: 10.1016/j.clindermatol.2016.05.021
141. Salviano-Silva A, Petzl-Erler ML, Boldt ABW. CD59 polymorphisms are associated with gene expression and different sexual susceptibility to pemphigus foliaceus. *Autoimmunity* (2017) 50:377–85. doi: 10.1080/08916934.2017.1329830
142. Hebert HL, Bowes J, Smith RL, Mchugh NJ, Barker J, Griffiths CEM, et al. Polymorphisms in IL-1B distinguish between psoriasis of early and late onset. *J Invest Dermatol.* (2014) 134:1459–62. doi: 10.1038/jid.2013.485
143. Sadik CD, Bischof J, Van Beek N, Dieterich A, Benoit S, Sardy M, et al. Genomewide association study identifies GALC as susceptibility gene for mucous membrane pemphigoid. *Exp Dermatol.* (2017) 26:1214–20. doi: 10.1111/exd.13464
144. Malheiros D, Panepucci RA, Roselino AM, Araujo AG, Zago MA, Petzl-Erler ML. Genome-wide gene expression profiling reveals unsuspected molecular alterations in pemphigus foliaceus. *Immunology* (2014) 143:381–95. doi: 10.1111/imm.12315
145. Ludwig RJ, Vanhoorelbeke K, Leypoldt F, Kaya Z, Bieber K, Mclachlan SM, et al. Mechanisms of autoantibody-induced pathology. *Front Immunol.* (2017) 8:603. doi: 10.3389/fimmu.2017.00603
146. Ono S, Egawa G, Kitoh A, Dainichi T, Otsuka A, Nakajima S, et al. Local inflammation exacerbates cutaneous manifestations in a murine autoimmune pemphigus model. *J Allergy Clin Immunol.* (2017) 139:2026–8.e2025. doi: 10.1016/j.jaci.2016.12.959
147. Arakawa M, Dainichi T, Ishii N, Hamada T, Karashima T, Nakama T, et al. Lesional Th17 cells and regulatory T cells in bullous pemphigoid. *Exp Dermatol.* (2011) 20:1022–4. doi: 10.1111/j.1600-0625.2011.01378.x
148. Takahashi H, Kuwana M, Amagai M. A single helper T cell clone is sufficient to commit polyclonal naive B cells to produce pathogenic IgG in experimental pemphigus vulgaris. *J Immunol.* (2009) 182:1740–5. doi: 10.4049/jimmunol.182.3.1740
149. Nishimoto S, Kotani H, Tsuruta S, Shimizu N, Ito M, Shichita T, et al. Th17 cells carrying TCR recognizing epidermal autoantigen induce psoriasis-like skin inflammation. *J Immunol.* (2013) 191:3065–72. doi: 10.4049/jimmunol.1300348
150. Schmidt T, Solimani F, Pollmann R, Stein R, Schmidt A, Stulberg I, et al. TH1/TH17 cell recognition of desmoglein 3 and bullous pemphigoid antigen 180 in patients with lichen planus. *J. Allergy Clin. Immunol.* (2018) doi: 10.1016/j.jaci.2018.02.044. [Epub ahead of print].
151. Gal B, Dulic S, Kiss M, Groma G, Kovacs L, Kemeny L, et al. Increased circulating anti-alpha6-integrin autoantibodies in psoriasis and psoriatic arthritis but not in rheumatoid arthritis. *J Dermatol.* (2017) 44:370–4. doi: 10.1111/1346-8138.13667
152. Nishie W. Update on the pathogenesis of bullous pemphigoid: an autoantibody-mediated blistering disease targeting collagen XVII. *J Dermatol Sci.* (2014) 73:179–86. doi: 10.1016/j.jdermsci.2013.12.001
153. Mezentsev A, Nikolaev A, Bruskin S. Matrix metalloproteinases and their role in psoriasis. *Gene* (2014) 540:1–10. doi: 10.1016/j.gene.2014.01.068
154. Dainichi T, Kurono S, Ohyama B, Ishii N, Sanzen N, Hayashi M, et al. Anti-laminin gamma-1 pemphigoid. *Proc Natl Acad Sci USA.* (2009) 106:2800–5. doi: 10.1073/pnas.0809230106
155. Chan LS, Ahmed AR, Anhalt GJ, Bernauer W, Cooper KD, Elder MJ, et al. The first international consensus on mucous membrane pemphigoid: definition, diagnostic criteria, pathogenic factors, medical treatment, and prognostic indicators. *Arch Dermatol.* (2002) 138:370–9. doi: 10.1001/archderm.138.3.370
156. Mcfadden JP, Powles A, Kimber I, Fry L. Psoriasis and basement-membrane laminin. *Br J Dermatol.* (2013) 169:718–9. doi: 10.1111/bjd.12400
157. Wu K, Higashi N, Hansen ER, Lund M, Bang K, Thestrup-Pedersen K. Telomerase activity is increased and telomere length shortened in T cells from blood of patients with atopic dermatitis and psoriasis. *J Immunol.* (2000) 165:4742–7. doi: 10.4049/jimmunol.165.8.4742
158. Watanabe M, Natsuga K, Nishie W, Kobayashi Y, Donati G, Suzuki S, et al. Type XVII collagen coordinates proliferation in the interfollicular epidermis. *Elife* (2017) 6:e26635. doi: 10.7554/eLife.26635
159. Matsumura H, Mohri Y, Binh NT, Morinaga H, Fukuda M, Ito M, et al. Hair follicle aging is driven by transepidermal elimination of stem cells via COL17A1 proteolysis. *Science* (2016) 351:aad4395. doi: 10.1126/science.aad4395

20

Epidermolysis Bullosa Acquisita: The 2019 Update

Hiroshi Koga[1], *Catherine Prost-Squarcioni*[2], *Hiroaki Iwata*[3], *Marcel F. Jonkman*[4], *Ralf J. Ludwig*[5]* and *Katja Bieber*[5]

[1] Department of Dermatology, Kurume University School of Medicine, and Kurume University Institute of Cutaneous Cell Biology, Fukuoka, Japan, [2] Department of Dermatology, APHP, Avicenne Hospital, Referral Center for Autoimmune Bullous Diseases, Bobigny, France, [3] Department of Dermatology, Hokkaido University Graduate School of Medicine, Sapporo, Japan, [4] Department of Dermatology, Center for Blistering Diseases, University Medical Center Groningen, University of Groningen, Groningen, Netherlands, [5] Lübeck Institute of Experimental Dermatology, University of Lübeck, Lübeck, Germany

***Correspondence:**
Ralf J. Ludwig
ralf.ludwig@uksh.de

Epidermolysis bullosa acquisita (EBA) is an orphan autoimmune disease. Patients with EBA suffer from chronic inflammation as well as blistering and scarring of the skin and mucous membranes. Current treatment options rely on non-specific immunosuppression, which in many cases, does not lead to a remission of treatment. Hence, novel treatment options are urgently needed for the care of EBA patients. During the past decade, decisive clinical observations, and frequent use of pre-clinical model systems have tremendously increased our understanding of EBA pathogenesis. Herein, we review all of the aspects of EBA, starting with a detailed description of epidemiology, clinical presentation, diagnosis, and current treatment options. Of note, pattern analysis via direct immunofluorescence microscopy of a perilesional skin lesion and novel serological test systems have significantly facilitated diagnosis of the disease. Next, a state-of the art review of the current understanding of EBA pathogenesis, emerging treatments and future perspectives is provided. Based on pre-clinical model systems, cytokines and kinases are among the most promising therapeutic targets, whereas high doses of IgG (IVIG) and the anti-CD20 antibody rituximab are among the most promising "established" EBA therapeutics. We also aim to raise awareness of EBA, as well as initiate basic and clinical research in this field, to further improve the already improved but still unsatisfactory conditions for those diagnosed with this condition.

Keywords: epidermolysis bullosa acquisita, animal models, diagnosis, treatment, pathogenesis

EPIDEMIOLOGY

The incidence of most autoimmune blistering diseases is increasing. Although the incidence of epidermolysis bullosa acquisita (EBA) is not known in detail, it is estimated to be rare. The most common autoimmune subepidermal blistering disease, bullous pemphigoid (BP), is reported to have an annual estimated incidence between 2.4 and 21.7 per million (1, 2). By contrast, the estimated incidence of EBA is reported to be <0.5 per million (3–7). In South Korea, the incidence and prevalence of EBA is estimated to be higher than that of previous reports (8), but the exact epidemiologic data have not been surveyed. In Germany, the EBA prevalence has recently been determined to be 2.8 cases per million (9). This ethnical difference may be due to the reported association of EBA with the human leukocyte antigen (HLA) class II (10–12). EBA occurs at any age; the onset age in previous case reports exhibit a wide range from 1 to 94 years old (13–15). Two onset age peaks are reported; the second and seventh decades (9).

CLINICAL PRESENTATION

Several clinical EBA manifestations have been described: (i) the classical/mechano-bullous form and (ii) the non-classical/non-mechano-bullous forms (16). The latter includes BP-like EBA that meets the clinical criteria of both EBA and BP, mucous membrane (MM)-EBA that is clinically defined by predominant mucous membrane lesions, IgA-EBA that is defined by the IgA class of immune deposits, and Brunsting-Perry-like EBA (**Figure 1**). Few patients may have a MM-IgA-EBA. The relative frequencies of these different clinical forms of EBA reported in the few series in the literature (17–21) depend on the morphological and/or serological diagnostic means available to the authors (**Table 1**). The two most common presentations of EBA are the classical/mechano-bullous and the BP-like forms.

It should be recognized that in an individual EBA patient, clinical presentation may change over time. Notably, patients may switch from a BP-like form to a classical/mechanobullous form or when mucous membrane lesions appear secondarily from a BP-like form to a MM-EBA (22).

Regardless of the clinical form, patients present with cutaneous-mucous fragility, which is easily suspected when the lesions are on trauma-prone areas. Bullous lesions or erosions that are linear or with angular contours can also provide evidence of this fragility (**Figure 2**). Questioning the patient can confirm that bullous lesions appear immediately or a few hours after a trauma which can be minimal. This fragility can be quantified by applying an analogical visual scale. Because in EBA the subepidermal cleavage is deep on the dermal side of the basement membrane zone (BMZ), the cutaneous blisters can persist for a long time, collapsing and becoming flaccid before their rupture; they can also be haemorrhagic.

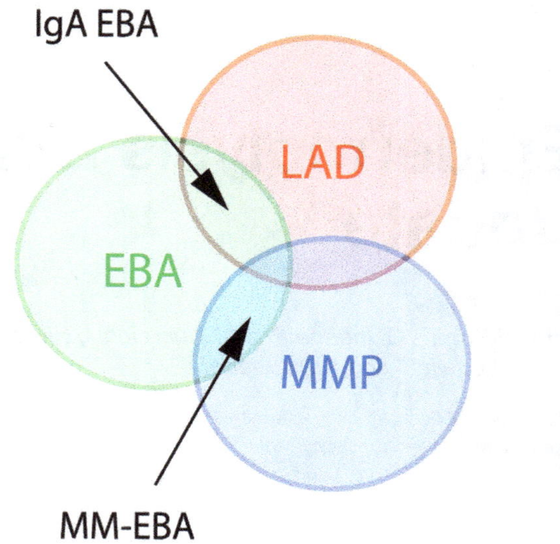

FIGURE 1 | Diagram of different clinical forms of EBA. LAD, linear IgA disease. MMP, mucous membrane pemphigoid; EBA, epidermolysis bullosa acquisita; MM-EBA, mucous membrane EBA.

CLASSICAL/MECHANO-BULLOUS EBA

Two cases of an adult-onset, acquired blistering disease resembling patients with hereditary dystrophic epidermolysis bullosa were reported by Elliott (23). Other similar cases were described in early decades of the twentieth century (24, 25). The first to actually coin the term "epidermolysis bullosa acquisita" was probably Hundley and Smith (26). A landmark paper by Roenigk and colleagues was published in 1971, who described three new cases of EBA, reviewed the world literature and proposed the first diagnostic criteria for classical/mechano-bullous EBA (27).

The criteria of Roenigk were modified once immunological tests for EBA diagnosis had been developed. Advanced clinical criteria of the classical/mechanobullous form have been published in 2017 (16). Current clinical diagnostic criteria for the classical/mechanobullous form are skin fragility, blisters, or erosions on non-inflamed or scarred skin, scarring and milium formation, preferably located at trauma-prone sites and the extensor skin surface (dorsal hands, elbows, knees, Achilles tendon, feet) with possible nail dystrophy and scarring alopecia (**Figure 2**). Fibrosis of the hands and fingers leading to a mitten-like deformity may occur in patients with severe disease reminiscent of hereditary dystrophic epidermolysis bullosa. Mucosal involvement may also occur, but it is not predominant.

BP-LIKE EBA

BP-like form of EBA was first described by Gammon et al. (28). This occurred shortly after the demonstration by Nieboer

Abbreviations: 17-AAG, tanespimycin; 17-DMAG, 17-imethylaminoethylamino-17-demethoxygeldanamycin; ABQOL, autoimmune bullous disease quality of life; AIBD, autoimmune blistering disease; AKT, protein kinase B; APC, antigen-presenting cell; AZA, azathioprine; BLT, leukotriene B4 receptor; BMZ, basement membrane zone; BP, bullous pemphigoid; C, complement factor; CARD9, caspase recruitment domain-containing protein 9; CD, cluster of differentiation; CDNP, cell-derived nanoparticles; COL, collagen; CPA, cyclophosphamide; CR, complete remission; CSA, cyclosporine; CXCR, CXC-chemokin receptor; DDS, diaminodiphenyl sulfone; DEJ, dermal-epidermal junction; DIF, direct immunofluorescence; DMF, dimethylfumarate; EBA, epidermolysis bullosa acquisita; ECP, extracorporeal photochemotherapy; ELISA, enzyme-linked immunosorbent assay; EndoS, endoglycosidase S; ERK, extracellular signal-regulated kinase; FcgR, Fc gamma receptor; FcRn, neonatal Fc receptor; Flii, flightless I; FOAM, fluorescent overlay antigen mapping; G0, agalactosylated antibodies; GM-CSF, granulocyte-macrophage colony-stimulating factor; HLA, human leukocyte antigen; Hsp, heat-shock protein; i.p., intraperitoneal; IA, immunoadsorption; IC, immune complexes; IEM, immunoelectron microscopy; IFN, interferon; Ig, immunoglobulin; IIF, indirect immunofluorescence microscopy; IL, interleukin; IVIG, high-dose intravenous immunoglobulin; JAK2, janus kinase 2; LAD, linear IgA bullous disease; LTB4, leukotriene B4; MHC, major histocompatibility complex; MIP1a, macrophage inflammatory protein1a; MM-EBA, mucous membrane EBA; MMF, mycophenolate mofetil; MMP, mucous membrane pemphigoid; MMPs, matrix metalloproteases; MTX, methotrexate; NADPH, nicotinamide adenine dinucleotide phosphate; NC, non-collagenous; NCF1, neutrophil cytosolic factor 1; NKT, natural killer T cells; p.o., per os; PI3K, phosphatidylinositol-4,5-bisphosphate 3-kinase; PR, partial remission; RORa, retinoid-related orphan receptor-alpha; ROS, reactive oxygen species; RTX, rituximab; SLE, systemic lupus erythematodes; SSS, NaCl-split skin; SYK, Spleen tyrosine kinase; TABQOL, treatment-based autoimmune bullous disease quality of life; Th, T-helper; TNF-α, tumor necrosis factor α; Treg, regulatory T cells; Trem1, triggering receptor expressed on myeloid cells-1.

TABLE 1 | Clinical variants of EBA in the series of the literature.

References	Years of study	n	Classica/ mechano-bullous	Brunsting-Perry like	Bullous pemphigoid like	Mucous membrane EBA	IgA EBA
Briggaman (17)	<1985	12	4 (30%)	0	5 (40%)	1 (8%)	2 (17%)
Kim (18)	1994–2009	30	11 (36.7%)	2 (6.7%)	14 (46.7%)	2 (6.7%)	1 (3.3%)
Buijsrogge (19)	2002–2008	38	13 (34%)	1 (2.6%)	13 (34%)	2 (5.2%)	9 (24%)
Iranzo (20)	1985–2012	12	5 (42%)	1 (8.3%)		4[a] (33%)	
Seta (21)	1983–2013	77	42 (56%)	1 (1.2%)	21[b] (27%)	11[c] (14%)	2 (2.4%)

[a]2 patients had the mixed form, [b]1 had a prurigo-like form, [c]11 had mucous membrane-EBA, including 2 with isolated IgA deposits.

et al. (29) and Yaoita et al. (30) that EBA autoantibodies are deposited in the anchor fibrils zone, which allowed for a definite diagnosis by immunoelectron microscopy (IEM), even though the clinic was (based on the criteria by Roenigk) atypical. Indeed, patients with a BP-like form of EBA have generally profuse skin lesions suggestive of a BP in some areas and an EBA in others (17, 31, 32). The patients have pruritus, tense bullae and erosions on inflamed erythematous or urticarial skin as well as trauma-induced bullous lesions surrounded by normal skin (**Figure 2**). The lesions are on the trunk and folds but also on limb extensor areas and distal extremities. The face can be affected. Mucosal involvement is also possible, but it is not predominant. Finally, lesions heal most often leaving atrophic scars and milia cysts as in the mechanobullous form.

MM-EBA

The high frequency of mucosal lesions in EBA, in particular tongue and lip involvement, was highlighted by Dahl (33). Currently, MM-EBA cases are defined as EBA that mainly affects mucous membranes with a squamous epithelium (16, 33–35), such as the mucous membrane of the mouth, pharynx, esophagus, epiglottis, conjunctiva, genitalia, anus, and respiratory tract in malpighian metaplasia, especially the trachea and bronchi. Only one of these sites can be involved and remain so for a long time before a second localization appears in the case of inadvertent discontinuation of the treatment, a decrease in dose or no treatment (36). These cases are frequently misdiagnosed.

As on the skin, bullous lesions of mucous membranes rupture late in MM-EBA. Thus, intact blisters are frequently seen on mucous membranes in comparison to mucous membrane pemphigoid (MMP), in which they are rare (**Figure 2**). The erosions on the mucous membranes are similar in MM-EBA and classical MMPs, except in the esophagus where they can be linear, caused by mucous membrane fragility and the passage of the fibroscope (37). The cicatricial lesions (atrophic scars, synechiae, and stenosis) are identical in MM-EBA and MMP. The cicatricial lesions have mild consequences in the mouth, genitals and anus, but cause severe impairment in the esophagus, larynx, trachea, bronchi, and conjunctiva, which dictate more aggressive treatment and multidisciplinary management.

Esophageal stenosis, usually as a web located at the upper esophagus, causes the most severe damage to the esophagus. Esophageal stenosis causes dysphagia, weight loss and, at worst, malnutrition and/or false routes and pulmonary infection (34, 36–50).

Severe lesions at the nose and throat are perforation of the nasal septum and/or stenosis of nostrils, choanal, pharynx, and larynx (39, 51–53). Involvement of the trachea and bronchi may also rarely occur (51, 54). Scarring of the larynx or trachea are potentially life-threatening because this may lead to asphyxiation if tracheostomy is not performed. In general, mucous membrane lesions in EBA patients are, however, asymptomatic in 30% of cases (51).

Few case reports and small series of ocular involvement in EBA have been reported (13, 33, 34, 55–64). Patients presented the involvement of at least two other sites. Interestingly, in MM-EBA, immune deposits of IgA are present in half of the cases and the only Ig class in a third. Patients displayed a fibrosing conjunctivitis that might worsen and eventually cause blindness.

The frequency of esophageal, nasal and throat, and conjunctival involvement was, respectively, 6, 11, and 25% of 39 EBA cases in a French series (65). Bladder involvement has also been reported in one case (66).

In addition to MM-EBA, the involvement of mucous membranes in "skin-predominant" EBA is common (34). Hence, after the diagnosis of EBA, an interdisciplinary approach is needed for both diagnosis and treatment.

IGA-EBA

Currently, IgA-EBA is defined as an EBA that presents with linear IgA deposits at the BMZ. IgA-EBA may resemble linear IgA bullous disease with erythematous cutaneous arciform lesions and a few scars and milium cysts, in particular in children. However, it IgA-EBA may also develop into a more severe clinical manifestation, especially with scarring at mucosal

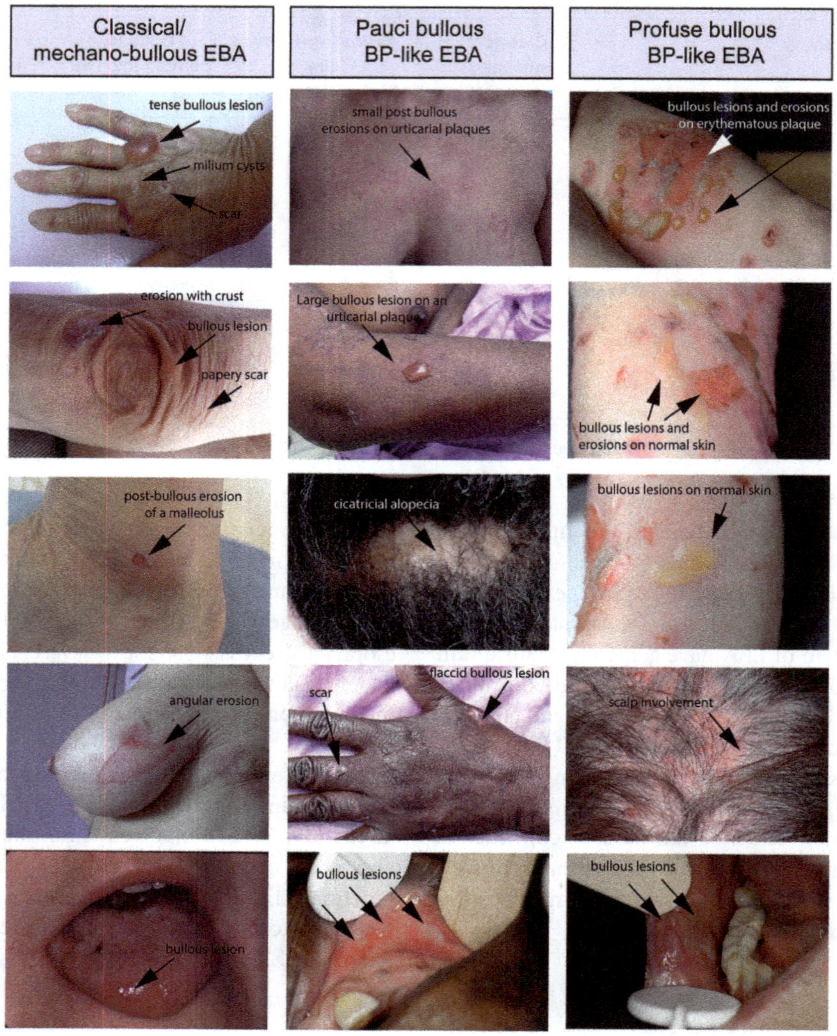

FIGURE 2 | Different clinical forms of EBA. All patients were documented at the first visit in a center for auto-immune bullous disease. **(Left)** Patient with a classical/mechanobullous form of EBA: lesions are preferably localized to the extensor skin surfaces and trauma-prone sites, i.e., dorsal hands knees elbows and ankles. Tense or flaccid bullous lesions are surrounded by non-inflamed skin; erosions are covered or not by crusts; one erosion with angular contours had been induced by adhesive plaster; old lesions have healed with milium formation and/or are atrophic papery scar. **(Middle)** Patient with a BP-like form of EBA, with little blistering: urticarial plaques with small or large bullous lesions as in BP, but location of lesions on extensor areas of limbs, hands and scalp, and scars and extensor areas of the face (not shown) and limbs (atypical for BP). **(Right)** Patient with a BP-like form of EBA, with extensive blistering: bullous lesions and erosions on erythematous skin in flexural areas of limbs (tight and arm) as in BP but also bullous lesions and erosions on normal skin and involvement of extensor area of the limbs and scalp, atypical for a BP involvement of the scalp (not shown) and both flexural and extensor areas of limbs extremities with bullous lesions and erosions on erythematous but also normal skin. The tongue and the lips are the most frequent sites of mucosal lesions in all EBA variants. Other mucosal lesions (not shown) are possible regardless of the variant of EBA The involvement of nasal and buccal mucous membrane are visible in all EBA variants.

sites, as reported in 30% of the 82 cases in the Vodegel literature review, including 4% with severe ocular involvement (16, 19, 67, 68).

BRUNSTING-PERRY TYPE EBA

Patients with Brunsting-Perry type EBA present only cutaneous lesions, without erythematous or urticarial plaques, which predominate in the head and neck and heal leaving very atrophic scars. Review of seven of the eight cases reported in the literature has recently been published by Asfour et al. (69–76).

NON-INFLAMMATORY VS. INFLAMMATORY FORMS OF EBA

The definition of inflammatory and non-inflammatory forms of EBA varies with the authors in the literature (17–21): (i) for most of them but one, the non-inflammatory form of EBA overlays the classical/non-mechano-bullous form; (ii) Buijsrogge et al. included the Brunsting-Perry like type in the mechano-bullous phenotype (19); (iii) for Briggaman et al. (17) who were the first to describe the inflammatory form of EBA, and for Kim et al. (18), the inflammatory form of EBA is synonymous to the BP-like form; (iv) for Buijsrogge et al. (19); and Iranzo et al. (20), all the patients who have not a mechano-bullous phenotype form, have an inflammatory phenotype and (v), for Seta et al. (21), inflammatory lesions are characteristic of the BP-like form of EBA but can also be seen in some patients with MM-EBA or IgA EBA.

The authors of the consensus conference (16) agreed on the following: (i) BP-like EBA are usually inflammatory forms of EBA, (ii) MM-EBA may be inflammatory forms of EBA, (iii) IgA-EBA may be inflammatory forms of EBA, (iv) Brunsting-Perry-like EBA are usually non-inflammatory forms of EBA, and (v) Brunsting-Perry-like EBA are not classical/mechano-bullous forms of EBA.

QUALITY OF LIFE IN EBA AND ASSOCIATED DISORDERS

In general, EBA has a significant impact on the quality of life, which is now to be measured by generalized scores and the "autoimmune bullous disease quality of life" (ABQOL) and "treatment-based autoimmune bullous disease quality of life" (TABQOL) scores created specifically for autoimmune bullous diseases (77, 78).

Many systemic diseases have been reported to be associated with EBA, such as amyloidosis, thyroiditis, multiple endocrinopathy syndrome, rheumatoid arthritis, pulmonary fibrosis, chronic lymphocytic leukemia, thymoma, and diabetes [review in Gupta et al. (22)]. Most of these reports are, however, anecdotal. The only unarguable association of EBA with other diseases is with chronic inflammatory bowel diseases, in particular Crohn's disease, which has been reported to be present in 25% of EBA patients (65, 79). In B-cell lymphomas, presence of circulating and tissue-bound auto-antibodies to type VII collagen (COL7) has also been described in association with a frequency of 6% in 100 EBA cases, but the patients did not have clinical features suggestive of EBA (80). Furthermore, EBA associated with systemic lupus erythematosus, but not fulfilling the criteria of bullous erythematosus systemic lupus, are described (81, 82).

DIAGNOSIS

If clinically suspected, the minimal diagnostic criteria for EBA diagnosis are the detection of linear immunoglobulin- or C3- deposits along the dermal-epidermal junction in a perilesional skin biopsy with detection of a u-serrated pattern of Ig-binding.

Routine histopathology from a lesional skin (or mucous membrane) biopsy does not allow to distinguish EBA from other subepidermal AIBD. It shows: (i) initially, papillary oedema and vacuolar alteration along the dermo-epidermal junction and at a later stage, a subepidermal or subepithelial cleavage, (ii) a great variability in the magnitude and/or quality of the inflammatory infiltrate, (iii) milia cysts and fibrosis in older lesions (**Figure 3**).

Definite diagnosis can be performed by either of the following methods: (i) serration pattern analysis of linear immunoglobulin deposits in the perilesional skin biopsy, (ii) fluorescent overlay antigen mapping (FOAM), (iii) immunoelectron microscopy, and/or (iv) detection of circulating antibodies against COL7.

If possible and needed, more than one of the above may be used to diagnose or exclude EBA. In addition, serology, i.e., detection of circulating anti-COL7 antibodies, should be performed, and, if positive, can serve as a biomarker of disease severity (83).

Diagnosis of EBA can be made by indirect immunofluorescence microscopy (IIF) using 1 M NaCl-split skin (SSS) as a substrate (84). Here, binding of antibodies to the dermal site (floor) of the blister is observed. By immunoblot analysis, binding to the 290-kDa antigen by the patient IgG is detected. The newly developed COL7 ELISA has a sensitivity of 45%. Combining SSS and ELISA reaches a sensitivity of 50%. Thus, half of the patients with EBA are sero-negative (85), and thus a negative serological finding does not exclude EBA as a differential diagnosis.

In serological negative cases, direct immunofluorescence (DIF) on sodium chloride-separated skin biopsy might reveal the diagnosis. Specifically, the diagnosis can be made using DIF serration pattern analysis, which shows distinct, EBA-specific, linear u-serrated immune-depositions at the BMZ (86). DIF serration pattern analysis by n-vs.-u may consider require expertise, which can be studied online: "n-vs.-u UMCG" (https://www.umcg.nl/NL/UMCG/Afdelingen/dermatologie/Wetenschappelijk_Onderzoek/NversusU/Paginas/default.aspx.

Direct Immunodetection of Perilesional Skin Biopsies

All pemphigoid diseases are characterized by a linear deposition of immunoglobulins and/or complement along the epidermal basement membrane zone (**Figure 4A**). These antibodies are directed against various hemidesmosomal proteins: (i) type XVII collagen (BP180) in BP, MMP, pemphigoid gestationis, lichen planus pemphigoides, and LAD, (ii) BP230 in BP, (iii) laminin-332 in anti-laminin-332 pemphigoid, (iv) integrin β4 in ocular MMP, and (v) p200 in anti-p200 pemphigoid. Moreover, in EBA and bullous systemic lupus erythematosus (SLE), antibodies against COL7, present in the sublamina densa, also give rise to a linear deposition pattern (87).

If in suspected pemphigoid disease, a linear Ig- and/or C3- deposition is observed, it is important to determine the targeted autoantigen. In most variants of BP and in EBA, the deposits consist of IgG and complement. Mixed IgG/IgA depositions are usually encountered, especially in mucosal dominant pemphigoid. In some patients, IgA is the only present Ig-subtype, leading to a diagnosis of LAD or IgA EBA (67, 88, 89). However, in mucosal dominant pemphigoid with mixed IgA/IgG depositions, the IgG component may be faint, which sometimes result in a misdiagnosis of LAD. In very few patients, linear IgM deposition may be present in addition to IgG and C3. Even less cases have been described with linear IgM deposition only (90, 91).

Bullous SLE is characterized by antibodies against COL7 in patients fulfilling the diagnostic criteria for SLE. In bullous SLE, in addition to, or superimposed on a linear IgG deposition,

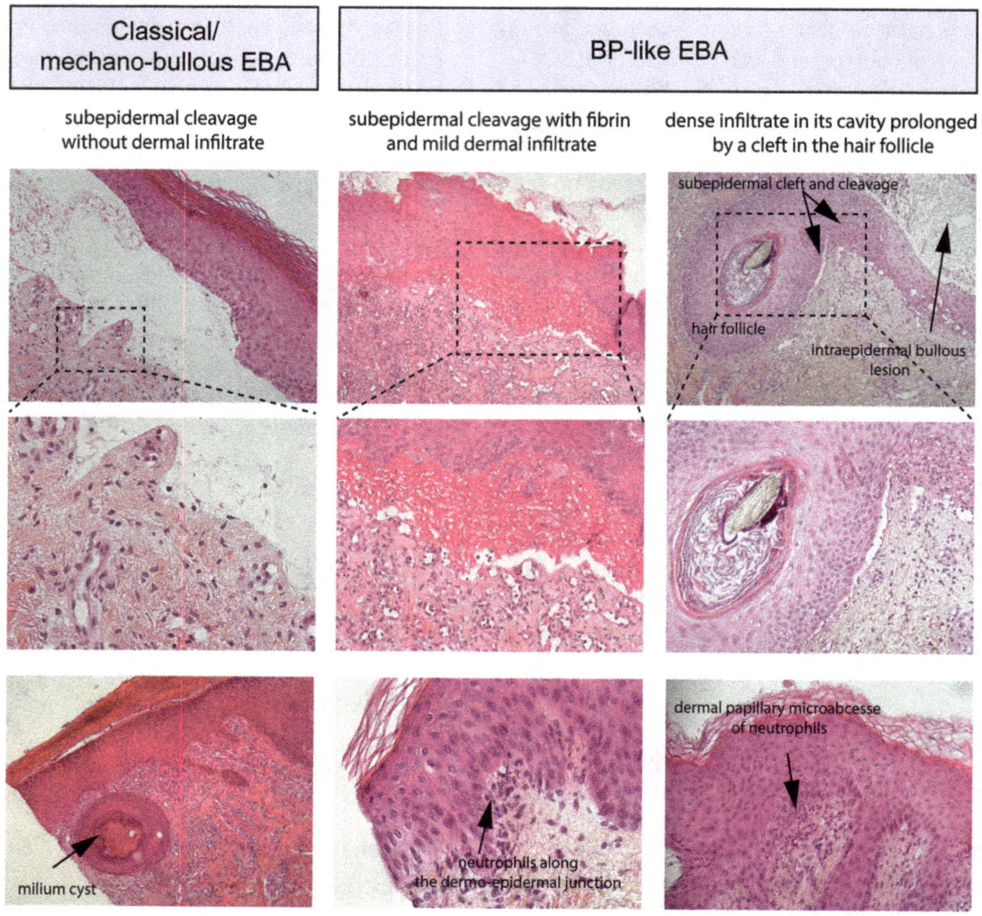

FIGURE 3 | Standard histology. **(Left)** Histological study of lesional skin biopsies in a patient with a classical/mechanobullous form of EBA, subepidermal cleavage without dermal infiltrate; bottom, milium cyst in the dermis. **(Middle)** Patient with a BP-like form of EBA, subepidermal cleavage with fibrin in the blister cavity and mild dermal infiltrate. Bottom, Neutrophils along the dermo-epidermal junction **(Right)** Patient with a BP-like form of EBA, one intraepidermal bullous lesion and one subepidermal bullous lesion with dense infiltrate in its cavity prolonged by a cleft in the hair follicle; bottom, a dermal papillary microabcesse of neutrophils.

a biopsy might show a lupus band, which is characterized by granular deposition of immunoglobulins and complement, in coincidence with epidermal anti-nuclear antibodies.

In most pemphigoid patients, a linear-serrated pattern can be discerned in direct IF microscopy of a peri-lesional skin biopsy. This serration pattern can be divided into an n-serrated and a u-serrated pattern (**Figure 4A**). The identification of these particular patterns allows to differentiate between (i) sublamina densa binding diseases caused by autoantibodies against COL7, e.g., EBA and bullous SLE and (ii) blistering diseases with binding above the lamina densa with antibodies against hemidesmosomal components, e.g., BP, pemphigoid gestationis, MMP, anti-p200 pemphigoid, and anti-laminin 332 pemphigoid. The u- and n-serrated patterns form based on the molecular architecture of the dermal-epidermal junction (DEJ): Specifically, if autoantibodies against COL7 are present, the immunodeposits are located between the rootlets of the basal keratinocytes, leading to the EBA-associated u-serrated pattern (**Figure 4A**). If, however, immune-depositions are located above the lamina densa, they trail the plasma membrane in the basal cell rootlets, resulting in the n-serrated pattern (**Figure 4A**). If it is not possible to determine the serration pattern, which occurs in few cases, it is recommended wise to cut thinner sections or obtain an additional peri-lesional skin biopsy.

However, if diagnosis of EBA cannot be established based on the serration pattern, the level of antibody deposition can be determined by fluorescent overlay antigen mapping (FOAM), which is based on the visualization of a targeted antigen relative to a known topographic marker. For instance, in **Figure 4B**, red staining is used for BP180 as a topographic reference, whereas green staining corresponds to IgA deposits. In the case of IgA-EBA, separate patterns of IgA deposits (green) and BP180 (red) can be seen with red staining on the dermal side (89). FOAM can be performed using a standard immunofluorescence microscope. However, confocal microscopy usually yields better results.

Direct immunoelectron microscopy provides a more detailed location of the deposition site, i.e., the lamina densa and/or sublamina densa at the DEJ (29). This location is distinct from that in other AIBDs (29, 30, 92).

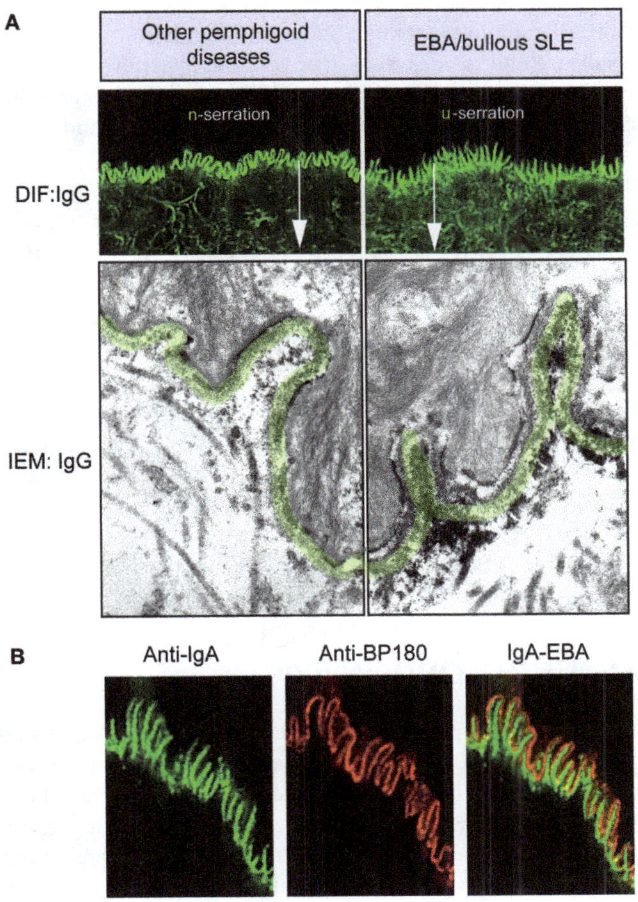

FIGURE 4 | Diagnosis of EBA by direct immunofluorescence. **(A)** All pemphigoid variants are characterized by linear deposition of immunoglobulins and/or complement along the epidermal basement membrane zone. Serration pattern can be separated in an n-serrated pattern (blistering diseases with binding above the lamina densa with antibodies against hemidesmosomal components, e.g., BP, pemphigoid gestationis, mucous membrane pemphigoid, anti-p200 pemphigoid, and anti-laminin 332 pemphigoid, exept MM-EBA) and a u-serrated pattern (sublamina densa binding diseases caused by autoantibodies against COL7, e.g., EBA and bullous SLE). **(B)** In some cases, it is not possible to determine the serration pattern, especially in mucosal biopsies. In these cases, the level of the deposition of antibodies can be determined by fluorescent overlay antigen mapping (FOAM). FOAM is a technique that is based on the possibility of visualizing a targeted antigen relative to a topographic marker. For instance, using red staining, it is used for BP180 as a topographic reference marker, and green staining is used for IgA deposits. In the case of IgA-EBA, separate patterns of IgA deposits (green) and BP180 (red) can be observed with red staining on the dermal side.

Indirect Immunofluorescence on Salt-Split Skin

Diagnosis of EBA can be made by indirect immunofluorescence (IIF) using 1 M NaCl-split skin (SSS) as a substrate. Here, antibody binding of to the dermal site (floor) of the blister is observed. By immunoblot analysis binding to the 290-kDa antigen of patient immunoglobulin is detected (84). Using SSS as a substrate, IIF shows IgG binding on the dermal side of the split. IgG binding can therefore be easily distinguished from BP and, in some cases, MMP, in which the immunoglobulins bind on the epidermal side of the split.

COL7-SPECIFIC SEROLOGICAL ANALYSES BY ELISA

For the serological diagnosis of EBA, three different assays are available: (i) an enzyme-linked immunosorbent assay (ELISA) that uses the non-collagenous (NC)1 and NC2 domains of COL7 (15, 93–95), (ii) an ELISA that is based on the NC1 domain alone (83), and (iii) an indirect IF test employing the NC1 domain (83). If they can be detected, serum levels anti-COL7 IgG correlate with disease activity (96). However, no correlation has been detected between the antibody specificity and the clinical phenotype (97).

THERAPY

First, the treatment of EBA remains challenging because no randomized control trials have been documented due to its rare prevalence (98, 99). Similar to other AIBDs, systemic corticosteroids are widely accepted as a first choice in the treatment of EBA. Initial doses range from 0.5 to 2.0 mg/kg/day (87). With systemic corticosteroids, steroid-sparing agents, including colchicine, diaminodiphenyl sulfone (DDS, dapsone), methotrexate (MTX), azathioprine (AZA), cyclosporine (CSA), mycophenolate mofetil (MMF), and cyclophosphamide (CPA), have been reported in treatment of EBA. Other therapeutic options, including high-dose intravenous Immunoglobulin (IVIG), rituximab (RTX), plasmapheresis and immunoadsorption (IA), and extracorporeal photochemotherapy (ECP) also have been reported (98, 100).

A retrospective analysis included 30 cases from the EBA cohort study regarding treatment and outcome (18). In this cohort study, the median time to remission was 9 months, and complete remission (CR) was observed in 33, 33, and 45% at 1 year, 3 years, and 6 years follow-up, respectively. Relapse sometimes occurs while receiving therapy, while a rate of relapse has not been reported in cohort studies.

Very recently, we collected information that included the treatment of EBA cases who met current diagnostic criteria published between 1971 and 2016 (101). Among all the reported treatments, we found IVIG and RTX to be associated with CR. Based on this retrospective analysis and previous reports in other autoimmune bullous diseases as a reference, each treatment is shortly summarized below.

COLCHICINE

In EBA, colchicine is usually used at 1–2 mg/day. Of note, colchicine monotherapy (2 mg/day) has been reported (20, 102). By some experts, colchicine is considered a first line EBA treatment, especially for mild cases due to the relatively minor side effects compared with other therapeutic choices (103–105). There is currently no controlled study reporting the efficacy of this treatment, and no experimental data are available.

Hence, colchicine is a triable treatment for mild cases, and it should be considered if other immunosuppressant treatments are ineffective.

DIAMINODIPHENYL SULFONE (DDS, KNOWN AS DAPSONE)

Based on expert opinion, DDS is considered a safe and relatively effective first line treatment (18). Although DDS monotherapy (100 mg/day) has been reported with CR in single IgA-EBA cases (67), 25–150 mg/day of DDS is usually used as an adjuvant therapy with systemic corticosteroids. Adverse effects, haemolysis, methemoglobinemia, agranulocytosis, peripheral neuropathy, and psychosis might be observed (106). A rare adverse effect called "dapsone syndrome" should be considered. Some experts recommend that this therapy can be effective (105, 107). Similar to BP (108), DDS appears to have a corticosteroid-sparing effect in EBA.

METHOTREXATE (MTX)

Usually, MTX is used in combination with systemic corticosteroid with/without other immunosuppressants at 20–25 mg weekly. A retrospective review for MTX in the treatment of pemphigus and pemphigoid has reported the use of 5–50 mg weekly of MTX. Adverse effects, including nausea, anemia, and infection sometimes led to the discontinuation of treatment (109). In EBA, no case-series study has focused on the efficacy of MTX. Based on the efficacy in BP (109), MTX may be a viable treatment for EBA as a corticosteroid-sparing agent.

AZATHIOPRINE (AZA)

In EBA, AZA was the most frequently used immunosuppressant as an adjuvant therapy (101). Two types of adverse effects have been reported; non-dose-related adverse effects, including pancreatitis, fever, rash, malaise, nausea, diarrhea, and hepatitis, and dose-related adverse effects, including leucopoenia and some forms of hepatitis (110). Like MTX, no case-series study has focused on the efficacy of AZA in EBA. Based on the efficacy in BP (108), AZA may not be a beneficial treatment for EBA, and further analysis is needed.

CYCLOSPORINE (CSA)

CSA is mainly used as an adjuvant therapy (101). Renal dysfunction, hypertension, headache, tremor, paraesthesia, hypertrichosis, and hyperlipidaemia may be observed as adverse effects, and most persistent renal dysfunction is related to prolonged therapy or doses >5 mg/kg/day (111).

MYCOPHENOLATE MOFETIL (MMF)

In our recent, retrospective analysis (101), 1–3 g/day of MMF was used in combination with systemic corticosteroids. A randomized clinical trial of methylprednisolone plus-AZA vs. -MMF therapy in pemphigus showed a slightly lower frequency of adverse effects, including hypertension, hyperglycaemia, and infection in the MMF-treated group, although it was not a significant difference (112). The results from the randomized control study in pemphigus suggested that 2 g/day offered a better risk–benefit profile than 3 g/day (113). In a case-series study, EBA cases were successfully treated with MMF as a steroid-sparing agent (114). Hence, MMF could be a steroid-sparing agent in EBA.

CYCLOPHOSPHAMIDE (CPA)

There has been no case-series study focused on the efficacy of CPA in EBA, and relativity fewer reports have examined treatment with CPA compared with other immunosuppressants. Therefore, CPA appears to be a therapeutic option when other immunosuppressants cannot control the disease, but limited data is available (101).

HIGH-DOSE INTRAVENOUS IMMUNOGLOBULIN (IVIG)

In our recent, retrospective analysis (101), 31 EBA cases were treated with IVIG, among which 24 cases providing information on the regimen of IVIG and outcome are summarized in **Table 2.** Ahmed et al. reported 10 cases treated with 2 g/kg/cycle (divided into 3 consecutive days) of IVIG in EBA with severe disease and non-responsive to conventional therapies (118). After 16–22 cycles of IVIG therapy, clinical remission was observed from 29 to 123 (mean 53.9) months without any other therapies. The main adverse effect was headache, which increased the intervals of each infusion in two cases, although no severe adverse effects were observed. These two cases are also well summarized in previous reports of IVIG treatment in EBA. In most cases, 2 g/kg/cycle for 3 days or 400 mg/kg/day for 5 sequential days were used with clinical improvement. In experimental mouse studies of EBA and BP, beneficial effects of IVIG have been demonstrated (128–131). Recently, a randomized double-blind trial of IVIG was reported in BP showing a lower disease activity score in the IVIG-treated group compared with placebo (132). Therefore, IVIG is an effective treatment in severe or intractable cases of EBA.

RITUXIMAB (RTX)

Rituximab, a humanized anti-CD20 monoclonal antibody, was used in 10 cases with a protocol of 375 mg/m^2 weekly for 4 weeks (in most cases) and was associated with CR in our recent, retrospective analysis (101), which is summarized in **Table 3.** In pemphigus, another regimen, 1,000 mg every 2 weeks on day 0 and day 14 twice and 500 mg at 12 and 18 months, showed good efficacy in an open-label randomized trial (140). A recent study reported 4 EBA patients treated with 1,000 mg of RTX every 2 weeks twice, similar to the regimen in pemphigus with PR and CR outcomes in each case and no response in 2

TABLE 2 | Reports of IVIG treatment in EBA.

Reported year	Reference	Age	Sex	Phenotype of EBA	Treatments prior to IVIG	Regimen of IVIG	Concomitant-started treatment	Outcome
2013	(115)	37	f	BP-like	Corticosteroid, colchicine, DDS	2 g/kg/cycle		No response
2013	(116)	20	f	BP-like	Corticosteroid, DDS	500 mg/kg/day, 4 days	colchicine (1 mg/day)	CR
2013	(117)	2	m	BP-like	Corticosteroid	400 mg/kg/day, 4 days	DDS (1 mg/kg/day)	PR
2011	(118)	55	f	BP-like	Corticosteroid, AZA	2 g/kg/cycle divided in 3 days		CR
2011	(118)	61	m	Mechanobullous	Corticosteroid, DDS	2 g/kg/cycle divided in 3 days		CR
2011	(118)	37	m	Mechanobullous	Corticosteroid, DDS	2 g/kg/cycle divided in 3 days		CR
2011	(118)	55	f	Mechanobullous	Corticosteroid, DDS	2 g/kg/cycle divided in 3 days		CR
2011	(118)	47	f	Mechanobullous	Corticosteroid	2 g/kg/cycle divided in 3 days		CR
2011	(118)	50	f	Mechanobullous	DDS, MMF, MTX	2 g/kg/cycle divided in 3 days		CR
2011	(118)	73	m	Mechanobullous	Corticosteroid, DDS	2 g/kg/cycle divided in 3 days		CR
2011	(118)	75	f	Mechanobullous	Corticosteroid, DDS	2 g/kg/cycle divided in 3 days		CR
2011	(118)	59	m	BP-like	Colchicine, CSA	2 g/kg/cycle divided in 3 days		CR
2011	(118)	62	f	BP-like	Colchicine, MTX, MFM	2 g/kg/cycle divided in 3 days		CR
2007	(119)	70	m	Unknown	Corticosteroid, AZA, DDS, CSA	2 g/kg/cycles		PR
2007	(120)	65	m	Mechanobullous (+p200 pemphigoid)	Corticosteroid, DDS, CSA, MMF	400 mg/kg/day, 5 days		PR
2007	(121)	58	f	Unknown	Corticosteroid, AZA, MMF, CSA	2 g/kg/cycles		no response
2006	(63)	22	m	Unknown	Corticosteroid, DDS	2 g/kg/cycle divided in 3 days		PR (4 cycles later)
2006	(122)	54	f	Mechanobullous	Corticosteroid, AZA, colchicine,	2 g/kg/cycle divided in 5 days		PR (4 cycles later)
2002	(123)	43	f	Both	None	400 mg/kg/day, 5 days		CR (PR after 1 cycle)
2000	(124)	37	m	BP-like	Corticosteroid	1.2 g/kg/cycle divided in 2–3 days		CR (after 9 months)
1998	(46)	59	m	Mechanobullous	Corticosteroid, DDS, MTX, CSA, CPA, IA	400 mg/kg/day, 5 days		CR
1997	(125)	29	m	BP-like	Corticosteroid, AZA, DDS, PE, colchicine, CSA	40 mg/kg/day, 5 days		CR (after 4 cycles)
1995	(126)	55	m	BP-like	Corticosteroid, AZA, DDS, colchicine	400 mg/kg/day, 5 days		CR (after 9 cycles)
1993	(127)	16	m	Both	Corticosteroid, CSA	400 mg/kg/day, 4 days every 2 weeks		CR

BP, bullous pemphigoid; DDS, diaminodiphenyl sulfone; MTX, methotrexate; AZA, azathioprine; CSA, cyclosporine; MMF, mycophenolate mofetil; CPA, cyclophosphamide; IVIG, high-dose intravenous immunoglobulin; PE, plasma exchange; CR, complete remission; PR, partial remission.

cases (141). In EBA animal models, depletion of B cells at the induction of experimental disease showed that B cells, in addition to developing into plasma cells, serve as important antigen-presenting cells. Specifically, if anti-CD20 treatment was applied at the time of immunization, development of antigen-specific CD4+ T cells was significantly hampered in immunization-induced EBA (142). Hence, RTX seems to be a promising treatment option for EBA. Further controlled clinical studies are

TABLE 3 | Reports of RTX in EBA.

Reported year	Reference	Age	Sex	Phenotype of EBA	Treatments prior to RTX	Regimen of IRTX	Concomitant-started treatment	Outcome
2013	(133)	71	f	Unknown	corticosteroid, DDS	375 mg/m^2, every week, 4 w, 4 cycles	IA	CR (after 18 weeks)
2012	(134)	68	f	Mechanobullous	Corticosteroid, colchicine, MTX, DDS, AZA	375 mg/m^2, every week, 4 w		CR (after 16 weeks)
2010	(43)	50	m	Mechanobullous	Corticosteroid, MMF, colchicine, IVIG, AZA	375 mg/m^2, every week, 4 w		CR (over 4 months)
2010	(135)	71	f	BP-like	Corticosteroid, DDS, colchicine	375 mg/m^2 every week, 4 w, 1 cycle	IA	CR (within 16 weeks)
2009	(136)	54	f	Mechanobullous	Corticosteroid, dapsone, aza, CSA, CPA, IVIG, MMF	375 mg/m^2, every week, 4 w, 3 cycles		PR (CR for skin involvements)
2007	(137)	75	f	BP-like	Corticosteroid, AZA, MMF	375 mg/m^2, every week, 4 w		PR (for 10 months)
2007	(138)	67	m	Mechanobullous	Corticosteroid, AZA, CSA, DDS, MTX, CPA, ECP	375 mg/m^2, every week, 4 w	IA	PR
2007	(138)	42	m	Mechanobullous	Corticosteroid, AZA, CSA, DDS, MTX, CPA, IVIG	375 mg/m^2, every week, 4 w	IA	PR
2007	(121)	58	f	Mechanobullous	Corticosteroid, AZA, MMF, CSA, IVIG	375 mg/m^2, every week, 4 w		PR (after 1 week)
2006	(139)	46	m	BP-like	Corticosteroid, DDS, AZA, IA, colchicine	375 mg/m^2, every week, 4 w		CR (after 11 weeks)

DDS, diaminodiphenyl sulfone; MTX, methotrexate; AZA, azathioprine; CSA, cyclosporine; MMF, mycophenolate mofetil; CPA, cyclophosphamide; IVIG, high-dose intravenous immunoglobulin; RTX, rituximab; PE, plasma exchange; IA, immunoadsorption; ECP, extracorporeal photochemotherapy, CR, complete remission; PR, partial remission.

required to determine which regimen of RTX is most effective in EBA.

PLASMAPHERESIS AND IMMUNOADSORPTION (IA)

Although plasmapheresis has been used for the treatment of pemphigus and pemphigoid, including EBA, it makes the shift to IA because of its advantages compared with plasmapheresis: (i) selective removal of immunoglobulin from the circulation; (ii) no requirement for the substitution of plasma components, such as human albumin or fresh frozen plasma; (iii) two to three times more processing capacity per treatment session than plasmapheresis; and (iv) fewer side-effects, such as infections and allergic reactions (90). Interestingly, there are several reports of combination therapy with IA and RTX in EBA that might provide an effective treatment protocol in EBA (133, 135, 138). Kolesnik et al. (133) and Kubisch et al. (135) reported that each patient was treated with IA for 3 consecutive days followed by IA every week and 375 mg/m^2 of RTX on the day after IA for 4 weeks, leading CR after 18 months and CR within 16 weeks, respectively. Niedermeier et al. (138) reported 2 intractable cases treated with 2 cycles of IA for 4 consecutive days at 4-week intervals followed by RTX (375 mg/m^2, every week for 4 w), leading to PR. Interestingly, antigen-specific immunoadsorption, i.e., where only autoantibodies specific for the respective autoantigen are removed from the circulation, are in pre-clinical development (143, 144).

EXTRACORPOREAL PHOTOCHEMOTHERAPY (ECP)

ECP has been reported in the treatment of Sezary syndrome, mycosis fungoides, and autoimmune bullous diseases (145). There are several reports of the use of ECP in refractory EBA with outcomes of CR and PR in 3 cases, respectively, and no response in 1 case (61, 100, 146, 147). The mode of action of ECP in the treatment of EBA is still unknown, although one report has shown a decrease in circulating antibody detected by immunofluorescence and an increase in suction blister time (100). Despite the low number of published EBA patients, due to the reported success rates, ECP should be considered a therapeutic option in patients with refractory EBA.

OTHERS

Daclizumab, a humanized monoclonal antibody against the a-subunit of the high-affinity interleukin-2 receptor also known as the Tac antigen or CD25, was reported in the treatment of EBA (148), in which only one of 3 cases showed clinical improvement. Sulfasalazine was used in a patient with EBA associated with Crohn's disease, resulting in no improvement of the skin lesion (149). The usefulness of doxycycline has been reported in BP (150). Doxycycline and another tetracycline, minocycline, were found in the literature on EBA cases, although its usefulness remains unclear in EBA treatment (151–153).

PROGNOSIS

EBA is a chronic disease characterized by exacerbations and remissions over the course of months to years. Although data on the prognostic factors in EBA are lacking in the literature, the experts admit that the prognosis of EBA depends on its severity at the time of diagnosis and propose treatment accordingly.

Analogous to BP (154, 155) and MMP (35), an EBA is considered severe if the patient has 10 or more cutaneous bullous lesions and/or 3 or more instances of mucosal sites and/or conjunctival, laryngo-tracheal or esophageal involvement. Otherwise, the EBA is classified as moderate or minimal. The MMP-DAI (disease activity index) score (156) can be used to quantify the extent of the disease, but the cut-offs between the severe, moderate, and minimal forms of EBA have not been established to date.

The goal of the treatment is to obtain control of the disease followed by CR, i.e., the absence of active lesions (erythema, urticaria, bullous lesions, and erosions) without worsening of the cicatricial lesions, which are irreversible.

A CR off treatment of EBA is not possible since a long-term maintenance treatment is recommended. CR under minimal treatment may occur after months to years in mild or moderate forms (unpublished data), but minimal skin fragility without bullous lesions can persist for several months to years. The milium cysts may eventually disappear.

The prognosis has been reserved in severe forms, as evidenced by the publication of numerous case reports in therapeutic failure. Indeed, in some patients, the disease may progress quickly with periods of severe exacerbation and rapid scarring. The cicatricial lesions (synechiae, stenosis, joint contractures) may engage the functional prognosis and be life-threatening. In a retrospective study of 30 patients with EBA, all of whom were initially treated with a combination of methylprednisolone, dapsone, and colchicine (six who did not respond were subsequently treated with other immunosuppressants), 8 of 24 patients (33 percent) achieved complete remission and 5 of 24 (21 percent) achieved partial remission within 1 year (18). The prognosis of these severe forms could improve because of recent publications demonstrating the therapeutic success of intravenous immunoglobulins and rituximab (see above). The overall prognosis and response to treatment may be more favorable in children than in adults (157, 158).

Taken together, these findings underline the need for an early diagnosis, multidisciplinary care by experienced practitioner and prompt implementation of appropriate treatment to improve the prognosis of EBA.

PATHOGENESIS

COL7 as the Autoantigen in EBA

Nearly a century after the first description of EBA, the carboxyl terminus of COL7 was identified as the autoantigen in EBA. Since that time, it has been shown that most patients develop autoantibodies that bind to epitopes located within the NC1 domain of COL7 (159–162), whereas antibody reactivity to either the collagenous domain (163) or the NC2 domain (164) is detected in a very small minority of patients. No correlation was detected between antibody specificity and clinical phenotype (159). In a recent multicentre study with 95 EBA patients, NC1/NC2 ELISA showed a higher sensitivity (97.9%) than NC1 ELISA (89.5%), supporting a considerable number of patients with antibodies against NC2 (95).

Interestingly, the humoral autoimmune response toward COL7 encompasses almost all IgG subclasses. Most commonly, COL7 autoantibodies are IgG, but in ~10% of EBA patients, IgA autoantibodies against COL7 are detected. Few cases of IgE- and IgM-COL7-reactive immunoglobulins have been described (101). The nature and/or cause of this broad immunoglobulin isotype reactivity against COL7 is, however, unknown.

GENETIC AND ENVIRONMENTAL FACTORS CONTRIBUTE TO TOLERANCE LOSS IN EBA

As with most autoimmune diseases, the exact cause of the disease is unknown. With regard to EBA, the data indicate a certain genetic predisposition as well as a contribution of environmental factors to EBA pathogenesis. Due to the small number of EBA cases, it is difficult to study the influence of certain environmental factors or infections. EBA susceptibility is associated with genes in and outside the major histocompatibility complex (MHC) locus. Specifically, an association with the MHC locus (HLA-DR2) has been documented in humans in two independent studies (10, 11). The association with the MHC locus is also supported by animal studies, where an association of susceptibility to immunization-induced EBA is linked to the H2s locus (165). Evidence for the involvement of genes outside the MHC locus arises from one case of coincident EBA in members of a family provided further support for the genetic control of EBA (166). The contribution of genes outside the MHC locus is again underscored by corresponding observations in experimental EBA (165, 167, 168). First, when C57Bl6/J mice are immunized with COL7, they develop autoantibodies but no clinical disease. When mice on the same genetic background lack expression of the inhibitory Fc gamma receptor (FcγR) IIB, they also develop clinically overt blistering (165, 168). Similarly, mice carrying the EBA-associated H2s allele develop severe clinical disease when on the B6 genetic background but only moderate disease when on the C57BL/10 background (165, 169). To pinpoint the mutations associated with EBA susceptibility, mice of an advanced, autoimmune-prone intercross line were immunized with COL7. Herein, one third of the mice developed clinical disease, while the remaining mice remained phenotypically healthy (170, 171) Classical quantitative trait loci mapping identified several genes outside the MHC that were associated with either the onset or severity of clinical disease (170). However, the number of genes is still too large to pinpoint the association with clinical disease to single genes, yet in a nutshell, it provides evidence for a genetic basis of EBA susceptibility.

In addition to genetic factors, animal models of EBA clearly indicated an influence of resident microbial communities in disease pathogenesis (172, 173) (**Figure 5**). By the use of outbred mice in immunization-induced EBA, it could be shown that Firmicutes were the most abundant (54%), followed by

Proteobacteria (21%), Actinobacteria (12%), and Bacteroidetes (6%), which is similar to previous studies in the skin. At the genus level, Staphylococcus (36%), Corynebacterium (9%), and Ralstonia (8%) were most abundant (172). Ellebrecht et al. used the same model to show skin community changes before and after immunization. Among SJL/J mice that were immunized with COL7, only 80% of the mice developed disease, whereas the others remained healthy. Interestingly, the specific antibody concentrations and binding of antibodies to the DEJ were unaffected. By contrast, immunized mice that did not develop clinical phenotypes showed a greater alpha diversity, compared to mice that developed EBA symptoms after immunization (173).

THE AFFERENT PHASE: CD4 T CELL-DEPENDENT PRODUCTION OF AUTO-ANTIBODIES AGAINST COL7

EBA is characterized and causes autoantibodies directed against COL7. Unfortunately, little human data are available for this relevant and complex phase of pathogenesis, which includes the interaction of various immune cells, such as antigen-presenting cells, autoreactive B cells, T cells and neutrophils, and subsequently leads to antibody production. Regarding human data, COL7-specific T cells (isolated from the blood) can be detected EBA patients (174, 175), but most data concerning the interaction of these cell in the afferent phase has been derived from animal models (167).

In the immunization-induced EBA model, T-cell-deficient mice do not develop COL7-specific antibodies and, consequently, clinical disease development, indicating that autoantibody production in this model is T cell-dependent. Furthermore, disease susceptibility could be restored in T cell-deficient SJL/J mice by T cells transfer from COL7-immunized wild-type mice (176). To delineate T-cell subsets involved in the generation of anti-COL7 antibodies in this model of immunization-induced EBA, CD4+ and CD8+ T cells were depleted for 2 weeks, starting at immunization. Depletion of CD4+ T cells led to a delay of both autoantibody production and the clinical disease onset. By contrast, CD8+ T cells depletion at the same time period did not impact production of COL7-specific autoantibodies or clinical disease (142). Therefore, in experimental EBA, CD4+ T are required for induction of autoantibody production. Since only few and specific inbred mouse strains developed clinically overt disease after COL7 immunization, the autoantibody response of clinically healthy vs. diseased mice after immunization was contrasted. Here, complement-fixing antibodies were linked to clinical EBA manifestation (169). Furthermore, by determination of the IgG isotype of the autoantibodies, a Th1 polarization of the immune response was noted. In addition, an increase in the Interferon (IFN)-γ/Interleukin (IL)-4 ratio in the draining lymph nodes of EBA-susceptible mice compared with EBA-resistant strains was observed (169). Regarding the involvement of neutrophils in autoantibody production, GM-CSF-deficient mice generated less COL7-specific autoantibodies, which was paralleled by reduced neutrophil numbers in peripheral lymph nodes, draining the immunized site. The same effect was observed in neutrophil-depleted wild-type mice (177).

To further address which antigen-presenting cells are required the formation of antigen-specific CD4+ T cells, B cells were depleted in mice and subsequently immunized with COL7. In the absence of B cells, the antigen-specific CD4+ T-cell response was completely abolished. Furthermore, depletion of dendritic cells and macrophages had similar effects. Hence, the development of COL7-specific CD4+ T cells requires the presence of APC—specifically B cells, dendritic cells, and macrophages (142) (**Figure 5**). More interestingly, the absence of T_{reg} cells in scurfy mice cells led to blistering via the formation of pathogenic autoantibodies, demonstrating a critical involvement of these cell types in the afferent phase of EBA (178, 179).

In contrast to T cells, autoreactive B cells are almost exclusively found in the peripheral lymph nodes in the immunization-induced EBA mouse model (180, 181), which may be due to missing expression of homing-associated CXCR3 and CXCR4 chemokine receptors. In immunization-induced EBA, COL7-specific plasma cells have a half-life of ~7 weeks. This resembles an intermediate between short- and long-living plasma cells (180). A similar intermediate plasma cell type is most likely also present in patients because autoantibody titers in patients with autoimmune bullous diseases slowly decline over a period of 8–12 weeks after B cell-depleting rituximab treatment (182).

An important molecular requirement for autoantibody production in experimental EBA is heat-shock protein 90 (Hsp90). Specifically, pharmacological HSP90 inhibition suppressed autoantibody production in immunization-induced EBA. In the same model, HSP90 blockade impaired the onset of clinical disease manifestation when injected prior to immunization with COL7. Furthermore, clinical disease progression was ameliorated when the compounds were applied in therapeutic experimental settings. Interestingly, B cell development was unaffected by the HSP90 inhibition, while T-cell proliferation was impaired. Overall, this identified T cells as targets of HSP90 inhibition in experimental EBA (174).

CIRCULATION AND PATHOGENICITY OF AUTOANTIBODIES AGAINST COL7

Targeting the Half-Life of Anti-COL7 Autoantibodies

After (auto)-antibodies are present in the circulation, their half-life is controlled by the neonatal Fc receptor (FcRn). FcRn is constructed as a heterodimer, consisting of an alpha-chain and a beta-2-microglobulin light chain (183). Among other functions, FcRn protects IgG from catabolism (184). Inhibition of the FcRn leads to the enhanced clearance of IgG, including autoantibodies. In antibody transfer-induced animal models of EBA (167), disease induction in mice is completely blocked (128, 185). However, this protection can be overridden by the transfer of large amounts of antibodies (185). Similarly, treatment of experimental EBA or other pemphigoid diseases with high doses of IgG (IVIG), which by saturation also inhibits the FcRn, reduces circulating autoantibody titers and leads to disease improvement

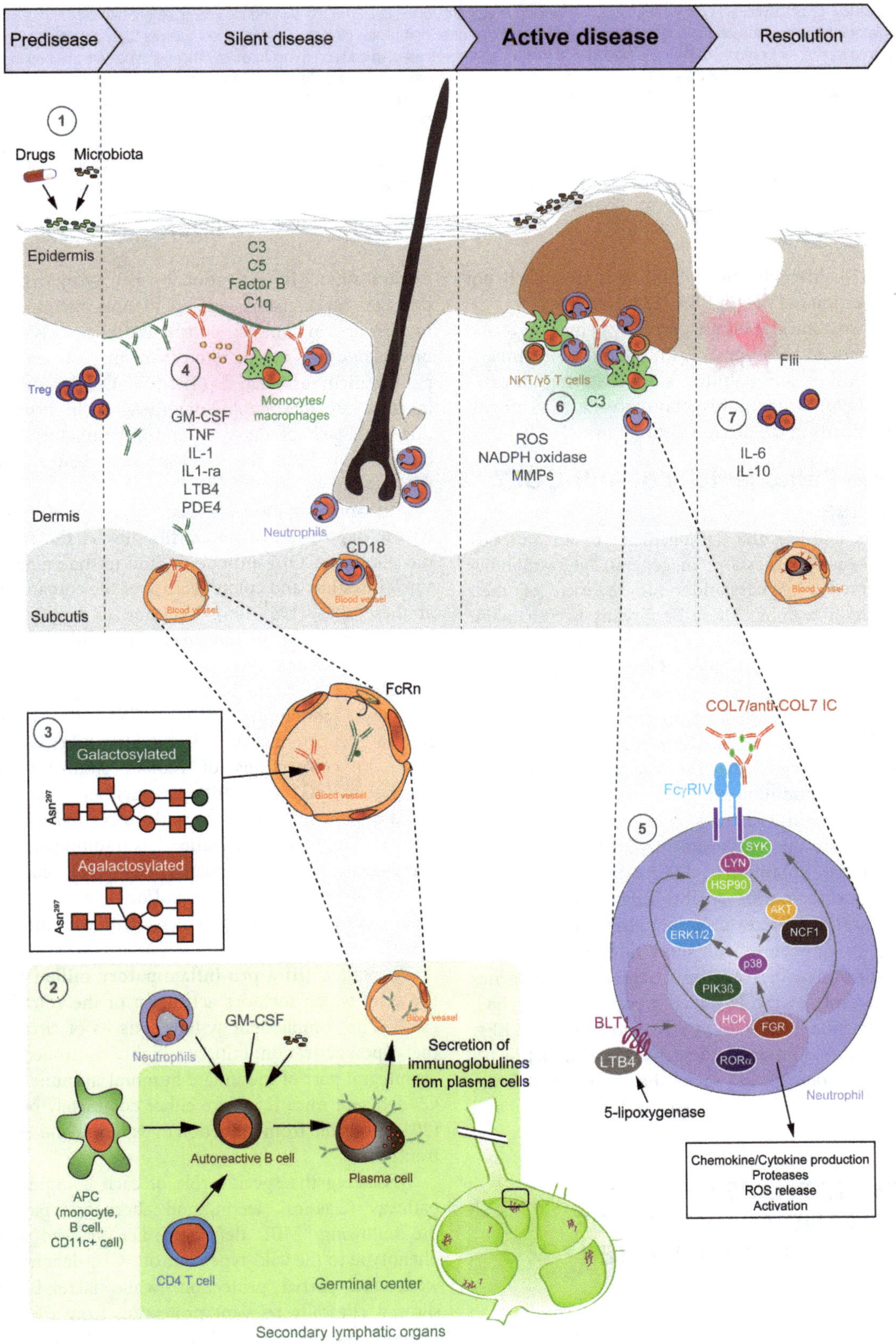

FIGURE 5 | Pathogenesis of EBA. (1) Genetic factors and the skin microbiome promote a tolerance loss. (2) This phenomenon is mediated by the interaction of APCs with autoreactive B and T cells, leading to clonal expansion and differentiation into plasma cells. Autoantibodies against COL7 are released into the blood circulation and effector organs. (3) During inflammation, galactosylation of antibodies may differ. High galactosylation of IgG is crucial for these anti-inflammatory properties,

(Continued)

FIGURE 5 | whereas low galactosylation is pro-inflammatory. (4) Binding of autoantibodies to DEJ in the skin induces complement deposition, pro-inflammatory cytokine and mediator release and subsequently leukocyte extravasation. (5) Immune complexes bind in a Fc-dependent manner to neutrophils and induce a signaling cascade leading to activation, including the (6) release of ROS and matrix metalloproteases. In addition to neutrophils, other cell types are involved in split formation, as shown for monocytes/macrophages, NKT and γδ T cells. By contrast, T_{reg} cells have an inhibitory effect on EBA progression. (7) Resolution of autoantibody-induced tissue injury. T_{reg}, regulatory T cell; NKT, natural killer cell; C, complement; GM-CSF, granulocyte-macrophage colony-stimulating factor; IL, interleukin; LTB4, leukotriene B4; PDE4, phosphodiesterase 4; ROS, reactive oxygen species; NADPH, nicotinamide adenine dinucleotide phosphate; MMPs, matrix metalloproteinases; APC, antigen-presenting cell; CD, cluster of differentiation; SYK, spleen tyrosine kinase; Lyn, tyrosine-Protein Kinase Lyn; HSP, heat shock protein; AKT, protein kinase B; NCF1, neutrophil cytosolic factor 1; ERK, extracellular signal-regulated kinase; PI3K, phosphatidylinositol-4,5-bisphosphate 3-kinase; HCK, tyrosine-protein kinase HCK; FGR, tyrosine-protein kinase FGR; RORα, retinoid-related orphan receptor-alpha; BLT1, leukotriene B4 receptor 1; LTB4, leukotriene B4.

(128, 129, 186, 187), although FcRn inhibition is most likely not the only mode of action of IVIG in EBA (131, 188, 189).

Interestingly, two clinical trials are currently being conducted to evaluate the safety and efficacy of FcRn inhibitory treatments in patients with other autoimmune skin blistering diseases (NCT03334058) (190). Hence, this may become a treatment option for EBA patients in the not too distant future (167).

Targeting the Pathogenicity of Anti-COL7 Autoantibodies

In addition to its half-life, the pathogenicity of an antibody can also affect disease progression. In general, IgG antibodies have one conserved N-glycosylation site in each of their constant heavy chain regions. These Fc glycans have a major impact on their structure as well as their effector functions. Non-galactosylated (agalactosylated; G0) IgG antibodies have long been thought to have pro-inflammatory effector functions in autoimmune patients with rheumatoid arthritis. In contrast, sialylated IgGs mediate anti-inflammatory effects. Recent evidence also suggests that pro-inflammatory immune responses, including autoimmune reactions, mainly induce antigen-specific G0 IgGs, whereas tolerance leads to the generation of immunosuppressive, galactosylated, and sialylated IgGs. Under normal conditions, differentially glycosylated IgGs clearly mediate their pro- or anti-inflammatory effector functions as immune complexes in an antigen-specific manner (191) (**Figure 5**). In agreement with these findings, the use of EndoS, an endoglycosidase derived from Streptococcus pyogenes that selectively hydrolyses the N-linked glycan of native IgG, impaired split formation at the DEJ in skin cryosections. In EBA mouse models, EndoS abrogated clinical disease induction in mice (192, 193). This observation raises the possibility that the glycosylation status of IgG can also affect the onset, severity and progression of disease.

THE EFFERENT PHASE OF EBA: ATTRACTION AND ACTIVATION OF LEUKOCYTES LEADS TO BLISTER FORMATION

Based on the current understanding of EBA pathogenesis (**Figure 5**), the effector phase of EBA, i.e., autoantibody-induced inflammation and blistering, can be divided into (**i**) autoantibody binding to COL7, (**ii**) complement activation and the formation of a pro-inflammatory milieu, (**iii**) leukocyte extravasation, (**iv**) activation by Fcγ receptors, and (**v**) tissue damage. Mechanisms leading to non-inflammatory blistering in EBA are, in contrast, poorly understood. With the increased understanding of pathomechanisms of epitope-dependent pathogenicity-associated (194), non-inflammatory BP, new insights into mechanobullous EBA can be expected. However, due to a lack of data on non-inflammatory mechanisms of blistering in EBA, the following text relates to inflammatory EBA.

Autoantibody-induced tissue injury in EBA is initiated by **(i) the deposition of autoantibodies at the DEJ**. Apart from the skin anti-COL7 antibodies bind to the esophagus, stomach, small intestine, and colon because of the autoantigen expression at these sites (195, 196). Yet, not all isotypes of anti-COL7 have the potential to induce dermal-epidermal separation: *Ex vivo*, only human IgG1 and IgG3, but not IgG2 and IgG4, are capable to cause blistering (197). Furthermore, immune complexes containing IgA1 or IgA2 COL7 autoantibodies activate neutrophils and also induce subepidermal blistering when in cryosections of human skin. Of note, and in contrast to IgG1 autoantibodies, neither IgA1 nor IgA2 leads to complement deposition at the dermal-epidermal junction. Because complement activation has traditionally been thought a prerequisite for blister induction, this may be compensated by so far unknown soluble factors and/or by a stronger activation of neutrophil granulocytes when engaging IgA immune complexes (198).

Thereafter, **(ii) a pro-inflammatory milieu is generated** in the skin, which includes activation of the complement system (199). The complement system consists of circulating proteins that, upon activation, initiate a highly controlled cascade that is an integral part of the innate humoral immune response (200). C5-deficient mice (168) are either completely or (168) partially (201) protected from induction of experimental EBA by antibody transfer.

Dissecting the specific role of each complement activation pathway (classical, lectin, and alternative pathway) showed the following: MBL deficient mice showed a similar EBA phenotype to the wild-type controls. C1q-deficient mice showed weak and partial protection, while factor-B-deficient mice showed clinically relevant protection from EBA induction by antibody transfer (199). This identified the alternative pathway of the complement system as a main driver of skin blistering and inflammation in antibody transfer-induced EBA (202). Downstream of C5, C5ar1-deficient mice are significantly protected from experimental EBA, whereas C6-deficient mice developed widespread blistering disease, excluding the membrane attack complex as a pharmacological target for EBA. In line, pharmacological blockade of C5, factor B, or C5aR1 led to a significant improvement of the blistering phenotype in antibody transfer-induced EBA (202, 203).

In addition to the complement system, the lipid mediator leukotriene B4 (LTB4) is a potent granulocyte chemoattractant (204, 205) and activator (206) and is abundant in the blister fluids of bullous pemphigoid patients, but its pathogenic significance for pemphigoid diseases had been unknown until recently. LTB4 is biosynthesized from arachidonic acid through sequential enzymatic conversion by 5-lipoxygenase and LTA4-hydrolase. The 5-lipoxygenase is most abundant in neutrophils, and it is activated upon cell stimulation by, for example, immune complexes or the complement fragment C5a (207). Mice deficient in 5-lipoxygenase, a key enzyme in LTB4 biosynthesis, or BLT1-deficient mice are completely resistant to the induction of experimental EBA by antibody transfer (208). In addition to complement and lipid mediators, several cytokines have been identified to modulate the effector phase of EBA. Cytokines that are differentially regulated in experimental EBA (209) or cytokines associated with those functional data (210) are summarized in **Table 4** (171, 224).

The pro-inflammatory milieu induces the **(iii) attraction of different leukocyte populations** (**Table 5**). Unfortunately, the composition of these cells has not been investigated thus far in EBA patients, but it is known from BP patients that the infiltrate includes cells such as lymphocytes, histiocytes, eosinophils, neutrophils, and mast cells (228, 229). Subsequent mechanistic studies using the antibody transfer-induced model have uncovered neutrophils as the major culprits responsible for blister formation (208). The recruitment of neutrophils into the skin is mediated by CD18- and ICAM-1 (216, 230–232). In addition, CD18 crucially regulates neutrophil adhesion as an indispensable step leading to tissue damage (233).

Concerning the functional role of T cells, it was recently demonstrated that T cells can enhance neutrophil recruitment into the site of inflammation by modulating the expression of the cell surface integrin CD18 on neutrophils. Interestingly, this effect was neither mediated by CD4 nor CD8 cells, but rather γδT and NKT cells (225). Interestingly, blockade of T_{reg} led to a dramatic worsening of the clinical disease manifestation in antibody transfer-induced EBA (224).

In addition to granulocytes and lymphocytes, macrophages/monocytes may be involved in the blister formation in EBA. However, the blockade of these cells is technically difficult and does not effectively impair disease progression (142). Nevertheless, more studies are needed because macrophages/monocytes are able to produce high amounts of reactive oxygen species (ROS) after immune complex stimulation and induce *ex vivo* split formation in human skin sections (214). Furthermore, the application of high concentrations of anti-COL7 IgG has been shown to induce mast cell activation, but mast cell deficient mice develop experimental EBA just like wild type animals, indicating that mast cells do not contribute to the immune-mediated tissue injury (234–236). Concerning the role of additional cell types in inflammation, a possible role of plasma cells (227) has been discussed, but further studies are needed to unravel the cellular orchestration responsible for the lesional sites.

After extravasation from the blood into the skin, **(iv) myeloid effector cells bind to the skin-bound immune complexes** in a FcγR-dependent fashion (**Table 6**). In EBA the full IgG molecule of the autoantibodies, but not their corresponding F(ab)2 fragments, are pathogenic. Specifically, only the full anti-COL7 IgG elicits dermal-epidermal separation when, together with PMN, incubated on cryosections of human skin (248). Likewise, and unlike the full IgG, F(ab′)2 fragments of anti-COL7 IgG do not induce clinical EBA manifestation when injected into mice (168). The central role of these Fc-FcγR interactions for mediating skin inflammation and subepidermal blistering in experimental EBA is further supported by the complete protection of mice toward EBA induction when injected with chicken anti-mouse COL7 IgY, which is known not bind to murine complement and Fc receptors (249). In addition, the therapeutic effects observed when blocking these interactions, i.e., using soluble CD32/SM101 (231), highlights the key role of Fc-FcγR interactions in EBA pathogenesis. Furthermore, IgG glycosylation has been shown to have preventive and therapeutic effects in mouse models of chronic inflammatory diseases, including EBA (191). Further studies eluted on the differential contribution of the different FcγR (250). In mice, three different activating FcγR and one inhibitory FcγR are described: FcγRI, FcγRIII, and FcγRIV are activating FcγR, all with specific binding avidities toward IgG. The FcγRIIB is the only inhibitory FcγR (250). Of note, an increased expression of FcγRIV has been demonstrated in the skin of mice with experimental EBA (181). Subsequent functional studies identified the FcγRIV as the key mediator of tissue injury in EBA. By contrast, blockade of FcγRI, FcγRIII, or both receptors in combination had no effect on the induction of experimental EBA by antibody transfer. In FcγRIIB deficient mice enhanced blistering was observed in antibody transfer-induced EBA, as well as BP (181, 251), indicating a protective role of this FcRγ in experimental EBA. In human *ex vivo* models of BP, FcγRIIA, and FcγRIIIB contributed to the autoantibody-induced tissue damage (252). Once the neutrophils are bound to the immune complexes, a multifaceted signaling cascade is initiated (**Table 6**). This involves activation of the retinoid-related orphan receptor (ROR)α (230), heat shock protein (HSP)90 (241), phosphodiesterase 4 (240), phosphatidylinositol-4,5-bisphosphate 3-kinase (PI3K) β and δ (238, 239), p38, AKT, ERK1/2 (244), the spleen tyrosine kinase SYK (171, 245), and src kinases (247), as well as CARD9 (246)—which have been reviewed in detail elsewhere (253). The exact temporal and spatial order of these signaling events is currently unknown. Ultimately, the signaling cascade leads to the activation of myeloid effector cells, specifically release of ROS and proteases, both of which are required for subepidermal blistering in EBA (216, 225).

Recently the contribution of cytokines in EBA pathogenesis has been eluted both on the morphological, as well as the functional level (254). Because biologics targeting cytokines are already in clinical use—although, with few exceptions such

TABLE 4 | Mediators of the EBA effector phase.

Target	Function	References
C5	C5-deficient mice are partially or completely protected from EBA inducing by antibody transfer	(201, 211)
C1q/factor B	Respective knock-out mice are partially protected from EBA inducing by antibody transfer	(203)
IgG glycosylation	Enzymatic removal of terminal IgG N-glycosylation renders anti-COL7 antibodies non-pathogenic in antibody transfer-induced EBA	(192, 193)
Galactosylated IgG	Immune complexes with highly galactosylated immune complexes inhibit pro-inflammatory signaling of the C5aR1 through dectin-1 and Fc gamma receptor IIB, resulting in a protection from antibody transfer-induced EBA	(202)
IL-6	In antibody transfer-induced EBA, IL-6 has anti-inflammatory effects, through up-regulation of IL-1ra	(209)
CXCR-1/2	Blockade of the CXCR-1/2 ligands impairs induction of EBA by antibody transfer and slows disease progression when applied in therapeutic settings in immunization-induced EBA	(212)
GM-CSF	Blockade of GM-CSF impairs induction of EBA by antibody transfer and slows disease progression when applied in therapeutic settings in immunization-induced EBA	(177)
IL-1/IL-1ra	Both anti-IL1β or IL-1ra (anakinra) treatment impair the induction of EBA by antibody transfer. Additionally, anakinra halts disease progression when applied therapeutically in immunization-induced EBA	(213)
TNFa	Blockade of TNF impairs induction of EBA by antibody transfer and halts disease progression when applied in therapeutic settings in immunization-induced EBA	(214)
LTB4	Blockade of either LTB4 biosynthesis or its' receptor completely protects mice from EBA induction by antibody transfer	(208)
IL-17A/E	IL17R-deficient mice are partially protected from EBA inducing by antibody transfer	(215)
NADPH oxidase	Neutrophil cytosolic factor 1-deficient mice, lacking functional NADPH oxidase, -deficient mice are completely protected from EBA inducing by antibody transfer	(216)
Elastase	Elastase is required for the induction of subepidermal blisters *ex vivo*	(217)
Flii	Blockade of Flii protects mice from EBA induction by antibody transfer	(218–220)
MIP1α	Increased expression, but no effect on clinical phenotype	(221)
S100	Increased expression, but no effect on clinical phenotype	(222)
Trem1	Increased expression, but no effect on clinical phenotype	(223)

C, complement factor; IgG, immunoglobulin G; IL, interleukin; COL7, type VII collagen; CXCR, CXC-chemokin receptor; GM-CSF, granulocyte-macrophage colony-stimulating factor; TNF, tumor necrosis factor; LTB, leukotriene; NADPH, nicotinamide adenine dinucleotide phosphate; Flii, flightless I; MIP1α, macrophage inflammatory protein1α; Trem1, Triggering receptor expressed on myeloid cells-1.

TABLE 5 | Cell lineage in the effector phase.

Cell type	Function	References
Neutrophils	Neutrophil depletion partially protects from EBA induction by antibody transfer	(208, 216)
NKT/γδ T cells	Depletion of NK or γδ T cells partially protects from EBA induction by antibody transfer	(225)
T_{regs}	Depletion of T_{regs} worsens the clinical disease manifestation in antibody transfer-induced EBA	(224)
Keratinocytes	Upon binding of COL7 antibodies, pro-inflammatory mediators are released from keratinocytes	(209, 226)
IL-10$^+$ B lineage cells	IL-10, derived from IL-10+ B cells impairs neutrophil functions and impairs clinical disease manifestation in immunization-induced EBA	(227)
Monocytes/macrophages	Monocytes/macrophages induce subpeidermal splits *ex vivo*, and depletion of all myeloid cells completely protects from EBA induction by passive antibody transfer, while selective depletion of neutrophils confers partial protection	(214, 216)

NKT, natural killer T cells; T_{regs}, regulatory T cells; IL, interleukin.

as rituximab and omalizumab, for other indications (255)—we here highlight their contribution for EBA pathogenesis. Several cytokines have been shown to contribute to blister formation in experimental EBA (**Table 4**). IL-6 acts as a pro-inflammatory cytokine in various autoimmune diseases (256, 257). Hence, IL-6 has emerged as a potential target for the treatment of autoimmune diseases, and IL-6-targeting therapies are licensed for rheumatoid arthritis and juvenile idiopathic arthritis (256). In EBA patients and in experimental EBA models, serum IL-6 levels are elevated. Unexpectedly, mice lacking IL-6 expression show an increased clinical phenotype in experimental EBA compared with controls. Furthermore, treatment with recombinant IL-6 leads to a dose-dependent reduction of clinical disease manifestation in EBA induced by antibody transfer. Thus, in experimental EBA, IL-6 has a profound anti-inflammatory activity (209). At the molecular level, the protective effect of IL-6 is mediated by the IL-6-dependent release of IL-1ra (213). In line, IL-1R–deficient mice or wild-type mice treated with either the

TABLE 6 | Receptors and signaling in the efferent phase of EBA.

Target	Function	References
FcγRs	Activating FcγR promote skin inflammation in experimental EBA, while the inhibitory FcγRIIB confers protection from induction of EBA by antibody transfer	(181)
FcRn	The FcRn controls the half-live of IgG. This FcRn-deficient mice are partially protected from EBA induction by antibody transfer	(185)
CD18	CD18-deficient mice are completely protected from EBA induced by antibody transfer	(216)
CD11b	CD11b-deficient develop a more severe clinical phenotype in antibody transfer-induced EBA.	(237)
C5aR1	C5aR1-deficient mice are almost completely protected from EBA induced by antibody transfer	(202, 203)
CXCR1/2	Pharmacological CXCR1/2 inhibition prevents disease progression in immunization-induced EBA	(212)
BLT1	BLT41-deficient mice are almost completely protected from EBA induced by antibody transfer	(208)
PI3Kβ	PI3Kβ-deficient mice are partially protected from EBA induction by antibody transfer, through inhibition of neutrophil activation	(238)
PI3Kδ	Pharmacological inhibition of PI3Kδ impairs induction of EBA by antibody transfer and has therapeutic effects in immunization-induced EBA	(239)
Phosphodiesterase 4	Pharmacological inhibition of PDE4 impairs induction of EBA by antibody transfer and has therapeutic effects in immunization-induced EBA	(240)
RORα	RORα-deficient mice are completely protected from EBA induced by antibody transfer	(230)
HSP90	HSP90 is involved in both loss of tolerance to COL7, as well as to antibody-induced tissue damage in experimental EBA	(241, 242)
JAK2	Pharmacological inhibition of JAK2 impairs induction of EBA by antibody transfer and has therapeutic effects in immunization-induced EBA	(243)
AKT, ERK, p38	Pharmacological inhibition of these targets impairs induction of EBA by antibody transfer (ERK, p38) or impairs subepidermal splitting *ex vivo* (all)	(244)
SYK	Pharmacological inhibition of SYK or SYK-deficient mice are completely protected from EBA induction by antibody transfer	(171, 245)
CARD9	CARD9-deficient mice are partially protected from EBA induction by antibody transfer	(246)
Src kinases	Hck, Fgr and Lyn-tripple-deficient mice are partially protected from EBA induction by antibody transfer	(247)
TREM1	See **Table 5**	(223)
Caspase 1	Caspase-1/11-deficient mice develop antibody transfer-induced EBA similarity to wild type littermate controls	(213)

FcγR, Fc gamma receptor; FcRn, neonatal Fc receptor; BLT, leukotriene B4 receptor; CXCR, CXC-chemokin receptor; PI3K, Phosphatidylinositol-4,5-Bisphosphate 3-kinase; RORα, retinoid-related orphan receptor-alpha; HSP90, heat-shock protein 90; JAK2, Janus kinase 2; AKT, protein kinase B; ERK, extracellular signal-regulated kinase; SYK, spleen tyrosine kinase; CARD9, Caspase recruitment domain-containing protein 9; SRC, tyrosine-protein kinase SRC; HCK, tyrosine-protein kinase HCK; LYN, tyrosine-protein kinase LYN; TREM1, Triggering receptor expressed on myeloid cells-1.

IL-1R antagonist Anakinra or a IL-1β function blocking antibody are also partially protected from the EBA-inducing effects of anti-COL7 IgG. Mechanistically, IL-1β increases ICAM-1 expression on endothelial cells, suggesting that IL-1β supports recruitment of inflammatory cells into the skin. Interestingly, these effects of IL-1 were independent of caspase-1 because of caspase-1/11–deficient mice showed a similar phenotype to wild type control animals when injected with anti-COL7 IgG (213).

Additionally, the evaluation of cytokines affecting neutrophil functions, such as IL-8 (CXCL1 and CXCL2 in the mouse) and GM-CSF in experimental EBA, showed an increased expression. To evaluate if the increased expression is of functional relevance these cytokines were inhibited by either antibodies of mice lacking expression of the respective cytokine(s). Treatment with allosteric CXCR1 and 2 inhibitors (DF2156A) impaired the induction of skin blistering in antibody transfer-induced EBA.

In a therapeutic setting, the administration of DF2156A improves the clinical manifestation of EBA after disease onset in immunization-induced EBA (212). For the evaluation of GM-CSF, anti-COL7 IgG was injected into GM-CSF-deficient mice or wild type mice treated with a function-blocking GM-CSF antibody. The induction of experimental EBA was impaired if the function of GM-CSF was blocked in comparison to appropriate controls. *In vitro* studies have demonstrated the requirement of GM-CSF for neutrophil recruitment from bone marrow into the blood and from the blood into the skin. Furthermore, GM-CSF preactivates neutrophils, leading to an enhancement of immune complex-induced neutrophil activation. In a therapeutic setting, the blockade of GM-CSF in mice with already established immunization-induced EBA has demonstrated beneficial therapeutic effects (177, 213). In addition to these cytokines, increased expression of TNF has been observed in experimental EBA, and prophylactic blockade of TNF and therapeutic use of etanercept in the immunization-induced EBA model impair the induction and progression of experimental EBA (214). By contrast, increased expression of CCL3/MIP1α is a mandatory cytokine for disease development (221).

THE RESOLUTION PHASE OF EBA

For most autoimmune bullous diseases, the location of blisters differs over time, indicating a frequent, but unfortunately overall insufficient, healing process in the skin (**Figure 5**). Flightless I (Flii), an actin remodeling protein, has been shown to modulate the resolution of skin blistering in experimental models of EBA. *In vivo*, the induction of EBA leads to increased cutaneous Flii expression, resulting in impaired Claudin-1 and Claudin-4 tight junction protein expression, as well as a delay in the recovery from blistering (218, 258). Overexpression of Flii produces severe blistering post-induction of EBA, while decreased Flii reduces blister severity, elevates integrin expression, and improves COL7 production. In addition, topically applied Flii neutralizing antibodies improve the healing of blistered skin in murine EBA (218–220, 259).

An interesting experiment could show a protective effect of IL-10-positive plasma cells toward the neutrophil-dependent inflammation in EBA. After the start of skin inflammation, plasmacytosis is induced by injection of goat anti-mouse IgD serum and provides protection from skin inflammation and neutrophil infiltration for at least another 3 weeks. Suppression of EBA skin inflammation is abrogated by the co-injection of a neutralizing IL-10 receptor antibody. Despite its anti-inflammatory effect, plasmacytosis neither reduces the numbers of autoreactive COL7-specific plasma cells nor the autoantibodies that trigger the disease (227). These observations point toward a significant contribution of pathways that are involved in the resolution of cutaneous involvement. Therefore, EBA may manifest not only when many pro-inflammatory stimuli are present but also when the balance of pro-inflammatory, anti-inflammatory, and resolving pathways are unbalanced, driving the cells toward pro-inflammatory mechanisms.

CD11b is an integrin family member that pairs with CD18 to form the CR3 heterodimer. CD11b is expressed on the surface of many leukocytes, including monocytes, neutrophils, natural killer cells, granulocytes, and macrophages. Unexpectedly, in the antibody transfer-induced model of EBA, CD11b-deficient mice develop more severe disease symptoms than wild-type mice in the late phase of the disease. Furthermore, compared to wild-type controls, CD11b-deficient mice express increased levels of circulating IFN-γ and IL-4, suggesting an anti-inflammatory role for CD11b in the resolution phase of experimental autoimmune diseases, such as EBA (237).

EMERGING TREATMENTS

The current (unsatisfactory) treatment options for EBA have been outlined above. An increasing understanding of EBA pathogenesis indicates new potential therapeutic targets that interfere in different phases of disease progression, including the generation of autoantibodies, maintaining autoantibodies in the circulation, and autoantibody-induced tissue injury.

Due to the lack of clinical studies, we categorized the emerging treatments into three categories:

TREATMENTS DESCRIBED IN CASE REPORTS

Several case reports are known for the treatment of EBA using ECP (145) and Daclizumab (148). Furthermore, anti-C1s mAb, a mouse monoclonal IgG2a antibody, inhibits the activation of C1s, which is a serine protease of the classical complement system. TNT003 completely blocks complement classical pathway activation by the reduction of C4a and C5a production induced by incubation of the sera from patients with BP on cryosections of human skin (260). The disease induction of experimental EBA is also complement-dependent. This finding suggests that TNT003 might work even in EBA. A "humanized version" of TNT003, TNT009 is currently evaluated in a phase I clinical trial in BP patients (NCT02502903) and data reported on congresses indicates a favorable safety, as well as efficacy in some patients. Sulfasalazine was used in a patient with EBA associated with Crohn's disease, resulting in no improvement of the skin lesion (149). The utility of doxycycline has been reported in BP (150). Doxycycline and another tetracycline, minocycline, have been described in the literature in EBA cases, although their usefulness remains unclear (151–153).

TREATMENTS APPLIED IN THERAPEUTIC SETTINGS IN EXPERIMENTAL EBA

Due to the low incidence, clinical studies with EBA patients are not performed. Therefore, animal models are indispensable for investigating the pathogenesis of EBA and other autoimmune blistering diseases and to test new target substances for treatment; these models include the transfer of autoantibodies to experimental animals, adoptive transfer of autoantibody-producing B cells to immune-deficient mice and construction of transgenic mice that produce autoantibodies (167). Although animal models have many benefits, as described above, both the advantages and disadvantages of each model should be considered. Although the models duplicate the clinical, histopathological, ultrastructural, and immunological features of the human disease, these systems are mostly completely murine, and it is possible that findings in mice will not translate to humans.

The most important mouse model to test treatments applied in therapeutic settings is the immunization-induced EBA model (167, 168). Immunization with parts of the NC1 domain of COL7 with an adjuvant induces anti-COL7 IgG production in mice. The susceptibility of experimental EBA is closely associated with the H2s haplotype in mice (165). During a time period of 4–6 weeks, the mice develop antibodies against mCOL7 that bind to the DEJ and induce neutrophil activation and blistering. Using the immunization-induced EBA model, the pathomechanisms of blistering and potential therapeutic options have been studied, and more importantly, this model is used to test potential new drug candidates and therapeutics (167). Successfully applied drugs are summarized in **Table 7**.

TABLE 7 | Experimental treatments in pre-clinical immunization-induced EBA.

Medication	Target	Impact on disease	Application	References
Methylprednisolone	Multiple	Impair EBA progression	i.p.	(129, 212)
DF2156A	CXCR1/2	Halting EBA progression	p.o.	(212)
IVIG	Multiple	Impair EBA progression	i.p.	(129)
Anti-GM-CSF	GM-CSF	Impair EBA progression	i.p.	(177)
Etanercept	TNFα	Impair EBA progression	i.p.	(214)
EndoS	Fc glycosylation	Halting EBA progression	i.p.	(192)
sCD32/SM101	FcγR	Impair EBA progression	i.p	(231)
Anakinra	IL-1	Improvement	i.p.	(213)
17-DMAG	HSP90	Improvement	i.p.	(174)
17-AAG	HSP90	Impair EBA progression	top	(242)
TCBL-145	HSP90	Improvement	i.p.	(174)
Dimethylfumarate	Multiple	Improvement	p.o.	(261)
goat anti-mouse IgD serum	Induction of IL10 plasma cells	Impair EBA progression	i.p.	(227)
Calcitriol treatment	Vitamin D	Impair EBA progression	p.o.	(262)
LAS191954	PI3Kδ	Improvement	p.o.	(239)
Roflumilast	PDE4	Halting EBA progression	p.o.	(240)

CXCR1/2, CXC-chemokin receptor; GM-CSF; granulocyte-macrophage colony-stimulating factor; TNF, tumor necrosis factor; EndoS, endoglycosidase S; FcγR, Fc gamma receptor; IL, interleukin; 17-DMAG, 17-dimethylaminoethylamino-17-demethoxygeldanamycin; HSP90, heat shock protein 90; 17-AAG, Tanespimycin (17-N-allylamino-17-demethoxygeldanamycin); TCBL-145, D-Tyr-Phe-D-Trp-Leu-AMB (AMB: NH-CH_2-CH_2-$CH(CH_3)_2$); PI3K, phosphoinositide 3-kinase; p.o., per os; i.p., intraperitoneal; top, topical.

TREATMENTS APPLIED IN PREVENTIVE SETTINGS IN EXPERIMENTAL EBA

Beneath the validation of potential drug candidates in the therapeutic setting in immunization-induced EBA, some authors have also investigated several drugs in antibody transfer-induced EBA. In this model, rabbit sera or whole rabbit IgG immunized with COL7 NC1 domain are injected into mice. These mice develop clinical and histological subepidermal blistering within a few days. The antibody transfer models are used to investigate the cellular and molecular basis of blistering and to investigate preventive effects of several therapeutic options. The use of antibody transfer models enables examination of the effector phase of EBA. Testing novel drugs or investigating the pathogenesis of EBA is straightforwardly done because clinical symptoms are visible days after starting the experiment. However, similar to most animal models, the situation in human patients is only partially reflected—mostly, because the signaling cascade and the interaction of different cell types vary among human and mice. Additionally, induced disease may last less than a few days after the transfer of antibodies. Furthermore, the loss of tolerance and the generation of autoantibodies cannot be studied in models based on antibody transfer. Therefore, the investigation of potential drug candidates should always be performed in addition to immunization-induced EBA in a therapeutic setting.

Complement

Complement activation has been described as a prerequisite for blister formation. In the antibody-transfer model, blister induction is completely dependent on complement C5 because C5-deficient mice or mice injected with F(ab)2 fragments of the immune IgGs are devoid of blisters. This finding indicates that the complement system can be targeted in animal models. Targeting therapies for complement system factor B, C5, and C5R ameliorate disease severity in antibody-transfer models (199, 201, 203, 211, 260). Interestingly, in antibody transfer-induced BP, C5ar1$^{(-/-)}$ mice are protected from disease development, whereas the extent of skin lesions is increased in C5ar2$^{(-/-)}$ animals.

SYK

SYK is a non-receptor cytoplasmic enzyme that is mainly expressed in hematopoietic cells. SYK regulates cellular responses to extracellular antigens or antigen-immunoglobulin complexes. In EBA pathogenesis, myeloid SYK is a central player in driving inflammation in prototypical autoantibody-transfer models. The SYK inhibitor (BAY61-3606) protects mice from inflammation in antibody-transfer EBA (171, 245).

Cell-Derived Nanoparticles (CDNPs)

CDNPs are intercellular protein complexes, such as annexin A1, annexin A5, actin, *14-3-3ε*, *14-3-3ζ*, galectin-3, and heat-shock proteins 27 and 70. CDNPs play a therapeutic role against viral infections, cancer and in the experimental EBA model. Mice that receive anti-COL7 IgG develop skin lesions. Treatment with CDNPs significantly reduces the affected skin lesions and increases IL-4 expression (263).

LTB4

LTB4 is a potent chemoattractant and activator of myeloid cells, particularly of neutrophils. The 5-lipoxygenase–deficient and BLT1-deficient mice exhibit neither any clinical nor histological signs of disease in the antibody-transfer model. The 5-lipoxygenase inhibitor (zileuton) targeting the LTB4/BLT1 pathway ameliorates disease severity by ~50% in antibody-transfer models (208).

Flii I

Flii is a member of the gelsolin family of actin remodeling proteins in regulating cell adhesion and intracellular signaling. Flii expression is increased in the epidermis during development and during epidermal stratification to maintain barrier functions, such as tight junctions. Topical application of Flii-neutralizing antibody significantly reduces the clinical severity of blistering and histological separations in antibody-transfer EBA mice. In addition, the barrier function measured by transepidermal water loss (TEWL) is significantly decreased in Flii-neutralizing antibody-treated mice (218, 219).

IL-6 (Protective)

IL-6 is a proinflammatory cytokine and plays a role during the transition from innate to acquired immunity. In the initial immune response to pathogen, IL-6 attracts neutrophils to the affected tissue. In addition, IL-6 plays a crucial role in B- and T-cell differentiation. Elevated IL-6 concentrations are observed in many inflammatory diseases and often correlate with disease activity. IL-6 expression is increased in the skin of EBA patients. Interestingly, the EBA severity is enhanced in IL-6-deficient mice in an experimental model. Furthermore, treatment with recombinant IL-6 dose-dependently impairs the induction of experimental EBA (209).

Galactosylated Immunoglobulins

Antibody-transfer EBA model activation is FcgR-dependent in blister formation. Immune-complexes induce the classical complement pathway via Fc fragment. The mouse IgG1 subclass preferentially binds to inhibitory FcgRIIB and suppresses the inflammatory response. Glycosylation of Asn297 in the IgG Fc fragment plays an important role in complement activation. Highly galactosylated immune-complex treatment reduces the development of cutaneous lesions in an antibody-transfer model (202).

CARD9

Caspase recruitment domain-containing protein 9 (CARD9) is an intracellular adapter protein that is expressed in myeloid-lineage cells. CARD9 plays a critical role in host defense against pathogens in both mice and humans. Card9 deficient mice are significantly protected against skin blistering in antibody-transfer EBA. In this setting, CARD9 is required for development of the inflammatory response. These pieces of evidence suggest a therapeutic target in EBA (246).

Signal Transduction by Scr Kinases

Src family kinases, such as Hck, Fgr, and Lyn, play roles in malignant transformation and tumor progression, and therefore they can be targets of cancer therapy. In addition, Src family kinases are present in many types of immune cells. It is known that Src family kinases have a role in integrin signal transduction in neutrophils and macrophages. Hck, Fgr, and Lyn-deficient mice are completely protected in antibody-transfer EBA (247).

T Cells

T_{regs} are of importance in modulating host responses to tumors and infections and in inhibiting the development of autoimmunity and allergies. T cell-deficient mice are protected from induction of skin lesions in antibody-transfer EBA. In particular, specific depletion of T_{regs} increases disease progression in antibody transfer-induced EBA. In a similar experimental setting, NKT-deficient mice and γδT cell-deficient mice are protected against the induction of experimental EBA (224, 225).

Signal Transduction by p38, MAPK AKT

In the antibody-transfer model, neutrophils are crucial for inducing clinical disease. Neutrophil activation is mediated by the phosphorylation of ERK1/2, p38 MAPK, and Akt. Methylprednisolone inhibits the phosphorylation of Akt, ERK1/2, and p38 MAPKs in neutrophils. Chemical inhibitors of Akt (Akt inhibitor VIII), ERK1/2 (U0126), and p38 MAPK (SB203580) statistically suppress *ex-vivo* dermal-epidermal separation. In addition, ERK1/2 (U0126), and p38 MAPK (SB203580) demonstrate an ~10% reduction of disease severity compared with the control (244).

RORα

RORα is a steroid nuclear hormone receptor and a transcription factor. Experimental EBA shows strain-dependent disease severity. To elucidate the strain-dependency, RORα is found to be a risk gene for the antibody-transfer model. The RORα agonist SR3335 impairs blister formation in both types of antibody-transfer EBA (230).

Signal Transduction by PI3Kβ

PI3Ks play major roles in the signaling pathways that link cell surface receptors to the control of cell function. There are four defined isoforms of PI3Ks. In particular, PI3Kβ is widely expressed and blocks arterial thrombus formation. PI3Kβ-deficient mice are protected from the development of blisters in the antibody-transfer EBA model.

Others

This antibody-transfer mouse model can be used to validate or, at least as important exclude novel therapeutic targets in EBA. For example, TREM1, MIP1a, CD11b, caspase 1/11, and S100, which are all increasingly expressed in experimental EBA, have no impact on disease manifestation (213, 221–223, 237).

CONCLUSIONS

Since the first description of EBA over 100 years ago, our understanding of this serious disease has dramatically improved. The knowledge of the cellular and molecular mechanisms led to the development of new therapies, some of which have been successfully tested in preclinical models and in concept studies in bullous pemphigoid patients. In the future, new drug targets will evolve to improve the treatment and living standards of people with EBA.

AUTHOR CONTRIBUTIONS

All authors listed have made a substantial, direct and intellectual contribution to the work, and approved it for publication.

REFERENCES

1. Kridin K. Subepidermal autoimmune bullous diseases: overview, epidemiology, and associations. *Immunol Res.* (2018) 66:6–17. doi: 10.1007/s12026-017-8975-2
2. Kridin K, Ludwig RJ. The growing incidence of bullous pemphigoid: overview and potential explanations. *Front Med.* (2018) 5:220. doi: 10.3389/fmed.2018.00220
3. Bertram F, Brocker EB, Zillikens D, Schmidt E. Prospective analysis of the incidence of autoimmune bullous disorders in Lower Franconia, Germany. *J Dtsch Dermatol Ges.* (2009) 7:434–40. doi: 10.1111/j.1610-0387.2008.06976.x
4. Wong SN, Chua SH. Spectrum of subepidermal immunobullous disorders seen at the National Skin Center, Singapore: a 2-year review. *Br J Dermatol.* (2002) 147:476–80. doi: 10.1046/j.1365-2133.2002.04919.x
5. Nanda A, Dvorak R, Al-Saeed K, Al-Sabah H, Alsaleh QA. Spectrum of autoimmune bullous diseases in Kuwait. *Int J Dermatol.* (2004) 43:876–81. doi: 10.1111/j.1365-4632.2004.02292.x
6. Bernard P, Vaillant L, Labeille B, Bedane C, Arbeille B, Denoeux JP, et al. Incidence and distribution of subepidermal autoimmune bullous skin diseases in three French regions. Bullous Diseases French Study Group. *Arch Dermatol.* (1995) 131:48–52. doi: 10.1001/archderm.1995.01690130050009
7. Zillikens D, Wever S, Roth A, Weidenthaler-Barth B, Hashimoto T, Brocker EB. Incidence of autoimmune subepidermal blistering dermatoses in a region of central Germany. *Arch Dermatol.* (1995) 131:957–8. doi: 10.1001/archderm.131.8.957
8. Lee CW. Prevalences of subacute cutaneous lupus erythematosus and Epidermolysis bullosa acquisita among Korean/Oriental populations. *Dermatology* (1998) 197:187.
9. Hubner F, Recke A, Zillikens D, Linder R, Schmidt E. Prevalence and age distribution of pemphigus and pemphigoid diseases in Germany. *J Invest Dermatol.* (2016) 136:2495–98. doi: 10.1016/j.jid.2016.07.013
10. Gammon WR, Heise ER, Burke WA, Fine JD, Woodley DT, Briggaman RA. Increased frequency of HLA-DR2 in patients with autoantibodies to epidermolysis bullosa acquisita antigen: evidence that the expression of autoimmunity to type VII collagen is HLA class II allele associated. *J Invest Dermatol.* (1988) 91:228–32. doi: 10.1111/1523-1747.ep12470317
11. Zumelzu C, Le Roux-Villet C, Loiseau P, Busson M, Heller M, Aucouturier F, et al. Black patients of African descent and HLA-DRB1*15:03 frequency overrepresented in epidermolysis bullosa acquisita. *J Invest Dermatol.* (2011) 131:2386–93. doi: 10.1038/jid.2011.231
12. Lee CW, Kim SC, Han H. Distribution of HLA class II alleles in Korean patients with epidermolysis bullosa acquisita. *Dermatol* (1996) 193:328–9.
13. Caux F, Kirtschig G, Lemarchand-Venencie F, Venencie PY, Hoang-Xuan T, Robin H, et al. IgA-epidermolysis bullosa acquisita in a child resulting in blindness. *Br J Dermatol.* (1997) 137:270–5. doi: 10.1046/j.1365-2133.1997.18191915.x
14. Trigo-Guzman FX, Conti A, Aoki V, Maruta CW, Santi CG, Resende Silva CM, et al. Epidermolysis bullosa acquisita in childhood. *J Dermatol.* (2003) 30:226–9. doi: 10.1111/j.1346-8138.2003.tb00376.x
15. Marzano AV, Cozzani E, Fanoni D, De Pita O, Vassallo C, Berti E, et al. Diagnosis and disease severity assessment of epidermolysis bullosa acquisita by ELISA for anti-type VII collagen autoantibodies: an Italian multicentre study. *Br J Dermatol.* (2013) 168:80–4. doi: 10.1111/bjd.12011
16. Prost-Squarcioni C, Caux F, Schmidt E, Jonkman MF, Vassileva S, Kim SC, et al. International Bullous Diseases Group: consensus on diagnostic criteria for epidermolysis bullosa acquisita. *Br J Dermatol.* (2017) 179:30–41. doi: 10.1111/bjd.16138
17. Briggaman RA, Gammon WR, Woodley DT. Epidermolysis bullosa acquisita of the immunopathological type (dermolytic pemphigoid). *J Invest Dermatol.* (1985) 85:79s–84s. doi: 10.1111/1523-1747.ep12275505
18. Kim JH, Kim YH, Kim SC. Epidermolysis bullosa acquisita: a retrospective clinical analysis of 30 cases. *Acta Derm Venereol.* (2011) 91:307–12. doi: 10.2340/00015555-1065
19. Buijsrogge JJ, Diercks GF, Pas HH, Jonkman MF. The many faces of epidermolysis bullosa acquisita after serration pattern analysis by direct immunofluorescence microscopy. *Br J Dermatol.* (2011) 165:92–8. doi: 10.1111/j.1365-2133.2011.10346.x
20. Iranzo P, Herrero-Gonzalez JE, Mascaro-Galy JM, Suarez-Fernandez R, Espana A. Epidermolysis bullosa acquisita: a retrospective analysis of 12 patients evaluated in four tertiary hospitals in Spain. *Br J Dermatol.* (2014) 171:1022–30. doi: 10.1111/bjd.13144
21. Seta V, Aucouturier F, Bonnefoy J, Le Roux-Villet C, Pendaries V, Alexandre M, et al. Comparison of 3 type VII collagen (C7) assays for serologic diagnosis of epidermolysis bullosa acquisita (EBA). *J Am Acad Dermatol.* (2016) 74:1166–72. doi: 10.1016/j.jaad.2016.01.005
22. Gupta R, Woodley DT, Chen M. Epidermolysis bullosa acquisita. *Clin Dermatol.* (2012) 30:60–9. doi: 10.1016/j.clindermatol.2011.03.011
23. Elliott GT. Two cases of epidermolysis bullosa. *J Cutan Genitourin Dis.* (1895) 13:10.
24. Kablitz R. *Ein Beitrag Zur Frage der Epidermolysis bullosa (heriditaria et acquisita).* Dissertation, Rostock (1904).
25. Wise F, Lautman MF. Epidermolysis bullosa beginning in adult life. the acquired for of the disease, with the report of a case and review of the literature. *J Cutan Dis.* (1915) 33:44.
26. Hundley JL, Smith DC. Epidermolysis bullosa acquisita. *South Med J.* (1941) 34:364. doi: 10.1097/00007611-194104000-00004
27. Roenigk HH Jr, Ryan JG, Bergfeld WF. Epidermolysis bullosa acquisita. Report of three cases and review of all published cases. *Arch Dermatol.* (1971) 103:1-10. doi: 10.1001/archderm.1971.04000130003001
28. Gammon WR, Briggaman RA, Wheeler CE Jr. Epidermolysis bullosa acquisita presenting as an inflammatory bullous disease. *J Am Acad Dermatol.* (1982) 7:382–7. doi: 10.1016/S0190-9622(82)80319-8
29. Nieboer C, Boorsma DM, Woerdeman MJ, Kalsbeek GL. Epidermolysis bullosa acquisita. Immunofluorescence, electron microscopic and immunoelectron microscopic studies in four patients. *Br J Dermatol.* (1980) 102:383–92. doi: 10.1111/j.1365-2133.1980.tb06550.x
30. Yaoita H, Briggaman RA, Lawley TJ, Provost TT, Katz SI. Epidermolysis bullosa acquisita: ultrastructural and immunological studies. *J Invest Dermatol.* (1981) 76:288–92. doi: 10.1111/1523-1747.ep12526124
31. Gammon WR. Epidermolysis bullosa acquisita. *Semin Dermatol.* (1988) 7:218–24.
32. Woodley DT, Briggaman RA, Gammon WT. Review and update of epidermolysis bullosa acquisita. *Semin Dermatol.* (1988) 7:111–22.
33. Dahl MG. Epidermolysis bullosa acquisita–a sign of cicatricial pemphigoid? *Br J Dermatol.* (1979) 101:475–84. doi: 10.1111/j.1365-2133.1979.tb00030.x

34. Luke MC, Darling TN, Hsu R, Summers RM, Smith JA, Solomon BI, et al. Mucosal morbidity in patients with epidermolysis bullosa acquisita. *Arch Dermatol.* (1999) 135:954–9. doi: 10.1001/archderm.135.8.954
35. Chan LS, Ahmed AR, Anhalt GJ, Bernauer W, Cooper KD, Elder MJ, et al. The first international consensus on mucous membrane pemphigoid: definition, diagnostic criteria, pathogenic factors, medical treatment, and prognostic indicators. *Arch Dermatol.* (2002) 138:370–9. doi: 10.1001/archderm.138.3.370
36. Schattenkirchner S, Lemann M, Prost C, Caux F, Guigui B, Cadot M, et al. Localized epidermolysis bullosa acquisita of the esophagus in a patient with Crohn's disease. *Am J Gastroenterol.* (1996) 91:1657–9.
37. Zehou O, Raynaud JJ, Le Roux-Villet C, Alexandre M, Airinei G, Pascal F, et al. Oesophageal involvement in 26 consecutive patients with mucous membrane pemphigoid. *Br J Dermatol.* (2017) 177:1074–85. doi: 10.1111/bjd.15592
38. Schattenkirchner S, Eming S, Hunzelmann N, Krieg T, Smola H. Treatment of epidermolysis bullosa acquisita with mycophenolate mofetil and autologous keratinocyte grafting. *Br J Dermatol.* (1999) 141:932–3. doi: 10.1046/j.1365-2133.1999.03176.x
39. Delgado L, Aoki V, Santi C, Gabbi T, Sotto M, Maruta C. Clinical and immunopathological evaluation of epidermolysis bullosa acquisita. *Clin Exp Dermatol.* (2011) 36:12–8. doi: 10.1111/j.1365-2230.2010.03845.x
40. Tokuda Y, Amagai M, Yaoita H, Kawachi S, Ito T, Matsuyama I, et al. A case of an inflammatory variant of epidermolysis bullosa acquisita: chronic bullous dermatosis associated with nonscarring mucosal blisters and circulating IgG anti-type-VII-collagen antibody. *Dermatol* (1998) 197:58–61.
41. Miyagawa S, Iida T, Hachisuka H, Yamashina Y, Shirai T. Epidermolysis bullosa acquisita with oesophageal stenosis. *Br J Dermatol.* (1992) 127:172–6. doi: 10.1111/j.1365-2133.1992.tb08052.x
42. Taniuchi K, Inaoki M, Nishimura Y, Mori T, Takehara K. Nonscarring inflammatory epidermolysis bullosa acquisita with esophageal involvement and linear IgG deposits. *J Am Acad Dermatol.* (1997) 36:320–2. doi: 10.1016/S0190-9622(97)80408-2
43. Meissner C, Hoefeld-Fegeler M, Vetter R, Bellutti M, Vorobyev A, Gollnick H, et al. Severe acral contractures and nail loss in a patient with mechano-bullous Epidermolysis bullosa acquisita. *Eur J Dermatol.* (2010) 20:543–4. doi: 10.1684/ejd.2010.1002
44. Moura EG, Couto-Junior DS, Alvarado-Escobar H, da Costa-Martins B, Sallum RA, Artifon EL, et al. Epidermolysis bullosa acquisita complicated by esophageal stenosis. endoscopic treatment with thermoplastic dilators and intralesional steroid injection. *Rev Gastroenterol Mex.* (2011) 76:279–85.
45. Stewart MI, Woodley DT, Briggaman RA. Epidermolysis bullosa acquisita and associated symptomatic esophageal webs. *Arch Dermatol.* (1991) 127:373–7. doi: 10.1001/archderm.1991.01680030093013
46. Harman KE, Whittam LR, Wakelin SH, Black MM. Severe, refractory epidermolysis bullosa acquisita complicated by an oesophageal stricture responding to intravenous immune globulin. *Br J Dermatol.* (1998) 139:1126–7. doi: 10.1046/j.1365-2133.1998.2576m.x
47. Chua S, Dodd H, Saeed IT, Chakravarty K. Dysphagia in a patient with lupus and review of the literature. *Lupus* (2002) 11:322–4. doi: 10.1191/0961203302lu195cr
48. Shipman AR, Agero AL, Cook I, Scolyer RA, Craig P, Pas HH, et al. Epidermolysis bullosa acquisita requiring multiple oesophageal dilatations. *Clin Exp Dermatol.* (2008) 33:787–9. doi: 10.1111/j.1365-2230.2008.02875.x
49. Tu J, Kumarasinghe PW. Epidermolysis bullosa acquisita with moderately severe Dysphagia due to esophageal strictures. *Indian J Dermatol.* (2011) 56:224–7. doi: 10.4103/0019-5154.80428
50. Ishii N, Furumura M, Hamada T, Mori O, Ohzono A, Ueda A, et al. Oesophageal involvement in epidermolysis bullosa acquisita. *Br J Dermatol.* (2015) 172:288–90. doi: 10.1111/bjd.13224
51. Alexandre M, Brette MD, Pascal F, Tsianakas P, Fraitag S, Doan S, et al. A prospective study of upper aerodigestive tract manifestations of mucous membrane pemphigoid. *Medicine* (2006) 85:239–52. doi: 10.1097/01.md.0000231954.08350.52
52. Kiniwa Y, Ashida A, Ohashi A, Kitoh R, Fukuda S, Hashimoto T, et al. A case of epidermolysis bullosa acquisita associated with laryngeal stenosis. *Acta Derm Venereol.* (2012) 92:93–4. doi: 10.2340/00015555-1163
53. Benton EC, Bhogal B, Oakley R, Groves RW. Beware the blistering patient with dysphonia. *Clin Exp Dermatol.* (2013) 38:691–2. doi: 10.1111/ced.12009
54. Poirier E, Soued I, Alexandre M, Boussoura S, Lamberto C, Uzunhan Y, et al. Pemphigoide des muqueuses avec sténose laryngée ou trachéale. In: *Annual Meeting of the Société Française de Dermatologie.* Paris, December 2014. (2014) 141 (Hs12):S262.
55. Lang PG Jr, Tapert MJ. Severe ocular involvement in a patient with epidermolysis bullosa acquisita. *J Am Acad Dermatol.* (1987) 16:439–43. doi: 10.1016/S0190-9622(87)70057-7
56. Zierhut M, Thiel HJ, Weidle EG, Steuhl KP, Sonnichsen K, Schaumburg-Lever G. Ocular involvement in epidermolysis bullosa acquisita. *Arch Ophthalmol.* (1989) 107:398–401. doi: 10.1001/archopht.1989.01070010408035
57. Zambruno G, Manca V, Kanitakis J, Cozzani E, Nicolas JF, Giannetti A. Linear IgA bullous dermatosis with autoantibodies to a 290 kd antigen of anchoring fibrils. *J Am Acad Dermatol.* (1994) 31:884–8. doi: 10.1016/S0190-9622(94)70252-7
58. Aclimandos WA. Corneal perforation as a complication of epidermolysis bullosa acquisita. *Eye* (1995) 9(Pt 5):633–6. doi: 10.1038/eye.1995.153
59. Hoang-Xuan T, Robin H, Heller M, Caux F, Prost C. Epidermolysis bullosa acquisita diagnosed by direct immunoelectron microscopy of the conjunctiva. *Ophthalmology* (1997) 104:1414–20. doi: 10.1016/S0161-6420(97)30122-5
60. Bauer JW, Schaeppi H, Metze D, Muss W, Pohla-Gubo G, Hametner R, et al. Ocular involvement in IgA-epidermolysis bullosa acquisita. *Br J Dermatol.* (1999) 141:887–92. doi: 10.1046/j.1365-2133.1999.03163.x
61. Camara A, Becherel PA, Bussel A, Lagrange S, Chosidow O, Joly P, et al. Resistant acquired bullous epidermolysis with severe ocular involvement: the success of extracorporeal photochemotherapy. *Ann Dermatol Venereol.* (1999) 126:612–5.
62. Dantas PE, Nishiwaki-Dantas MC, Seguim MH, Cursino JW. Bilateral corneal involvement in epidermolysis bullosa acquisita. *Cornea* (2001) 20:664–7. doi: 10.1097/00003226-200108000-00022
63. Letko E, Bhol K, Anzaar F, Perez VL, Ahmed AR, Foster CS. Chronic cicatrizing conjunctivitis in a patient with epidermolysis bullosa acquisita. *Arch Ophthalmol.* (2006) 124:1615–8. doi: 10.1001/archopht.124.11.1615
64. Cox NH, Bearn MA, Herold J, Ainsworth G, Liu C. Blindness due to the IgA variant of epidermolysis bullosa acquisita, and treatment with osteo-odonto-keratoprosthesis. *Br J Dermatol.* (2007) 156:775–7. doi: 10.1111/j.1365-2133.2006.07739.x
65. Le Roux-Villet C, Prost-Squarcioni C. Epidermolysis bullosa acquisita: clinical, histological and immunologicalanalysis of 39 cases. *Ann Dermatol Venereol.* (2002) 129(Suppl. 1):S71–2.
66. Lee CW. Epidermolysis bullosa acquisita associated with vesicular cystitis. *Br J Dermatol.* (1988) 119:101–5. doi: 10.1111/j.1365-2133.1988.tb07109.x
67. Vodegel RM, de Jong MC, Pas HH, Jonkman MF. IgA-mediated epidermolysis bullosa acquisita: two cases and review of the literature. *J Am Acad Dermatol.* (2002) 47:919–25. doi: 10.1067/mjd.2002.125079
68. Gottlieb J, Ingen-Housz-Oro S, Alexandre M, Grootenboer-Mignot S, Aucouturier F, Sbidian E, et al. Idiopathic linear IgA bullous dermatosis: prognostic factors based on a case series of 72 adults. *Br J Dermatol.* (2017) 177:212–22. doi: 10.1111/bjd.15244
69. Lee CW, Jun KM. Epidermolysis bullosa acquisita presenting with localized facial blisters. *Clin Exp Dermatol.* (1992) 17:363–5. doi: 10.1111/j.1365-2230.1992.tb00234.x
70. Joly P, Ruto F, Thomine E, Delpech A, Balguerie X, Tron F, et al. Brunsting-Perry cicatricial bullous pemphigoid: a clinical variant of localized acquired epidermolysis bullosa? *J Am Acad Dermatol.* (1993) 28:89–92. doi: 10.1016/0190-9622(93)70016-M
71. Kurzhals G, Stolz W, Maciejewski W, Karpati S, Meurer M, Breit R. Localized cicatricial pemphigoid of the Brunsting-Perry type with transition into disseminated cicatricial pemphigoid. report of a case proved by preembedding immunogold electron microscopy. *Arch Dermatol.* (1995) 131:580–5. doi: 10.1001/archderm.1995.01690170082012
72. Choi GS, Lee ES, Kim SC, Lee S. Epidermolysis bullosa acquisita localized to the face. *J Dermatol.* (1998) 25:19–22. doi: 10.1111/j.1346-8138.1998.tb02339.x

73. Woodley DT. Epidermolysis bullosa acquisita. In: Freedberg IM, Eisen AZ, Wolff K, editors. *Dermatology in General Medicine*. New York, NY: Mc Graw Hill (2003). p. 609–16.
74. Tanaka N, Dainichi T, Ohyama B, Yasumoto S, Oono T, Iwatsuki K, et al. A case of epidermolysis bullosa acquisita with clinical features of Brunsting-Perry pemphigoid showing an excellent response to colchicine. *J Am Acad Dermatol.* (2009) 61:715–9. doi: 10.1016/j.jaad.2008.12.020
75. Minato H, Ishii N, Fukuda S, Wakasa T, Wakasa K, Sogame R, et al. Heterogeneity of Brunsting-Perry type pemphigoid: a case showing blister formation at the lamina lucida, immune deposition beneath the lamina densa and autoantibodies against the 290-kD polypeptide along the lamina densa. *J Dermatol.* (2011) 38:887–92. doi: 10.1111/j.1346-8138.2010.01172.x
76. Asfour L, Chong H, Mee J, Groves R, Singh M. Epidermolysis bullosa acquisita (brunsting-perry pemphigoid variant) localized to the face and diagnosed with antigen identification using skin deficient in type VII collagen. *Am J Dermatopathol.* (2017) 39:e90–6. doi: 10.1097/DAD.0000000000000829
77. Sebaratnam DF, Hanna AM, Chee SN, Frew JW, Venugopal SS, Daniel BS, et al. Development of a quality-of-life instrument for autoimmune bullous disease: the Autoimmune Bullous Disease Quality of Life questionnaire. *JAMA Dermatol.* (2013) 149:1186–91. doi: 10.1001/jamadermatol.2013.4972
78. Tjokrowidjaja A, Daniel BS, Frew JW, Sebaratnam DF, Hanna AM, Chee S, et al. The development and validation of the treatment of autoimmune bullous disease quality of life questionnaire, a tool to measure the quality of life impacts of treatments used in patients with autoimmune blistering disease. *Br J Dermatol.* (2013) 169:1000–6. doi: 10.1111/bjd.12623
79. Chen M, O'Toole EA, Sanghavi J, Mahmud N, Kelleher D, Weir D, et al. The epidermolysis bullosa acquisita antigen (type VII collagen) is present in human colon and patients with crohn's disease have autoantibodies to type VII collagen. *J Invest Dermatol.* (2002) 118:1059–64. doi: 10.1046/j.1523-1747.2002.01772.x
80. Aractingi S, Bachmeyer C, Prost C, Caux F, Flageul B, Fermand JP. Subepidermal autoimmune bullous skin diseases associated with B-cell lymphoproliferative disorders. *Medicine* (1999) 78:228–35. doi: 10.1097/00005792-199907000-00003
81. Camisa C, Sharma HM. Vesiculobullous systemic lupus erythematosus. report of two cases and a review of the literature. *J Am Acad Dermatol.* (1983) 9:924–33. doi: 10.1016/S0190-9622(83)70210-0
82. Gammon WR, Briggaman RA. Bullous SLE: a phenotypically distinctive but immunologically heterogeneous bullous disorder. *J Invest Dermatol.* (1993) 100:28S—34S. doi: 10.1111/1523-1747.ep12355210
83. Komorowski L, Muller R, Vorobyev A, Probst C, Recke A, Jonkman MF, et al. Sensitive and specific assays for routine serological diagnosis of epidermolysis bullosa acquisita. *J Am Acad Dermatol.* (2013) 68:e89–95. doi: 10.1016/j.jaad.2011.12.032
84. Gammon WR, Kowalewski C, Chorzelski TP, Kumar V, Briggaman RA, Beutner EH. Direct immunofluorescence studies of sodium chloride-separated skin in the differential diagnosis of bullous pemphigoid and epidermolysis bullosa acquisita. *J Am Acad Dermatol.* (1990) 22:664–70. doi: 10.1016/0190-9622(90)70094-X
85. Terra JB, Jonkman MF, Diercks GF, Pas HH. Low sensitivity of type VII collagen enzyme-linked immunosorbent assay in epidermolysis bullosa acquisita: serration pattern analysis on skin biopsy is required for diagnosis. *Br J Dermatol.* (2013) 169:164–7. doi: 10.1111/bjd.12300
86. Meijer JM, Atefi I, Diercks GFH, Vorobyev A, Zuiderveen J, Meijer HJ, et al. Serration pattern analysis for differentiating epidermolysis bullosa acquisita from other pemphigoid diseases. *J Am Acad Dermatol.* (2018) 78:754–59 e6. doi: 10.1016/j.jaad.2017.11.029
87. Schmidt E, Zillikens D. Pemphigoid diseases. *Lancet* (2013) 381:320–32. doi: 10.1016/S0140-6736(12)61140-4
88. Wilson BD, Beutner EH, Kumar V, Chorzelski TP, Jablonska S. Linear IgA bullous dermatosis. an immunologically defined disease. *Int J Dermatol.* (1985) 24:569–74. doi: 10.1111/j.1365-4362.1985.tb05575.x
89. Vodegel RM, de Jong MC, Meijer HJ, Weytingh MB, Pas HH, Jonkman MF. Enhanced diagnostic immunofluorescence using biopsies transported in saline. *BMC Dermatol.* (2004) 4:10. doi: 10.1186/1471-5945-4-10
90. Schmidt E, Klinker E, Opitz A, Herzog S, Sitaru C, Goebeler M, et al. Protein A immunoadsorption: a novel and effective adjuvant treatment of severe pemphigus. *Br J Dermatol.* (2003) 148:1222–9. doi: 10.1046/j.1365-2133.2003.05302.x
91. Suchniak JM, Diaz LA, Lin MS, Fairley JA. IgM-mediated epidermolysis bullosa acquisita. *Arch Dermatol.* (2002) 138:1385–6. doi: 10.1001/archderm.138.10.1385
92. Caux F. Diagnosis and clinical features of epidermolysis bullosa acquisita. *Dermatol Clin.* (2011) 29:485–91. doi: 10.1016/j.det.2011.03.017
93. Saleh MA, Ishii K, Kim YJ, Murakami A, Ishii N, Hashimoto T, et al. Development of NC1 and NC2 domains of type VII collagen ELISA for the diagnosis and analysis of the time course of epidermolysis bullosa acquisita patients. *J Dermatol Sci.* (2011) 62:169–75. doi: 10.1016/j.jdermsci.2011.03.003
94. Marzano AV, Cozzani E, Biasin M, Russo I, Alaibac M. The use of Biochip immunofluorescence microscopy for the serological diagnosis of epidermolysis bullosa acquisita. *Arch Dermatol Res.* (2016) 308:273–6. doi: 10.1007/s00403-016-1632-0
95. Schmidt T, Hoch M, Lotfi Jad SS, Solimani F, Di Zenzo G, Marzano AV, et al. Serological diagnostics in the detection of IgG autoantibodies against human collagen VII in epidermolysis bullosa acquisita: a multicentre analysis. *Br J Dermatol.* (2017) 177:1683–92. doi: 10.1111/bjd.15800
96. Kim JH, Kim YH, Kim S, Noh EB, Kim SE, Vorobyev A, et al. Serum levels of anti-type VII collagen antibodies detected by enzyme-linked immunosorbent assay in patients with epidermolysis bullosa acquisita are correlated with the severity of skin lesions. *J Eur Acad Dermatol Venereol.* (2013) 27:e224–30. doi: 10.1111/j.1468-3083.2012.04617.x
97. Vorobyev A, Ludwig RJ, Schmidt E. Clinical features and diagnosis of epidermolysis bullosa acquisita. *Expert Rev Clin Immunol.* (2017) 13:157–69. doi: 10.1080/1744666X.2016.1221343
98. Witte M, Koga H, Hashimoto T, Ludwig RJ, Bieber K. Discovering potential drug-targets for personalized treatment of autoimmune disorders - what we learn from epidermolysis bullosa acquisita. *Expert Opin Ther Targets* (2016) 20:985–98. doi: 10.1517/14728222.2016.1148686
99. Ludwig RJ. Clinical Presentation, Pathogenesis, Diagnosis, and Treatment of Epidermolysis Bullosa Acquisita. *ISRN Dermatol.* (2013) 2013:812029. doi: 10.1155/2013/812029
100. Gordon KB, Chan LS, Woodley DT. Treatment of refractory epidermolysis bullosa acquisita with extracorporeal photochemotherapy. *Br J Dermatol.* (1997) 136:415–20. doi: 10.1111/j.1365-2133.1997.tb14957.x
101. Iwata H, Vorobyev A, Koga H, Recke A, Zillikens D, Prost-Squarcioni C, et al. Meta-analysis of the clinical and immunopathological characteristics and treatment outcomes in epidermolysis bullosa acquisita patients. *Orphanet J Rare Dis.* (2018) 13:153. doi: 10.1186/s13023-018-0896-1
102. Megahed M, Scharffetter-Kochanek K. Epidermolysis bullosa acquisita–successful treatment with colchicine. *Arch Dermatol Res.* (1994) 286:35–46. doi: 10.1007/BF00375841
103. Dasgeb B, Kornreich D, McGuinn K, Okon L, Brownell I, Sackett DL. Colchicine: an ancient drug with novel applications. *Br J Dermatol.* (2018) 178:350–6. doi: 10.1111/bjd.15896
104. Cunningham BB, Kirchmann TT, Woodley D. Colchicine for epidermolysis bullosa acquisita. *J Am Acad Dermatol.* (1996) 34:781–4. doi: 10.1016/S0190-9622(96)90013-4
105. Ishii N, Hamada T, Dainichi T, Karashima T, Nakama T, Yasumoto S, et al. Epidermolysis bullosa acquisita: what's new? *J Dermatol.* (2010) 37:220–30. doi: 10.1111/j.1346-8138.2009.00799.x
106. Zhu YI, Stiller MJ. Dapsone and sulfones in dermatology: overview and update. *J Am Acad Dermatol.* (2001) 45:420–34. doi: 10.1067/mjd.2001.114733
107. Hashimoto T, Ishii N, Ohata C, Furumura M. Pathogenesis of epidermolysis bullosa acquisita, an autoimmune subepidermal bullous disease. *J Pathol.* (2012) 228:1–7. doi: 10.1002/path.4062
108. Sticherling M, Franke A, Aberer E, Glaser R, Hertl M, Pfeiffer C, et al. An open, multicentre, randomized clinical study in patients with bullous pemphigoid comparing methylprednisolone and azathioprine with methylprednisolone and dapsone. *Br J Dermatol.* (2017) 177:1299–305. doi: 10.1111/bjd.15649
109. Gurcan HM, Ahmed AR. Analysis of current data on the use of methotrexate in the treatment of pemphigus and pemphigoid. *Br J Dermatol.* (2009) 161:723–31. doi: 10.1111/j.1365-2133.2009.09246.x

110. Fraser AG, Orchard TR, Jewell DP. The efficacy of azathioprine for the treatment of inflammatory bowel disease: a 30 year review. *Gut* (2002) 50:485–9. doi: 10.1136/gut.50.4.485
111. Ryan C, Amor KT, Menter A. The use of cyclosporine in dermatology: part II. *J Am Acad Dermatol.* (2010) 63:949–72. doi: 10.1016/j.jaad.2010.02.062
112. Beissert S, Werfel T, Frieling U, Bohm M, Sticherling M, Stadler R, et al. A comparison of oral methylprednisolone plus azathioprine or mycophenolate mofetil for the treatment of pemphigus. *Arch Dermatol.* (2006) 142:1447–54. doi: 10.1001/archderm.142.11.1447
113. Beissert S, Mimouni D, Kanwar AJ, Solomons N, Kalia V, Anhalt GJ. Treating pemphigus vulgaris with prednisone and mycophenolate mofetil: a multicenter, randomized, placebo-controlled trial. *J Invest Dermatol.* (2010) 130:2041–8. doi: 10.1038/jid.2010.91
114. Sami N. Mycophenolate mofetil (MMF) in the treatment of epidermolysis bullosa acquisita (EBA) long-term follow-up. *JAAD Case Rep.* (2015) 1:321–3. doi: 10.1016/j.jdcr.2015.07.007
115. Barreiro-Capurro A, Mascaro-Galy JM, Iranzo P. Retrospective study of the clinical, histologic, and immunologic features of epidermolysis bullosa acquisita in 9 patients. *Actas Dermosifiliogr.* (2013) 104:904–14. doi: 10.1016/j.ad.2013.05.005
116. Gual A, Guilabert A, Iranzo P, Flores G, Diaz LA, Mascaro JM Jr. IgG autoantibody subclass analysis as a tool to differentiate epidermolysis bullosa acquisita with overlapping features of bullous systemic lupus erythematosus. *J Am Acad Dermatol.* (2013) 69:e34–6. doi: 10.1016/j.jaad.2013.01.025
117. Baican A, Chiriac G, Torio-Padron N, Sitaru C. Childhood epidermolysis bullosa acquisita associated with severe dental alterations: a case presentation. *J Dermatol.* (2013) 40:410–1. doi: 10.1111/1346-8138.12107
118. Ahmed AR, Gurcan HM. Treatment of epidermolysis bullosa acquisita with intravenous immunoglobulin in patients non-responsive to conventional therapy: clinical outcome and post-treatment long-term follow-up. *J Eur Acad Dermatol Venereol.* (2012) 26:1074–83. doi: 10.1111/j.1468-3083.2011.04205.x
119. Busch JO, Sticherling M. Epidermolysis bullosa acquisita and neuroendocrine pancreatic cancer - coincidence or pathogenetic relationship? *J Dtsch Dermatol Ges.* (2007) 5:916–8. doi: 10.1111/j.1610-0387.2007.06338.x
120. Pastar Z, Rados J, Lipozencic J, Dobric I, Marinovic B, Ishii N, et al. Case of concurrent epidermolysis bullosa acquisita and anti-p200 pemphigoid-how to treat it? *Int J Dermatol.* (2007) 46:295–8. doi: 10.1111/j.1365-4632.2006.02969.x
121. Crichlow SM, Mortimer NJ, Harman KE. A successful therapeutic trial of rituximab in the treatment of a patient with recalcitrant, high-titre epidermolysis bullosa acquisita. *Br J Dermatol.* (2007) 156:194–6. doi: 10.1111/j.1365-2133.2006.07596.x
122. Campos M, Silvente C, Lecona M, Suarez R, Lazaro P. Epidermolysis bullosa acquisita: diagnosis by fluorescence overlay antigen mapping and clinical response to high-dose intravenous immunoglobulin. *Clin Exp Dermatol.* (2006) 31:71–3. doi: 10.1111/j.1365-2230.2005.01989.x
123. Gourgiotou K, Exadaktylou D, Aroni K, Rallis E, Nicolaidou E, Paraskevakou H, et al. Epidermolysis bullosa acquisita: treatment with intravenous immunoglobulins. *J Eur Acad Dermatol Venereol.* (2002) 16:77–80. doi: 10.1046/j.1468-3083.2002.00386.x
124. Jappe U, Zillikens D, Bonnekoh B, Gollnick H. Epidermolysis bullosa acquisita with ultraviolet radiationsensitivity. *Br J Dermatol.* (2000) 142:517–20. doi: 10.1046/j.1365-2133.2000.03368.x
125. Kofler H, Wambacher-Gasser B, Topar G, Weinlich G, Schuler G, Hintner H, et al. Intravenous immunoglobulin treatment in therapy-resistant epidermolysis bullosa acquisita. *J Am Acad Dermatol.* (1997) 36:331–5. doi: 10.1016/S0190-9622(97)80411-2
126. Mohr C, Sunderkotter C, Hildebrand A, Biel K, Rutter A, Rutter GH, et al. Successful treatment of epidermolysis bullosa acquisita using intravenous immunoglobulins. *Br J Dermatol.* (1995) 132:824–6. doi: 10.1111/j.1365-2133.1995.tb00735.x
127. Meier F, Sonnichsen K, Schaumburg-Lever G, Dopfer R, Rassner G. Epidermolysis bullosa acquisita: efficacy of high-dose intravenous immunoglobulins. *J Am Acad Dermatol.* (1993) 29:334–7. doi: 10.1016/0190-9622(93)70189-Z
128. Li N, Zhao M, Hilario-Vargas J, Prisayanh P, Warren S, Diaz LA, et al. Complete FcRn dependence for intravenous Ig therapy in autoimmune skin blistering diseases. *J Clin Invest.* (2005) 115:3440–50. doi: 10.1172/JCI24394
129. Hirose M, Tiburzy B, Ishii N, Pipi E, Wende S, Rentz E, et al. Effects of intravenous immunoglobulins on mice with experimental epidermolysis bullosa acquisita. *J Invest Dermatol.* (2015) 135:768–75. doi: 10.1038/jid.2014.453
130. Sasaoka T, Ujiie H, Nishie W, Iwata H, Ishikawa M, Higashino H, et al. Intravenous IgG reduces pathogenic autoantibodies, serum IL-6 levels, and disease severity in experimental bullous pemphigoid models. *J Invest Dermatol.* (2018) 138:1260–67. doi: 10.1016/j.jid.2018.01.005
131. Kamaguchi M, Iwata H, Mori Y, Toyonaga E, Ujiie H, Kitagawa Y, et al. Anti-idiotypic antibodies against BP-IgG prevent type XVII collagen depletion. *Front Immunol.* (2017) 8:1669. doi: 10.3389/fimmu.2017.01669
132. Amagai M, Ikeda S, Hashimoto T, Mizuashi M, Fujisawa A, Ihn H, et al. A randomized double-blind trial of intravenous immunoglobulin for bullous pemphigoid. *J Dermatol Sci.* (2017) 85:77–84. doi: 10.1016/j.jdermsci.2016.11.003
133. Kolesnik M, Becker E, Reinhold D, Ambach A, Heim MU, Gollnick H, et al. Treatment of severe autoimmune blistering skin diseases with combination of protein A immunoadsorption and rituximab: a protocol without initial high dose or pulse steroid medication. *J Eur Acad Dermatol Venereol.* (2014) 28:771–80. doi: 10.1111/jdv.12175
134. Kim JH, Lee SE, Kim SC. Successful treatment of epidermolysis bullosa acquisita with rituximab therapy. *J Dermatol.* (2012) 39:477–9. doi: 10.1111/j.1346-8138.2011.01360.x
135. Kubisch I, Diessenbacher P, Schmidt E, Gollnick H, Leverkus M. Premonitory epidermolysis bullosa acquisita mimicking eyelid dermatitis: successful treatment with rituximab and protein A immunoapheresis. *Am J Clin Dermatol.* (2010) 11:289–93. doi: 10.2165/11533210-000000000-00000
136. Saha M, Cutler T, Bhogal B, Black MM, Groves RW. Refractory epidermolysis bullosa acquisita: successful treatment with rituximab. *Clin Exp Dermatol.* (2009) 34:e979–80. doi: 10.1111/j.1365-2230.2009.03608.x
137. Wallet-Faber N, Franck N, Batteux F, Mateus C, Gilbert D, Carlotti A, et al. Epidermolysis bullosa acquisita following bullous pemphigoid, successfully treated with the anti-CD20 monoclonal antibody rituximab. *Dermatol* (2007) 215:252–5. doi: 10.1159/000106585
138. Niedermeier A, Eming R, Pfutze M, Neumann CR, Happel C, Reich K, et al. Clinical response of severe mechanobullous epidermolysis bullosa acquisita to combined treatment with immunoadsorption and rituximab (anti-CD20 monoclonal antibodies). *Arch Dermatol.* (2007) 143:192–8. doi: 10.1001/archderm.143.2.192
139. Schmidt E, Benoit S, Brocker EB, Zillikens D, Goebeler M. Successful adjuvant treatment of recalcitrant epidermolysis bullosa acquisita with anti-CD20 antibody rituximab. *Arch Dermatol.* (2006) 142:147–50. doi: 10.1001/archderm.142.2.147
140. Joly P, Maho-Vaillant M, Prost-Squarcioni C, Hebert V, Houivet E, Calbo S, et al. First-line rituximab combined with short-term prednisone versus prednisone alone for the treatment of pemphigus (Ritux 3): a prospective, multicentre, parallel-group, open-label randomised trial. *Lancet* (2017) 389:2031–40. doi: 10.1016/S0140-6736(17)30070-3
141. Lamberts A, Euverman HI, Terra JB, Jonkman MF, Horvath B. Effectiveness and safety of rituximab in recalcitrant pemphigoid diseases. *Front Immunol.* (2018) 9:248. doi: 10.3389/fimmu.2018.00248
142. Iwata H, Bieber K, Tiburzy B, Chrobok N, Kalies K, Shimizu A, et al. B cells, dendritic cells, and macrophages are required to induce an autoreactive CD4 helper T cell response in experimental epidermolysis bullosa acquisita. *J Immunol.* (2013) 191:2978–88. doi: 10.4049/jimmunol.1300310
143. Langenhan J, Dworschak J, Saschenbrecker S, Komorowski L, Schlumberger W, Stocker W, et al. Specific immunoadsorption of pathogenic autoantibodies in pemphigus requires the entire ectodomains of desmogleins. *Exp Dermatol.* (2014) 23:253–9. doi: 10.1111/exd.12355
144. Mersmann M, Dworschak J, Ebermann K, Komorowski L, Schlumberger W, Stocker W, et al. Immunoadsorber for specific apheresis of autoantibodies in the treatment of bullous pemphigoid. *Arch Dermatol Res.* (2016) 308:31–8. doi: 10.1007/s00403-015-1606-7

145. Woodley DT, Remington J, Chen M. Autoimmunity to type VII collagen: epidermolysis bullosa acquisita. *Clin Rev Allergy Immunol.* (2007) 33:78–84. doi: 10.1007/s12016-007-0027-6
146. Baroudjian B, Le Roux-Villet C, Brechignac S, Alexandre M, Caux F, Prost-Squarcioni C, et al. Long-term efficacy of extracorporeal photochemotherapy in a patient with refractory epidermolysis bullosa acquisita. *Eur J Dermatol.* (2012) 22:795–7. doi: 10.1684/ejd.2012.1840
147. Miller JL, Stricklin GP, Fine JD, King LE, Arzubiaga MC, Ellis DL. Remission of severe epidermolysis bullosa acquisita induced by extracorporeal photochemotherapy. *Br J Dermatol.* (1995) 133:467–71. doi: 10.1111/j.1365-2133.1995.tb02680.x
148. Egan CA, Brown M, White JD, Yancey KB. Treatment of epidermolysis bullosa acquisita with the humanized anti-Tac mAb daclizumab. *Clin Immunol.* (2001) 101:146–51. doi: 10.1006/clim.2001.5113
149. Labeille B, Gineston JL, Denoeux JP, Capron JP. Epidermolysis bullosa acquisita and Crohn's disease. a case report with immunological and electron microscopic studies. *Arch Intern Med.* (1988) 148:1457–9. doi: 10.1001/archinte.1988.00380060221040
150. Williams HC, Wojnarowska F, Kirtschig G, Mason J, Godec TR, Schmidt E, et al. Doxycycline versus prednisolone as an initial treatment strategy for bullous pemphigoid: a pragmatic, non-inferiority, randomised controlled trial. *Lancet* (2017) 389:1630–8. doi: 10.1016/S0140-6736(17)30560-3
151. Cavailhes A, Balme B, Gilbert D, Skowron F. Successful use of combined corticosteroids and rituximab in the treatment of recalcitrant epidermolysis bullosa acquisita. *Ann Dermatol Venereol.* (2009) 136:795–9. doi: 10.1016/j.annder.2009.02.007
152. Kawase K, Oshitani Y, Mizutani Y, Shu E, Fujine E, Seishima M. Inflammatory epidermolysis bullosa acquisita effectively treated with minocycline. *Acta Derm Venereol.* (2014) 94:6145–6. doi: 10.2340/00015555-1804
153. Nagano T, Tani M, Hiramatsu Y, Kohriyama K, Ishihara K, Nei M, et al. A case of epidermolysis bullosa acquisita with bleeding tendency due to factor VIII inhibitor (acquired haemophilia). *Br J Dermatol.* (2004) 151:716–7. doi: 10.1111/j.1365-2133.2004.06150.x
154. Joly P, Roujeau JC, Benichou J, Delaporte E, D'Incan M, Dreno B, et al. A comparison of two regimens of topical corticosteroids in the treatment of patients with bullous pemphigoid: a multicenter randomized study. *J Invest Dermatol.* (2009) 129:1681–7. doi: 10.1038/jid.2008.412
155. Murrell DF, Daniel BS, Joly P, Borradori L, Amagai M, Hashimoto T, et al. Definitions and outcome measures for bullous pemphigoid: recommendations by an international panel of experts. *J Am Acad Dermatol.* (2012) 66:479–85. doi: 10.1016/j.jaad.2011.06.032
156. Murrell DF, Marinovic B, Caux F, Prost C, Ahmed R, Wozniak K, et al. Definitions and outcome measures for mucous membrane pemphigoid: recommendations of an international panel of experts. *J Am Acad Dermatol.* (2015) 72:168–74. doi: 10.1016/j.jaad.2014.08.024
157. Callot-Mellot C, Bodemer C, Caux F, Bourgault-Villada I, Fraitag S, Goudie G, et al. Epidermolysis bullosa acquisita in childhood. *Arch Dermatol.* (1997) 133:1122–6. doi: 10.1001/archderm.1997.03890450070008
158. Edwards S, Wakelin SH, Wojnarowska F, Marsden RA, Kirtschig G, Bhogal B, et al. Bullous pemphigoid and epidermolysis bullosa acquisita: presentation, prognosis, and immunopathology in 11 children. *Pediatr Dermatol.* (1998) 15:184–90. doi: 10.1111/j.1525-1470.1998.tb01311.x
159. Vorobyev A, Ujiie H, Recke A, Buijsrogge JJ, Jonkman MF, Pas HH, et al. Autoantibodies to multiple epitopes on the non-collagenous-1 domain of type VII collagen induce blisters. *J Invest Dermatol.* (2015) 135:1565–73. doi: 10.1038/jid.2015.51
160. Lapiere JC, Woodley DT, Parente MG, Iwasaki T, Wynn KC, Christiano AM, et al. Epitope mapping of type VII collagen. identification of discrete peptide sequences recognized by sera from patients with acquired epidermolysis bullosa. *J Clin Invest.* (1993) 92:1831–9. doi: 10.1172/JCI116774
161. Gammon WR, Murrell DF, Jenison MW, Padilla KM, Prisayanh PS, Jones DA, et al. Autoantibodies to type VII collagen recognize epitopes in a fibronectin-like region of the noncollagenous (NC1) domain. *Journal Invest Dermatol.* (1993) 100:618–22. doi: 10.1111/1523-1747.ep12472291
162. Chen M, Doostan A, Bandyopadhyay P, Remington J, Wang X, Hou Y, et al. The cartilage matrix protein subdomain of type VII collagen is pathogenic for epidermolysis bullosa acquisita. *Am J Pathol.* (2007) 170:2009–18. doi: 10.2353/ajpath.2007.061212
163. Ishii N, Yoshida M, Ishida-Yamamoto A, Fritsch A, Elfert S, Bruckner-Tuderman L, et al. Some epidermolysis bullosa acquisita sera react with epitopes within the triple-helical collagenous domain as indicated by immunoelectron microscopy. *Br J Dermatol.* (2009) 160:1090–3. doi: 10.1111/j.1365-2133.2008.08952.x
164. Ishii N, Yoshida M, Hisamatsu Y, Ishida-Yamamoto A, Nakane H, Iizuka H, et al. Epidermolysis bullosa acquisita sera react with distinct epitopes on the NC1 and NC2 domains of type VII collagen: study using immunoblotting of domain-specific recombinant proteins and postembedding immunoelectron microscopy. *Br J Dermatol.* (2004) 150:843–51. doi: 10.1111/j.1365-2133.2004.05933.x
165. Ludwig RJ, Recke A, Bieber K, Muller S, Marques Ade C, Banczyk D, et al. Generation of antibodies of distinct subclasses and specificity is linked to H2s in an active mouse model of epidermolysis bullosa acquisita. *J Invest Dermatol.* (2011) 131:167–76. doi: 10.1038/jid.2010.248
166. Noe MH, Chen M, Woodley DT, Fairley JA. Familial epidermolysis bullosa acquisita. *Dermatol Online J.* (2008) 14:2. Available online at: https://escholarship.org/uc/item/14b7543k
167. Bieber K, Koga H, Nishie W. *In vitro* and *in vivo* models to investigate the pathomechanisms and novel treatments for pemphigoid diseases. *Exp Dermatol.* (2017) 26:1163–70. doi: 10.1111/exd.13415
168. Sitaru C, Chiriac MT, Mihai S, Buning J, Gebert A, Ishiko A, et al. Induction of complement-fixing autoantibodies against type VII collagen results in subepidermal blistering in mice. *J Immunol.* (2006) 177:3461–8. doi: 10.4049/jimmunol.177.5.3461
169. Hammers CM, Bieber K, Kalies K, Banczyk D, Ellebrecht CT, Ibrahim SM, et al. Complement-fixing anti-type VII collagen antibodies are induced in Th1-polarized lymph nodes of epidermolysis bullosa acquisita-susceptible mice. *J Immunol.* (2011) 187:5043–50. doi: 10.4049/jimmunol.1100796
170. Ludwig RJ, Muller S, Marques A, Recke A, Schmidt E, Zillikens D, et al. Identification of quantitative trait loci in experimental epidermolysis bullosa acquisita. *J Invest Dermatol.* (2012) 132:1409–15. doi: 10.1038/jid.2011.466
171. Samavedam UK, Mitschker N, Kasprick A, Bieber K, Schmidt E, Laskay T, et al. Whole-genome expression profiling in skin reveals SYK as a key regulator of inflammation in experimental epidermolysis bullosa acquisita. *Front Immunol.* (2018) 9:249. doi: 10.3389/fimmu.2018.00249
172. Srinivas G, Moller S, Wang J, Kunzel S, Zillikens D, Baines JF, et al. Genome-wide mapping of gene-microbiota interactions in susceptibility to autoimmune skin blistering. *Nat Commun.* (2013) 4:2462. doi: 10.1038/ncomms3462
173. Ellebrecht CT, Srinivas G, Bieber K, Banczyk D, Kalies K, Kunzel S, et al. Skin microbiota-associated inflammation precedes autoantibody induced tissue damage in experimental epidermolysis bullosa acquisita. *J Autoimmun.* (2016) 68:14–22. doi: 10.1016/j.jaut.2015.08.007
174. Kasperkiewicz M, Müller R, Manz R, Magens M, Hammers CM, Somlai C, et al. Heat-shock protein 90 inhibition in autoimmunity to type VII collagen: evidence that nonmalignant plasma cells are not therapeutic targets. *Blood* (2011) 117:6135–42. doi: 10.1182/blood-2010-10-314609
175. Bieber K, Ernst AL, Tukaj S, Holtsche MM, Schmidt E, Zillikens D, et al. Analysis of serum markers of cellular immune activation in patients with bullous pemphigoid. *Exp Dermatol.* (2017) 26:1248–52. doi: 10.1111/exd.13382
176. Sitaru AG, Sesarman A, Mihai S, Chiriac MT, Zillikens D, Hultman P, et al. T cells are required for the production of blister-inducing autoantibodies in experimental epidermolysis bullosa acquisita. *J Immunol.* (2010) 184:1596–603. doi: 10.4049/jimmunol.0901412
177. Samavedam UK, Iwata H, Muller S, Schulze FS, Recke A, Schmidt E, et al. GM-CSF modulates autoantibody production and skin blistering in experimental epidermolysis bullosa acquisita. *J Immunol.* (2014) 192:559–71. doi: 10.4049/jimmunol.1301556
178. Haeberle S, Wei X, Bieber K, Goletz S, Ludwig RJ, Schmidt E, et al. Regulatory T-cell deficiency leads to pathogenic bullous pemphigoid antigen 230 autoantibody and autoimmune bullous disease. *J Allergy Clin Immunol.* (2018) S0091-6749:30614-6. doi: 10.1016/j.jaci.2018.04.006
179. Muramatsu K, Ujiie H, Kobayashi I, Nishie W, Izumi K, Ito T, et al. Regulatory T-cell dysfunction induces autoantibodies to bullous pemphigoid

antigens in mice and human subjects. *J Allergy Clin Immunol.* (2018) S0091-6749:30615-8. doi: 10.1016/j.jaci.2018.03.014

180. Tiburzy B, Szyska M, Iwata H, Chrobok N, Kulkarni U, Hirose M, et al. Persistent autoantibody-production by intermediates between short-and long-lived plasma cells in inflamed lymph nodes of experimental epidermolysis bullosa acquisita. *PLoS ONE* (2013) 8:e83631. doi: 10.1371/journal.pone.0083631
181. Kasperkiewicz M, Nimmerjahn F, Wende S, Hirose M, Iwata H, Jonkman MF, et al. Genetic identification and functional validation of FcgammaRIV as key molecule in autoantibody-induced tissue injury. *J Pathol.* (2012) 228:8–19. doi: 10.1002/path.4023
182. Nagel A, Hertl M, Eming R. B-cell-directed therapy for inflammatory skin diseases. *J Invest Dermatol.* (2009) 129:289–301. doi: 10.1038/jid.2008.192
183. Martin WL, West AP Jr, Gan L, Bjorkman PJ. Crystal structure at 2.8 A of an FcRn/heterodimeric Fc complex: mechanism of pH-dependent binding. *Mol Cell* (2001) 7:867–77. doi: 10.1016/S1097-2765(01)00230-1
184. Kuo TT, Baker K, Yoshida M, Qiao S-W, Aveson VG, Lencer WI, et al. Neonatal Fc receptor: from immunity to therapeutics. *J Clin Immunol.* (2010) 30:777–89. doi: 10.1007/s10875-010-9468-4
185. Sesarman A, Sitaru AG, Olaru F, Zillikens D, Sitaru C. Neonatal Fc receptor deficiency protects from tissue injury in experimental epidermolysis bullosa acquisita. *J Mol Med.* (2008) 86:951–9. doi: 10.1007/s00109-008-0366-7
186. Liu Z, Roopenian DC, Zhou X, Christianson GJ, Diaz LA, Sedmak DD, et al. Beta2-microglobulin-deficient mice are resistant to bullous pemphigoid. *J Exp Med.* (1997) 186:777–83. doi: 10.1084/jem.186.5.777
187. Rath T, Baker K, Pyzik M, Blumberg RS. Regulation of immune responses by the neonatal fc receptor and its therapeutic implications. *Front Immunol.* (2014) 5:664. doi: 10.3389/fimmu.2014.00664
188. Schwab I, Mihai S, Seeling M, Kasperkiewicz M, Ludwig RJ, Nimmerjahn F. Broad requirement for terminal sialic acid residues and FcgammaRIIB for the preventive and therapeutic activity of intravenous immunoglobulins *in vivo*. *Eur J Immunol.* (2014) 44:1444–53. doi: 10.1002/eji.201344230
189. Ishii N, Hashimoto T, Zillikens D, Ludwig RJ. High-dose intravenous immunoglobulin (IVIG) therapy in autoimmune skin blistering diseases. *Clin Rev Allergy Immunol.* (2010) 38:186–95. doi: 10.1007/s12016-009-8153-y
190. Werth VP, Culton D, Blumberg L, Humphries J, Blumberg R, Hall R. 538 FcRn blockade with SYNT001 for the treatment of pemphigus. *J Invest Dermatol.* (2018) 138:S92. doi: 10.1016/j.jid.2018.03.546
191. Collin M, Ehlers M. The carbohydrate switch between pathogenic and immunosuppressive antigen-specific antibodies. *Exp Dermatol.* (2013) 22:511–4. doi: 10.1111/exd.12171
192. Hirose M, Vafia K, Kalies K, Groth S, Westermann J, Zillikens D, et al. Enzymatic autoantibody glycan hydrolysis alleviates autoimmunity against type VII collagen. *J Autoimmun.* (2012) 39:304–14. doi: 10.1016/j.jaut.2012.04.002
193. Mihai S, Albert H, Ludwig RJ, Iwata H, Bjorck L, Collin M, et al. *In vivo* enzymatic modulation of IgG antibodies prevents immune complex-dependent skin injury. *Exp Dermatol.* (2017) 26:691–6. doi: 10.1111/exd.13163
194. Wada M, Nishie W, Ujiie H, Izumi K, Iwata H, Natsuga K, et al. Epitope-dependent pathogenicity of antibodies targeting a major bullous pemphigoid autoantigen collagen XVII/BP180. *J Invest Dermatol.* (2016) 136:938–46. doi: 10.1016/j.jid.2015.11.030
195. Ishii N, Recke A, Mihai S, Hirose M, Hashimoto T, Zillikens D, et al. Autoantibody-induced intestinal inflammation and weight loss in experimental epidermolysis bullosa acquisita. *J Pathol.* (2011) 224:234–44. doi: 10.1002/path.2857
196. Paller AS, Queen LL, Woodley DT, Lane AT, Gammon WR, Briggaman RA. Organ-specific, phylogenetic, and ontogenetic distribution of the epidermolysis bullosa acquisita antigen. *J Invest Dermatol.* (1986) 86:376–9. doi: 10.1111/1523-1747.ep12285623
197. Recke A, Sitaru C, Vidarsson G, Evensen M, Chiriac MT, Ludwig RJ, et al. Pathogenicity of IgG subclass autoantibodies to type VII collagen: induction of dermal-epidermal separation. *J Autoimmun.* (2010) 34:435–44. doi: 10.1016/j.jaut.2009.11.003
198. Recke A, Trog LM, Pas HH, Vorobyev A, Abadpour A, Jonkman MF, et al. Recombinant human IgA1 and IgA2 autoantibodies to type VII collagen induce subepidermal blistering *ex vivo*. *J Immunol.* (2014) 193:1600–8. doi: 10.4049/jimmunol.1400160
199. Mihai S, Chiriac MT, Takahashi K, Thurman JM, Holers VM, Zillikens D, et al. The alternative pathway of complement activation is critical for blister induction in experimental epidermolysis bullosa acquisita. *J Immunol.* (2007) 178:6514–21. doi: 10.4049/jimmunol.178.10.6514
200. Klos A, Tenner AJ, Johswich K-O, Ager RR, Reis ES, Köhl J. The role of the anaphylatoxins in health and disease. *Mol Immunol.* (2009) 46:2753–66. doi: 10.1016/j.molimm.2009.04.027
201. Iwata H, Witte M, Samavedam UK, Gupta Y, Shimizu A, Ishiko A, et al. Radiosensitive hematopoietic cells determine the extent of skin inflammation in experimental epidermolysis bullosa acquisita. *J Immunol.* (2015) 195:1945–54. doi: 10.4049/jimmunol.1501003
202. Karsten CM, Pandey MK, Figge J, Kilchenstein R, Taylor PR, Rosas M, et al. Anti-inflammatory activity of IgG1 mediated by Fc galactosylation and association of FcγRIIB and dectin-1. *Nat Med.* (2012) 18:1401–06. doi: 10.1038/nm.2862
203. Mihai S, Hirose M, Wang Y, Thurman JM, Holers VM, Morgan BP, et al. Specific inhibition of complement activation significantly ameliorates autoimmune blistering disease in mice. *Front Immunol.* (2018) 9:535. doi: 10.3389/fimmu.2018.00535
204. Afonso PV, Janka-Junttila M, Lee YJ, McCann CP, Oliver CM, Aamer KA, et al. LTB4 is a signal-relay molecule during neutrophil chemotaxis. *Dev Cell.* (2012) 22:1079–91. doi: 10.1016/j.devcel.2012.02.003
205. Lammermann T, Afonso PV, Angermann BR, Wang JM, Kastenmuller W, Parent CA, et al. Neutrophil swarms require LTB4 and integrins at sites of cell death *in vivo*. *Nature* (2013) 498:371–5. doi: 10.1038/nature12175
206. Peters-Golden M, Henderson WR Jr. Leukotrienes. *N Engl J Med.* (2007) 357:1841–54. doi: 10.1056/NEJMra071371
207. Sadik CD, Kim ND, Iwakura Y, Luster AD. Neutrophils orchestrate their own recruitment in murine arthritis through C5aR and FcgammaR signaling. *Proc Natl Acad Sci USA.* (2012) 109:E3177–85. doi: 10.1073/pnas.1213797109
208. Sezin T, Krajewski M, Wutkowski A, Mousavi S, Chakievska L, Bieber K, et al. The leukotriene B4 and its receptor BLT1 act as critical drivers of neutrophil recruitment in murine bullous pemphigoid-like epidermolysis bullosa acquisita. *J Invest Dermatol.* (2017) 137:1104–13. doi: 10.1016/j.jid.2016.12.021
209. Samavedam UK, Kalies K, Scheller J, Sadeghi H, Gupta Y, Jonkman MF, et al. Recombinant IL-6 treatment protects mice from organ specific autoimmune disease by IL-6 classical signalling-dependent IL-1ra induction. *J Autoimmun.* (2013) 40:74–85. doi: 10.1016/j.jaut.2012.08.002
210. Ludwig RJ, Vanhoorelbeke K, Leypoldt F, Kaya Z, Bieber K, McLachlan SM, et al. Mechanisms of autoantibody-induced pathology. *Front Immunol.* (2017) 8:603. doi: 10.3389/fimmu.2017.00603
211. Sitaru C, Mihai S, Otto C, Chiriac MT, Hausser I, Dotterweich B, et al. Induction of dermal-epidermal separation in mice by passive transfer of antibodies specific to type VII collagen. *J Clin Invest.* (2005) 115:870–8. doi: 10.1172/JCI200521386
212. Hirose MBL, Zimmer D, Götz J, Westermann J, Allegretti M, Moriconi A, et al. The allosteric CXCR1/2 inhibitor DF2156A improves experimental epidermolysis bullosa acquisita. *J Genet Syndr Gene Ther.* (2013) 2013:9. doi: 10.4172/2157-7412.S3-005
213. Sadeghi H, Lockmann A, Hund AC, Samavedam UK, Pipi E, Vafia K, et al. Caspase-1-independent IL-1 release mediates blister formation in autoantibody-induced tissue injury through modulation of endothelial adhesion molecules. *J Immunol.* (2015) 194:3656–63. doi: 10.4049/jimmunol.1402688
214. Hirose M, Kasprick A, Beltsiou F, Dieckhoff Schulze K, Schulze FS, Samavedam UK, et al. Reduced skin blistering in experimental epidermolysis bullosa acquisita after anti-TNF treatment. *Mol Med.* (2016) 22:918–26. doi: 10.2119/molmed.2015.00206
215. Wannick M, Yu X, Iwakura Y, Ludwig R, Petersen F, Hölscher C. The role of IL-17A in the pathogenesis of Epidermolysis bullosa acquisita. In: *Experimental Dermatology Conference abstract in Inflammatory Skin Disease Summit - The Translational Revolution.* Vienna (2014).
216. Chiriac MT, Roesler J, Sindrilaru A, Scharffetter-Kochanek K, Zillikens D, Sitaru C. NADPH oxidase is required for neutrophil-dependent

autoantibody-induced tissue damage. *J Pathol.* (2007) 212:56–65. doi: 10.1002/path.2157
217. Shimanovich I, Mihai S, Oostingh GJ, Ilenchuk TT, Brocker EB, Opdenakker G, et al. Granulocyte-derived elastase and gelatinase B are required for dermal-epidermal separation induced by autoantibodies from patients with epidermolysis bullosa acquisita and bullous pemphigoid. *J Pathol.* (2004) 204:519–27. doi: 10.1002/path.1674
218. Kopecki Z, Yang GN, Arkell RM, Jackson JE, Melville E, Iwata H, et al. Flightless I over-expression impairs skin barrier development, function and recovery following skin blistering. *J Pathol.* (2014) 232:541–52. doi: 10.1002/path.4323
219. Kopecki Z, Ruzehaji N, Turner C, Iwata H, Ludwig RJ, Zillikens D, et al. Topically applied flightless I neutralizing antibodies improve healing of blistered skin in a murine model of epidermolysis bullosa acquisita. *J Invest Dermatol.* (2013) 133:1008–16. doi: 10.1038/jid.2012.457
220. Kopecki Z, O'Neill GM, Arkell RM, Cowin AJ. Regulation of focal adhesions by flightless i involves inhibition of paxillin phosphorylation via a Rac1-dependent pathway. *J Invest Dermatol.* (2011) 131:1450–9. doi: 10.1038/jid.2011.69
221. Kasperkiewicz M, Kalies K, Pagel R, Bieber K, Zillikens D, Ludwig RJ. CCL3/MIP1alpha represents a biomarker but not a mandatory cytokine for disease development in experimental epidermolysis bullosa acquisita. *J Dermatol Sci.* (2017) 88:248–50. doi: 10.1016/j.jdermsci.2017.06.019
222. Akbarzadeh R, Yu X, Vogl T, Ludwig RJ, Schmidt E, Zillikens D, et al. Myeloid-related proteins-8 and−14 are expressed but dispensable in the pathogenesis of experimental epidermolysis bullosa acquisita and bullous pemphigoid. *J Dermatol Sci.* (2016) 81:165–72. doi: 10.1016/j.jdermsci.2015.12.001
223. Drager S, Kalies K, Sidronio TB, Witte M, Ludwig RJ, Bieber K. Increased TREM-1 expression in inflamed skin has no functional impact on the pathogenesis of cutaneous disorders. *J Dermatol Sci.* (2017) 88:152–5. doi: 10.1016/j.jdermsci.2017.05.016
224. Bieber K, Sun S, Witte M, Kasprick A, Beltsiou F, Behnen M, et al. Regulatory T cells suppress inflammation and blistering in pemphigoid diseases. *Front Immunol.* (2017) 8:1628. doi: 10.3389/fimmu.2017.01628
225. Bieber K, Witte M, Sun S, Hundt JE, Kalies K, Drager S, et al. T cells mediate autoantibody-induced cutaneous inflammation and blistering in epidermolysis bullosa acquisita. *Sci Rep.* (2016) 6:38357. doi: 10.1038/srep38357
226. Schmidt E, Ambach A, Bastian B, Brocker EB, Zillikens D. Elevated levels of interleukin-8 in blister fluid of bullous pemphigoid compared with suction blisters of healthy control subjects. *J Am Acad Dermatol.* (1996) 34:310–2. doi: 10.1016/S0190-9622(96)80146-0
227. Kulkarni U, Karsten CM, Kohler T, Hammerschmidt S, Bommert K, Tiburzy B, et al. IL-10 mediates plasmacytosis-associated immunodeficiency by inhibiting complement-mediated neutrophil migration. *J Allergy Clin Immunol.* (2016) 137:1487–97 e6. doi: 10.1016/j.jaci.2015.10.018
228. Hussein MR, Ali FM, Omar AE. Immunohistological analysis of immune cells in blistering skin lesions. *J Clin Pathol.* (2007) 60:62–71. doi: 10.1136/jcp.2006.037010
229. Ambach A, Zillikens D, Klingert B, Hartmann AA, Burg G. Immune phenotyping of mononuclear infiltrate in bullous pemphigoid. *Hautarzt* (1992) 43:81–5.
230. Sadeghi H, Gupta Y, Moller S, Samavedam UK, Behnen M, Kasprick A, et al. The retinoid-related orphan receptor alpha is essential for the end-stage effector phase of experimental epidermolysis bullosa acquisita. *J Pathol.* (2015) 237:111–22. doi: 10.1002/path.4556
231. Iwata H, Pipi E, Mockel N, Sondermann P, Vorobyev A, van Beek N, et al. Recombinant soluble CD32 suppresses disease progression in experimental epidermolysis bullosa acquisita. *J Invest Dermatol.* (2015) 135:916–9. doi: 10.1038/jid.2014.451
232. Engineer L, Dow EC, Braverman IM, Ahmed AR. Epidermolysis bullosa acquisita and multiple myeloma. *J Am Acad Dermatol.* (2002) 47:943–6. doi: 10.1067/mjd.2002.113682
233. Yu X, Akbarzadeh R, Pieper M, Scholzen T, Gehrig S, Schultz C, et al. Neutrophil adhesion is a prerequisite for antibody-mediated proteolytic tissue damage in experimental models of epidermolysis bullosa acquisita. *J Invest Dermatol.* (2018) 138:1990–8. doi: 10.1016/j.jid.2018.03.1499
234. Kasprick A, Yu X, Scholten J, Hartmann K, Pas HH, Zillikens D, et al. Conditional depletion of mast cells has no impact on the severity of experimental epidermolysis bullosa acquisita. *Eur J Immunol.* (2015) 45:1462–70. doi: 10.1002/eji.201444769
235. Yu X, Kasprick A, Hartmann K, Petersen F. The role of mast cells in autoimmune bullous dermatoses. *Front Immunol.* (2018) 9:386. doi: 10.3389/fimmu.2018.00386
236. Fang H, Zhang Y, Li N, Wang G, Liu Z. The autoimmune skin disease bullous pemphigoid: the role of mast cells in autoantibody-induced tissue injury. *Front Immunol.* (2018) 9:407. doi: 10.3389/fimmu.2018.00407
237. Deng F, Chen Y, Zheng J, Huang Q, Cao X, Zillikens D, et al. CD11b-deficient mice exhibit an increased severity in the late phase of antibody transfer-induced experimental epidermolysis bullosa acquisita. *Exp Dermatol.* (2017) 26:1175–8. doi: 10.1111/exd.13434
238. Kulkarni S, Sitaru C, Jakus Z, Anderson KE, Damoulakis G, Davidson K, et al. PI3Kbeta plays a critical role in neutrophil activation by immune complexes. *Sci Signal.* (2011) 4:ra23. doi: 10.1126/scisignal.2001617
239. Koga H, Kasprick A, Lopez R, Auli M, Pont M, Godessart N, et al. Therapeutic effect of a novel PI3Kδ inhibitor in experimental epidermolysis bullosa acquisita. *Front Immunol.* (2018) 9:1558. doi: 10.3389/fimmu.2018.01558
240. Koga H, Recke A, Vidarsson G, Pas HH, Jonkman MF, Hashimoto T, et al. PDE4 inhibition as potential treatment of epidermolysis bullosa acquisita. *J Invest Dermatol.* (2016) 136:2211–20. doi: 10.1016/j.jid.2016.06.619
241. Tukaj S, Hellberg L, Ueck C, Hansel M, Samavedam U, Zillikens D, et al. Heat shock protein 90 is required for *ex vivo* neutrophil-driven autoantibody-induced tissue damage in experimental epidermolysis bullosa acquisita. *Exp Dermatol.* (2015) 24:471–3. doi: 10.1111/exd.12680
242. Tukaj S, Bieber K, Kleszczynski K, Witte M, Cames R, Kalies K, et al. Topically applied Hsp90 blocker 17AAG inhibits autoantibody-mediated blister-inducing cutaneous inflammation. *J Invest Dermatol.* (2017) 137:341–9. doi: 10.1016/j.jid.2016.08.032
243. Samavedam UKS, Scheuber J, Seavey MM, Koga H, Witte M, Schulze FS, et al. Therapeutic efficacy of a novel selective JAK2 inhibitor (CEP-33779) in organ-specific, autoantibody-induced tissue injury. *J Invest Dermatol.* (2014) 2014:S16.
244. Hellberg L, Samavedam UK, Holdorf K, Hansel M, Recke A, Beckmann T, et al. Methylprednisolone blocks autoantibody-induced tissue damage in experimental models of bullous pemphigoid and epidermolysis bullosa acquisita through inhibition of neutrophil activation. *J Invest Dermatol.* (2013) 133:2390–9. doi: 10.1038/jid.2013.91
245. Nemeth T, Virtic O, Sitaru C, Mocsai A. The Syk tyrosine kinase is required for skin inflammation in an *in vivo* mouse model of epidermolysis bullosa acquisita. *J Invest Dermatol.* (2017) 137:2131–9. doi: 10.1016/j.jid.2017.05.017
246. Nemeth T, Futosi K, Sitaru C, Ruland J, Mocsai A. Neutrophil-specific deletion of the CARD9 gene expression regulator suppresses autoantibody-induced inflammation *in vivo*. *Nat Commun.* (2016) 7:11004. doi: 10.1038/ncomms11004
247. Kovacs M, Nemeth T, Jakus Z, Sitaru C, Simon E, Futosi K, et al. The Src family kinases Hck, Fgr, and Lyn are critical for the generation of the *in vivo* inflammatory environment without a direct role in leukocyte recruitment. *J Exp Med.* (2014) 211:1993–2011. doi: 10.1084/jem.20132496
248. Sitaru C, Kromminga A, Hashimoto T, Brocker EB, Zillikens D. Autoantibodies to type VII collagen mediate Fcgamma-dependent neutrophil activation and induce dermal-epidermal separation in cryosections of human skin. *Am J Pathol.* (2002) 161:301–11. doi: 10.1016/S0002-9440(10)64182-X
249. Sesarman A, Mihai S, Chiriac MT, Olaru F, Sitaru AG, Thurman JM, et al. Binding of avian IgY to type VII collagen does not activate complement and leucocytes and fails to induce subepidermal blistering in mice. *Br J Dermatol.* (2008) 158:463–71. doi: 10.1111/j.1365-2133.2007.08388.x
250. Nimmerjahn F, Ravetch JV. Fcgamma receptors as regulators of immune responses. *Nat Rev Immunol.* (2008) 8:34–47. doi: 10.1038/nri2206
251. Schulze FS, Beckmann T, Nimmerjahn F, Ishiko A, Collin M, Kohl J, et al. Fcgamma receptors III and IV mediate tissue destruction in a novel adult mouse model of bullous pemphigoid. *Am J Pathol.* (2014) 184:2185–96. doi: 10.1016/j.ajpath.2014.05.007

252. Yu X, Holdorf K, Kasper B, Zillikens D, Ludwig RJ, Petersen F. FcgammaRIIA and FcgammaRIIIB are required for autoantibody-induced tissue damage in experimental human models of bullous pemphigoid. *J Invest Dermatol.* (2010) 130:2841–4. doi: 10.1038/jid.2010.230
253. Ludwig RJ. Signalling and targeted therapy of inflammatory cells in epidermolysis bullosa acquisita. *Exp Dermatol.* (2017) 26:1179–86. doi: 10.1111/exd.13335
254. Ludwig RJ, Schmidt E. Cytokines in autoimmune bullous skin diseases. Epiphenomena or contribution to pathogenesis? *G Ital Dermatol Venereol.* (2009) 144:339–49.
255. Reichert JM. Marketed therapeutic antibodies compendium. *MAbs* (2012) 4:413–5. doi: 10.4161/mabs.19931
256. Tanaka T, Narazaki M, Kishimoto T. IL-6 in inflammation, immunity, and disease. *Cold Spring Harb Perspect Biol.* (2014) 6:a016295. doi: 10.1101/cshperspect.a016295
257. Luo Y, Zheng SG. Hall of fame among pro-inflammatory cytokines: interleukin-6 gene and its transcriptional regulation mechanisms. *Front Immunol.* (2016) 7:604. doi: 10.3389/fimmu.2016.00604
258. Kopecki Z, Arkell RM, Strudwick XL, Hirose M, Ludwig RJ, Kern JS, et al. Overexpression of the Flii gene increases dermal-epidermal blistering in an autoimmune ColVII mouse model of epidermolysis bullosa acquisita. *J Pathol.* (2011) 225:401–13. doi: 10.1002/path.2973
259. Kopecki Z, Ludwig RJ, Cowin AJ. Cytoskeletal regulation of inflammation and its impact on skin blistering disease epidermolysis bullosa acquisita. *Int J Mol Sci.* (2016) 17:1116. doi: 10.3390/ijms17071116
260. Kasprick A, Holtsche MM, Rose EL, Hussain S, Schmidt E, Petersen F, et al. The anti-C1s antibody TNT003 prevents complement activation in the skin induced by bullous pemphigoid autoantibodies. *J Invest Dermatol.* (2018) 138:458–61. doi: 10.1016/j.jid.2017.08.030
261. Muller S, Behnen M, Bieber K, Moller S, Hellberg L, Witte M, et al. Dimethylfumarate impairs neutrophil functions. *J Invest Dermatol.* (2015) 136:117–26. doi: 10.1038/JID.2015.361
262. Tukaj S, Bieber K, Witte M, Ghorbanalipoor S, Schmidt E, Zillikens D, et al. Calcitriol treatment ameliorates inflammation and blistering in mouse models of epidermolysis bullosa acquisita. *J Invest Dermatol.* (2018) 138:301–9. doi: 10.1016/j.jid.2017.09.009
263. Kunz N, Hauenschild E, Maass S, Kalies KU, Klinger M, Barra M, et al. Nanoparticles prepared from porcine cells support the healing of cutaneous inflammation in mice and wound re-epithelialization in human skin. *Exp Dermatol.* (2017) 26:1199–206. doi: 10.1111/exd.13450

Permissions

All chapters in this book were first published by Frontiers; hereby published with permission under the Creative Commons Attribution License or equivalent. Every chapter published in this book has been scrutinized by our experts. Their significance has been extensively debated. The topics covered herein carry significant findings which will fuel the growth of the discipline. They may even be implemented as practical applications or may be referred to as a beginning point for another development.

The contributors of this book come from diverse backgrounds, making this book a truly international effort. This book will bring forth new frontiers with its revolutionizing research information and detailed analysis of the nascent developments around the world.

We would like to thank all the contributing authors for lending their expertise to make the book truly unique. They have played a crucial role in the development of this book. Without their invaluable contributions this book wouldn't have been possible. They have made vital efforts to compile up to date information on the varied aspects of this subject to make this book a valuable addition to the collection of many professionals and students.

This book was conceptualized with the vision of imparting up-to-date information and advanced data in this field. To ensure the same, a matchless editorial board was set up. Every individual on the board went through rigorous rounds of assessment to prove their worth. After which they invested a large part of their time researching and compiling the most relevant data for our readers.

The editorial board has been involved in producing this book since its inception. They have spent rigorous hours researching and exploring the diverse topics which have resulted in the successful publishing of this book. They have passed on their knowledge of decades through this book. To expedite this challenging task, the publisher supported the team at every step. A small team of assistant editors was also appointed to further simplify the editing procedure and attain best results for the readers.

Apart from the editorial board, the designing team has also invested a significant amount of their time in understanding the subject and creating the most relevant covers. They scrutinized every image to scout for the most suitable representation of the subject and create an appropriate cover for the book.

The publishing team has been an ardent support to the editorial, designing and production team. Their endless efforts to recruit the best for this project, has resulted in the accomplishment of this book. They are a veteran in the field of academics and their pool of knowledge is as vast as their experience in printing. Their expertise and guidance has proved useful at every step. Their uncompromising quality standards have made this book an exceptional effort. Their encouragement from time to time has been an inspiration for everyone.

The publisher and the editorial board hope that this book will prove to be a valuable piece of knowledge for researchers, students, practitioners and scholars across the globe.

List of Contributors

Magdalena Kraft and Margitta Worm
Department of Dermatology, Venerology and Allergology, Allergy-Center-Charité, Charité-Universitätsmedizin Berlin, Berlin, Germany

Emiliano Antiga, Lavinia Quintarelli, Alice Verdelli, Diletta Bonciani, Veronica Bonciolini and Marzia Caproni
Section of Dermatology, Department of Health Sciences, University of Florence, Florence, Italy

Mareike Witte, Detlef Zillikens and Enno Schmidt
Department of Dermatology, University of Lübeck, Lübeck, Germany

Daniela Kugelmann, Vera Rötzer, Desalegn Tadesse Egu, Michael Tobias Fuchs and Franziska Vielmuth
Chair of Vegetative Anatomy, Institute of Anatomy, Medical Faculty, Ludwig-Maximilians-Universität München, Munich, Germany

Hilda Vargas-Robles and Michael Schnoor
Department of Molecular Biomedicine, Cinvestav-IPN, Mexico City, Mexico

Klemens Rottner
Division of Molecular Cell Biology, Zoological Institute, Technische Universität Braunschweig, Braunschweig, Germany
Department of Cell Biology, Helmholtz Centre for Infection Research, Braunschweig, Germany

Volker Spindler
Chair of Vegetative Anatomy, Institute of Anatomy, Medical Faculty, Ludwig-Maximilians-Universität München, Munich, Germany
Department of Biomedicine, University of Basel, Basel, Switzerland

Duerna Tie, Xia Da and Eishin Morita
Department of Dermatology, Shimane University Faculty of Medicine, Izumo, Japan

Nanako Yamada and Osamu Yamamoto
Division of Dermatology, Department of Medicine of Sensory and Motor Organs, Faculty of Medicine, Tottori University, Yonago, Japan

Jinmin Lee and Aimee S. Payne
Department of Dermatology, University of Pennsylvania, Philadelphia, PA, United States

Victoria P. Werth
Department of Dermatology, University of Pennsylvania, Philadelphia, PA, United States
Corporal Michael J. Crescenz VAMC, Philadelphia, PA, United States

Russell P. Hall III
Department of Dermatology, Duke University, Durham, NC, United States

Rüdiger Eming
Department of Dermatology and Allergology, Philipps-Universität Marburg, Marburg, Germany

Janet A. Fairley
Department of Dermatology, University of Iowa, Iowa City, IA, United States

David C. Fajgenbaum
Orphan Disease Center, Perelman School of Medicine, University of Pennsylvania, Philadelphia, PA, United States

Karen E. Harman
Centre of Evidence Based Dermatology, University of Nottingham, Nottingham, United Kingdom

Neil J. Korman
Department of Dermatology, University Hospitals Cleveland Medical Center, Case Western Reserve University, Cleveland, OH, United States

Dedee F. Murrell
Department of Dermatology, University of New South Wales, Sydney, NSW, Australia

Philippe Musette
Department of Dermatology, Rouen University Hospital, Rouen, France

Haley B. Naik
Program for Clinical Research, Department of Dermatology, University of California, San Francisco, San Francisco, CA, United States

Christian D. Sadik
Department of Dermatology, Allergy, and Venereology, University of Lübeck, Lübeck, Germany

Jun Yamagami
Department of Dermatology, Keio University, Tokyo, Japan

Marc L. Yale
International Pemphigus and Pemphigoid Foundation, Sacramento, CA, United States

Hideyuki Ujiie, Norihiro Yoshimoto, Ken Natsuga, Ken Muramatsu and Wataru Nishie
Department of Dermatology, Hokkaido University Graduate School of Medicine, Sapporo, Japan

Farzan Solimani, Robert Pollmann, Thomas Schmidt, Dario Didona, Julia Pickert, Rüdiger Eming and Michael Hertl
Department of Dermatology and Allergology, Philipps-University, Marburg, Germany

Ansgar Schmidt
Institute of Pathology, Philipps-University, Marburg, Germany

Norito Ishii
Department of Dermatology, Kurume University School of Medicine, and Kurume University Institute of Cutaneous Cell Biology, Kurume, Japan
Institute of Cutaneous Cell Biology, Kurume University, Kurume, Japan

Björn Tackenberg
Department of Neuroimmunology, Philipps-University, Marburg, Germany

Andreas Kirschbaum
Department of Surgery, Philipps-University, Marburg, Germany

Takashi Hashimoto
Department of Surgery, Philipps-University, Marburg, Germany
Osaka City University Graduate School of Medicine, Osaka, Japan

Giulia Di Lullo
Tumor Immunology Unit, Division of Immunology, Transplantation and Infectious Diseases, Istituto di Ricovero e Cura a Carattere Scientifico (IRCCS) San Raffaele Scientific Institute, Milan, Italy

Valentina Calabresi, Feliciana Mariotti and Giovanni Di Zenzo
Laboratory of Molecular and Cell Biology, IDI-IRCCS, Rome, Italy

Giovanna Zambruno
Genetic and Rare Diseases Research Division, Bambino Gesù Children's Hospital, IRCCS, Rome, Italy

Antonio Lanzavecchia
Institute for Research in Biomedicine, Università della Svizzera italiana, Bellinzona

Delphine Giusti, Grégory Gatouillat and Bach Nga Pham
Laboratory of Dermatology, Faculty of Medicine of Reims, University of Champagne-Ardenne, Reims, France
Laboratory of Immunology, Reims University Hospital, University of Champagne-Ardenne, Reims, France

Estela Bini, Kevin Didier, Sébastien Le Jan, Stéphane Nesmond and Celine Muller
Laboratory of Dermatology, Faculty of Medicine of Reims, University of Champagne-Ardenne, Reims, France

Christine Terryn
PICT Platform, University of Reims Champagne-Ardenne, Reims, France

Anne Durlach
Laboratory of Pathology, Reims University Hospital, Reims, France

Philippe Bernard
Laboratory of Dermatology, Faculty of Medicine of Reims, University of Champagne-Ardenne, Reims, France
Department of Dermatology, Reims University Hospital, University of Champagne-Ardenne, Reims, France

Frank Antonicelli
Laboratory of Dermatology, Faculty of Medicine of Reims, University of Champagne-Ardenne, Reims, France
Department of Biological Sciences, Immunology, UFR Odontology, University of Reims Champagne-Ardenne, Reims, France

Mariya Y. Radeva, Elias Walter and Jens Waschke
Department I, Institute of Anatomy and Cell Biology, Ludwig-Maximilians-Universität (LMU) Munich, Munich, Germany

Ramona Alexandra Stach
Department of Dermatology, University Medical Center Tübingen, Eberhard Karls University, Tübingen, Germany

Amir S. Yazdi
Department of Dermatology, University Medical Center Tübingen, Eberhard Karls University, Tübingen, Germany
Department of Dermatology, RWTH Aachen, Aachen, Germany

Nicolas Schlegel
Department of General, Visceral, Vascular and Paediatric Surgery, Julius-Maximilians-Universität, Würzburg, Germany

Ofer Sarig
Department of Dermatology, Tel-Aviv Sourasky Medical Center, Tel-Aviv, Israel

Eli Sprecher
Department of Dermatology, Tel-Aviv Sourasky Medical Center, Tel-Aviv, Israel
Department of Human Molecular Genetics and Biochemistry, Sackler Faculty of Medicine, Tel-Aviv University, Tel-Aviv, Israel

Roberto Maglie
Department of Dermatology and Allergology, Philipps University, Marburg, Germany
Surgery and Translational Medicine, Section of Dermatology, University of Florence, Florence, Italy
Section of Dermatology, Departement of Health Sciences, University of Florence, Florence, Italy

Dyah A. M. Oktarina
Department of Dermatology, Centre for Blistering Diseases, University Medical Centre Groningen, University of Groningen, Groningen, Netherlands
Department of Dermatology and Venereology, Faculty of Medicine, Public Health and Nursing, Universitas Gadjah Mada, Yogyakarta, Indonesia

Ena Sokol, Duco Kramer, Marcel F. Jonkman and Hendri H. Pas
Department of Dermatology, Centre for Blistering Diseases, University Medical Centre Groningen, University of Groningen, Groningen, Netherlands

Vivien Hébert, Maud Maho-Vaillant, Marie-Laure Golinski and Pascal Joly
INSERM U1234, Normandie University, Rouen, France
Department of Dermatology, Rouen University Hospital, Normandie University, Rouen, France

Marie Petit, Gaëtan Riou, Olivier Boyer and Sébastien Calbo
INSERM U1234, Normandie University, Rouen, France

Céline Derambure
INSERM U1245, Normandie University, Rouen, France

Irina Condrat
Department of Dermatology and Venerology, Medical Center - University of Freiburg, Faculty of Medicine, University of Freiburg, Freiburg, Germany
Department of Dermatology, Iuliu Hatieganu University of Medicine and Pharmacy, Cluj Napoca, Romania

Yinghong He and Cristina Has
Department of Dermatology and Venerology, Medical Center - University of Freiburg, Faculty of Medicine, University of Freiburg, Freiburg, Germany

Rodica Cosgarea
Department of Dermatology, Iuliu Hatieganu University of Medicine and Pharmacy, Cluj Napoca, Romania

Kentaro Izumi
Department of Dermatology, Hokkaido University Graduate School of Medicine, Sapporo, Japan
Lübeck Institute of Experimental Dermatology, Center for Research on Inflammation of the Skin, University of Lübeck, Lübeck, Germany

Hiroshi Shimizu
Department of Dermatology, Hokkaido University Graduate School of Medicine, Sapporo, Japan

Schauer, Maja Mockenhaupt, Leena Bruckner-Tuderman and Dimitra Kiritsi
Department of Dermatology, Medical Center - University of Freiburg, Faculty of Medicine, University of Freiburg, Freiburg, Germany,

Teruki Dainichi
Department of Dermatology, Kyoto University Graduate School of Medicine, Kyoto, Japan

Kenji Kabashima
Department of Dermatology, Kyoto University Graduate School of Medicine, Kyoto, Japan
Singapore Immunology Network and Institute of Medical Biology, Agency for Science, Technology and Research (A*STAR), Singapore, Singapore

Hiroshi Koga
Department of Dermatology, Kurume University School of Medicine, and Kurume University Institute of Cutaneous Cell Biology, Fukuoka, Japan

Catherine Prost-Squarcioni
Department of Dermatology, APHP, Avicenne Hospital, Referral Center for Autoimmune Bullous Diseases, Bobigny, France

Hiroaki Iwata
Department of Dermatology, Hokkaido University Graduate School of Medicine, Sapporo, Japan

Ralf J. Ludwig and Katja Bieber
Lübeck Institute of Experimental Dermatology, University of Lübeck, Lübeck, Germany

Index

Printed in the USA
CPSIA information can be obtained
at www.ICGtesting.com
LVHW080037211023
761596LV00010BA/1797